Peter BARNES

Peter BARNES

New Drugs for Asthma, Allergy and COPD

Progress in Respiratory Research

Vol. 31

Series Editor   *Chris T. Bolliger*, Cape Town

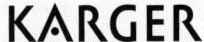

Basel · Freiburg · Paris · London · New York ·
New Delhi · Bangkok · Singapore · Tokyo · Sydney

New Drugs for Asthma, Allergy and COPD

Volume Editors　*Trevor T. Hansel,* London
　　　　　　　　Peter J. Barnes, London

195 colour figures and 72 tables, 2001

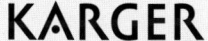

Basel · Freiburg · Paris · London · New York ·
New Delhi · Bangkok · Singapore · Tokyo · Sydney

Trevor T. Hansel
Clinical Studies Unit
National Heart and Lung Institute
Imperial College
London (UK)

Peter J. Barnes
Department of Thoracic Medicine
National Heart and Lung Institute
Imperial College
London (UK)

Library of Congress Cataloging-in-Publication Data

New drugs for asthma, allergy and COPD / volume editors, Trevor T. Hansel, Peter J. Barnes.
 p. ; cm. – (Progress in respiratory research, ISSN 1422–2140 ; vol. 31)
 Includes bibliographical references and indexes.
 ISBN 3805568622 (alk paper : hard cover)
 1. Respiratory agents. 2. Antiasthmatic agents. 3. Lungs – Diseases, Obstructive – Chemotherapy.
 I. Hansel, T.T. (Trevor T.), 1956- II. Barnes, Peter J., 1946- III. Series.
 [DNLM: 1. Asthma – drug therapy. 2. Anti-Asthmatic Agents – therapeutic use. 3. Hypersensitivity – drug therapy.
 4. Lung Diseases, obstructive – drug therapy.   WF 553 N5321 2001]
 RM388.N49 2001
 615′.72–dc21
                                                                                                                      00-050644

Bibliographic Indices. This publication is listed in bibliographic services, including Current Contents® and Index Medicus.

Drug Dosage. The authors and the publisher have exerted every effort to ensure that drug selection and dosage set forth in this text are in accord with current recommendations and practice at the time of publication. However, in view of ongoing research, changes in government regulations, and the constant flow of information relating to drug therapy and drug reactions, the reader is urged to check the package insert for each drug for any change in indications and dosage and for added warnings and precautions. This is particularly important when the recommended agent is a new and/or infrequently employed drug.

All rights reserved. No part of this publication may be translated into other languages, reproduced or utilized in any form or by any means, electronic or mechanical, including photocopying, recording, microcopying, or by any information storage and retrieval system, without permission in writing from the publisher.

© Copyright 2001 by S. Karger AG,
P.O. Box, CH–4009 Basel (Switzerland)
www.karger.com
Printed in Switzerland on acid-free paper by
Reinhardt Druck, Basel
ISBN 3–8055–6862–2, ISSN 1422–2140

Contents

VIII Foreword

IX Preface

General Aspects

2 **The Need for New Therapy**
Barnes, P.J.; Hansel, T.T. (NHLI, Imperial College, London)

6 **Current Therapy for Asthma**
Barnes, P.J. (NHLI, Imperial College, London)

11 **Current Therapy for COPD**
Pauwels, R. (Ghent University Hospital, Ghent)

15 **Pharmacogenetics**
Hall, I.P. (University Hospital, Nottingham); Hansel, T.T. (NHLI, Imperial College, London)

20 **Delivery of Biologics to the Lung**
Cipolla, D.; Farr, S.; Gonda, I.; Otulana, B. (Aradigm Corporation, Hayward, Calif.)

24 **Immunopathology: Comparison of COPD and Asthma**
Jeffery, P.K. (NHLI, Imperial College, London)

30 **Monitoring Lung Function**
Pride, N. (NHLI, Imperial College, London)

35 **Airway Hyperresponsiveness**
Sterk, P.J. (Leiden University Medical Centre, Leiden)

39 **Airways Remodelling**
Holgate, S.T.; Davies, D.E. (University of Southampton, Southampton)

44 **Exhaled Breath Analysis**
Kharitonov, S.A.; Barnes, P.J. (NHLI, Imperial College, London)

48 **Clinical Studies on New Drugs**
Hansel, T.T.; Barnes, P.J. (NHLI, Imperial College, London)

Bronchodilators

54 **Bronchodilators: An Overview**
Anderson, G.P. (University of Melbourne, Melbourne); Rabe, K.F. (Leiden University Center, Leiden)

60 **Long-Acting β_2-Agonists**
Johnson, M.; Hagan, G.W.E. (GlaxoWellcome, Uxbridge)

64 **Single-Isomer β-Agonists**
Handley, D.A. (Sepracor, Marlborough, Mass.); Morley, J. (Haldane Research, Huntingdon); Nelson, H.S. (National Jewish Medical and Research Center, Denver, Colo.)

68 **Dual D_2 Dopamine Receptor and β_2-Adrenoceptor Agonists for the Modulation of Sensory Nerves in COPD**
Newbold, P.; Jackson, D.M.; Young, A.; Dougall, I.G.; Ince, F.; Rocchiccioli, K.M.S.; Holt, P.R. (AstraZeneca, Loughborough)

72 **Anticholinergics: Tiotropium**
Disse, B.; Witek, T.J., Jr. (Boehringer Ingelheim, Ingelheim and Ridgefield, Conn.)

77 **Potassium Channel Openers**
Agents for the Treatment of Airway Hyperreactivity
Fozard, J.R.; Manley, P.W. (Novartis Pharma Ltd., Basel)

81 **Urodilatin**
Forssmann, K.; Meyer, M.; Forssmann, W.G. (CardioPep Pharma GmbH and IPF PharmaCeuticals GmbH, Hannover)

Steroids

86 **Steroids: An Overview**
Dahl, R.; Nielsen, L.P. (University of Aarhus, Aarhus)

91 **Ciclesonide: An On-Site-Activated Steroid**
Dietzel, K.; Engelstätter, R.; Keller, A. (Byk Gulden Pharmaceuticals, Konstanz)

94 **Soft Steroids**
Axelsson, B.; Brattsand, R. (AstraZeneca, Lund)

98 **Dissociated Steroids**
Brown, T.J.; Belvisi, M.G.; Foster, M.L. (Aventis Pharmaceuticals, Dagenham)

102 **Oestradiol Metabolites**
Effects on Airway Remodelling
Stewart, A.G.; Vlahos, R.; Fernandes, D.J.; Hughes, R.A. (University of Melbourne, Melbourne)

Leukotriene Inhibitors

108 **Leukotriene Inhibitors: An Overview**
O'Byrne, P.M. (McMaster University, Hamilton); Drazen, J.M. (Harvard Medical School, Boston, Mass.)

111 Cysteinyl Leukotriene Antagonists
McMillan, R.M. (AstraZeneca, Macclesfield)

115 5-Lipoxygenase Inhibitors
Dahlén, S.-E. (Karolinska Institutet, Stockholm)

121 LTB$_4$ Antagonism
Jennewein, H.M.; Anderskewitz, R.; Meade, C.J.; Pairet, M.; Birke, F. (Boehringer Ingelheim, Ingelheim)

Mediator Inhibitors and Agonists

128 H$_1$-Antihistamines
De Vos, C.; Rihoux, J.P. (UCB Pharma SA, Brussels)

133 Histamine H$_3$ Antagonists
McLeod, R.L.; Egan, R.W.; Cuss, F.M. (Schering-Plough, Kenilworth, N.J.); Bolser, D.C. (University of Gainesville, Gainesville, Fla.); Hey, J.A. (Schering-Plough, Kenilworth, N.J.)

137 Kinin Receptor Antagonists
Meini, S.; Maggi, C.A. (Menarini Ricerche SpA, Florence)

141 Endothelin Antagonists
Hay, D.W.P.; Compton, C.H. (SmithKline Beecham Pharmaceuticals, King of Prussia, Pa., and Harlow)

145 Tachykinin Antagonists
Hay, D.W.P. (SmithKline Beecham Pharmaceuticals, King of Prussia, Pa.)

151 Antioxidants
MacNee, W. (University of Edinburgh, Edinburgh)

156 Selective iNOS Inhibitors
Manning, P.T.; Thompson, J.M. (Searle, St. Louis, Mo., and Skokie, Ill.); Currie, M.G. (Sepracor Inc., Marlborough, Mass.)

160 Mucus Regulation
Rogers, D.F. (NHLI, Imperial College, London)

165 P2Y Receptor Agonists
Role in Mucosal Hydration and Mucociliary Clearance
Pendergast, W.; Evans, R. (Inspire Pharmaceuticals, Inc., Durham, N.C.)

Protease Inhibitors

170 Tryptase Inhibition
Clark, J.M.; Van Dyke, R.E.; Kurth, M.C. (Axys Pharmaceuticals, Inc., S. San Francisco, Calif.)

173 Neutrophil Elastase Inhibitors
Smith, R.A. (GlaxoWellcome, Stevenage); Stockley, R.A. (Queen Elizabeth Hospital, Birmingham); Hodgson, S.T. (GlaxoWellcome, Stevenage)

177 Macrophage Metalloelastase Inhibitors
Martin, R.L. (Roche Bioscience, Palo Alto, Calif.); Shapiro, S.D. (Washington University, St. Louis, Mo.); Tong, S.E.; Van Wart, H.E. (Roche Bioscience, Palo Alto, Calif.)

Allergen- and IgE-Directed Therapies

182 Allergen, IgE and Mast-Cell-Directed Responses: An Overview
Larché, M.; Kay, A.B. (NHLI, Imperial College, London)

186 Allergen Immunotherapy
Wilson, D.R.; Durham, S.R. (NHLI, Imperial College, London)

191 Peptide Immunotherapy
Oldfield, W.L.G.; Kay, A.B.; Larché, M. (NHLI, Imperial College, London)

195 Recombinant Allergens
Valenta, R.; Kraft, D. (University of Vienna, Vienna)

201 Anti-IgE Antibody
Boushey, H.A. (University of California, San Francisco, Calif.); Fick, R. (Genentech, Inc., S. San Francisco, Calif.); Fahy, J.V. (University of California, San Francisco, Calif.)

206 CD23
Conrad, D.H. (Virginia Commonwealth University, Richmond, Va.)

T Cell Immunomodulation

212 T Cell Immunomodulation: An Overview
Koulis, A.; Robinson, D.S. (NHLI, Imperial College, London)

217 Costimulatory Molecules in T Cell Activation
Coyle, A.J.; Gutierrez-Ramos, J.-C. (Millennium Pharmaceuticals Inc., Cambridge, Mass.)

222 GATA-3: A Th2-Selective Target
Ray, A.; Ray, P. (Yale University, New Haven, Conn.)

226 Mycobacterial Immunization
Agents to Limit Asthma
Hopkin, J.M. (University of Wales, Swansea)

229 CpG Oligodeoxynucleotides
Kline, J.N.; Krieg, A.M. (University of Iowa, Iowa City, Iowa, and Coley Pharmaceutical Group, Wellesley, Mass.)

233 CD8 T Cells: Potential Therapeutic Targets?
Out, T.A. (Academic Medical Center and CLB Sanquin Blood Supply Foundation, Amsterdam); de Pater-Huijsen, F.L.; Jansen, H.M. (Academic Medical Center, Amsterdam); Corrigan, C.J. (Guy's, King's and St. Thomas' School of Medicine, London)

237 Macrocyclic Immunosuppressants
Keller, T.H.; Hersperger, R.; Della Cioppa, G. (Novartis, Horsham and Basel)

Cytokine-Directed Therapy

242 Cytokines: An Overview
Chung, K.F. (NHLI, Imperial College, London)

247 TNF Antagonism
McDonnell, N.D.; Abbott, N.M.; Mohler, K.M. (Immunex Corp., Seattle, Wash.); Hansel, T.T. (NHLI, Imperial College, London); Kips, J.C. (Ghent University Hospital, Ghent)

251 GM-CSF Antagonists
Williams, W.V. (SmithKline Beecham, Philadelphia, Pa.)

256 Interleukin-4 Antagonism
Borish, L. (University of Virginia, Charlottesville, Va.); Agosti, J.M. (Immunex Corporation, Seattle, Wash.)

260 Interleukin-13 Antagonism
Donaldson, D.D. (Wyeth-Ayerst, Andover, Mass.); Elias, J.A. (Yale University, New Haven, Conn.); Wills-Karp, M. (Johns Hopkins University, Baltimore, Md.)

265 Interleukin-5 Antagonism
Leckie, M.J. (NHLI, Imperial College, London); Walker, C. (Novartis Research Centre, Horsham)

269 Interleukin-10
Narula, S.; Cuss, F. (Schering-Plough Research Institute, Kenilworth, N.J.)

274 Interleukin-12, Interleukin-18 and Interferon-γ
Bryan, S. (NHLI, Imperial College, London); Kobayashi, M. (Wyeth-Ayerst, Andover, Mass.); Sur, S. (University of Texas, Galveston, Tex.)

Chemokine Receptor Inhibition

280 Chemokines: An Overview
Sabroe, I.; Williams, T.J. (Imperial College, South Kensington)

284 Chemokine Receptors on Th1 and Th2 Cells
Sinigaglia, F. (Roche Milano Ricerche, Milan); Fabbri, L.M. (University of Modena, Modena); D'Ambrosio, D. (Roche Milano Ricerche, Milan)

288 CCR-3 Antagonists
Bryan, S.A. (NHLI, Imperial College, London); Ponath, P.D. (LeukoSite, Inc., Cambridge, Mass.); Wilhelm, R.S. (Roche Bioscience, Palo Alto, Calif.)

293 Interleukin-8 Receptor (CXCR2) Antagonists
Sarau, H.M.; Widdowson, K.L.; Palovich, M.R.; White, J.R.; Underwood, D.C.; Griswold, D.E. (SmithKline Beecham Pharmaceuticals, King of Prussia, Pa.)

Adhesion Molecule Inhibitors

298 Adhesion Molecule Antagonism: An Overview
Bochner, B.S. (Johns Hopkins University, Baltimore, Md.)

302 Small-Molecule VLA-4 Antagonists
Adams, S.P.; Lobb, R.R. (Biogen Inc., Cambridge, Mass.)

306 Selectin Antagonists
Therapeutics for Airway Inflammation
Berens, K.L.; Vanderslice, P.; Dupré, B.; Dixon, R.A.F. (Texas Biotechnology Corporation, Houston, Tex.)

310 ICAM-1 and VCAM-1 Antagonists
Richards, I.M.; Slatter, V.K. (Pharmacia Corporation, Kalamazoo, Mich.)

Inhibition of Cell Signalling

316 Eosinophil G-Protein-Coupled Receptor Signalling: An Overview
Lindsay, M.A.; De Souza, P.M.; Lynch, O.T.; Giembycz, M.A. (NHLI, Imperial College, London)

321 Phosphodiesterase 4 Inhibitors
Torphy, T.J.; Compton, C.H.; Marks, M.J. (SmithKline Beecham, King of Prussia, Pa., Harlow, and Collegeville, Pa.); Sturton, G. (Bayer plc, Slough)

Therapies Acting on Transcription

328 Therapies Acting on Transcription: An Overview
Caramori, G.; Adcock, I.M. (NHLI, Imperial College, London)

332 Chromatin Modification
Urnov, F.D.; Wolffe, A.P. (Sangamo Biosciences, Richmond, Calif.)

337 Activator Protein-1 and Nuclear Factor-Kappa B
Bennett, B.L.; Manning, A.M. (Signal Pharmaceuticals, Inc., San Diego, Calif.)

342 Inhibition of p38 MAP Kinase
Underwood, D.C.; Griswold, D.E. (SmithKline Beecham Pharmaceuticals, King of Prussia, Pa.)

346 STAT6
Role in IL-4-Mediated Signaling
Schaefer, G.; Venkataraman, C.; Schindler, U. (Tularik, Inc., S. San Francisco, Calif.)

350 Retinoids
Belloni, P.N. (Roche Bioscience, Palo Alto, Calif.)

Genetic Therapy

358 Asthma and COPD Genetics and Genomics: An Overview
Morrison, J.F.J. (AstraZeneca, Macclesfield)

361 Respirable Antisense Oligonucleotides
Nyce, J.W. (EpiGenesis Pharmaceuticals, Inc., Princeton, N.J.)

365 Antisense Therapy
Bennett, C.F. (Isis Pharmaceuticals, Inc., Carlsbad, Calif.)

370 Ribozyme Therapy
Sandberg, J.A.; Lee, P.A.; Usman, N. (Ribozyme Pharmaceuticals, Inc., Boulder, Colo.)

374 Gene Therapy
Kolb, M.; Gauldie, J. (McMaster University, Hamilton)

379 Author Index

381 Subject Index

388 Abbreviations

Foreword

For this first volume written in the new millennium I decided to go for a book on new drugs for asthma and COPD which would be of interest to many doctors involved in the treatment of these diseases. When looking for someone to edit this 31st volume of the series 'Progress in Respiratory Research' I was fortunate enough to get Trevor T. Hansel and Peter J. Barnes interested. During our initial meeting in Madrid in September 1999, I told them that I would be interested in 'real' progress in drug research and not in a book which would be outdated by the time it is printed. After some moments of hesitation they said that this would mean involvement of a lot of researchers from pharmaceutical companies together with clinicians, and what about conflicts of interest!? When I replied that this mix represented the real world, and was exactly what I wanted, they promised to think about it and get back to me. After a short period they announced their concept of putting together a book with 80 ultra concise chapters addressing every possible drug from established, commercially available substances to compounds in their early testing phase.

The final product exceeds my wildest expectations. Trevor and Peter managed to rally a fantastic group of authors, whose names reflect a 'who's who' in the field. The chapters rarely exceed 4 printed pages, limiting the information to the essentials. The book is lavishly illustrated with 72 tables and 195 colour figures, which have been edited by Trevor to obtain uniformity; that means an eosinophil looks the same in every figure of the book!

This book will serve as a key reference of current and future developments in the treatment of asthma, allergy, and COPD; it will appeal to the practising physician as well as to the pulmonologist with a special pharmacological interest. Get it and enjoy it!

Chris T. Bolliger
Series Editor

Preface

Asthma and COPD have now become amongst the commonest diseases in the world, and both are increasing. There have been major advances in our understanding of asthma and significant improvement in asthma management, particularly with the early and more widespread use of inhaled corticosteroids. Yet, despite effective therapy for asthma, there is a pressing need for new and more specific therapies that control the disease or even cure the underlying disease process. Progress in understanding and treating COPD has been much slower, mainly because the disease has been relatively neglected. None of the treatments available today prevent the relentless progression of COPD and there is an urgent need to develop novel approaches.

The aim of this book is to offer a state-of-the-art description of the exciting progress in research and development that is being made with new therapies for asthma, allergy and COPD. We are very aware that many large tomes that contain review chapters by leading scientific and clinical authorities are already available on allergic and respiratory diseases. On this basis, our major intention was to link the biotechnology and pharmaceutical industry with academic and clinical opinion. In order to develop better therapies, we rely on this partnership, since the modern-day reality is that novel drug discovery and production generally occur from within the industry.

We have been amazed by the enthusiastic response from our colleagues in the pharmaceutical industry in providing as much information as they can about early developments with their novel potential therapies. By way of introduction to these contributions, we have overviews written by leading academic clinical scientists. With over 200 authors, and a total of 80 chapters, we hope

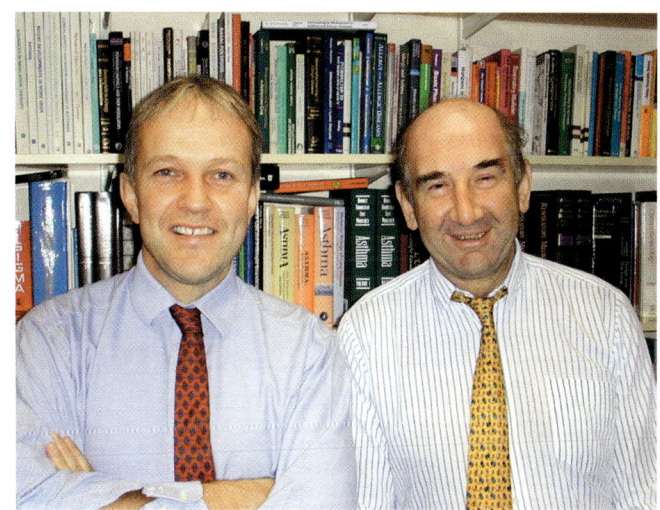

T.T.H. *P.J.B.*

to provide concise and highly condensed information. In this way we have tried to have specialists from the industry writing on their own fields of interest. This is a rapidly advancing field, and this format of segmented brief chapters has allowed us to put information on the internet, and should permit provision of regular updates.

The book has 14 sections that range from an introduction covering general aspects of drug development for asthma and COPD to a review of currently available small-molecular-weight synthetic medicinal chemical classes: bronchodilators, corticosteroids, anti-leukotrienes, and mediator and protease inhibitors. We then proceed from allergen and IgE-directed therapies to T cell immunomodulation and cytokine-directed therapy, to chemokine receptor and adhesion molecule inhibition, to therapy directed against cell signalling and transcription, before looking at future prospects for genetic therapy.

A considerable team has been involved in producing this volume, and we are very grateful for the vision of Chris Bolliger, Editor of *Progress in Respiratory Research*, who always wanted us to go for something 'completely different'! In addition, we have found the entire staff at Karger Medical Publishers, Basel, a superbly professional group of people to interact with.

We hope that you will find this book interesting and helpful, and that it will give as much enjoyment to you, the reader, as we have had in its design and editing. Finally, and most importantly of all, we hope that this book will help in the process of finding better therapy for patients with allergic and respiratory diseases.

Trevor T. Hansel
Peter J. Barnes

General Aspects

The Need for New Therapy

Peter J. Barnes   Trevor T. Hansel

Department of Thoracic Medicine, National Heart and Lung Institute, Imperial College, London, UK

Summary

The perspectives for new therapies in asthma and COPD are quite different. In asthma we already have relatively cheap and safe therapies that are effective in controlling the disease, so that the need for new treatments is somewhat limited. However, important advances can still be made to improve long-term therapy for patients with more severe persistent asthma, as well as acute therapy for emergency exacerbations of asthma, while in the future there is the prospect of allergen immunotherapy causing disease modification and even cure. In COPD, however, both bronchodilator and anti-inflammatory therapy is less effective, and there are currently no therapies that reduce the progression of the disease. Driven by the urgent need for new therapies, a shift in resources from discovery of drugs for asthma to COPD is taking place.

Asthma

New Asthma Treatments. Asthma therapy has been revolutionized over the last decade by the earlier and more widespread use of inhaled corticosteroids. Short-acting β_2-agonists are very effective in relief of symptoms and the introduction of long-acting inhaled β_2-agonists has greatly improved asthma control. Fixed-combination inhalers of corticosteroid with long-acting bronchodilators have recently been introduced and provide highly effective control of asthma for the majority of patients. This treatment is simple and very convenient for patients, so it is likely to dominate asthma therapy in the foreseen future. However, there are some areas of asthma therapy where improvements may be possible through the development of improved existing treatments or introduction of novel therapies [1] (fig. 1).

Problems with Existing Treatments. Although current asthma therapy is effective and well tolerated, there are some limitations [2]. Inhaled corticosteroids are very effective in controlling asthma in most patients [3]. However, there are still concerns about side effects, particularly in children and in patients with severe asthma who require high doses. Many patients are reluctant to take inhaled corticosteroids because of the fear of adverse effects of steroids; the general public has 'corticophobia' as a result of stories in the press about side effects of oral corticosteroids and anabolic steroids. Local side effects of inhaled corticosteroid, particularly dysphonia, may be a problem in some patients, such as lecturers and singers. The dose of inhaled corticosteroids that most patients require for asthma control is relatively low so that systemic side effects are unlikely. However, a recent community study suggests that there was a linear relationship between the cumulative dose of inhaled steroid used and the risk of fracture [4].

Inhaled β_2-agonists, while highly effective as bronchodilators, also have side effects in some patients, particularly the elderly. Tremor and palpitations can be distressing in some patients, but can usually be avoided by reducing the dose or frequency and adding an anticholinergic inhaler. Tolerance to the bronchodilator effects of β_2-agonists is a potential problem, but although there is a small reduction in the protective effect of β_2-agonists against challenges, such as allergen and exercise, this is of relatively small degree and is not progressive [5].

Theophylline is a useful treatment for patients with severer asthma, but at the doses that are needed for bronchodilatation, side effects are relatively common. However, lower doses of theophylline are also effective in asthma control and avoid many of the problems with side effects. The side effects of existing anti-asthma therapies are due to their non-pulmonary effects, since corticosteroids, β_2-agonists and theophylline have effects on many different cell types. This suggests that it may be necessary to develop more specific therapies, targeted at specific abnormalities in allergic inflammation, in order to reduce the risk of adverse effects [6].

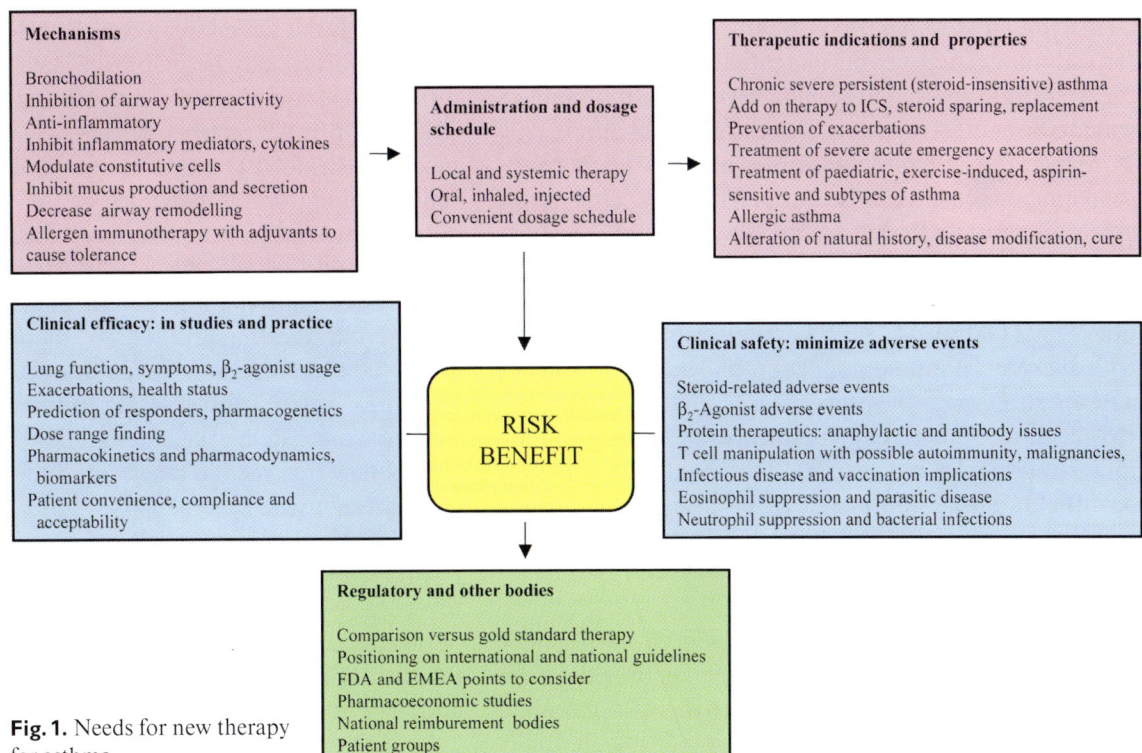

Fig. 1. Needs for new therapy for asthma.

Severe and Emergency Asthma. Most asthmatic patients can be controlled on inhaled corticosteroid with or without a long-acting inhaled β$_2$-agonist and in patients with severer disease with the addition of theophylline and an anticholinergic bronchodilator. However, about 5% of patients have severe asthma and require high doses of inhaled corticosteroids and in approximately 1% of patients by maintenance doses of oral corticosteroids [7]. These patients have the potential for improvement since they usually respond to even higher doses of oral corticosteroid. These steroid-dependent patients are relatively steroid-resistant, while occasionally patients have complete resistance to the effects of corticosteroids [8, 9]. These patients, while comprising only ~5% of all asthmatic patients, account for over 50% of medical costs [10], and it should be stressed that admissions to hospital following severe exacerbations of asthma generally result in a 4-day hospital stay. Some new form of treatment is needed for these patients with severe asthma that is independent of the molecular mechanisms of action of corticosteroids and several possible approaches are discussed in this volume.

Inhaled versus Oral Therapy. The most effective currently available therapies for asthma, corticosteroids and β$_2$-agonists, are given by inhalation to reduce or avoid side effects due to the systemic actions of these non-specific therapies. However, it is difficult to develop inhaled drugs, and patients may find it difficult to use inhalers. Oral therapy for asthma may have advantages as it would be easier to take and this may improve compliance [11]. Anti-leukotrienes, which are much less effective in the control of asthma than inhaled corticosteroids, have proved popular with patients as they are available as a once- or twice-daily tablet. Another important advantage of oral therapy that inhibits allergic inflammation is that it will control concomitant allergic diseases such as rhinitis and atopic dermatitis that commonly coincide with asthma [6].

Disease Modification. Although inhaled corticosteroids are very effective at controlling asthma, symptoms recur when inhaled corticosteroids are withdrawn and there is an increase in markers of inflammation [12, 13]. This indicates that corticosteroids suppress inflammation in asthmatic airways, but do not change the underlying unknown driving mechanism, so that when steroids are discontinued, the inflammation and asthma symptoms recur. The concept of disease-modifying drugs is well established in rheumatology. It implies that a treatment will alter the disease process and maintain disease control even when discontinued. So far this has not been established for any existing asthma therapy, but it is possible that new treatments aimed at upstream immunological pathways may have the potential for disease modification.

A Cure for Asthma? No currently available treatment for asthma is curative, but potentially a cure is possible through strategies that prevent or reverse the immunological abnormalities in atopy. There are several approaches to reduce the preponderance of Th2 cells in atopy by switching the balance in favour of Th1 cells. This can be achieved in animals by exposure to bacterial products such as BCG, *Mycobacterium vaccae* or unmethylated cytosine-guanosine dinucleotide-containing oligonucleotides (CpG ODN) [14–16]. This suggests that vaccination with allergens, immunomodulators and adjuvants may be a future strategy for the prevention or cure of asthma [17]. However, the long-term consequences of altering the immune response are not yet certain and clinical studies may be difficult. Initial studies with BCG vaccination in young children are equivocal and more studies are needed [18].

COPD

Compared to asthma, COPD has been surprisingly neglected in terms of mechanistic research, drug development, and therapeutic advances. Yet this is a common disease with an increasing prevalence that is potentially treatable with novel therapies.

Size of the Problem. It is estimated that approximately 14 million people in the USA are currently affected by COPD. In the US Third National Health and Nutrition Examination Survey (NHANESIII) study airflow obstruction was found in approximately 14% of white male smokers compared to approximately 3% in non-smokers, with slightly lower figures in white women and blacks [19]. COPD is now the fourth leading cause of death in the USA and the only common cause of death that is increasing. This is pobably a gross underestimate, as COPD is likely to be contributory to other common causes of death. There has been an increase in COPD prevalence and mortality, even in industrialized countries, and COPD now represents a major world-wide health problem. The World Health Organization global impact of disease analysis predicts that COPD will rise from its current ranking of 12th most prevalent disease world-wide to 5th position, and from the 6th commonest cause of death to 3rd by 2020 [20]. Reasons for the dramatic increase in COPD include reduced mortality from other causes, such as cardiovascular diseases, in industrialized countries and infectious diseases in developing countries, with a marked increase in cigarette smoking and environmental pollution in developing countries.

The Neglect of COPD. There are several reasons why COPD has been relatively neglected in terms of new drug development. Firstly, COPD has been perceived as 'untreatable' fixed airflow obstruction. Secondly, patients with COPD have been treated with anti-asthma therapies, but these drugs may be inappropriate in a disease with a different pathophysiology, involving different cells, mediators and inflammatory effects [21]. Thirdly, since in most patients COPD is the result of long-term heavy cigarette smoking it has been felt to be the 'fault' of the patient. Fourthly, there has been little interest in the molecular and cell biology of COPD to identify new therapeutic targets and there are no satisfactory animal models for early drug testing [22]. Lastly, there are uncertainties about how to test new drugs for COPD, which may require long-term studies in large numbers of patients and a lack of surrogate markers to monitor the short-term efficacy of new treatments. However, some progress is under way and there are several classes of drug that are now in preclinical and clinical development [23, 24].

Problems with Existing Therapies. COPD is poorly reversible with current therapies. Bronchodilators are the only treatments which provide symptomatic benefit, but the effects of bronchodilators are less than seen in asthma, and high doses are required to achieve a maximal effect. Long-acting inhaled β_2-agonists have been an important advance, and the new once-daily inhaled anticholinergic drug, tiotropium bromide, is likely to be an important advance [25–27]. But bronchodilators do not change the natural history of COPD and do not reduce the accelerated decline in lung function that is typical of the disease [28]. Indeed, apart from quitting smoking, no currently available therapies alter the progression of COPD.

Because COPD involves a chronic inflammation of the airways and lung parenchyma, it was assumed that inhaled corticosteroid would be effective in reducing disease progression. However, several large long-term studies have now demonstrated that even high doses of inhaled corticosteroids are ineffective [29–31]. This is probably because corticosteroids are ineffective in suppressing the inflammation of COPD, in contrast to their marked efficacy in asthma [32, 33]. This means that new classes of anti-inflammatory drugs must be sought.

New Therapies for COPD. In order to develop novel therapies for COPD, there is a need to understand the disease better at a cellular and molecular level [34]. Our current understanding of COPD suggests several possible targets, including mediator inhibitors, anti-proteases, and novel classes of anti-inflammatory drugs. An example of a new class of drug that appears to be promising in COPD are phosphodiesterse-4 inhibitors, which target different aspects of the inflammatory process to corticosteroids [35]. It is likely that several new classes of drug will be developed for the treatment of COPD and many of these are discussed in this volume. There is also a need to find drugs that prevent exacerbations which account for a large proportion of health care spending in COPD. Exacerbations are poorly understood but it is clear that many are not due to bacterial infections, as previously assumed.

Conclusions

Asthma and COPD are amongst the commonest chronic diseases world-wide and there is evidence that both diseases are increasing. This represents an enormous and growing therapeutic market and there is therefore an opportunity for development of new drugs. Asthma is now well treated with existing therapies, but there is a need to find better treatment for patients with severe disease and emergency exacerbations, who represent a small proportion of patients but disproportionate medical costs. There is also a need to find an oral therapy that is as safe and effective as inhaled corticosteroids, and to find treatments that are disease-modifying or curative. By contrast, COPD is poorly treated with currently available drugs and there is a need to find new classes of drug that slow the progression of the disease and reduce exacerbations. More research into the underlying cellular and molecular mechanisms in COPD is needed in order to identify new targets.

References

1 Barnes PJ: New treatments for asthma. Eur J Int Med 2000;11:9–20.
2 Barnes PJ: Current therapies for asthma: Promise and limitations. Chest 1997;111:17S–22S.
3 Barnes PJ, Pedersen S, Busse WW: Efficacy and safety of inhaled corticosteroids: An update. Am J Respir Crit Care Med 1998;157:S1–S53.
4 Wong CA, Walsh LJ, Smith CJ, Wisniewski AF, Lewis SA, Hubbard R, et al: Inhaled corticosteroid use and bone-mineral density in patients with asthma. Lancet 2000;355:1399–1403.
5 Pauwels RA, Lofdahl C-G, Postma DS, Tattersfield AE, O'Byrne PM, Barnes PJ, et al: Effect of inhaled formoterol and budenoside on exacerbations of asthma. N Engl J Med 1997; 337:1412–1418.
6 Barnes PJ: Therapeutic strategies for allergic diseases. Nature 1999;402:B31–B38.
7 Barnes PJ, Woolcock AJ: Difficult asthma. Eur Respir J 1998;12:1209–1218.
8 Barnes PJ, Greening AP, Crompton GK: Glucocorticoid resistance in asthma. Am J Respir Crit Care Med 1995;152:125S–140S.
9 Szefler SJ, Leung DY: Glucocorticoid-resistant asthma: Pathogenesis and clinical implications for management. Eur Respir J 1997;10:1640–1647.
10 Barnes PJ, Jonsson B, Klim J: The costs of asthma. Eur Respir J 1996;9:636–642.
11 Kelloway JS, Wyatt RA, Adlis SA: Comparison of patients' compliance with prescribed oral and inhaled asthma medications. Arch Intern Med 1994;154:1349–1352.
12 Vathenen AS, Knox AJ, Wisniewski A, Tattersfield AE: Time course of change in bronchial reactivity with an inhaled corticosteroid in asthma. Am Rev Respir Dis 1991;143:1317–1321.
13 Jatakanon A, Lim S, Barnes PJ: Changes in sputum eosinophils predict loss of asthma control. Am J Respir Crit Care Med 2000;161:64–72.
14 Herz U, Gerhold K, Gruber C, Braun A, Wahn U, Renz H, et al: BCG infection suppresses allergic sensitization and development of increased airway reactivity in an animal model. J Allergy Clin Immunol 1998;102:867–874.
15 Wang CC, Rook GA: Inhibition of an established allergic response to ovalbumin in BALB/c mice by killed *Mycobacterium vaccae*. Immunology 1998;93:307–313.
16 Sur S, Wild JS, Choudhury BK, Sur N, Alam R, Klinman DM: Long term prevention of allergic lung inflammation in a mouse model of asthma by CpG oligodeoxynucleotides. J Immunol 1999;162:6284–6293.
17 Holt PG: A potential vaccine strategy for asthma and allied atopic diseases during infancy. Lancet 1994;344:456–458.
18 Hopkin JM: Atopy, asthma and mycobacteria. Thorax 2000;55:443–445.
19 Center for Disease Control: Vital and health statistics: Current estimates from the National Health Interview Survey, 1995. DHHS Publ No 96-1527, 1998.
20 Lopez AD, Murray CC: The global burden of disease, 1990–2020. Nat Med 1998;4:1241–1243.
21 Barnes PJ: Mechanisms in COPD: Differences from asthma. Chest 2000;117:10S–14S.
22 Barnes PJ: Novel approaches and targets for treatment of chronic obstructive pulmonary disease. Am J Respir Crit Care Med 1999;160:S72–S79.
23 Barnes PJ: New therapies for chronic obstructive pulmonary disease. Thorax 1998;53:137–147.
24 Barnes PJ: Chronic obstructive pulmonary disease: New opportunities for drug development. Trends Pharmacol Sci 1998;19:415–423.
25 Disse B, Speck GA, Rominger KL, Witek TJ, Hammer R: Tiotropium (Spiriva): Mechanistical considerations and clinical profile in obstructive lung disease. Life Sci 1999;64:457–464.
26 Barnes PJ: The pharmacological properties of tiotropium. Chest 2000;117:63S–66S.
27 Littner MR, Ilowite JS, Tashkin DP, Friedman M, Serby CW, Menjoge SS, et al: Long-acting bronchodilation with once-daily dosing of tiotropium (Spiriva) in stable chronic obstructive pulmonary disease. Am J Respir Crit Care Med 2000;161:1136–1142.
28 Anthonisen NR, Connett JE, Kiley JP, Altose MD, Bailey WC, Buist AS, et al: Effects of smoking intervention and the use of an inhaled anticholinergic bronchodilator on the rate of decline of FEV_1. JAMA 1994;272:1497–1505.
29 Vestbo J, Sorensen T, Lange P, Brix A, Torre P, Viskum K: Long-term effect of inhaled budesonide in mild and moderate chronic obstructive pulmonary disease: A randomised controlled trial. Lancet 1999;353:1819–1823.
30 Pauwels RA, Lofdahl CG, Laitinen LA, Schouten JP, Postma DS, Pride NB, et al: Long-term treatment with inhaled budesonide in persons with mild chronic obstructive pulmonary disease who continue smoking. N Engl J Med 1999;340:1948–1953.
31 Burge PS, Calverley PMA, Jones PW, Spencer S, Anderson JA, Maslen T: Randomised, double-blind, placebo-controlled study of fluticasone propionate in patients with moderate to severe chronic obstructive pulmonary disease; the ISOLDE trial. Br Med J, in press.
32 Keatings VM, Jatakanon A, Worsdell YM, Barnes PJ: Effects of inhaled and oral glucocorticoids on inflammatory indices in asthma and COPD. Am J Respir Crit Care Med 1997;155:542–548.
33 Culpitt SV, Nightingale JA, Barnes PJ: Effect of high dose inhaled steroid on cells, cytokines and proteases in induced sputum in chronic obstructive pulmonary disease. Am J Respir Crit Care Med 1999;160:1635–1639.
34 Barnes PJ: Recent advances in chronic obstructive pulmonary disease. N Engl J Med, in press.
35 Torphy TJ, Barnette MS, Underwood DC, Griswold DE, Christensen SB, Murdock RD, et al: Ariflo (SB 207499), a second generation phosphodiesterase 4 inhibitor for the treatment of asthma and COPD: From concept to clinic. Pulm Pharmacol Ther 1999;12:131–136.

Peter J. Barnes
Department of Thoracic Medicine
National Heart and Lung Institute
Imperial College, Dovehouse Street
London SW3 6LY (UK)
Tel. +44 171 351 3050, Fax +44 171 351 5675
E-Mail p.j.barnes@lc.ac.uk

Current Therapy for Asthma

Peter J. Barnes

Department of Thoracic Medicine, National Heart and Lung Institute, Imperial College, London, UK

Summary

Currently available therapy for asthma is highly effective and is able to control the majority of patients so that they can lead a normal life. National and international guidelines for the treatment of asthma are generally based on use of inhaled β_2-agonists together with inhaled corticosteroids. Advances in therapy have been due to the introduction of more effective and safer treatments and to changes in the way that these treatments are administered to patients. This represented an important change in strategy from the treatment of symptoms as they arose largely with bronchodilator therapy to control and prevent symptoms with anti-inflammatory treatments.

The earlier and more widespread use of inhaled corticosteroids has revolutionized asthma therapy over the last 10 years, with improvement in asthma control, a reduction in asthma morbidity and almost certainly a decrease in mortality [1]. In most countries, guidelines for asthma therapy have now been introduced and these form the framework of modern management, with a stepwise escalation in therapy [2, 3]. Asthma therapies are now classified as relievers that provide rapid relief of symptoms (short-acting β_2-agonists, anticholinergics) that are used as needed and controllers which provide long-term control of symptoms that are used as a regular treatment (corticosteroids, theophylline, long-acting inhaled β_2-agonists, cromones, anti-leukotrienes and immunomodulators) (table 1).

General Issues

Aims of Therapy. Therapy should be aimed at controlling symptoms so that normal life is possible. If currently available treatment is used correctly, it is likely that the vast majority of adults with asthma can lead normal lives and participate in normal leisure activities. Therapy of asthma should aim to:

- minimize (ideally abolish) symptoms
- restore normal or best possible lung function
- prevent severe attacks
- prevent the slow decline in lung function
- prevent death

These aims should be achieved by using the minimum of treatment with the lowest incidence of side effects, but it is important to remember that severe asthma is associated with a high morbidity and mortality, so that side effects of drugs may be acceptable in patients with severer disease. The aims of asthma therapy should be more than alleviation of symptoms, since effective therapies are now available to control all but the most severe asthma. An important aim of therapy is to control symptoms so that normal life is possible. This includes the normal participation in sporting activities and the ability to work normally. Now that home monitoring of PEF is recommended for some patients with more difficult asthma, an additional aim of therapy is to keep the PEF at the best possible level. This is particularly important in patients who may have a poor perception of the severity of their asthma and who tolerate severe impairment of lung function. Asthma

Table 1. Asthma therapy

Reliever	Controllers
Short-acting β_2-agonists	Inhaled corticosteroids
Anticholinergics	Long-acting inhaled β_2-agonists
	Theophylline
	Cromones
	Anti-leukotrienes
	Immunomodulators

exacerbations should be regarded as a failure in therapy, and an important aim of therapy is to prevent such attacks, if necessary by changing treatment. Since poorly controlled asthma may lead to a progressive decline in lung function, it is also hoped that more effective control of airway inflammation may prevent the progressive increase in airway obstruction which occurs in patients with severe asthma, and that it will also prevent death from asthma.

Diagnosis. An objective diagnosis of asthma should be made, based on a documented bronchodilator response (>12% increase in FEV_1), a 15% improvement with corticosteroid therapy or variability in PEF over time of >20%. Bronchial provocation tests (methacholine or histamine challenge and exercise challenge) have little place in routine diagnosis, but may be useful in patients who present with cough or exercise-induced symptoms.

Environmental Control. Avoidance of factors that worsen asthma control is an important part of management. Patients should quit smoking, which may interfere with the anti-inflammatory effects of corticosteroids. Parents of asthmatic children should also stop smoking. Most asthmatic patients are atopic and environmental allergen exposure should be avoided as much as possible. There are several strategies to avoid exposure to house dust mite and furry pets (especially cats), although complete avoidance of house dust mites is very difficult in temperate climates. Occupational exposure to allergens and sensitizers should be avoided where relevant.

Pharmacological Therapy

Short-Acting β_2-Agonists. Beta-agonists are by far the most effective bronchodilators and are well tolerated when given by inhalation. Beta-agonists work as functional antagonists on airway smooth muscle and therefore prevent and reverse bronchoconstriction irrespective of the mechanism. They also inhibit mast cell mediator release and are effective in preventing exercise- and allergen-induced asthma. However, they do not suppress chronic airway inflammation and do not reduce airway hyperresponsiveness and are therefore not adequate alone to treat persistent asthma. Side effects are not usually a problem when β_2-agonists are administered by inhalation, but become more frequent with oral and intravenous administrations. The commonest adverse effects are muscle tremor and palpitations, which are more common in elderly patients. There were concerns that inhaled β_2-agonists may be associated with increased asthma mortality, but it now seems that the association between a high dose of β_2-agonist and mortality is more a reflection of severe and unstable asthma, which has higher risk of death [4]. Evidence that regular use of short-acting inhaled β_2-agonists resulted in poorer control of asthma [5] has now been refuted by studies showing that there is no difference between 'as required' and 'four times a day' salbutamol in either mild or severer asthma [6, 7]. However, short-acting inhaled β_2-agonists are best given as required as this is a useful measure of how well asthma is controlled. Regular use of short-acting inhaled β_2-agonists four times a day have now been superseded by the use of long-acting inhaled β_2-agonists twice daily, which give more effective symptom control [8]. There have also been concerns about the development of tolerance to the bronchodilator effects of β_2-agonists. However, although a reduction in the protective effect of short-acting β_2-agonists has been demonstrated, this is not progressive and most of the protective effect is preserved [9].

Long-Acting β_2-Agonists. Inhaled salmeterol and formoterol give bronchodilatation and bronchoprotection lasting over 12 h and are therefore suitable for twice daily dosing [8]. Like short-acting β_2-agonists, they have no effect on chronic inflammation and therefore should not be used without corticosteroids. Inhaled long-acting β_2-agonists give better asthma control than increasing the dose of inhaled corticosteroids in moderate and severe asthma and also reduce mild and severe exacerbations [10–12]. Salmeterol and formoterol have a similar duration of action, but there are pharmacological differences. Formoterol is a nearly full agonist whereas salmeterol is a partial agonist and this may account for the small degree of bronchodilator tolerance seen with formoterol. Formoterol has a more rapid onset of action than salmeterol and therefore may be useful as relief medication. Oral β_2-agonists are not normally recommended, but a long-acting oral β_2-agonist bambuterol is as effective as salmeterol in controlling symptoms, although side effects may be more common [13].

Anticholinergics. Inhaled anticholinergic drugs (ipratropium bromide, oxitropium bromide) are less effective bronchodilators than β_2-agonists in asthma. They are used as additional bronchodilators in patients already treated with β_2-agonists. As they are additive to β_2-agonists, they may be used to reduce the dose in patients who have side effects from β_2-agonists.

Theophylline. Theophylline has been used in asthma treatment for over 50 years but has become less popular as β_2-agonists are more effective bronchodilators and the high doses needed for bronchodilatation are frequently associated with side effects, such as nausea and headaches [14]. However, more recent studies have demonstrated that theophylline exerts anti-asthma effects at lower concentrations (5–10 mg/l) and these concentrations have few side effects [15]. At these concentrations, theophylline gives better improvement in asthma control than increasing the dose of inhaled corticosteroids [16].

Inhaled Corticosteroids. Inhaled corticosteroids are by far the most effective treatment currently available for the treatment of asthma [17]. They are effective in virtually every patient and at all ages. They are a rational approach to the treatment of asthma, in which there is chronic eosinophilic inflammation in the airways that is suppressed by corticosteroids. Inhaled corticosteroids are now used much earlier in treatment and are recommended in any patient who has symptoms or needs to use a β_2-agonist more than three times a week. Inhaled corticosteroids improve asthma control, reduce exacerbations and almost certainly reduce mortality. In addition, early use of inhaled corticosteroids may prevent irreversible changes in lung function that occur in some patients with asthma [18, 19]. Several inhaled corticosteroids are currently used in asthma and differ mainly in terms of their pharmacokinetic characteristics. Beclomethasone dipropionate and triamcinolone are absorbed from the gastrointestinal tract to a greater extent than fluticasone propionate or budesonide, so the latter are preferred when higher doses are needed or in the treatment of children. Side effects of inhaled corticosteroids are not a problem at the doses that most patients require for asthma control. Local side effects include dysphonia and oral candidiasis and may be reduced by using a large volume spacer or changing to a dry powder inhaler. All currently used inhaled corticosteroids are absorbed from the lung and so have systemic effects. However, at the doses that most patents require, systemic side effects such as stunting of growth in children and osteoporosis in adults are not a problem [17]. The dose-response to inhaled corticosteroids is relatively flat [20] and rather than increasing to high doses, it is preferable to add another class of drug (long-acting inhaled β_2-agonist or theophylline) in most patients.

Oral Corticosteroids. Oral corticosteroids are mainly used as short course (5–10 days) to treat exacerbations of asthma. Approximately 1% of patients with severe asthma may require maintenance oral steroids to control asthma. The lowest dose possible should be used to avoid side effects. Prednisolone and prednisone are the preferred steroids.

Cromones. Sodium cromoglycate (cromolyn) and nedocromil sodium are controller drugs that have a relatively weak effect. They are only effective in a proportion of patients with mild disease and the response to these drugs is unpredictable. They are effective in preventing bronchoconstriction induced by exercise and allergens, but are not very effective in long-term control of asthma, partly because of their short duration of action. They are safe and sodium cromoglycate has been used particularly in children, but low doses of inhaled corticosteroids are now preferred.

Anti-Leukotrienes. Anti-leukotrienes are the first new class of drug introduced for asthma in over 30 years. They include 5-lipoxygenase inhibitors (zileuton) and leukotriene receptor antagonists (zafirlukast, montelukast, pranlukast). These drugs have an inhibitory effect on exercise- and allergen-induced bronchoconstriction, but also have some anti-inflammatory effects. Numerous clinical studies have shown that they have anti-asthma effects, including improvement in lung function, symptoms, β_2-agonist use and a reduction in exacerbations [21]. A major advantage is that they are active orally and do not have any major class-specific side effects. However, they are less effective than inhaled corticosteroids and are not a substitute in mild asthma. They are used as add-on therapy, although they are relatively ineffective in patients with severe asthma.

Steroid-Sparing Therapies. In the small proportion of patients who require maintenance oral corticosteroids therapy there are some treatments that can be used to reduce the requirement for oral corticosteroids [22]. These treatments include methotrexate, cyclosporin A and oral gold. All of these treatments have marginal efficacy and often have side effects that are worse than those of oral corticosteroids. They should only be continued if there is objective evidence of benefit.

Immunotherapy. Desensitizing injections against specific allergens have been popular in the treatment of allergies, including asthma. However, in asthma this treatment is not very effective [23] and there is a risk of a severe reaction, including a fatal exacerbation. Since safe and more effective therapies are readily available, this treatment cannot be recommended until safer immunotherapy treatments (such as specific peptides) are developed [24].

Treatment Strategies

Asthma guidelines advocate a stepwise increase in asthma therapy, depending on the assumed severity of asthma and the response to treatment (fig. 1). In the British Guidelines there are 5 steps in therapy (fig. 2), whereas in the Global Initiative for Asthma Guidelines, 4 levels of therapy are recognized [2, 3].

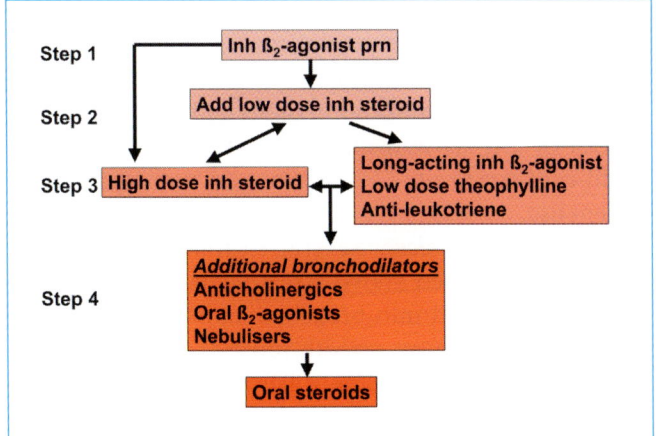
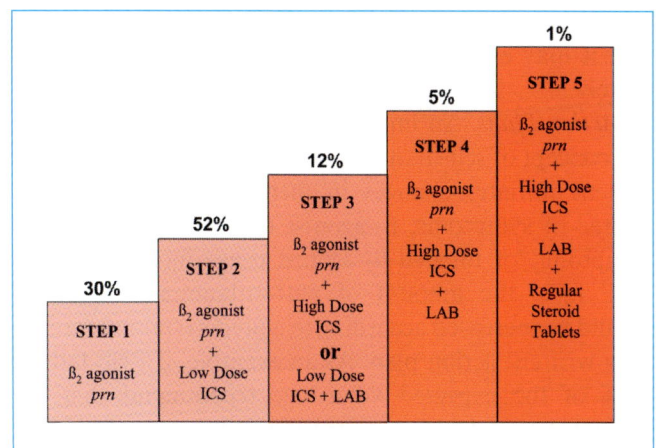
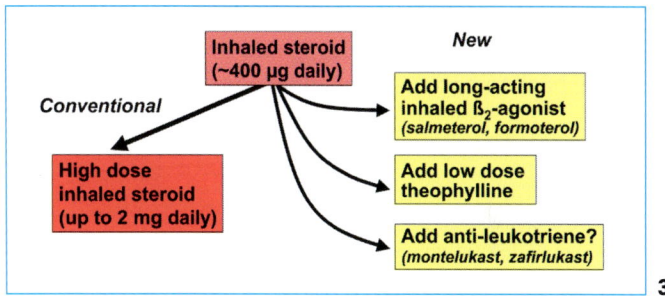

Fig. 1. Guidelines for asthma therapy.
Fig. 2. Stepwise treatment of asthma according to the British Thoracic Society Guidelines. The percentages of patients at each step in the guidelines from a community study is also shown. ICS = Inhaled corticosteroid; LAB = long-acting β_2-agonist.
Fig. 3. Treatment choices at step 3.

Step 1: Mild Episodic Asthma. For patients with mild episodic asthma, a short inhaled β_2-agonist should be used for symptomatic control only and should not be used as a regular therapy. The frequency of use of the β_2-agonist inhaler is a good guide to the degree of asthma control and any patient who requires to use an inhaler on a daily basis or who wakes at night because of asthma should be started on an inhaled anti-inflammatory drug.

Step 2: Mild Persistent Asthma. Patients with mild persistent asthma should be started on an inhaled anti-inflammatory agent. For most patients this should be an inhaled corticosteroid. In children, cromoglycate is an option, but this is less effective than an inhaled corticosteroid and should only be used when there is a reluctance to use an inhaled steroid. A patient may be started on either low-dose inhaled steroid (e.g. beclomethasone dipropionate (BDP), budesonide 50–200 µg or fluticasone propionate (FP) 50–100 µg twice daily). More rapid control is achieved by starting with a higher dose (800 µg daily) and once control is achieved by slowly reducing the dose.

Step 3: Moderate Persistent Asthma. If asthma is not controlled on low-dose inhaled corticosteroids, the previously recommended strategy was to increase the dose (up to 2,000 µg daily for BDP and budesonide or 1,000 µg daily for FP). An alternative approach is to add another class of controller drug. This may be a long-acting inhaled β_2-agonist, low-dose theophylline or possibly an anti-leukotriene [10–12, 16, 25] (fig. 3). Fixed-combination inhalers with a corticosteroid and long-acting β_2-agonist have now been developed and these are more convenient to the patient and may improve compliance.

Step 4: Severe Persistent Asthma. A small proportion of patients is not controlled on high-dose inhaled corticosteroid with the addition of another controller. In these patients an additional bronchodilator (anticholinergic or theophylline) should be tried, and nebulized bronchodilators are sometimes necessary. In patients with brittle asthma, subcutaneous β_2-agonists may be useful [26].

In some patients, asthma is only controlled by oral steroids, but the minimum dose should be used. It is usual to use prednisone or prednisolone as a single oral dose in the morning to reduce adrenal suppression and side effects.

Step-Down. It is very important to reduce treatment as asthma comes under control, so that the patient is on the minimal therapy required. The requirement for anti-inflammatory therapy may vary from time to time. Thus during the pollen season, sensitive patients usually need to increase the dose of inhaled steroids to prevent the onset of symptoms. If a patient is virtually asymptomatic for 6 months, it is reasonable to gradually reduce the dose of inhaled steroids (by ~25% of dose every 3 months), and it may even be possible to withdraw steroids completely.

Action Plans. An important part of asthma therapy is the concept of self-management of the disease, so that the patient initiates changes in therapy, according to the degree of symptoms, β_2-agonist use or PEF. If asthma symptoms, or inhaled β_2-agonist usage increases or the PEF falls, the amount of anti-inflammatory therapy should be increased according to a predetermined (preferably written) action plan. As an example, if PEF falls to 70% of the expected value, we recommend that the patient should double the dose of inhaled steroids. If PEF falls to 50% of expected value, a short course of oral steroids is needed. This should be prednisone/prednisolone 30–40 mg orally each morning and given until the PEF comes back to normal, then either continued for 2 further days or tailed off by 5 mg daily. If the PEF falls to 30% of the expected value then urgent medical attention should be sought. The use of this sort of action plan has been shown to reduce asthma admissions and improve overall control of asthma and quality of life [27]. Convenient credit-card size printed action plans are now available for patient use.

Therapeutic Choices. Several treatments for asthma have been discussed above. Treatments for asthma can broadly be divided into bronchodilators, which act *predominantly* on airway smooth muscle, and anti-inflammatory, prophylactic or controller therapies, which control asthma symptoms when taken regularly. There are advantages and disadvantages to each treatment and it is important to consider convenience of use and potential side effects. Cost of therapy is also an important consideration, particularly in developing countries.

References

1 Barnes PJ: Inhaled glucocorticoids for asthma. N Engl J Med 1995;332:868–875.
2 British Thoracic Society: BTS guidelines for the management of chronic obstructive pulmonary disease. Thorax 1997;52(supp 15):S1–S28.
3 Global Initiative for Asthma: Global strategy for asthma management and prevention. NHLBI/WHO Workshop Report, Publ 95-3659, 1995.
4 Suissa S, Ernst P, Boivin J-F, Horwitz RI, Habbick B, Cockroft D, et al: A cohort analysis of excess mortality in asthma due to use of inhaled β-agonists. Am J Respir Crit Care Med 1994;149:604–610.
5 Sears MR, Taylor DR, Print CG, Lake DG, Li Q, Flannery EM, et al: Regular inhaled beta-agonist treatment in bronchial asthma. Lancet 1990;336:1391–1396.
6 Drazen JM, Israel E, Boushey HA, Chinchilli VM, Fahy JV, Fish JE, et al: Comparison of regularly scheduled with as needed use of albuterol in mild asthma. N Engl J Med 1996;335:841–847.
7 Dennis SM, Sharp SJ, Vickers MJ, Frost CD, Crompton GK, Barnes PJ, Lee TH: The effects of regular inhaled salbutamol on asthma control. Lancet 2000;355:1675–1679.
8 Boulet L-P: Long versus short-acting β₂-agonists. Drugs 1994;47:207–222.
9 O'Connor BJ, Aikman SL, Barnes PJ: Tolerance to the non-bronchodilator effects of inhaled β₂-agonists. N Engl J Med 1992;327:1204–1208.
10 Greening AP, Ind PW, Northfield M, Shaw G: Added salmeterol versus higher-dose corticosteroid in asthma patients with symptoms on existing inhaled corticosteroid. Lancet 1994;344:219–224.
11 Woolcock A, Lundback B, Ringdal N, Jacques L: Comparison of addition of salmeterol to inhaled steroids with doubling the dose of inhaled steroids. Am J Respir Crit Care Med 1996; 153:1481–1488.
12 Pauwels RA, Lofdahl C-G, Postma DS, Tattersfield AE, O'Byrne PM, Barnes PJ, et al: Effect of inhaled formoterol and budesonide on exacerbations of asthma. N Engl J Med 1997; 337:1412–1418.
13 Crompton GK, Ayres JG, Basran G, Schiraldi G, Brusasco V, Eivindson A, et al: Comparison of oral bambuterol and inhaled salmeterol in patients with symptomatic asthma and using inhaled corticosteroids. Am. J. Respir Crit Care Med 1999;159:824–828.
14 Weinberger M, Hendeles L: Theophylline in asthma. N Engl J Med 1996; 334:1380–1388.
15 Barnes PJ, Pauwels RA: Theophylline in asthma: Time for reappraisal? Eur Respir J 1994;7:579–591.
16 Evans DJ, Taylor DA, Zetterstrom O, Chung KF, O'Connor BJ, Barnes PJ: A comparison of low-dose inhaled budesonide plus theophylline and high-dose inhaled budesonide for moderate asthma. N Engl J Med 1997;337:1412–1418.
17 Barnes PJ, Pedersen S, Busse WW: Efficacy and safety of inhaled corticosteroids: An update. Am J Respir Crit Care Med 1998;157:S1–S53
18 Haahtela T, Järvinsen M, Kava T, Kiviranta K, Koskinen S, Lemtonen K, et al: Effects of reducing or discontinuing inhaled budesonide in patients with mild asthma. N Engl J Med 1994;331:700–705.
19 Agertoft L, Pedersen S: Effects of long-term treatment with an inhaled corticosteroid on growth and pulmonary function in asthmatic children. Respir Med 1994;5:369–372.
20 Busse WW, Chervinsky P, Condemi J, Lumry WR, Petty TL, Rennard S, et al: Budesonide delivered by Turbuhaler is effective in a dose-dependent fashion when used in the treatment of adult patients with chronic asthma. J Allergy Clin Immunol 1998;101:457–463.
21 Drazen JM, Israel E, O'Byrne PM: Treatment of asthma with drugs modifying the leukotriene pathway. N Engl J Med 1999;340:197–206.
22 Hill SJ, Tattersfield AE: Corticosteroid sparing agents in asthma. Thorax 1995;50:577–582.
23 Creticos PS, Reed CE, Norman PS, Khoury J, Adkinson NF, Buncher R, et al: Ragweed immunotherapy in adult asthma. N Engl J Med 1996; 334:501–506.
24 Barnes PJ. Immunotherapy for asthma: Is it worth it? N Engl J Med 1996; 334:531–532.
25 Laviolette M, Malmstrom K, Lu S, Chervinsky P, Pujet JC, Peszek I, et al: Montelukast added to inhaled beclomethasone in treatment of asthma. Am J Respir Crit Care Med 1999;160:1862–1868.
26 Ayres JG, Miles JF, Barnes PJ: Brittle asthma. Thorax 1998;53:315–321.
27 Lahdensuo A, Haahtela T, Herrala J, Kava T, Kiviranta K, Kuusisto P, et al: Randomised comparison of cost effectiveness of guided self-management and traditional treatment of asthma in Finland. BMJ. 1998;316:1138–1139.

Peter J. Barnes
Department of Thoracic Medicine
National Heart and Lung Institute
Imperial College, Dovehouse Street
London SW3 6LY (UK)
Tel. +44 171 351 3050, Fax +44 171 351 5675
E-Mail p.j.barnes@lc.ac.uk

Current Therapy for COPD

Romain Pauwels

Department of Respiratory Diseases, Ghent University Hospital, Ghent, Belgium

Summary

The management of COPD aims at relieving symptoms, improving quality of life and preventing further deterioration. Managing COPD will therefore need a broader approach than pure pharmacological treatment, as reflected in the Global Initiative for Obstructive Lung Disease (GOLD) guidelines. The major risk factor of COPD is cigarette smoking, but other risk factors, including indoor pollution and occupational exposure might play a significant role. Chronic oxygen therapy prolongs survival in COPD patients with respiratory failure. Long-term studies looking at the influence of pharmacological treatments on the mortality of COPD are ongoing. Management approaches other than the avoidance of risk factors should therefore be regarded as symptomatic. The choice of treatment will mainly depend on the severity of the patient's COPD. The severity of the airflow limitation is certainly not the only, and very often not the major factor determining the severity of COPD in an individual patient. The airflow limitation in COPD is also largely irreversible. Therapeutic recommendations and choices should therefore take into account other patient characteristics besides the degree of airflow limitation.

Management Options in COPD

Avoidance of Risk Factors. Smoking Cessation. Smoking cessation is the single most effective intervention to stop the progressive worsening of COPD, and is the only intervention that has been shown to significantly influence the long-term evolution of the disease [1]. Smoking cessation is also the most cost-effective intervention. All available means should be used to help a patient stop smoking. These include individual and group counselling, nicotine substitution treatment (gum, patches, inhaler and nasal spray) and bupropion. Nicotine substitution therapy has been shown to approximately double the smoking cessation rate [2]. Bupropion treatment further increase the success rate of smoking intervention [3]. The individually tailored combination of these methods results in long-term smoking cessation in approximately one third of all COPD patients.

Occupational Exposures. Strategies aiming at reducing the burden of particles and gases should be applied at the workplace.

Indoor Air Pollution. The reduction of the inhalation of noxious particles and gases from indoor heating or cooking is very often dependent on the socio-economic conditions of the individual.

Education. Education in COPD is effective in obtaining smoking cessation, in increasing the effectiveness of and compliance with inhaler therapy, in improving the patient's response to exacerbations, and in discussions around advance directives and end of life issues. Education can be achieved through consultations with physicians and other health care workers or through more comprehensive pulmonary rehabilitation programs.

Pharmacological Treatment. Pharmacological treatment is used to prevent and control symptoms, to reduce the frequency and severity of acute exacerbations, to improve health and exercise tolerance. None of the existing medications has been shown to modify the long-term evolution of the airflow limitation in COPD. Several medications, such as the long-acting inhaled β_2-agonist salmeterol, the long-acting inhaled anticholinergic tiotropium, acetylcysteine and inhaled glucocorticosteroids, have been shown to decrease the frequency of exacerbations.

Bronchodilators. Bronchodilators are central to the symptomatic management of COPD. Anticholinergic agents, β_2-agonists and theophylline have been shown to improve the symptoms and the exercise tolerance in patients with COPD. They also partially reverse the airflow limitation but the improvement in symptoms and exercise tolerance is not necessarily associated with a significant improvement in spirometric measures. The choice between the different bronchodilators should be guided by the patient's symptomatic response and/or objective changes in airflow limitation. Inhaled therapy is usually preferred as first-line bronchodilator because of the safety concerns about theophylline. The rationale for combining different bronchodilators is not only the additional benefit but also avoiding side effects by not using higher doses of a single drug. The long-acting inhaled bronchodilators are at least as effective as the short-acting and more convenient [4, 5]. There are indications that they are more effective in preventing acute exacerbations [4].

Glucocorticosteroids. Prolonged treatment with inhaled glucocorticosteroids in COPD does not modify the long-term evolution of the airflow limitation [6, 7]. Such a treatment is only justifiable in symptomatic COPD patients with an objective improvement (at least 200 ml) of the postbronchodilator FEV_1 after a therapeutic trial for 6 weeks to 3 months or in COPD patients with an FEV_1 below 50% of predicted and repeated exacerbations [8]. The dose-response relationship and long-term safety of inhaled glucocorticosteroids in COPD are unknown. A response to a short course with oral glucocorticosteroids is a poor predictor of the long-term response to inhaled glucocorticosteroids [9].

The benefit-risk ratio of long-term treatment with oral glucocorticosteroids is so low that this treatment modality should be avoided in patients with COPD. An important side effect of long-term treatment with systemic glucocorticosteroids in COPD is steroid myopathy [10]. This myopathy contributes to the muscle weakness and decreased performance status in these patients.

Mucolytics. Mucolytics have been shown to improve symptoms in patients with COPD. They do not modify the airflow limitation.

Antioxidants. Antioxidants, in particular acetylcysteine, have been shown in a meta-analysis to reduce the frequency of acute exacerbations in COPD [11]. This meta-analysis is based on a number of rather small studies of limited duration. A larger scale 3-year study is currently ongoing.

Immunomodulators. One study showed a decrease in the severity but not in the frequency of exacerbations of COPD during treatment with OM-85 BV [12]. This study has not been confirmed.

Table 1. Factors determining Severity of COPD [15]

Severity of symptoms
Severity of airflow limitation
Frequency and severity of exacerbations
Presence of complications
Presence of respiratory failure
Presence of comorbid conditions
General health status
Number of medications needed to manage the disease

Vaccines. An influenza vaccine is recommended for all patients with COPD. These vaccines very significantly decrease morbidity and mortality due to influenza in these patients. The evidence for the systematic use of pneumococcal vaccine in COPD is less convincing.

Non-Pharmacological Treatment. Rehabilitation. The majority of COPD patients benefit from rehabilitation programs [13]. Improvements in symptoms and exercise tolerance have been amply documented. A comprehensive rehabilitation programme includes exercise training, nutritional counselling and education.

Oxygen Therapy. Long-term oxygen therapy is indicated for patients with advanced COPD and respiratory failure (PaO_2 <7.2 kPa or 55 mm Hg or PaO_2 between 7.2 and 8.0 kPa or 59 mm Hg and evidence of right heart failure or pulmonary hypertension or polycythaemia). Long-term administration of low concentrations of oxygen for at least 15 h per day has been shown to increase survival and improve exercise capacity and mental state in these patients.

Surgical Treatments. Bullectomy is indicated in selected patients with large bullae. Lung volume reduction surgery is a surgical procedure that still should be considered as experimental. Improvements in lung function parameters and quality of life have been documented in relatively small or non-randomized studies [14].

Management of Chronic COPD

The aim of chronic treatment in COPD is to prevent progression of the disease, exacerbations and decay of health and to improve symptoms, exercise tolerance, and quality of life. The management should be guided by the severity of the COPD and by the response to individual treatments; the severity of an individual's COPD being dependent on many factors (table 1). Tables 2–5 summarize the management recommendations from the Global Initiative for Obstructive Lung Disease (GOLD) guide-

Table 2. Definition of stage 0: at risk

Chronic symptoms	Avoidance of noxious agents
Cough	Smoking cessation
Sputum	Reduction of indoor pollution
No spirometric abnormalities	Reduction of occupational exposure

Table 3. Definition of stage I: mild

Chronic symptoms	Avoidance of noxious agents
Cough	Smoking cessation
Sputum	Reduction of indoor pollution
Dyspnea	Reduction of occupational exposure
$FEV_1/FVC < 70\%$	
$FEV_1 \geq 80\%$ predicted	Short-acting bronchodilator as needed

Table 4. Definition of stage II: moderate

$FEV_1/FVC < 70\%$	Avoidance of noxious agents
$30\% < FEV_1 < 80\%$ pred.	Smoking cessation
With or without chronic symptoms	Reduction of indoor pollution
	Reduction of occupational exposure
	Regular bronchodilator treatment
	Short-acting bronchodilator as needed
	Rehabilitation
	Consider inhaled steroids

Table 5. Definition of stage III: severe

$FEV_1/FVC < 70\%$	Avoidance of noxious agents
$FEV_1 < 30\%$ pred. or respiratory failure or right heart failure	Regular bronchodilator treatment
	Short-acting bronchodilator as needed
Chronic symptoms	Rehabilitation
	Consider inhaled steroids
	Long-term oxygen therapy if respiratory insufficiency
	Consider surgical alternatives

lines according to stages of severity [15]. The avoidance of risk factors is the major therapeutic intervention. The effect of smoking cessation cannot be underestimated and repeated efforts should be made to convince and help the patient. The bronchodilator therapy will be tailored to the individual symptoms and therapeutic response. The recommendations for the use of inhaled glucocorticosteroids have been discussed above.

Management of Acute Exacerbation of COPD

COPD is associated with acute exacerbations of symptoms. Exacerbations are often the primary reason for consultation for a patient with COPD. Increased breathlessness is usually the main symptom, but this can be associated with increased coughing and sputum and with change in the colour and/or viscosity of the sputum. Fever is rather rare unless associated with pneumonia. Exacerbations of COPD might be caused by respiratory infections, both viral and bacterial, and by an increase in air pollution. The cause of an exacerbation can very often not be identified.

Exacerbations of COPD are important clinical events for patients with COPD and require adequate medical attention. COPD exacerbations can lead to respiratory failure in patients with more advanced COPD. Repeated exacerbations are also associated with a more rapid decline in health status [8].

The treatment of an exacerbation of COPD is very much dependent on the severity of the exacerbation and the severity of the underlying COPD.

Mild to Moderate Exacerbation. A mild exacerbation can very often be managed by a temporary increase in the dose and frequency of the existing bronchodilator therapy or by the addition of a new bronchodilator. A course of antibiotics should be added if purulent sputum is present and the dyspnoea and sputum volume have increased [16]. The choice of antibiotic will depend on the local sensitivities of the most prevalent bacterial causes of COPD exacerbations: *Streptococcus pneumoniae, Hemophilus influenzae* and *Moraxella catharalis.*

Severe Exacerbation. Patients with severe symptoms during an exacerbation should receive treatment with bronchodilators, according to the recommendations given for mild to moderate exacerbations. A nebulizer or a pressurized metered-dose inhaler with a spacer should be used for the administration of higher doses of bronchodilators in subjects who are too short of breath to use the standard metered dose inhalers. The criteria for using antibiotics are the same as for milder exacerbations. Oral and systemic glucocorticosteroids have been shown to shorten the recovery from an exacerbation and help restore lung function more quickly [17, 18]. A dose of 40 mg of prednisolone per day for 10 days is recommended. Oxygen therapy should be given when hypoxaemia is suspected or documented. The oxygen concentration should be low, in order to avoid the risk of worsening hypercapnia. The oxygen concentration can be increased if blood gas monitoring is available. Indications for hospitalization of a patient with an acute exacerbation of COPD include a marked increase in the intensity of the symptoms, a background of severe COPD, the onset of new physical signs such as cyanosis or peripheral edema, the sudden onset of an arrhythmia, significant comorbidities, a change in mental status and older age [15]. In COPD patients with acute respiratory failure, temporary ventilatory support can be given by non-invasive means using either negative- or positive-pressure devices or by invasive mechanical ventilation [19].

References

1 Anthonisen NR, Connett JE, Kiley JP, Altose MD, Bailey WC, Buist AS, et al: Effects of smoking intervention and the use of an inhaled anticholinergic bronchodilator on the rate of decline of FEV_1. The Lung Health Study. JAMA 1994;272:1497–1505.

2 Silagy C, Mant D, Fowler G, Lodge M: Meta-analysis on efficacy of nicotine replacement therapies in smoking cessation. Lancet 1994; 343:139–142.

3 Jorenby DE, Leischow SJ, Nides MA, Rennard SI, Johnston JA, Hughes AR, et al: A controlled trial of sustained-release bupropion, a nicotine patch, or both for smoking cessation. N Engl J Med 1999;340:685–691.

4 Mahler DA, Donohue JF, Barbee RA, Goldman MD, Gross NJ, Wisniewski ME, et al: Efficacy of salmeterol xinafoate in the treatment of COPD. Chest 1999;115:957–965.

5 van Noord JA, Bantje TA, Eland ME, Korducki L, Cornelissen PJ: A randomised controlled comparison of tiotropium and ipratropium in the treatment of chronic obstructive pulmonary disease. The Dutch Tiotropium Study Group. Thorax 2000;55:289–294.

6 Pauwels RA, Lofdahl CG, Laitinen LA, Schouten JP, Postma DS, Pride NB, et al: Long-term treatment with inhaled budesonide in persons with mild chronic obstructive pulmonary disease who continue smoking. European Respiratory Society Study on Chronic Obstructive Pulmonary Disease. N Engl J Med 1999;340:1948–1953.

7 Vestbo J, Sorensen T, Lange P, Brix A, Torre P, Viskum K: Long-term effect of inhaled budesonide in mild and moderate chronic obstructive pulmonary disease: A randomised controlled trial. Lancet 1999;353:1819–1823.

8 Burge PS, Calverley PMA, Jones PW, Spencer S, Anderson JA, Maslen TK: Randomised, double blind, placebo controlled study of fluticasone propionate in patients with moderate to severe chronic obstructive pulmonary disease: The ISOLDE trial. Br Med J 2000;320:1297–1303.

9 Senderovitz T, Vestbo J, Frandsen J, Maltbaek N, Norgaard M, Nielsen C, et al: Steroid reversibility test followed by inhaled budesonide or placebo in outpatients with stable chronic obstructive pulmonary disease. The Danish Society of Respiratory Medicine. Respir Med 1999; 93:715–718.

10 Decramer M, Lacquet LM, Fagard R, Rogiers P: Corticosteroids contribute to muscle weakness in chronic airflow obstruction. Am J Respir Crit Care Med 1994;150:11–16.

11 Poole PJ, Black PN: Mucolytic agents for chronic bronchitis or chronic obstructive pulmonary disease. Cochrane Database Syst Rev 2000; CD001287.

12 Collet JP, Shapiro S, Ernst P, Renzi P, Ducruet T, Robinson A, et al: Effects of an immunostimulations in patients with chronic obstructive pulmonary disease. Am J Respir Crit Care Med 1997;156:1719–1724.

13 Goldstein RS, Gort EH, Stubbing D, Avendano MA, Guyatt GH: Randomised controlled trial of respiratory rehabilitation. Lancet 1994; 344:1394–1397.

14 Geddes D, Davies M, Koyoma H, Hansell D, Pastorino U, Pepper J, et al: Effect of lung-volume-reduction surgery in patients with severe emphysema. N Engl J Med 2000;343:239–245.

15 Global Initiative for Obstructive Lung Disease: Global Strategy for the Diagnosis, Management and Prevention of Chronic Obstructive Pulmonary Disease. National Heart, Lung and Blood Institute, Bethesda, 2000.

16 Anthonisen NR, Manfreda J, Warren CP, Hershfield ES, Harding GK, Nelson NA: Antibiotic therapy in exacerbations of chronic obstructive pulmonary disease. Ann Intern Med 1987;106:196–204.

17 Niewoehner DE, Erbland ML, Deupree RH, Collins D, Gross NJ, Light RW, et al: Effect of systemic glucocorticoids on exacerbations of chronic obstructive pulmonary disease. N Engl J Med 1999;340:1941–1947.

18 Davies L, Angus RM, Calverley PM: Oral corticosteroids in patients admitted to hospital with exacerbations of chronic obstructive pulmonary disease: A prospective randomised controlled trial. Lancet 1999;354:456–460.

19 Plant PK, Owen JL, Elliott MW: Early use of non-invasive ventilation for acute exacerbations of chronic obstructive pulmonary disease on general respiratory wards: A multicentre randomised controlled trial. Lancet 2000;355: 1931–1935.

Romain Pauwels, MD
Department of Respiratory Diseases
Ghent University Hospital, De Pintelaan 185
B–9000 Ghent (Belgium)
Tel. +32 92402611, Fax +32 92402341
E-Mail romain.pauwels@rug.ac.be

Pharmacogenetics

Ian P. Hall[a]   Trevor T. Hansel[b]

[a]Division of Therapeutics, University Hospital, Nottingham, and [b]National Heart and Lung Institute, Clinical Studies Unit, Imperial College, London, UK

Summary

This review deals with the evidence for variability in drug response due to genetic polymorphisms and speculates on potential use of genetic data in determining variability in drug response in patients with asthma and COPD. Polymorphism of the β_2-adrenoreceptor gene at a number of sites corresponding to amino acid positions 16 and 27 have been proposed as being functionally relevant. Genes for muscarinic M_2, histamine H_1 and glucocorticoid receptors and the 5-lipoxygenase promoter may also be relevant. The molecular genetics of COPD are less well understood, but genes for oxidative stress, TNF-α and nicotine metabolism have been implicated.

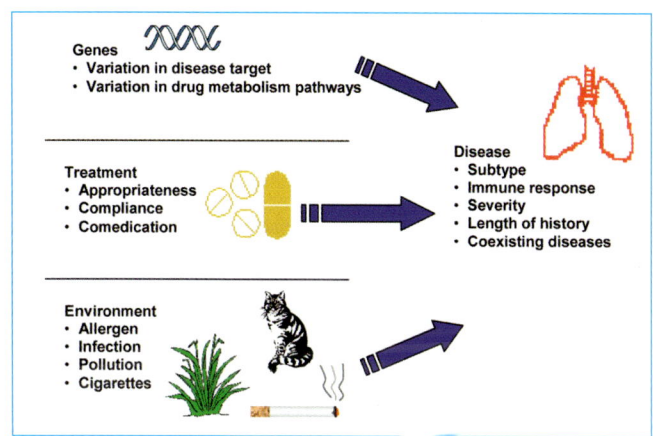

Fig. 1. Factors affecting treatment response.

Functional Genetic Polymorphism

As the human genome sequencing project has progressed, it has become increasingly clear that high rates of genetic polymorphism exist in the human genome. Whereas some mutations have clear deleterious effects, most polymorphisms have minor, if any, functional consequences. For a polymorphism to contribute to variability in drug responsiveness in the population at large, it would need to be at least reasonably common. Hence polymorphisms with an allelic frequency of 0.1% may be important in determining treatment response in very small numbers of individuals, but obviously cannot contribute to determining treatment response in large populations to any major extent. Intuitively, one would imagine that commoner polymorphisms would have smaller functional effects, although one area of research which remains to be explored in more depth is the possibility that a range of polymorphisms, each with relatively minor functional effects, could in combination contribute to a marked phenotypic change (fig. 1).

Genetic Variability

Current estimates of genetic polymorphism within the human genome for coding DNA are at 1 in 1,000 bp, and for non-coding DNA are at 1 in 500 bp. These figures, however, hide the large variability between different genes: for example, the β_2-adrenoceptor (see below) contains at least 17 polymorphisms within a region of 3 kb containing the gene and its major transcriptional controlling region.

Polymorphic Variation in Respiratory Drug Targets

Polymorphism screening has been performed for many of the immediate respiratory drug targets, although downstream targets such as components of signal transduction pathways and/or ion channels remain little studied.

Criteria for Assessing Pharmacogenetic Candidate Genes

- **Polymorphisms:** Does the candidate gene or its controlling region contain polymorphisms?
- **Coding region:** Is the polymorphism degenerate or non-degenerate (i.e. does it alter the amino acid sequence of the protein)?
- **Non-coding region:** Does the polymorphism interfere with known regulatory regions/splice-sites?
- Is the polymorphism **non-conservative**?
  Coding region: Conservative or non-conservative amino acid substitution?
  Non-coding region: Conservative or non-conservative base substitution?
- Are there **functional** data to suggest a functional effect for the polymorphism?
- Is there association in clinical studies of a relevant end-point with a given **allele/haplotype**?

Other Considerations for Pharmacogenetic Candidate Genes

- **Homozygotes versus heterozygotes**
  Autosomes contain a pair of genes at a given locus: individuals may be homozygous or heterozygous.
- **Nature of polymorphism**
  Most polymorphisms are single nucleotide polymorphisms and are hence b-iallelic, although some involve deletions or insertions which may introduce a frameshift in coding regions.
- **In vitro functional data**
  Most in vitro studies have used site directed mutagenesis to address the functionality of a given polymorphism. This effectively replicates the homozygous phenotype, but for common polymorphisms in the general population heterozygote individuals will predominate.
- **Linkage disequilibrium**
  When a given gene contains a number of polymorphic variants then additional difficulties are created. Over short regions of DNA linkage disequilibrium tends to be very strong, making it difficult to look at the effects of a given polymorphism in isolation.

β_2-Adrenoceptor. The human β_2-adrenoceptor remains the best studied candidate gene from a respiratory pharmacogenetic aspect [1, 2] (fig. 2). In all, 17 polymorphisms are known within the gene or its regulatory region, although functional data exist for only 4 sites.

Cys 19 Arg BUP. Preliminary functional data have suggested a role for the –47 C-T single nucleotide polymorphism (SNP). This alters the terminal amino acid of the short β upstream peptide (BUP), that has a role in transcriptional/translational inhibition of β_2-adrenoceptor expression in the airways. Translational inhibition is at least in part dependent on theariginine content of the peptide: the –47 C-T SNP increases the number of arginine residues in the peptide from 3 to 4. No clinical data currently exist on this polymorphism although in vitro studies suggest some reduction in β_2-adrenoceptor expression in transformed cell systems [3, 4].

Arg 16 Gly. The Gly 16 polymorphism results in increased receptor downregulation, following long-term exposure to agonist, both in recombinant cell systems and primary cultured airway smooth muscle. Clinical studies have suggested reduced response to β_2-agonists in individuals carrying Gly 16, with either tachyphylaxis to the bronchodilator effects of formoterol [5] or a reduced acute bronchodilator response to salbutamol in children [6]. A further study correlated the presence of Gly 16 with the nocturnal asthma phenotype [7]. The Gly 16 variant is frequent in the general population, having an allelic frequency of 60%.

Gln 27 Glu. In contrast, there are no good functional data to suggest a role for the Glu 27 polymorphism (which protects against downregulation) in determining treatment response. Weak linkage and association with reduced IgE and bronchial hyperreactivity have been observed in clinical studies, possibly due to linkage disequilibrium with the cytokine TH2 gene cluster close by on chromosome 5Q31 [8, 9]. Again, the allelic frequency is high at 50% for Glu 27 [10].

Thr 164 Ile. The Ile 164 variant of the β_2-adrenoceptor alters agonist binding and receptor sequestration following long-term stimulation [11, 12]. Because this polymorphism is close to the putative binding site for the lipophilic tail of salmeterol it is also possible that salmeterol binding may be altered in individuals carrying this variant of the receptor. Individuals carrying the Ile 164 variant will be expected to show reduced responses to β_2-agonists and potentially a different time course of action of salmeterol. However, this polymorphism is rare (allelic frequency 3%) and clinical studies have been limited, with homozygous individuals not studied to date.

Asthma Severity. In addition to the above studies, different β_2-adrenoceptor variants have not been found to be significantly associated with long-term disease control or fatal/near fatal asthma [13, 14]. However, studies have been complicated to some extent by the large number of β_2-adrenoceptor polymorphisms [15] and the linkage disequilibrium which exists [10].

Muscarinic M_2 Receptor. A screen by single strand conformational polymorphism (SSCP) and direct sequencing of the muscarinic M_2 receptor and a short region of the 5′ UTR and 3′ UTR revealed three changes from the published sequence. An A-insertion in the 3′ UTR at +1793 appeared to be present in all samples studied and hence

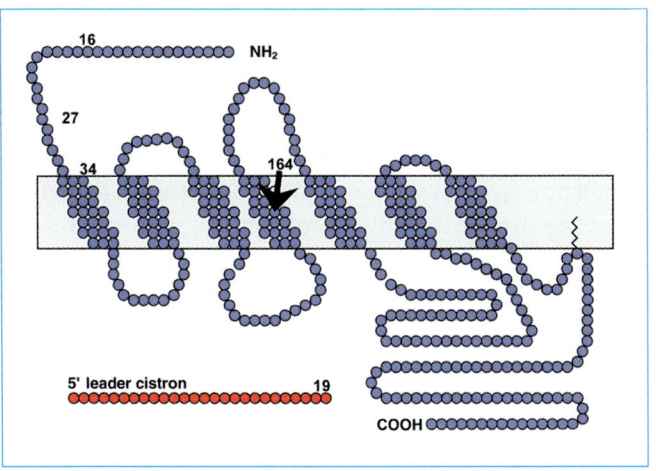

Nucleic acid position	Amino acid position	Wild type	Polymorphism (allele frequency)	Phenotype	Altered treatment response
–47	19 (5′ LC)	Arg	Cys (0.63)	⇑ expression	potential
46	16	Arg	Gly (0.61)	⇑ downregulation	yes
79	27	Gln	Glu (0.43)	⇓ downregulation	potential
491	164	Thr	Ile (0.05)	⇓ coupling	likely

Adapted from Liggett [1].

Fig. 2. β$_2$-Adrenoceptor polymorphism.

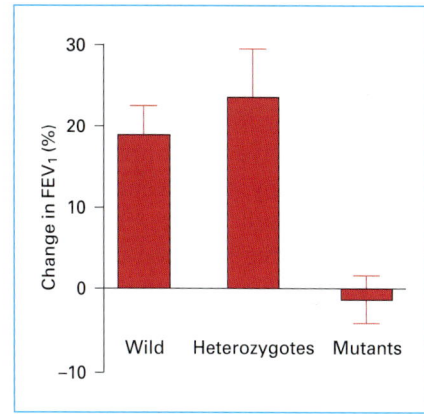

Fig. 3. 5LO promoter genotype and response to a 5LO inhibitor.

may represent an error in the database. The other two SNPs give rise to a degenerate polymorphism in the coding region (basepair +1197, T-C) and a common bi-allelic 3′ UTR polymorphism (+1196, T-A, allelic frequency 65% [16]. No functional data are available on these polymorphisms at present.

Histamine H$_1$ Receptor. Although not a primary target for asthma or COPD, anti-histamines acting via the H$_1$ receptor remain important in the management of atopic disease (e.g. allergic rhinitis). A limited screen (by SSCP) of the coding region of the H$_1$ receptor revealed one degenerate polymorphism (Gln 356 Gln), which is unlikely to be functionally relevant [17].

Glucocorticoid Receptor. The glucocorticoid receptor was one of the first to be sequenced to look for polymorphic variation. These studies were initiated by the observation that at least some asthmatics appear to be steroid insensitive. However, no genetic basis for steroid resistance was found at the receptor level [18]. More recently, a polymorphism which results in a single amino acid substitution (N-Asp 363 Ser) and a consequent gain of function has been described within the glucocorticoid receptor [19]. The possibility that this gain of function polymorphism might increase response to steroids or alter the extent of adrenal suppression profile following treatment with steroids deserves further study.

5-Lipoxygenase. Other than the β$_2$-adrenoceptor perhaps the best data on functionally important polymorphisms within respiratory drug targets comes from studies on the 5-lipoxygenase (5LO) promoter. This promoter contains a repeat transcription factor binding site for Sp1: the wild-type genotype containing 5 repeats [20]. Individuals have been observed with differing numbers of repeats, all of which appear to reduce transcriptional activity of the 5LO gene. In a large pharmacogenetic study performed retrospectively on a group of individuals in a phase III trial of the 5LO inhibitor ABT-761, individuals carrying genotypes which were predicted to give rise to lower levels of 5LO activity in the lungs were less responsive to the 5LO inhibitor [21] (fig. 3). Whether or not these polymorphisms may contribute to response to leukotriene receptor antagonists remains to be established.

Inflammation and Airway Hyperreactivity

Asthma commonly involves IgE-mediated allergic reactions to common aeroallergens that are the result of interactions between a number of genetic and environmental factors [22, 23]. In addition, a number of genes have now been associated with airway hyperreactivity (AHR). Through defining the genetic basis of asthma, atopy and AHR, it is hoped to provide better classification and new treatments. These genes may be important in predicting responders for biotechnology therapies directed specifically against IgE, eosinophils (anti-IL-5 and IL-4R), and AHR.

COPD

The molecular genetics of COPD are less well understood than asthma [24], although genes relating to oxidative stress [25], tumour necrosis factor-α [26] and nicotine metabolism have been implicated [27]. Depending on the type of therapy, these genes have the potential to exert pharmacogenetic effects. The phosphodiesterase isoenzymes are being screened as targets, but will be particularly challenging given the large number of genes within this gene family and the number of splice variants that can arise from individual gene members.

Pharmacoeconomics

The real test of the value of pharmacogenetic data will come in pharmacoeconomic studies assessing the value of prior knowledge of genotype to predict response before commencing treatment. Intuitively, it seems likely that this is unlikely to be feasible on a reactive basis, but with advances in DNA chip technology, it may be cost-effective on a pro-active basis. One possibility is that a pharmacogenetic profile for an individual could be established at a 'well-person check' which would potentially give information on the most effective drugs to be used, not just in respiratory disease, but in a range of other diseases which may develop in later life in that individual.

Phase II

The other setting in which pharmacogenetic information may be particularly important is in the context of small phase II clinical trials. If by chance such trials contain an excess of individuals with a given genotype, it would be easy to overestimate or underestimate the efficacy of the drug if the polymorphism has significant functional effects.

Conclusion

It is clear that significant genetic variation exists in many genes whose products are respiratory drug targets. Preliminary studies have been performed defining the extent of genetic variation in some of the primary targets, and reasonable functional data together with limited clinical studies have addressed the importance of these variants in determining treatment response. The available data on genetic polymorphism will increase markedly over the next few years and will need to be matched by a structured approach to looking at functional effects. Most polymorphisms are unlikely to have a sufficiently large clinical effect to be important in day-to-day management, but a small number of polymorphisms will exist which produce clinically important effects on treatment response.

References

1 Liggett SB: Molecular and genetic basis of β$_2$-adrenergic receptor function. J Allergy Clin Immunol 1999;103:S42–S46.
2 Hall IP: β$_2$-Adrenoceptor polymorphisms and asthma. Clin Exp Allergy 1999;29:1151–1154.
3 McGraw DW, Forbes SL, Kramer LA, Liggett SB: Polymorphisms of the 5′ leader cistron of the human β$_2$-adrenergic receptor regulate receptor expression. J Clin Invest 1998;102:1927–1932.
4 Scott MGH, Swan C, Wheatley AP, Hall IP: Identification of novel polymorphisms within the promoter region of the human β$_2$-adrenergic receptor gene. Br J Pharmacol 1999;126:841–844.
5 Tan KS, Hall IP, Dewar JC, Dow E, Lipworth BJ: Association between β$_2$-adrenoceptor (β$_2$-AR) polymorphism determines susceptibility to bronchodilator desensitisation in moderately severe stable asthmatics. Lancet 1997;350:995–999.
6 Martinez FD, Graves PD, Baldini M, et al: Association between genetic polymorphisms of the β$_2$-adrenoceptor and response to albuterol in children with and without a history of wheezing. J Clin Invest 1997;100:3184–3188.
7 Turki J, Pak J, Green SA, Martin RJ, Liggett SB. Genetic polymorphisms of the β$_2$-adrenergic receptor in nocturnal and non-nocturnal asthma. Evidence that Gly 16 correlates with the nocturnal phenotype. J Clin Invest 1995;95:1635–1641.
8 Hall IP, Wheatley A, Wilding P, Liggett SB: Association of the Glu27 β$_2$-adrenoceptor polymorphism with lower airway reactivity in asthmatic subjects. Lancet 1995;345:1213–1214.
9 Dewar JC, Wilkinson J, Wheatley A, Thomas NS, Doull I, Morton NE, Lio P, Harvey JF, Liggett SB, Holgate ST, Hall IP: The glutamine 27 β$_2$-adrenoceptor polymorphism is associated with elevated IgE levels in asthmatic families. J Allergy Clin Immunol 1997;100:261–265.
10 Dewar JC, Wheatley AP, Venn A, Morrison JFJ, Britton J, Hall IP: β$_2$-Adrenoceptor polymorphisms are in linkage disequilibrium, but are not associated with asthma in an adult population. Clin Exp Allergy 1998;28:442–448.
11 Liggett SB, Wagoner LE, Craft LL, Hornung RW, Hoit BD, McIntosh TC, Walsh RA: The Ile 164 β$_2$-adrenergic receptor polymorphism adversely affects the outcome of congestive heart failure. J Clin Invest 1998;102:1534–1539.
12 Green SA, Cole G, Jacinto M, Innis M, Liggett SB: A polymorphism of the human β$_2$-receptor within the fourth transmembrane domain alters ligand binding and functional properties of the receptor. J Biol Chem 1993;268:23116–23121.
13 Hancox RJ, Sears MR, Taylor DR: Polymorphism of the β$_2$-adrenoceptor and the response to long-term β$_2$-agonist therapy in asthma. Eur Resp J 1998;11:589–593.
14 Weir TD, Mallek N, Sandford AJ, Bai TR, Awadh N, Fitzgerald JM, Cockcroft D, James A, Liggett SB, Pare PD: β$_2$-Adrenergic receptor haplotypes in mild, moderate and fatal/near fatal asthma. Am J Respir Crit Care Med 1998;158:787–791.
15 Green SA, Turki J, Bejarna P, Hall IP, Liggett SB: Influence of β$_2$-adrenergic receptor genotypes on signal transduction in human airway smooth muscle cells. Am J Respir Cell Mol Biol 1995;13:25–33.
16 Fenech AG, Ebejer MJ, Felice AE, Ellul-Micallef R, Hall IP: Mutation screening of the human muscarinic M$_2$ receptor gene in Maltese asthmatic patients. Br J Pharmacol 1999;128:121P.

17 Dewar JC, Hall IP: A novel degenerate polymorphism in the human histamine H_1 receptor gene. Am J Respir Crit Care Med, in press.
18 Lane SJ, Arm JP, Staynov DZ, Lee TH: Chemical mutational analysis of the human glucocorticoid receptor cDNA in glucocorticoid-resistant bronchial asthma. Am J Respir Cell Mol Biol 1994; 11:42–48.
19 Huizenga NA, Koper JW, De Lange P, Pols HA, Stolk RP, Burger H, Grobbee DE, Brinkmann AO, De Jong FH, Lamberts SW: A polymorphism in the glucocorticoid receptor gene may be associated with increased sensitivity to glucocorticoids in vivo. J Clin Endocrinol Metab 1998;83:144–151.
20 In KH, Asano K, Beler D, Grosholz J, Finn PW, Silverman EK, et al: Naturally occurring mutations in the human 5-lipoxygenase gene promoter that modify transcription factor binding and reporter gene transcription. J Clin Invest 1997;99:1130–1137.
21 Drazen JM, Yandava CN, Dube L, Szczerback N, Hippensteel R, Pillari A, Israel E, Schork N, Silverman ES, Katz DA, Drajesk J: Pharmacogenetic association between ALOX5 promoter genotype and the response to anti-asthma treatment. Nat Genet 1999;22:168–170.
22 Cookson W: The alliance of genes and environment in asthma and allergy. Nature 1999; 402(suppl):B5-B11.
23 Wiesch DG, Meyers DA, Bleecker ER: Genetics of asthma. J Allergy Clin Immunol 1999; 104:895–901.
24 Barnes PJ: Molecular genetics of chronic obstructive pulmonary disease. Thorax 1999;54: 245–252.
25 Koyama H, Geddes DM: Genes, oxidative stress, and the risk of chronic obstructive pulmonary disease. Thorax 1998;53 S2:S10–S14.
26 Huang S-L, Su C-H, Chang S-C: Tumor necrosis factor-α gene polymorphism in chronic bronchitis. Am J Respir Crit Care Med 1997; 156:1436–1439.
27 Pianezza ML, Sellers EM and Tyndale RF: Nicotine metabolism defect reduces smoking. Nature 1998;393:750.

Ian P. Hall, University Hospital
Nottingham NG7 2UH (UK)
Tel. +44 115 970 9905, Fax +44 115 9422232
E-Mail Ian.Hall@nottingham.ac.uk

Delivery of Biologics to the Lung

David Cipolla Stephen Farr Igor Gonda Babatunde Otulana

Aradigm Corporation, Hayward, Calif., USA

Summary

Delivery of drugs by inhalation for the treatment of respiratory disease is well established. The primary advantage of local delivery is the achievement of efficacy while minimizing systemic side effects. With the respiratory tract as the target organ, biologics are likely to benefit even more by direct delivery because their transport between the blood circulation and the airway tissue and lumen is limited. This may result in better safety and efficacy, as well as improved economics since much lower doses may be effective compared to systemic administration. Protecting biologics against degradation during storage and aerosol generation may require the use of new types of formulations and inhalation systems with which they can be efficiently and reproducibly delivered. Examples of current clinical status of biologics delivered to the lung are provided.

The choice of delivery method to the lung depends on the target location, and the transport and clearance mechanisms specific to the drug of interest. The lung is a well-perfused organ, but ordinarily entry of high-molecular-weight substances from the blood circulation into the lung parenchyma and airway lumen is limited. Interestingly, the highly absorptive area of the small airways and alveoli can be accessed by direct deposition of the therapeutic substance, and this is explored for noninvasive delivery of macromolecules such as insulin for systemic activity [1]. This chapter, however, is limited to the direct delivery of biologics for local effects within the respiratory tract.

There are considerable therapeutic advantages with this organ-directed approach (table 1). Inhalation treatment of respiratory tract disease achieves rapidly high target site drug concentration in the lung and relatively low systemic exposure. For example, inhaled β-adrenergic agents provide rapid bronchodilation in asthma and are equipotent to oral doses approximately 20-fold greater [2]. Aerosolized doses of corticosteroids for asthma are orders of magnitude less than oral steroid doses, resulting in substantially less systemic adverse effects [3]. The ratio of lung to oropharyngeal deposition may determine the balance between desired (local) and undesired effects of these aerosols [4]. Pentamidine [5] and tobramycin [6], drugs used for the treatment of lung infections, are associated with serious systemic toxicity that can be minimized through their administration by inhalation. Even more localized delivery to specific airway segments that avoids toxicity at other sites can be achieved with a microspray guided via bronchoscope [7].

Table 1. Points to consider for the choice of pulmonary delivery system

Attribute	Reason for importance of the attribute
Stability of biologic during manufacture, development storage and aerosolization	Safety and efficacy
Efficiency of delivery to the lung	Safety, efficacy, convenience to patient, economics
Robust performance over realistic range of ambient conditions and the patients' ability to comply with proper technique	Safety and efficacy
Portability, frequency and duration of administration	Ease of use affecting patients' compliance with therapy

Methods of Direct Delivery of Biologics to the Lung

Key Factors Affecting Pulmonary Deposition of Inhaled Particles. In the majority of therapeutic applications, it is desirable to administer the drug to a large portion of the respiratory tract and in a manner convenient for self-administration by the patient. The major physical determinant of drug deposition in the respiratory tract following inhalation of an aerosol cloud is the aerodynamic size of the droplet or particle carrying the drug. This aerodynamic diameter depends on the physical size, shape and density of the particle [8]. The aerodynamics of delivery does not depend on the size of the drug molecule because the particle is typically orders of magnitude larger than the biological molecule. Oropharyngeal deposition is the primary cause of inefficiency and variability of conventional inhalation systems. To minimize this, particles in the aerodynamic size range 2–3 μm are to be used, and they need to be inhaled at a low inspiratory flow rate, followed, in some cases, by a brief breath-holding to avoid their exhalation. Correct breathing maneuvers are not easily achieved spontaneously, but desired reproducible breathing patterns can be obtained, e.g., with feedback using visual prompts leading to reproducible deposition [9].

Formulation Issues. The starting point for preclinical and clinical studies of a macromolecular drug is often the aqueous solution in which it was manufactured in purified form. Commercially viable formulations of parenteral and inhalation solutions of biologics are stable when refrigerated, and typically have adequate room temperature stability of ~ 30 days. Aggregation, the commonest degradation route for proteins, can be prevented frequently by the addition of small quantities of surfactant. Deamidation may be controlled by pH adjustment, and, similar to oxidation, does not necessarily have an impact on protein activity or safety [10]. If adequate stability cannot be achieved with an aqueous formulation, a 'dry powder' formulation may be attempted. Lyophilized proteins for injections do not have properties suitable for inhalation delivery without further processing and new methods of protein powder stabilization for aerosol delivery are therefore under development [10].

Delivery Systems. Nebulizers. A number of choices now exist to administer aqueous solutions of biologics. Conventional jet nebulizer systems consist of a source of compressed air and a single-use or reusable nebulizer. They can nebulize solutions and reconstituted powders. The aerosol output and particle size distribution are relatively independent of the formulation properties. Their disadvantages include long administration times, poor portability and variable and inefficient delivery [11]. Also, during nebulization, the vast majority of droplets is too large and refluxed within the nebulizer. Some biologics are degraded during this process [10]. Ultrasonic nebulizers run the additional risk of denaturing the biologic due to temperature increases during operation [11].

'Soft-Mist Inhalers'. New hand-held aerosol generators that utilize aqueous formulations overcome the key limitations of conventional nebulizers. Prevention of microbial growth in the aqueous formulation is essential and can be achieved in single use sterile dosage forms [10, 12]. Bulk drug reservoir systems may require addition of preservative to the formulation. The interaction of a preservative with the biologic may compromise the effectiveness of the preservative and the biochemical stability of the drug; very few suitable preservatives exist for respiratory products [10]. Aerosol generation using these novel aqueous delivery systems is accomplished by either mechanical extrusion of the formulation through nozzles, or with a vibrating orifice or ultrasonic mesh [10]. Mechanical extrusion of protein formulations in the AERx system through single-use nozzles, consisting of an array of micron-size holes, showed no loss of protein activity or integrity. In combination with the system's built-in breath control, 60–80% lung delivery of the loaded protein dose has been reported from in vitro and in vivo measurements [13, 14]. If a high concentration formulation is stable, a lung drug dose as high as 4 mg/puff can be achieved [15]. Somewhat lower efficiencies and doses/puff have been reported thus far for multidose reservoir systems currently in development [16, 17].

Propellant-Driven Metered Dose Inhalers (pMDI). Traditional pressurized metered dose- and dry powder-inhalers (pMDIs and DPIs) are inefficient and result in highly variable doses to the lung [10]. Further, the pMDI propellants are not suitable for the formulation of protein solutions. Suspension-based pMDIs would require special methods to manufacture the protein powders, which are yet to be investigated [10].

Dry-Powder Inhalers. Conventional DPI performance depends on the patient's breathing effort. New powder systems that deliver biologics at higher efficiencies and reproducibilities use power-assisted powder dispersion. They also utilize novel formulations with excipients for protection against degradation of the biologic during manufacture and storage [10]. The proportion of the excipient can be high, affecting the maximum drug dose/puff. Some excipients used in powder formulations such as sugars or salts cause bronchoconstriction in hyperresponsive subjects [10]. A powder formulation can be more stable at room temperature than an aqueous solution. Such formulations, however, may be sensitive to extremes of humidity that can result in physical and biochemical degradation of the product [10]. This may preclude the use of bulk drug reservoir DPIs, and necessitate the use of single-dose presentations.

The Spiros (Dura) device has a battery-driven propeller to disperse the drug powder. The lung dose with proteins is unknown for this system, but for albuterol it was 26 and 19% of the nominal dose at low and high inspiratory flow rates, respectively (coefficient of variation ~ 30%) [18]. The Inhale Therapeutics' DPI uses biologics stabilized in a glassy sugar matrix and compressed air to disperse the powder [10].

The use of physically larger solid particles carries some attraction because they are less cohesive and surface-adhesive, and therefore can be dispersed more efficiently with lower energy expenditure than smaller particles [8, 10]. Such particles may be able to deliver a higher dose/breath to the lung as long as they have appropriate aerodynamic behavior. Good penetration of larger particles with extremely low inspiratory flow rate was reported [19]. A new generation of large porous [20] and hollow [21] particles is being developed which have respirable aerodynamic size despite their larger physical size, due the reduction in density. They may provide in the future alternative strategies for biologic inhalation products.

Examples of Clinical Applications of Pulmonary Delivery of Biologics

Recombinant Human Deoxyribonuclease (Dornase alpha, rhDNase). Pulmozyme® (rhDNase, Genentech Inc.) for the treatment of cystic fibrosis, is currently the only biologic on the market for inhalation delivery. This compound has undergone extensive preclinical and clinical safety investigations [12]. Pulmozyme is approved for delivery by nebulizer, with each treatment taking typically 15–30 min. Recently, clinical development was initiated with rhDNase delivered by the AERx aqueous bolus delivery system with a view to shortening the delivery time and therefore enhancing compliance with the therapy [14].

Soluble IL-4 Receptor. Nuvance (Immunex), an IL-4 receptor, administered by inhalation via a nebulizer, is currently being studied for the treatment of asthma [22].

Anti-IgE Antibodies. While anti-IgE antibodies administered by injection showed efficacy in allergic asthmatic subjects [23], clinical trials with the inhaled product failed to demonstrate similar positive effects [24]. Whether delivery systems which are more efficient than conventional nebulizers would enhance the efficacy of the drug by inhalation is unknown at this time.

Human Alpha-1-Antitrypsin. Prolastin, human plasma-derived alpha-1-antitrypsin (A1AT; Bayer) is an injectable product for replacement therapy of A1AT in emphysema patients with congenitally low levels of serum A1AT. A1AT administration by inhalation was found to be safe using nebulizers [25].

Cystic Fibrosis Transmembrane Conductance Gene. Microspray delivery [7] with bronchoscope guidance was used to deliver the cystic fibrosis transmembrane conductance gene using an adenovirus vector in patients with cystic fibrosis. The greater localization of the gene vector by this method was presumed to result in better safety compared to administration of the vector by instillation [26].

Conclusions

We witnessed a remarkable growth in pulmonary delivery of biologics towards the end of the 20th century [27]. New delivery systems with the ability to deliver protein and gene therapies much more effectively and reproducibly are now in late-stage clinical testing which will provide the ultimate validation in terms of the safety and efficacy of these technologies. The beginning of the new millennium is marked by completion of the sequencing of the human genome that will accelerate the development of new therapeutic biologics. The scientists working in the discovery area will be able to select the most appropriate pulmonary delivery systems that match the properties of the therapeutic substance and, most importantly, the needs of the patients in the target population.

Acknowledgments

We would like to thank Drs. John Thipphawong (Aradigm Corporation) and Trevor Hansel (Imperial College) for the critical review and improvements of the manuscript.

References

1 Farr SJ, Gonda I, and Ličko V: Physicochemical and physiological factors influencing the effectiveness of inhaled insulin; in Dalby RN, Byron PR, Farr SJ (eds): Respiratory Drug Delivery VI. Buffalo Grove, Interpharm Press, 1998, pp 25–33.
2 Walter EH: Inhaled versus oral treatment with salbutamol. Res Clin Forums 1984;6:73–81.
3 Lipworth BJ: Systemic adverse effects of inhaled corticosteroid therapy: A systematic review and meta-analysis. Arch Intern Med 1999;159:941–955.
4 Borgstrom L: Local versus total systemic bioavailability as a means to compare different inhaled formulations of the same substance. J Aerosol Med 1998;11:55–63
5 Conte JE, Golden JA: Intrapulmonary and systemic pharmacokinetics of aerosolized pentamidine used for prophylaxis of pneumocystis pneumonia in patients infected with the human immunodeficiency virus. J Clin Pharmacol 1995;35:1166–1173.
6 Ramsey BW, Pepe MS, Quan JM, Otto KL, Montgomery AB, Williams-Warren J, Vasiljev KM, Borowitz D, Bowman CV, Marshall BS, Marshall S, Smith AL: Intermittent administration of inhaled tobramycin in patients with cystic fibrosis. N Engl J Med 1999;340:23–30.
7 Cipolla DC, Gonda I, Shak S, Kovesdi I, Crystal R, Sweeney TD: Coarse spray delivery to a localized region of the pulmonary airways for gene therapy. Hum Gene Ther 2000;11:361–371.
8 Gonda I: Physico-chemical principles in aerosol delivery; in Crommelin DJA, Midha KK (eds): Topics in Pharmaceutical Sciences 1991. Stuttgart, Medpharm Scientific Publishers, 1992, pp 95–115.
9 Farr SJ, Rowe AM, Rubsamen R, Taylor G: Aerosol deposition in the human lung following administration from a microprocessor controlled pressurised metered dose inhaler. Thorax 1995;50: 639–644.
10 Clark AR, Shire SJ: Formulation of proteins for pulmonary delivery; in McNally EJ (ed): Protein Formulation and Delivery. New York, Dekker, 2000, pp 201–234.
11 Cipolla D, Clark AR, Chan H, Gonda I, Shire SJ: Assessment of aerosol delivery systems for the recombinant human deoxyribonuclease I (rhDNase). STP Pharma Sciences 1994;4:50–62.
12 Gonda I: Deoxyribonuclease inhalation; in Adjei LA, Gupta PK (eds): Inhalation delivery of therapeutic peptides and proteins. New York, Dekker, 1997, pp 355–365.
13 Smaldone GC, Agosti J, Castillo R, Cipolla D, Blanchard J: Deposition of radiolabeled protein from AERx in patients with asthma (abstract 38). J Aerosol Med 1999;12:98.
14 Mudumba S, Khossravi M, Yim D, Rossi T, Pearce D, Hughes M, Cipolla D, Sweeney T: Delivery of rhDNase by the AERx pulmonary delivery system; in Dalby RN, Byron PR, Farr SJ (eds): Respiratory Drug Delivery VI. Buffalo Grove, Interpharm Press, in press.
15 Cipolla D, Boyd B, Evans R, Warren S, Taylor G, Farr S: Bolus administration of INS-365: Studying the feasibility of delivering high doses of drug using the AERx pulmonary delivery system; in Dalby RN, Byron PR, Farr SJ (eds): Respiratory Drug Delivery VI. Buffalo Grove, Interpharm Press, in press.
16 DeYoung LR, Chambers F, Narayan S, Wu C: The AeroDose multidose inhaler device design and delivery characteristics; in Dalby RN, Byron PR, Farr SJ (eds): Respiratory Drug Delivery VI. Buffalo Grove, Interpharm Press, 1998, pp 91–95.
17 Newman SP, Steed KP, Reader SJ, Hooper G, Zierenberg B: Efficient delivery to the lungs of flunisolide aerosol from a new portable hand-held multi-dose nebulizer. J Pharm Sci 1996; 85:960–964.
18 Hill M, Vaughan L, Dolovich M: Dose targeting for dry powder inhalers; in Dalby RN, Byron PR, Farr SJ (eds): Respiratory Drug Delivery V. Buffalo Grove, Interpharm Press, pp 197–208.
19 Anderson M, Svartenegren M, Camner P: Human tracheobronchial deposition and effect of a histamine aerosol inhaled by extremely slow inhalations. J Aerosol Sci 1999;30:289–297.
20 Vanbever R, Mintzes JD, Wang J, Nice J, Chen D, Batycky R, Langer R, Edwards DA: Formulation and physical characterization of large porous particles for inhalation. Pharm Res 1999;16:1735–1742.
21 Tarara TE, Dellamary LA, Smith DJ, Weers JG: Engineered hollow porous particles for inhalation. AAPS PharmSci Suppl 1999;1:2962.
22 Borish LC, Nelson HS, Lanz MJ, Claussen L, Whitmore JB, Agosti JM, Garrison L: Interleukin-4 receptor in moderate atopic asthma Am J Respir Crit Care Med 1999;160:1816–1823.
23 Patalano F: Injection of anti-IgE antibodies will suppress IgE and allergic symptoms. Allergy 1999;54:103–110.
24 Fahy JV, Cockroft DW, Boulet LP, et al: Effect of aerosolized anti-IgE (E25) on airway responses to inhaled allergen in asthmatic subjects. Am J Respir Crit Care Med 1999;160: 1023–1027.
25 Vogelmeier C, Kirlath I, Warrington S, Banik N: The intrapulmonary half-life and safety of aerosolized alpha-1-protease inhibitor in normal volunteers. Am J Respir Crit Care Med 1997;155:536–541.
26 Harvey B-G, Leopold PL, Hackett NR, Grasso TM, Williams PM, Tucker AL, Kaner RJ, Ferris B, Gonda I, Sweeney TD, Ramalingam R, Kovesdi I, Shak S, Crystal RG: Airway epithelial CFTR mRNA expression in cystic fibrosis patients after repetitive administration of a recombinant adenovirus. J Clin Invest 1999; 104:1245–1255.
27 Adjei LA, Gupta PK: Inhalation Delivery of Therapeutic Peptides and Proteins. New York, Dekker, 1997.

Igor Gonda, PhD
Aradigm Corporation, 3929 Point Eden Way
Hayward, CA 94545 (USA)
Tel +1 510 265 9000, Fax +1 510 265 0277
E-Mail gondai@aradigm.com

Immunopathology: Comparison of COPD and Asthma

Peter K. Jeffery

Imperial College School of Medicine at the National Heart and Lung Institute, London, UK

Summary

Both COPD and asthma are not disease entities, but rather each is a complex of conditions contributing to airflow obstruction. Three conditions may contribute to airflow limitation in COPD; (1) chronic bronchitis (mucous hypersecretion); (2) adult chronic bronchiolitis (small or peripheral airways disease) and (3) emphysema (defined anatomically by permanent, destructive enlargement of airspaces distal to terminal bronchioli without obvious fibrosis). The airways in chronic bronchitis and in COPD are markedly inflamed; however, in contrast to asthma, the predominant type of inflammatory cell and the main anatomic site of the lesion appear to differ. There is difficulty distinguishing subjects with COPD who may show a degree of reversibility and those older subjects with asthma whose reversible airflow obstruction has become more 'fixed'; moreover, mixtures of COPD and asthma may coexist in any one patient (fig. 1). The following synopsis focuses on the structural changes and the inflammation of conducting airways and lung in COPD and briefly makes comparisons with what is known in asthma.

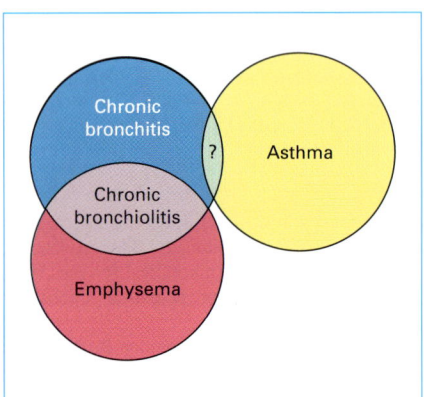

Fig. 1. Airflow limitation: simplified interrelationships between COPD and asthma.

Proximal Bronchi (Chronic Bronchitis)

Cough productive of sputum is the symptom most frequently experienced by smokers: cough is an effective mechanism for clearing large proximal airways (down to about the 6th generation of branching). Normally, respiratory tract secretions amount to less than 100 ml/day and have been suggested to consist primarily of glycosaminoglycans. Chronic irritation causes alterations to the biochemistry and flow of mucus and an increase in the number and activity of secretory cells: there is an enlargement of the mass of submucosal gland (by an increase in both the number and size of its cells) and an increase in the number of mucous cells (i.e. goblet cells) in the surface epithelium. Mucous gland enlargement and hyperplasia of goblet cells are the histological hallmarks of chronic bronchitis, although similar changes are also reported in asthma. However, in fatal asthma, in contrast to chronic bronchitis, the airways are occluded by a particularly tenacious mixture of exudate and mucus.

The normal presence of mucous gel is essential to mucociliary clearance – in normal healthy subjects the mucus is present as discrete flakes but in smoker's bronchitis it appears as a continuous sheet or 'blanket'. The appearance and increase of goblet cells in small airways (i.e., small bronchi and bronchioli of less than 2 mm in diameter) where goblet cells are normally absent or sparse

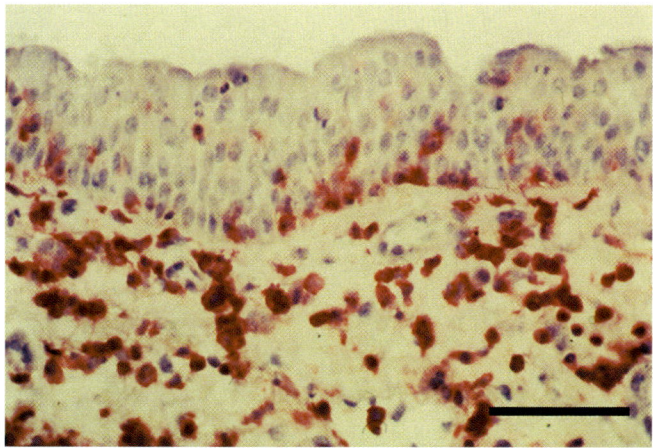

Fig. 2. Histological section of a mucosal biopsy taken by flexible fibre-optic bronchoscopy of a patient with an exacerbation of bronchitis. There are large numbers of CD45+ leukocytes infiltrating the subepithelium zone and fewer within the squamoid surface epithelium. Scale bar = 70 μm.

is a key alteration contributing to small airways disease and the development of COPD [1]. Epithelial changes in chronic bronchitis include epithelial atrophy, focal squamous metaplasia, ciliary abnormalities and decreases of ciliated cell number and mean ciliary length. In contrast, in asthma, there is patchy loss of surface epithelium, relatively uniform thickening and hyaline appearance of its reticular basement membrane, bronchial vessel dilatation, congestion and oedema and marked increase of bronchial smooth muscle [2, 3].

Smoking induces an inflammatory response: it alters the immunoregulatory balance of T-cell subsets in blood, BAL fluid, conducting airways and lung parenchyma [4, 5]. Smoking initiates a peripheral blood leukocytosis and a reversible decrease in the normally high CD4+ to CD8+ cell ratio in blood of heavy smokers (i.e. >50 pack-years). There is also a significant reduction of the CD4+ to CD8+ cell ratio in BAL fluid but not in blood of a group of milder smokers (14 pack-years). The increase in the number of BAL fluid and tissue CD8+ T-cells is positively associated with pack-years smoked [5, 6]. Histological examination of conducting airways (taken at resection for tumour) from smokers demonstrates that mucus hypersecretion shows a stronger association with inflammation than with the size of submucosal glands [7].

In bronchial biopsies of subjects with COPD there is infiltration of the mucosa by inflammatory cells [6, 8, 9] (fig. 2). In stable disease, this is associated with upregulation of cell surface adhesion molecules such as ICAM-1. In the surface epithelium, Fournier et al. [10] have demonstrated an increase in inflammatory cells of all types in smokers with chronic bronchitis and mild COPD by comparison with non-smokers. In the subepithelial zone of bronchitics there are significant increases in the numbers of CD45 (total leukocytes), CD3 (T cells), CD25 activated and VLA-1 (late activation) positive cells (presumed to be T cells) and of macrophages [8]. In smokers with COPD, T lymphocytes and neutrophils increase in the surface epithelium whilst T lymphocytes and macrophages increase in the subepithelium [9, 11–13]. In contrast to asthma, the predominant T cell subset in COPD is the CD8+ cell (and not the CD4+) which increases in number and proportion. Furthermore, the increase of CD8+ cells shows a negative association with FEV_1 expressed as a percentage of predicted [9].

Small Airways (Chronic Bronchiolitis)

Whilst the site of the lesion and diagnosis is, as yet, difficult to pinpoint by lung function, experimental physiologists [e.g. Hogg et al., 14] have indicated that the dominant site of airflow limitation lies in small bronchi and bronchioli of less than 3 mm in diameter. As the cross-sectional area of the bronchiolar zone of the lung is normally large in relation to the bronchial divisions, breathlessness and airflow limitation due to small airway disease are detectable only late in the course of the condition.

Ciliated and non-ciliated secretory cells are the main cell types in bronchioli [15] and, of them, the Clara cell is the major secretory cell type which functions also as the progenitor cell from which ciliated and mucous cells develop. It has been suggested that the Clara cell produces both a hypophase component of bronchiolar surfactant and a low-molecular-weight protease inhibitor (syn. antileukoprotease or bronchial mucosal protease inhibitor) [16], which normally prevents proteolysis of airway tissues. Replacement of Clara cells and their anti-elastase secretion thus predisposes the small airway to proteolytic digestion: such changes in respiratory bronchioli may underlie the development of emphysema of the centriacinar type (see below). In smokers, Clara cells are replaced by mucous cells and mucus appears in peripheral airways and its secretion is abnormally increased therein [17]. The increase in mucus at this distal site is difficult to clear by cough, leading to obstruction of small airways. Replacement of the normal surfactant lining by mucus leads to an abnormally high surface tension which results in small airway instability and predisposes to early airway closure during expiration [18].

In smokers dying suddenly of non-respiratory cause, there is inflammation in membranous and respiratory bronchioles as well as surrounding alveolitis consisting of pigmented macrophages [1, 19, 20]. These inflammatory changes to small airways appear to be related to clinical airflow obstruction in COPD [14, 21]. The same profile of CD8-predominant inflammation seen in the large airways also occurs deeper in the lung in both the small airways [13] and also the lung parenchyma [22, 23].

Histologically, one of the most consistently observed early effects of cigarette smoke in the airways of both man and experimental animals is a marked increase in the number of macrophages and neutrophils. The increase is seen also within the lung interstitium and alveolar space and can be detected in BAL fluid [20]. The associated early smoking-related structural changes have been described in studies comparing lungs of young smokers and controls of similar age in a group of subjects who had experienced sudden non-hospital deaths. In severely affected patients, the structural changes include: mucous metaplasia, bronchiolar smooth muscle hypertrophy, mural oedema, peribronchiolar fibrosis and an excess of airways less than 400 μm in diameter [1, 20, 24]. It is suggested that the primary lesion is persistent and progressive inflammation that leads to peribronchiolar fibrosis. The peribronchiolar inflammation and fibrosis may predispose to the development of centrilobular emphysema and may be responsible for the subtle abnormalities detected by tests of lung function. Associated loss of alveolar attachments to the airway perimeter (fig. 3a, b) contributes to loss of elastic recoil and favours increased airway tortuosity and early closure of bronchioli during expiration [25, 26].

Emphysema

Two main morphologic forms of emphysema are described, distinguished anatomically by the region of the acinus that is destroyed. *Centriacinar* (syn. centrilobular) emphysema is characterized by focal destruction restricted to respiratory bronchioli and the central portions of the acinus, each focus surrounded by areas of grossly normal lung parenchyma. This form of emphysema is usually most severe in the upper lobes of the lung (fig. 4). *Panacinar* (or panlobular) emphysema involves destruction of the walls, in a fairly uniform manner, of *all* the air spaces beyond the terminal bronchiolus. The panacinar form is characteristic of patients who develop smoking-related emphysema relatively early in life and, in contrast to the centriacinar form, has a tendency to involve the lower lobes more than the upper.

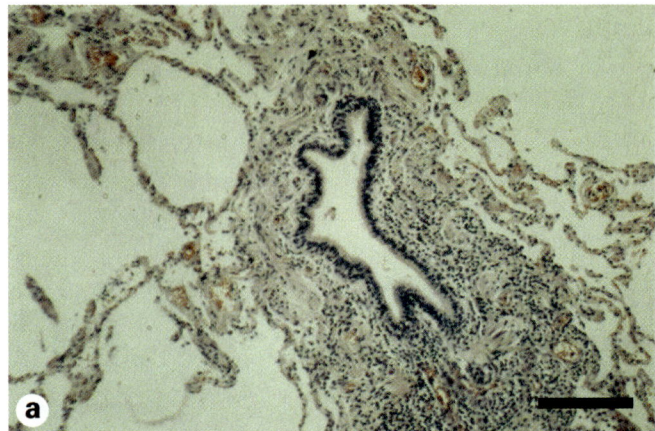

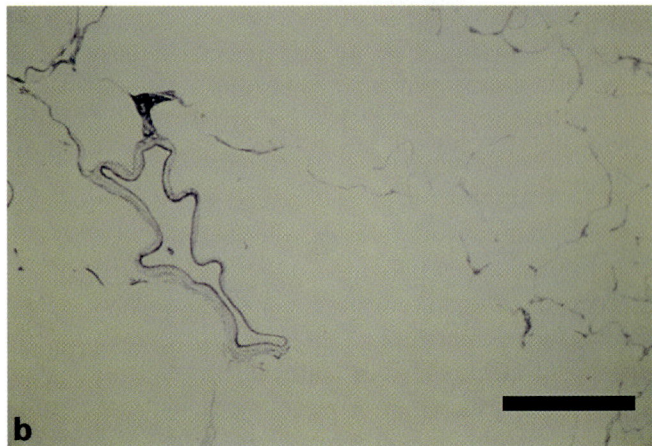

Fig. 3. Haematoxylin- and eosin-stained sections. **a** Transverse section of a small airway showing peribronchiolitis consisting mainly of lymphocytes (scale bar = 250 μm). **b** Emphysematous lung in which there is destruction of alveolar attachments to the bronchiolar wall, resulting in its tortuous appearance and early collapse during expiration. Scale bar = 1.0 mm.

The early changes of emphysema have been thought to include the appearance of small fenestrae in the alveolar septa which subsequently enlarge (an alteration which has been referred to as 'microscopic' emphysema) and subtle disruption to elastic fibres with accompanying loss of elastic recoil and subsequent bronchiolar and alveolar distortion, [27], (fig. 5a, b). These microscopic changes lead to loss, by destruction, of the elastic framework, of interalveolar septa and the macroscopic appearance of spaces greater than 1 mm in diameter. Recent data have shown that this destructive process is accompanied, paradoxically, by a net *increase* in the mass of collagen. This suggests that, contrary to the current internationally accepted

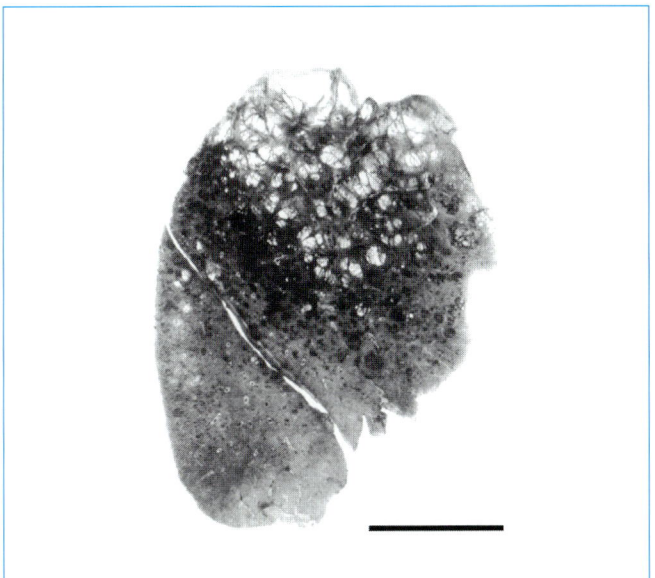

Fig. 4. Gross appearance of the cut surface of a lung in which the centriacinar emphysema is restricted to the upper aspects of each lobe. Scale bar = 10.0 cm. Courtesy of Prof. B. Heard.

definition of emphysema there is active alveolar wall fibrosis in emphysematous lungs [28].

The destruction of the respiratory zone in emphysema is considered to be the result of an inflammatory reaction involving neutrophils and release of neutrophil elastase which overwhelms the normal anti-protease protective screen [29, 30]. However, CD8+ T cells may also be directly involved in this process [31]. Similarly to the findings in the large conducting airways there are significant negative associations of the numbers of CD8+ cells and FEV_1 % of predicted in both the small (peripheral) conducting airways and lung parenchyma but the correlations (i.e. r values) are stronger than in the larger airways supporting the distal site as the major contributor to reduced lung function.

Differences and Similarities of COPD and Asthma

COPD and asthma seem to differ at the tissue level in a number of respects (tables 1, 2). But there are similarities also. Compared to normal healthy control tissue, there are a number of studies that report a small but significant increase in the number of tissue eosinophils in subjects with chronic bronchitis or COPD [7, 9, 32]. Sputum eosinophilia is also reported in cases of 'eosinophilic bronchitis', i.e. patients with chronic bronchitis but without a history of asthma and without bronchial hyperre-

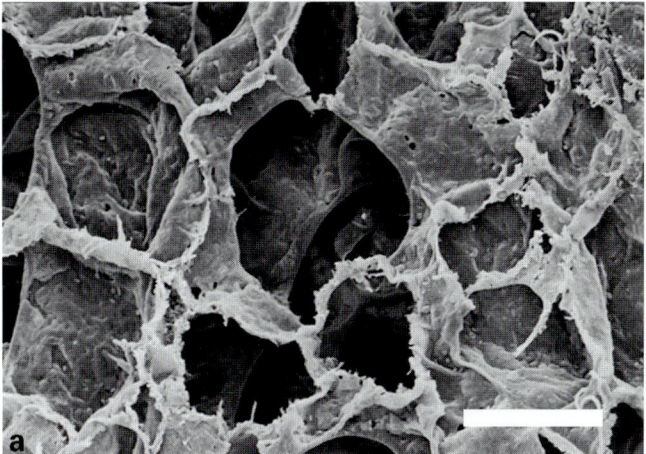
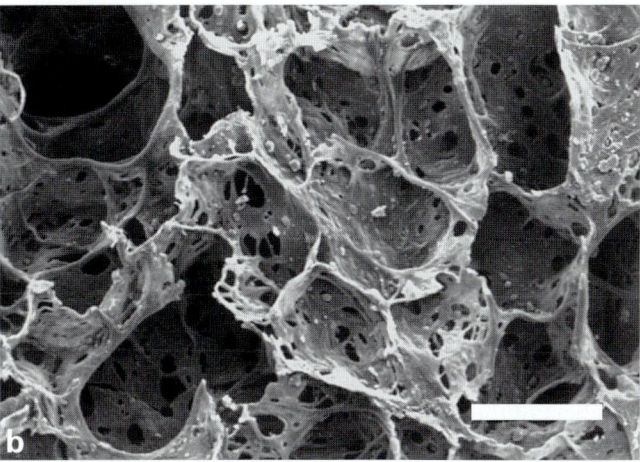

Fig. 5. Scanning electron micrographs of human lung alveolar tissue. **a** From a non-smoker, showing alveoli and the occasional 'pore of Kohn'. Scale bar = 150 μm. **b** From a smoker showing 'microscopic' emphysema and alveolar walls peppered by fenestrae too small to be seen by the naked eye. Such early lesions are considered to result in loss of lung elastic recoil. Scale bar = 150 μm.

Table 1. Fold increase in inflammatory cells in subjects with atopic asthma, smoker's chronic bronchitis (CB) and COPD versus healthy controls

	CB	COPD	Asthma
CD45+	2.2	2.3	2
CD3+	2.3	4.0	2
CD4+	±	2.8	2.5
CD8+	3	8.4	2
CD4+:CD8+	1:4	1:2	3:1
Neutrophil	±	2.2	–1.5
Eosinophil	1.7	3.5	93
Macrophage	4.5	8.6	±

Table 2. Simplified comparison of COPD and asthma

	COPD	Asthma
Airflow obstruction	progressive deterioration of lung function (? reversible component)	variable (± irreversible component)
Post mortem	excessive mucus (mucoid/purulent) small airway disease, emphysema	hyperinflation, airway plugs (exudate + mucus) no or little emphysema
Sputum	macrophage neutrophil (infective exacerbation)	eosinophilia, metachromatic cells Creola bodies
Surface epithelium	fragility undetermined	fragility/loss
Bronchiolar mucous cells	metaplasia/hyperplasia	mucous metaplasia is debated
Reticular basement membrane	variable or normal	homogeneously thickened and hyaline
Congestion/oedema	variable/fibrotic	present
Bronchial smooth muscle	enlarged mass (small airways)	enlarged mass (large airways)
Bronchial glands	enlarged mass (increased acidic glycoprotein)	enlarged mass (no change in mucin histochemistry)
Cellular infiltrate	predominantly CD3, CD8, CD68, CD25, VLA-1 and HLA-DR+, mild eosinophilia eosinophilia in exacerbations mast cell increase in smokers and COPD	predominantly CD3, CD4, CD25 (IL-2R)+ marked eosinophilia (activation) mast cell increase (decrease in severe/fatal)
Cytokines (ISH)	IL-4 and IL-5 gene expression RANTES only in exacerbations	IL-4, IL-5, eotaxin and RANTES gene expression

sponsiveness [33, 34]. Furthermore, the numbers of tissue eosinophils are markedly increased when there is an exacerbation of bronchitis [35]. Recently, we have found that inflammatory cells associated with mucus-secreting glands of bronchi (resected from smokers' lungs) demonstrate *gene* expression for both IL-4 and IL-5 and the numbers of these cells are significantly higher in subjects with chronic hypersecretion as compared with their asymptomatic controls [36]. Moreover, in exacerbations of bronchitis, lymphomononuclear cells are involved in the production of eosinophil chemoattractants including eotaxin and RANTES [37]. These and other data [38] emphasize the extent of similarity that may exist between an exacerbation of bronchitis in smokers with chronic bronchitis and non-smokers with asthma.

Conclusions

The involvement of activated lymphocytes seems to be a common theme in both asthma and COPD. However, the predominant lymphocyte subset in COPD and asthma appears to be distinct. The profound tissue eosinophilia of asthma does not normally appear in COPD unless there is an exacerbation of bronchitis. Whilst in COPD there is tissue destruction and remodelling in the lung parenchyma and bronchioli, this contrasts with the involvement of relatively large (proximal) airways in asthma. By rigorous recordings of clinical data in association with careful application of the histologic, cytologic, immunologic and molecular techniques now available, it is likely that biopsies of conducting airways will provide for differential diagnosis and the delineation of subtypes of patients with COPD or asthma. It is also likely that biopsies will help in monitoring disease progression and responsiveness to treatment. Comparative studies of the distinct patterns of interleukin and cytokine gene expression in smokers with COPD and smokers with asthma are now urgently needed: such studies will provide the basis for the rational development of novel therapies.

Acknowledgments

The author thanks Mr. Andrew Rogers for assistance with the illustrations and Dr. Mariusz Gizycki for his careful proofreading.

References

1 Cosio MG, Hale KA, Niewoehner DE: Morphologic and morphometric effects of prolonged cigarette smoking on the small airways. Am Rev Respir Dis 1980;122:265–271.
2 Dunnill MS, Massarella GR, Anderson JA: A comparison of the quantitative anatomy of the bronchi in normal subjects, in status asthmaticus, in chronic bronchitis, and in emphysema. Thorax 1969;24:176–179.
3 Jeffery PK: Pathology of Asthma. Br Med Bull 1992;48:23–39.
4 Miller LG, Goldstein G, Murphy M, Ginns LC: Reversible alterations in immunoregulatory T cells in smoking. Analysis by monoclonal antibodies and flow cytometry. Chest 1982;82:526–529.
5 Costabel U, Bross KJ, Reuter C, Ruhle K-H, Matthys H: Alterations in immunoregulatory T-cell subsets in cigarette smokers. A phenotypic analysis of bronchoalveolar and blood lymphocytes. Chest 1986;90:39–44.
6 Lams BE, Sousa AR, Rees PJ, Lee TH: Subepthelial immunopathology of large airways in smokers with and without chronic obstructive pulmonary disease. Eur Respir J 2000;15:512–516.
7 Mullen JBM, Wright JL, Wiggs BR, Pare PD, Hogg JC: Reassessment of inflammation of airways in chronic bronchitis. BMJ 1985;291:1235–1239.
8 Di Stefano A, Turato G, Maestrelli P, et al: Airflow limitation in chronic bronchitis is associated with T-lymphocyte and macrophage infiltration of the bronchial mucosa. Am J Respir Crit Care Med 1996;153:629–632.
9 O'Shaughnessy T, Ansari TW, Barnes NC, Jeffery PK: Inflammation in bronchial biopsies of subjects with chronic bronchitis: Inverse relationship of CD8+ T lymphocytes with FEV_1. Am J Resp Crit Care Med 1997;155:852–857.
10 Fournier M, Lebargy F, Le Roy Ladurie F, Lenormand E, Pariente R: Intraepithelial T-lymphocyte subsets in the airways of normal subjects and of patients with chronic bronchitis. Am Rev Respir Dis 1989;140:737–742.
11 O'Shaughnessy TC, Ansari TW, Barnes NC, Jeffery PK: Inflammatory cells in the airway surface epithelium of smokers with and without bronchitic airflow obstruction. Eur Respir J 1996;9 (suppl 23):14s.
12 Saetta M, Turato G, Facchini FM, et al: Inflammatory cells in the bronchial glands of smokers with chronic bronchitis. Am J Respir Crit Care Med 1997;156:1633–1639.
13 Saetta M: CD8+ T-lymphocytes in peripheral airways of smokers with chronic obstructive pulmonary disease. Am J Respir Crit Care Med 1998;157:822–826.
14 Hogg JC, Macklem PT, Thurlbeck WM: Site and nature of airway obstruction in chronic obstructive lung disease. N Engl J Med 1968;278:1355–1360.
15 Jeffery PK: Structural, immunologic, and neural elements of the normal human airway wall; In Busse WW, Holgate ST (eds): Asthma and rhinitis. Oxford, Blackwell, 1995:80–106.
16 Mooren HWD, Kramps JA, Franken C, Meijer CJLM, Dijkman JA: Localisation of a low-molecular weight bronchial protease inhibitor in the peripheral human lung. Thorax 1983;38:180–183.
17 Ebert RV, Hanks PB: Mucus secretion by the epithelium of the bronchioles of cigarette smokers. Br J Dis Chest 1981;75:277–282.
18 Macklem PT, Proctor DF, Hogg JC: The stability of peripheral airways. Respir Physiol 1970;8:191–203.
19 Wright JL, Hobson JE, Wiggs B, Pare PD, Hogg JC: Airway inflammation and peribronchiolar attachments in the lungs of nonsmokers, current and ex-smokers. Lung 1988;166:277–286.
20 Niewoehner DE, Klienerman J, Rice D: Pathologic changes in the peripheral airways of young cigarette smokers. N Engl J Med 1974;291:755–758.
21 Thurlbeck WM: Chronic airflow obstruction. Correlation of structure and function; in Petty TL (ed): Chronic Obstructive Pulmonary Disease, ed 2. Dekker, 1985:129–203.
22 Finkelstein R, Fraser RS, Ghezzo H, Cosio MG: Alveolar inflammation and its relation to Emphysema in Smokers. Am J Respir Crit Care Med 1995;152:1666–1672.
23 Saetta M, Baraldo S, Corbino L, et al: CD8+ cells in the lungs of smokers with chronic obstructive pulmonary disease. Am J Respir Crit Care Med 1999;160:711–717.
24 Hale KA, Ewing SL, Gosnell BA, Niewoehner DE: Lung disease in long-term cigarette smokers with and without chronic air-flow obstruction. Am Rev Respir Dis 1984;130:716–721.
25 Saetta M, Ghezzo H, Wong Dong Kim, et al: Loss of alveolar attachments in smokers. A morphometric correlate of lung function impairment. Am Rev Respir Dis 1985;132:894–900.
26 Linhartova A, Anderson AE Jr, Foraker AG: Further observations on luminal deformity and stenosis of nonrespiratory bronchioles in pulmonary emphysema. Thorax 1977;32:53–59.
27 Gillooly M, Lamb D: Microscopic emphysema in relation to age and smoking habit. Thorax 1993;48:491–495.
28 Lang MR, Fiaux GW, Gilooly M, Stewart JA, Hulmes DJS, Lamb D: Collagen content of alveolar wall tissue in emphysematous and non-emphysematous lungs. Thorax 1994;49:319–326.
29 Jeffery PK: Tobacco smoke-induced lung disease; in Cohen RD, Lewis B, Alberti KGMM, Denman AM (eds): The Metabolic and Molecular Basis of Acquired Disease. London, Ballière Tindall, 1990, pp 466–495.
30 MacNee W, Selby C: New perspectives on basic mechanisms in lung disease: 2. Neutrophil traffic in the lungs: Role of haemodynamics, cell adhesion and deformability. Thorax 1993;48:79–88.
31 Jeffery PK: Lymphocytes, chronic bronchitis and chronic obstructive pulmonary disease. Novartis Foundation Symposium, Chadwick, 2000, pp 149–168 in press.
32 Lacoste J-Y, Bousquet J, Chanez P, et al: Eosinophilic and neutrophilic inflammation in asthma, chronic bronchitis, and chronic obstructive pulmonary disease. J Allergy Clin Immunol 1993;92:537–548.
33 Gibson PG, Hargreaves FE, Girgis-Gabardo A, Morris M, Denburg JA, Dolovich J: Chronic cough with eosinophilic bronchitis and examination for variable airflow obstruction and response to corticosteroid. Allergy 1995;25:127–132.
34 Pizzichini E, Pizzichini MMM, Gibson P, et al: Sputum eosinophilia predicts benefit from prednisone in smokers with chronic obstructive bronchitis. Am J Respir Crit Care Med 1998;158:1511–1517.
35 Saetta M, Di Stefano A, Maestrelli P, et al: Airway eosinophilia and expression of interleukin-5 protein in asthma and in exacerbations of chronic bronchitis. Clin Exp Allergy 1996;26:766–774.
36 Zhu J, Majumdar S, Ansari T, et al: IL-4 and IL-5 mRNA in the bronchial wall of smokers. Am J Resp Crit Care Med 1999;159:A450.
37 Zhu J, Majumdar S, Turato G, Fabbri LM, Saetta M, Jeffery PK: Airway eosinophilia in bronchitis and gene expression for IL-4, Il-5 and eotaxin in bronchial biopsies. Eur Respir J 1999;14:A360s.
38 Chanez P, Vignola AM, O'Shaughnessy T, et al: Corticosteroid reversibility in COPD is related to features of asthma. Am J Respir Crit Care Med 1997;155:1529–1534.

Prof. P.K. Jeffery, DSc, PhD
Lung Pathology Unit
Royal Brompton Hospital
Sydney Street, London SW3 6NP (UK)
Tel. +44 171 351 8422, Fax +44 171 351 8435
E-Mail p.jeffery@ic.ac.uk

Monitoring Lung Function

Neil Pride

Department of Thoracic Medicine, National Heart and Lung Institute, Imperial College School of Medicine, London, UK

Summary

Measurement of airway function is central to the diagnosis and assessment of asthma and COPD. Many drug studies – particularly in asthma – have improvement in airway function as a major objective; even when this is not the case, airway function is almost always monitored to characterize the patients and to exclude confounding changes. Assessment of hyperinflation, exercise performance and alveolar structure/function are the most common additional aspects studied during drug trials. Many other aspects of lung function are sometimes relevant (e.g. blood gases and/or oximetry, tests of regional function (ventilation and perfusion scans), control of ventilation, skeletal and respiratory muscle function, pulmonary hypertension), but are not considered here.

Airway Function

Tests of Forced Expiration. The most widely used tests are based on forced expiration from the position of full inflation (total lung capacity, TLC) (table 1) [1–5]. Properly performed, these tests reflect the combined mechanical properties of the airways and lung parenchyma.

A forced expiratory vital capacity manoeuvre may be expressed either as change in volume versus time (spirometry, usually measuring the volume expired in the first second, FEV_1), as an instantaneous flow rate such as peak expiratory flow (PEF), or, as flow versus expired volume throughout the expiration (maximum expiratory flow-volume (MEFV) curve) (fig. 1). In disease there is a potential degree of freedom between change in FEV_1 and in PEF; furthermore PEF is more influenced by sub-optimal technique than FEV_1. Maximum expiratory flow rates at smaller lung volumes are achieved with relatively small expiratory pressures (perhaps 25% of maximum effort) and thus are termed effort-independent. In contrast, PEF

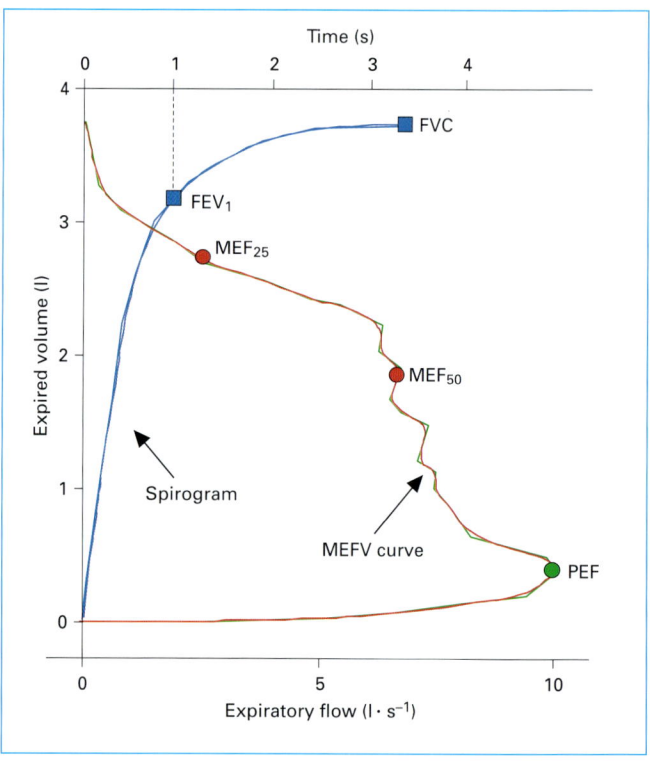

Fig. 1. FVC manoeuvre shown as expired volume versus time (spirogram) and expiratory flow versus expired volume (MEFV curve) in a normal subject. From the spirogram, FEV_1 and FVC are routinely recorded. PEF is the only flow rate commonly measured, usually with a mechanical indicator gauge calibrated in $l \cdot min^{-1}$. The detailed contour of the MEFV curve varies considerably between individuals, but is highly reproducible within an individual, making it useful for quality control of the manoeuvre and for detecting mild airflow obstruction. Early changes in the MEFV curve are a reduction in flow towards the end of expiration (MEF_{50}, MEF_{25}) and 'scooping' of the curve so that it becomes convex to the volume axis. These changes may have no effect on PEF or FVC and only a small effect on FEV_1.

Table 1. Tests of airway function

Test	Instrumentation[a]	Advantages	Disadvantages	Indication
Tests of forced expiration				
FEV_1, l	Spirometers which directly measure changes in volume (bulky, must accommodate at least 8 l) *or* flow-measuring devices (see MEFV curves below) (more portable but calibration less robust)	Simple, highly repeatable; 'tight' reference values Reflects airway and alveolar function over wide range of lung volumes	Relatively insensitive for studies of normal pharmacology	Most clinical studies of dilator and constrictor responses; 'gold standard'
PEF usually $l \cdot min^{-1}$	Mechanical indicator gauges (small, robust, need no power source, cheap) but linearity and stability of calibration can be a problem *or* flow-measuring devices (see MEFV curves below): absolute values may vary according to airflow resistance of device	Simplest; although it reflects large airway size in normals, obstruction in all size of airways reduces PEF in disease	More effort dependent and less reliable than FEV_1, especially in COPD	Home monitoring, exercise-induced responses; young children; most useful for changes within an individual
FVC, l	As for FEV_1	Indicates extent of airway closure/opening	Repeated forced expiration tiring, particularly in COPD where change in volume may continue for >6 s; usually parallels change in FEV_1	Examining airway closure
MEFV curves $l \cdot s^{-1}$	Flow measured with pneumotachograph, anemometer or turbine; change in volume derived by integrating flow *or* flow obtained by differentiating change in volume of a spirometer	Widely available; good quality control of repeatability	Repeated forced expiration tiring and may not add to FEV_1, FVC	Identifying mild airflow obstruction; measurements during forced inspiration can detect inspiratory obstruction
Measurement of airflow resistance during tidal breathing				
Airway resistance[b] $cm\, H_2O \cdot l^{-1} \cdot s$	Body plethysmograph; very bulky, expensive (3 pressure transducers) and requires skilled operator and calibration	Indicates tidal airway dimensions, usually combined with FRC	Complex equipment, repeatability poorer than tests of forced expiration, especially in severe obstruction	Best method for normal pharmacology; best alternative to spirometry for clinical responses; also indicates hyperinflation
Total respiratory resistance $cm\, H_2O \cdot l^{-1} \cdot s$	Forced oscillation of small volume change at mouth; less bulky and expensive and easier to operate	Indicates tidal airway dimensions during natural breathing	Not widely available, FRC not obtained (value includes chest wall resistance)	Alternative to body plethysmography

[a] A Buyers Guide published by the European Respiratory Society gives a full description of types, manufacturers and costs of spirometers. Eur Respir Buyers 2000;3:40–43, also available at www.ersnet.org.
[b] kPa in SI units: 1 kPa = 0.098 (~ 0.1) cm H_2O.

depends on the lung volume at which it is achieved (the closer to TLC the larger the PEF) and so is submaximal if the expiration is started slightly below TLC and/or there is a slow rise in the pressure generated by the expiratory (mainly abdominal) muscles [6]. Flow at all lung volumes is also reduced if the breath is held at TLC before commencing forced expiration [7].

Maximum expiratory flow is determined by the dynamic dimensions of the intrathoracic airways and by the recoil pressure of the lung (P_L) which provides an important part of the effective driving pressure for expiratory flow and also distends and stabilizes the intrapulmonary airways. In normal subjects at volumes close to TLC, resistance of the medium-size and small airways is low so PEF reflects central airway dimensions and P_L; as lung volume is reduced, total resistance rises due to narrowing of the medium-sized and small airways. FEV_1 in normal subjects is measured over a large portion of the forced vital capacity (FVC) (fig. 1) and reflects the lumped dimensions of all generations of airways.

Technical Factors, Instruments, Selection of 'Best' Tests and Repeatability. At present, most trials use FEV_1 (FVC) for laboratory measurements and PEF for home monitoring. Quality control for FEV_1 currently depends on regular calibration checks using a large syringe and inspection of the original spirogram. Computerized assessment based on the MEFV curve (time to PEF, sharpness of PEF, superimposition of descending part of successive MEFV curves, continuance to zero flow, time expiration is sustained) (fig. 1) can give real-time quality control to the operator and has been used in one large North American trial [8] and is likely to be widely adopted. Values should be expressed at body temperature (BTPS) not ambient room temperature. Manufacturers calibrate peak flow mechanical gauges but subsequently the most widely used check is to note the value obtained by a normal member of staff. Home PEF recording is subject to both technical and recording errors, although devices which electronically record the value and timing of PEF exist [9]. FEV_1 and FVC can also be monitored at home using portable devices which measure and integrate flow [10]. These devices are currently much more expensive than simple PEF gauges and usually lack the quality control possible in the laboratory, but many manufacturers are developing improved devices for home or office use.

Whichever technique or instrument is used, most experts recommend that maximum values from 3 technically satisfactory efforts should be used, provided the second best effort is within 5%. (Poor technique underestimates true values.) Repeatability of FEV_1 is better than that of PEF and other values from the MEFV curve [1, 2].

Reference Values for FEV_1. Values of FEV_1 depend on age, height, gender and ethnic group [1, 2, 11]. FEV_1 in non-smoking subjects reaches a maximum between 18 and 23 years; deterioration in FEV_1 at about 20 ml·year^{-1} begins in the late twenties and reaches 30 ml·year^{-1} in middle-aged and older adults. Decline in FEV_1 starts earlier in smokers and in middle age averages ~45 ml·year^{-1}. These rates of decline are small compared with random intra-individual variability so that it takes many years to establish reliable rates of decline (or treatment-induced changes in decline) [12] in an individual; a smoker susceptible to COPD is identified more easily by a low absolute value of FEV_1 in middle age.

Interpretation of Tests of Forced Expiration. In the early stages of smoking-induced airway disease and in asthma in clinical remission narrowing is confined to the smallest airways; PEF and FEV_1 (and resistance) remain within normal limits but maximum flow at small volume is usually reduced. When airway narrowing is more extensive, regardless of which size(s) of airways are most involved, resistance is increased and maximum flow reduced at *all* lung volumes. In severe airflow obstruction, the transition between PEF and subsequent maximum flow becomes larger (especially in COPD). Consequently, PEF falls proportionally less than FEV_1 as airflow obstruction worsens, while maximum flow at 50% or less of FVC falls proportionately more than PEF or FEV_1. These differences do not necessarily invalidate their use for monitoring airway function; nevertheless FEV_1 is the 'gold standard' for monitoring airway function (table 1). A reduced FEV_1 or PEF of itself is not certain evidence of airways obstruction; when lung volumes are reduced (as for instance after pneumonectomy), FEV_1 and PEF are also reduced. To diagnose obstruction, the FEV_1/FVC ratio also has to be reduced (<0.70 or <0.65 in subjects over 65 years); alternatively, the MEFV curve can be inspected for its characteristic convexity toward the volume axis. However, because FVC is difficult to repeat in COPD (forced expiration may take >10 s to complete), it is common to follow COPD by FEV_1 alone once the initial diagnosis has been confirmed. As the severity of asthma varies, there are changes in FVC as well as FEV_1; reductions in FVC usually parallel those in FEV_1 but indicate increased airway closure or near-closure, probably due to narrowing of small airways. Other attempts to localize the serial site of airway disease from tests based on forced expiration breathing air have had only limited success. Thus while PEF is particularly dependent on central intrathoracic airway dimensions in healthy subjects, this specificity is lost as airway narrowing (at any site in the tracheobronchial tree) progresses. This is fortunate: otherwise using PEF to monitor asthma would be very unreliable. In asthma, a reduced FEV_1 reflects solely airway changes, but loss of P_L due to emphysema also contributes in COPD.

Measurement of Airflow Resistance during Tidal Breathing. Measuring airway resistance indicates airway dimensions during tidal breathing (table 1); despite its greater physiological relevance, much less is known about normal values, changes with ageing, etc., chiefly because it is usually measured by whole-body plethysmography, which is only available in specialized lung function laboratories. Body plethysmography, however, is particularly useful for pharmacological studies in normal subjects or subjects with mild airflow obstruction, where a larger signal is obtained than with tests of forced expiration. As obstruction becomes more severe, it is difficult to define a single value of resistance and plethysmography becomes less useful. A simpler method of measuring resistance – forced oscillation – is becoming more widely available.

Diurnal Variation and Bronchodilator Responsiveness. Virtually all patients with airway obstruction, whether due to asthma or COPD, improve airway function after bronchodilators and also show diurnal variation in airway function (minimum at 4.00 h, maximum at 16.00 h). Hence repeated studies of airway function should be performed at a standard time of day. Home monitoring of PEF is usually performed on waking before bronchodilators are taken and in the early evening but more frequent measurements may be required to establish full circadian variability. Routine bronchodilator responses are usually measured after large doses of an inhaled β_2-adrenergic

Table 2. Tests of alveolar structure/function in asthma and COPD

Test	Instrumentation	Advantages	Disadvantages	Indication
TL_{CO}, ml·min^{-1}·mm Hg^{-1} and K_{CO}, ml·min^{-1}·mm Hg^{-1}·l^{-1}	Measure volume, expired helium and CO: standard equipment in lung function laboratories	Simple, indicates available perfused surface area of lung; can indicate microscopic emphysema	Reductions occur with many other diseases; uncertainty about extent of alveolar volume sampled	Simple assessment of alveolar function and/or pulmonary circulation in airway obstruction
Computerized tomography of lung, Hounsfield density units	Bulky, and expensive, but available in most hospitals; resolution and calibration improving, breath-hold time and radiation dose reducing	Density profile reflects pathology of emphysema; can measure lung volume	State of lung inflation needs to be controlled for comparative studies; 'density masks' detect gross, un- or poorly ventilated areas; radiation dose	Localization of emphysema (e.g. lung volume reduction surgery); identification and progression of emphysema

Conversion to SI units (mmol·min^{-1}·kPa^{-1}) is 0.335 times traditional units. Nomenclature and abbreviations are confusing, although technique is standard world-wide. CO transfer coefficient (K_{CO}; obtained simultaneously) may also be referred to as CO transfer per unit alveolar volume (TL/VA, DL/VA) although it is essentially the rate constant for CO uptake by the alveoli. See Hughes and Pride [5] for more details.

agonist, but in COPD, response to anticholinergics is also useful. Responses are commonly expressed as percent increase of baseline, but inevitably this is heavily influenced by initial values; it is better to express response as absolute increase (ml) or as percent of predicted value, which normalizes the absolute increase for height, age and gender of the subject. Effects of adding in a second bronchodilator are difficult to interpret fully unless a complete dose-response curve to the original bronchodilator is obtained to examine whether a plateau of airway response had been achieved. Action of a long-acting bronchodilator [13] may additionally be assessed by measuring trough function (usually on waking). If the trial drug is not an 'immediate' bronchodilator (for instance an anti-inflammatory agent) [14–16], the appropriate test is usually an improvement in post-bronchodilator airway function.

Hyperinflation

An increase in end-tidal lung volume – functional residual capacity (FRC) – usually accompanies airflow obstruction due to asthma and COPD [17]. Hyperinflation characteristically increases with increasing severity of obstruction, and in an individual further increases during exercise and is reduced by bronchodilators. Breathing tidally closer towards TLC widens the intrapulmonary airways, but the size of tidal volume is restricted and more negative inspiratory pressures are required, which may contribute to dyspnoea. Hyperinflation may be assessed by measuring FRC – either by body plethysmography, which has the advantage that both airway resistance and FRC are routinely measured, or by multi-breath helium dilution, which is available in most lung function laboratories. Alternatively, changes in FRC may be inferred simply by measuring inspiratory capacity (TLC – FRC) with a spirometer, because TLC does not appear to change as airway obstruction varies spontaneously or with drugs. Unfortunately, many spirometers can only be used for expiratory measurement.

Exercise Performance

Assessment of exercise ability is the most useful adjunct to tests of airway function. Exercise ability may be assessed by performance of a standard enforced task (bicycle or treadmill ergometry) or by measuring 6-min walk distance (which also tests motivation) [18] or walking with enforced acceleration (shuttle walk test) [19]. These assessments may be supplemented by visual analogue scales before and after exercise and questionnaires grading dyspnoea of effort and quality of life or health status [20, 21]. Airway function contributes to exercise performance but many other physiological factors play a part (hyperinflation, oxygenation, skeletal muscle strength and endurance, etc.) so there are many reasons why changes (or lack of changes) in airway function [22] may not be mirrored by corresponding changes in dyspnoea or exercise performance.

Assessment of Alveolar Structure and Function
(table 2)

Emphysema can be detected either by measuring associated specific mechanical properties (large TLC – detected by the same methods as those used to measure FRC –, or reduction in P_L, which requires placing a small oesophageal catheter) or by the simple single-breath CO transfer test (TL_{CO} or DL_{CO}), which is in routine use in lung function laboratories. Because TL_{CO} is measured during breathholding at TLC, the effects of uneven airway narrowing are minimized particularly when CO transfer coefficient (K_{CO}), which is the rate constant for CO uptake, is used. Whereas P_L, TL_{CO} and K_{CO} reflect the function of surviving, ventilated lung, qualitative assessment of CT imaging [23] (and gross pathology) emphasize the grossly emphysematous areas which have little or no surviving function, although recent attempts have been made to quantify lung surface area from complete CT density profiles [24]. Progression of emphysema is slow; estimates using CT densitometry suggest a loss of 1% of lung weight per annum in the accelerated form associated with α_1-antitrypsin deficiency [25] so that, similar to FEV_1, assessing progression in alveolar disease requires either a large number of subjects or long-term follow-up of smaller numbers to achieve an adequate signal-noise ratio. In asthma, alveolar structure and function remain normal.

Conclusions

Currently, most clinical studies in asthma and COPD are monitored by simple tests of forced expiration (spirometry measuring FEV_1 and FVC in the laboratory and mechanical gauges measuring PEF at home). Quality control of spirometry can be improved by concurrent recording of the maximum expiratory flow versus expired volume (MEFV) curve during the forced expiration. Measuring changes in exercise performance and hyperinflation provides additional information which may differ from that provided by spirometry. Future treatment of COPD is likely to be directed at alveolar disease as well as at the airway component; alveolar structure/function can be assessed by computed tomography and the standard single-breath carbon monoxide transfer test, which provide complementary information.

References

1 American Thoracic Society Statement: Standardization of Spirometry. 1994 update. Am J Respir Crit Care Med 1995;152:1107–1136.
2 European Respiratory Society: Standardised Lung Function Testing. Eur Respir J 1993;6(suppl 16):5–40.
3 British Thoracic Society: Guidelines for the measurement of respiratory function. Respir Med 1994;88:165–194.
4 Crapo RO: Pulmonary Function Testing. N Engl J Med 1994;331:25–30.
5 Hughes JMB, Pride NB (eds): Lung Function Tests: Physiological Principles and Clinical Applications. London, Saunders, 1999.
6 Lebowitz MD, Quanjer PH (eds): ERS Statement: Peak expiratory flow. Eur Respir J 1997;10(suppl 24):1–74S.
7 D'Angelo E, Prandl E, Milic-Emili J: Dependence of maximal flow-volume curves on time course of preceding inspiration. J Appl Physiol 1993;75:1155–1159.
8 Enright PL, Johnson LR, Connett JE, Voelker H, Buist AS: Spirometry in the Lung Health Study. 1. Methods and quality control. Am Rev Respir Dis 1991;143:1215–1223.
9 Higgs CM, Richardson RB, Lea DA, Lewis GT, Laszlo G: Influence of knowledge of peak flow on self-assessment of asthma: Studies with a coded peak flow meter. Thorax 1986;41:671–675.
10 Dirksen A, Madsen F, Pedersen OF, Vedel AM, Kok-Jensen A: Long-term performance of a hand held spirometer. Thorax 1996;51:973–976.
11 American Thoracic Society: Lung function testing: Selection of reference values and interpretative strategies. Am Rev Respir Dis 1991;144:1209–1218.
12 Scanlon PD, Connett JE, Waller LA, Altose MD, Bailey WC, Buist AS, Tashkin DP for the Lung Health Study Research Group: Smoking cessation and lung function in mild-to-moderate chronic obstructive pulmonary disease: The Lung Health Study. Am J Respir Crit Care Med 2000;161:381–390.
13 Littner MR, Ilowite JS, Tashkin DP, Friedman M, Serby CW, Menjoge SS, Witek TJ Jr: Long-acting bronchodilation with once-daily dosing of tiotropium (Spiriva) in stable chronic obstructive pulmonary disease. Am J Respir Crit Care Med 2000;161:1136–1142.
14 Pauwels RA, Lofdahl CG, Laitinen LA, Schouten JP, Postma DS, Pride NB, Ohlsson SV: Long-term treatment with inhaled budesonide in persons with mild chronic obstructive pulmonary disease who continue smoking. European Respiratory Society Study on Chronic Obstructive Pulmonary Disease. N Engl J Med 1999;340:1948–1953.
15 Burge PS, Calverley PMA, Jones PW, Spencer S, Anderson JA, Maslen TK: Randomised, double blind, placebo controlled study of fluticasone propionate in patients with moderate to severe chronic obstructive pulmonary disease: The ISOLDE trial. BMJ 2000;320:1297–1303.
16 Torphy TJ, Barnette MS, Underwood DC, Griswold DE, Christensen SB, Murdoch RD, Nieman RB, Compton CH: AriﬂoTM (SB 207499), a second-generation phosphodiesterase 4 inhibitor for the treatment of asthma and COPD: From concept to clinic. Pulm Pharmacol Ther 1999;12:131–135.
17 Gibson GJ: Pulmonary hyperinflation: A clinical overview. Eur Respir J 1996;9:2640–2649.
18 Enright PL, Sherrill DL: Reference equations for the six-minute walk in healthy adults. Am J Respir Crit Care Med 1998;158:1384–1387.
19 Revill SM, Morgan MDL, Singh SJ, Williams J, Hardman AE: The endurance shuttle walk: A new field test for the assessment of endurance capacity in chronic obstructive pulmonary disease. Thorax 1999;54:213–222.
20 Molken MR, Roos B, van Noord JA: An empirical comparison of the St George's respiratory questionnaire (SGRQ) and the chronic respiratory disease questionnaire (CRQ) in a clinical trial setting. Thorax 1999;54:995–1003.
21 Juniper EF: Health-related quality of life in asthma. Curr Opin Pulm Med 1999;5:105–110.
22 van Schayck CP: Is lung function really a good parameter in evaluating the long-term effects of inhaled corticosteroids in COPD? Eur Respir J 2000;15:238–239.
23 Gevenois PA, De Vuyst P, de M, V, Zanen J, Jacobovitz D, Cosio MG, Yernault JC: Comparison of computed density and microscopic morphometry in pulmonary emphysema. Am J Respir Crit Care Med 1996;154:187–192.
24 Coxson HO, Rogers RM, Whittall KP, D'yachkova Y, Pare PD, Sciurba FC, Hogg JC: A quantification of the lung surface area in emphysema using computed tomography. Am J Respir Crit Care Med 1999;159:851–856.
25 Dirksen A, Dijkman JH, Madsen F, Stoel B, Hutchison DCS, Ulrik CS, Skovgaard LT, Kok-Jensen A, Rudolphus A, Seersholm N, Vrooman HA, Reiber JHC, Hansen NC, Heckscher T, Viskum K, Stolk J: A randomised clinical trial of α_1-antitrypsin augmentation therapy. Am J Respir Crit Care Med 1999;160:1468–1472.

Neil Pride
Department of Thoracic Medicine
National Heart and Lung Institute
Imperial College School of Medicine
London SW3 6LY (UK)
Tel. +44 207 351 8920, Fax +44 207 351 8939
E-Mail n.pride@ic.ac.uk

Airway Hyperresponsiveness

Peter J. Sterk

Lung Function Laboratory, Department of Pulmonology, Leiden University Medical Centre,
Leiden, The Netherlands

Summary

Standardized bronchoprovocation tests are providing relevant pathophysiological and clinical information about patients with asthma and COPD. The responses to so-called 'indirect' challenges are largely dependent on the state of activation of inflammatory or resident cells within the airways, while 'direct' challenges are less variable and more influenced by chronic features of airway inflammation or remodelling. Hence, bronchoprovocation tests are providing complementary and integrated information about multiple pathophysiological pathways within the airways. Measurement of AHR warrants broader usage in clinical practice and in clinical studies with novel drugs for asthma.

Reasons to Measure AHR

AHR to bronchoconstrictor stimuli is a major pathophysiological feature of airways in diseases such as asthma and COPD. It is more and more realized that the integrative, physiological markers of airways disease might better reflect the complex acute and chronic pathophysiology than cellular or molecular biomarkers of inflammation. Interestingly, there is increasing evidence that monitoring AHR adds substantially to the benefits of long-term asthma management.

Pathogenesis

AHR can be defined as an increase in the ease and degree of airway narrowing in response to bronchoconstrictor stimuli in vivo. It can be measured by bronchoprovocation tests in the laboratory, which have been standardized to a great extent [1–3]. Bronchial challenge tests mimic the spontaneous variability in airway obstruction as observed in patients with asthma or COPD.

The understanding of the pathogenesis and pathophysiology of AHR has evolved rapidly during the past years. Epidemiological studies suggest that AHR has both a genetic and an environmental background. In children from a general population, it appears to be associated with parental asthma, atopy and early respiratory illness [4]. So far, the genetic predisposition of AHR has not been fully clarified. In clinical populations with asthma it was demonstrated that AHR to histamine is linked to loci on chromosome 5q, independently of linkage of serum IgE to the same chromosome [5]. In addition, environmental exposures, such as respiratory virus infections, allergens, and parental smoking might also contribute to induction of AHR. Even though there is no doubt that respiratory virus infections can temporarily worsen the degree of AHR in asthma [6], it remains to be established as to whether virus infections are causally involved [7].

Mechanisms of AHR

The underlying mechanisms of AHR are multiple, being associated both with acute as well as chronic airway inflammation. The major determinants of AHR seem to be the mechanical consequences of (sub)mucosal as well as adventitial inflammation on airway smooth muscle shortening and thereby on airway luminal diameter [8]. It essentially includes multiple mechanisms, including: acute inflammation and chronic airway wall remodelling [9], as well as primary or secondary changes in behaviour of the smooth muscle itself, including the occurrence of a difficult to reverse, contractile 'latch' state [10].

Acute airway obstruction can arise from smooth muscle contraction either with or without inflammatory changes in the airway wall. These inflammatory changes include hyperaemia, plasma exudate, oedema, or hypersecretion. In combination with smooth muscle contraction, such mucosal and peribronchial swelling will lead to excessive airway narrowing [11].

Table 1. Examples of challenge tests used in clinical research

Pharmacological challenges
- Histamine
- Methacholine
- AMP
- Bradykinin
- Leukotrienes
- Tachykinins

Physiological challenges
- Exercise
- Hypertonic saline (potentially combined with sputum induction) [15]
- Distilled water
- Cold air

Challenge with inducers of airways inflammation
- Allergen
- Ozone
- Occupational sensitizer
- Rhinovirus infection [16]

Challenge Agents

The interpretation of the presence and severity of AHR depends critically on the nature of the bronchoconstrictor challenge (table 1). Some bronchoconstrictors act directly and predominantly on the airway smooth muscle itself (e.g. methacholine, histamine), whereas other stimuli depend on the involvement of cellular or neurogenic mechanisms, indirectly leading to smooth muscle contraction and possibly to inflammatory changes in the airway wall (e.g. non-isotonic aerosols, cold/dry air, exercise, AMP, bradykinin, tachykinins, leukotrienes, sodium metabisulphite) [2].

It should be emphasized that airway inflammation is actually induced by challenge with sensitizing agents, particularly during late asthmatic reactions (e.g. allergens, occupational sensitizers) [2]. In addition, these challenges by themselves can also cause a transient worsening in airway responsiveness to other, non-sensitizing stimuli, which also occurs after respiratory virus infection [6]. Such measurements of allergen- or virus-induced AHR are highly suitable for pathophysiological research and so-called 'proof-of-concept' studies using new and experimental interventions in asthma [12, 13].

Based on the heterogeneity in pathophysiological pathways, it is not surprising that the results of the various challenge tests are only weakly correlated, and thereby not being interchangeable, each test implicitly providing different and perhaps complementary information on the multiple pathways leading to airway narrowing (see below).

Measurement of Responsiveness

The methods of measurement have been standardized internationally [1–3, 12–14]. The dose-response curves of pharmacological challenges are usually analysed in terms of position, the provocative concentration or dose leading to a certain change in lung function: PC_{20} or PD_{20} [2]. Because of the log-normal distribution of these variables, any differences between subjects, or any changes within subjects, are currently analysed in doubling doses. This refers to two-fold steps [2]. However, particularly in epidemiological studies, many subjects do not reach a 20% fall in FEV_1, so that we need other measures of AHR in those subjects in order to avoid censored data. One approach might be curve-fitting of the sigmoid log-dose response curve, or just using the so-called 'two-point' slope of the linear dose-response curve [17]. The latter indices have large advantages in epidemiological studies, but should be applied with caution [1].

Finally, there is little doubt that the maximal response on the dose-response curve is an essential outcome of bronchial challenge tests. The presence or absence of a plateau (excessive airway narrowing) and its level have successfully been used in drug trials. However, the level of expertise required for measuring this outcome precludes its application in multicentre studies [8]. As an indirect measure of excessive airway narrowing, the fall in FVC at the PC_{20} level is likely to be a promising alternative.

Relation with Airways Inflammation

AHR in asthma is associated with on-going airway inflammation. Hence, it can be regarded as a physiological surrogate marker of acute as well as airway chronic inflammation. This appears from cross-sectional and longitudinal relationships between e.g. the PC_{20} to methacholine and the number of activated eosinophils in bronchial biopsies and subepithelial collagen thickness in patients with moderately severe asthma [18].

Not surprisingly, the strength of such associations varies greatly between studies. This is because, fortunately (!), AHR is not identical to certain aspects of inflammation (fig. 1). It positively distinguishes itself from cellular or molecular markers of inflammation, namely that it integratively reflects multiple, variable as well as persistent features of inflammation, and even more than that [10, 19]. Not only in the bronchial (sub)mucosa, but also in the adventitia [9–11]. And not only in the large, central airways, but also in the small, peripheral airways [9–11]. This is a great advantage of this functional measurement in in vivo studies.

Fig. 1. When detecting and monitoring airway pathophysiology in asthma, the currently available methods do not provide similar information on the abnormalities within the airways. In each study one has to chose between information on specific, but limited inflammatory pathways, as opposed to general and more integrative information including the consequences of airway inflammation. Exhaled markers, cellular and molecular markers in sputum, 'indirect' challenges and 'direct' challenges are different in this respect. a = Inflammatory mediators and cytokines; b = cellular infiltration and activation; c = neurogenic activity; d = epithelial damage; e = submucosal gland hyperplasia; f = Collagen deposition in the subepithelial reticular layer; g = microvascular permeability internal and external of the smooth muscle layer; h = airway smooth muscle growth, contractility and latch; i = (peri)bronchial swelling by oedema, vascularity and fibrosis, and j = damage to alveolar attachments.

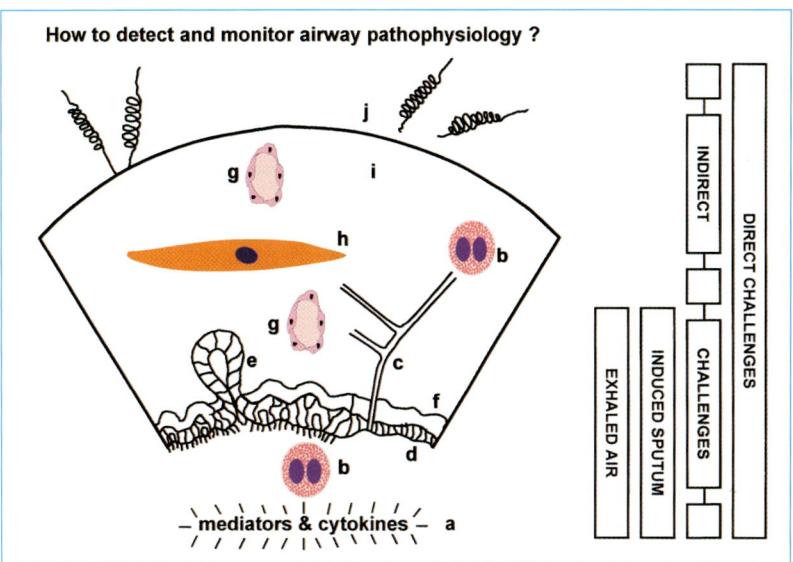

Direct or Indirect Challenges

It is often argued that the results by so-called 'indirect' challenge tests are a better reflection of airway inflammation than the response to 'direct' stimuli, such as histamine or methacholine. Indeed, the response to e.g. AMP is more sensitive than methacholine to allergen-induced inflammation or to inhaled steroid treatment [20] in asthma. Hence, it appears that AMP challenge can be a marker of acute and rapidly varying airway inflammation, probably reflecting cellular infiltration and activation. However, this might not be the feature of interest in long-term asthma monitoring. The relatively slow response of histamine or methacholine challenges to inhaled steroids might contain a more important message, namely the accompanying gradual improvement of e.g. oedema, hyperaemia, vascularity, smooth muscle growth and behaviour, or collagen deposition (fig. 1) [18]. Such features are often non-specifically referred to as airway remodelling [21], and are likely to be major determinants of methacholine responsiveness [9–11]. Hence, it can be postulated that the latter is particularly suitable in the long-term monitoring of asthma.

Asthma and COPD Management

AHR is closely associated with – but not identical to – the diagnosis of asthma [2]. It appears that pharmacological and exercise challenges are particularly suitable for the exclusion of asthma in the clinic, because of their high sensitivity and high negative predictive value. However, the tests are less useful to confirm the diagnosis, particularly in epidemiological studies, due to their moderate specificity and relatively low positive predictive value.

What is the benefit of monitoring AHR, on top of symptoms and lung function, in asthma management in clinical practice? This question requires long-term follow-up studies. Sont et al. [18] have recently completed a 2-year parallel follow-up study, in which they demonstrated that adding AHR to methacholine as a guide for asthma treatment improved the clinical as well as histopathological outcome. Hence, it appears that that monitoring asthma according to the current guidelines does *not* lead to optimal disease control, and that methacholine challenge tests appear to be a powerful adjunct measure to improve asthma control during long-term follow-up. It cannot be excluded that this also holds for COPD, because even in this disease AHR appears to be an independent predictor of long-term outcome [22].

Clinical Research

In view of the rapid progress in the development of new drugs for asthma, there is an on-going debate as to whether to include the measurements of AHR as an outcome variable in trials aimed to test a proof of concept and/or the clinical benefits of novel drugs. Based on the above, one would predict that AHR will provide complementary information as compared to cellular or molecular markers of inflammation in sputum, exhaled air or bronchial biopsies. And, equally important, it appears from long-term intervention trials that such information is clinically highly relevant.

The dissociation between simple measures of airway inflammation and AHR has been underlined by recent trials with anti-inflammatory interventions in asthma. First, it appeared that children with asthma who were uncontrolled despite high-dose therapy with inhaled steroids, still demonstrated AHR to histamine and AMP, whereas sputum eosinophil counts were already suppressed to nearly normal values [23]. Allergen avoidance on top of inhaled steroids in these children substantially improved AHR, which could not be demonstrated for sputum eosinophil counts [23]. This dissociation also occurs between AHR and sputum eosinophils during the occurrence of exacerbations despite high-dose steroid therapy in patients with severe asthma. Under those circumstances AHR to methacholine (but not to hypertonic saline) worsened, despite unchanged sputum eosinophil counts [24]. Hence, clinically relevant signals of inflammation are not being detected by some of the currently used measurements.

These results suggest that AHR is an indispensable outcome in the clinical research of asthma. This has been underlined by a recent study on the effects of single-dose treatment with a humanized, monoclonal antibody against IL-5 in atopic asthmatics. Despite being extremely effective in reducing the number of circulating and sputum eosinophils during a 16-week period, anti-IL-5 did not change AHR to histamine nor the late asthmatic response to inhaled allergen [25].

Conclusion

AHR comprises the common physiologic pathway for multiple (cellular and biochemical) abnormalities within the airways. Its association with airway remodelling, as opposed to acute inflammation only, appears to be the reason for its success in improving the clinical long-term management of asthma. Measurement of AHR in conjunction with biomarkers of inflammation is especially important in the early clinical phases of development of new therapies for asthma and COPD.

References

1 Chinn S: Methodology of bronchial responsiveness. Thorax 1998;53:984–988.
2 Sterk PJ, Fabbri LM, Quanjer PhH, et al: Airway responsiveness. Standardized challenge testing with pharmacological, physical and sensitizing stimuli in adults. Eur Respir J 1994; 6(suppl 16):53–83.
3 American Thoracic Society: Guidelines for methacholine and exercise challenge testing – 1999. Am J Respir Crit Care Med 2000;161: 309–329.
4 Peat JK, Salome CM, Woolcock AJ: Factors associated with bronchial hyperresponsiveness in Australian adults and children. Eur Respir J 1992;5:921–929.
5 Postma DS, Bleecker ER, Amelung PJ, Holroyd KJ, Xu J, Panhuysen CIM, Meyers DA, Levitt RC: Genetic susceptibility to asthma. Bronchial hyperresponsiveness coinherited with a major gene for atopy. N Engl J Med 1995;333:894–900.
6 Corne JM, Holgate ST: Mechanisms of virus induced exacerbations of asthma. Thorax 1997;52:380–389.
7 Wang S-Z, Forsyth KD: Asthma and respiratory syncytial virus infection in infancy: Is there a link? Clin Exp Allergy 1998;28:927–935.
8 Sterk PJ, Bel EH: Bronchial hyperresponsiveness: the need for a distinction between hypersensitivity and excessive airway narrowing. Eur Respir J 1989;2:267–274.
9 Paré PD, Bai TR: The consequences of chronic allergic inflammation. Thorax 1995;50:328–332.
10 King GC, Paré PD, Seow CY: The mechanics of exaggerated airway narrowing in asthma: The role of smooth muscle. Respir Physiol 1999;118:1–13.
11 Macklem PT: A theoretical analysis of the effect of airway smooth muscle load on airway narrowing. Am J Respir Crit Care Med 1996; 153:83–89.
12 Lötvall J, Inman M, O'Byrne PM: Measurements of airway hyperresponsiveness: New considerations. Thorax 1998;53:419–424.
13 Inman MD, Hamilton AL, Kerstjens HAM, Watson RM, O'Byrne PM: The utility of methacholine airway responsiveness measurements in evaluating anti-asthma drugs. J Allergy Clin Immunol 1998;101:342–348.
14 Inman MD, Watson R, Cockcroft DW, Wong BJO, Hargreave FE, O'Byrne PM: Reproducibility of allergen-induced early and late asthmatic responses. J Allergy Clin Immunol 1995; 95:1191–1195.
15 In 't Veen JCCM, de Gouw HWFM, Smits HH, Sont JK, Hiemstra PS, Sterk PJ, Bel EH: Repeatability of cellular and soluble markers of inflammation in induced sputum from patients with asthma. Eur Respir J 1996;9:2441–2447.
16 Grünberg K, Smits HH, Timmers MC, de Klerk EPA, Dolhain RJEM, Hiemstra PS, Sterk PJ: Experimental rhinovirus 16 infection. Effects on cell differentials and soluble markers in sputum in asthmatic subjects. Am J Respir Crit Care Med 1997;156:609–616.
17 Chinn S, Burney PGJ, Britton JR, Tattersfield AE, Higgins BG: Comparison of PD_{20} with two alternative measures of response to histamine challenge in epidemiological studies. Eur Respir J 1993;6:670–679.
18 Sont JK, Willems LNA, Bel EH, van Krieken JHJM, Vandenbroucke JP, Sterk PJ, and the AMPUL Study Group: The clinical control and histopathological outcome of asthma when using airway hyperresponsiveness as an additional guide of long-term treatment. Am J Respir Crit Care Med 1999;159:1043–1051.
19 Brusasco V, Crimi E, Pellegrino R: Airway hyperresponsiveness in asthma: Not just a matter of airway inflammation. Thorax 1998;53: 992–998.
20 O'Connor BJ, Ridge SM, Barnes PJ, Fuller RW: Greater effect of inhaled budesonide on adenosine 5′-monophosphate-induced than on sodium-metabisulfite-induced bronchoconstriction in asthma. Am Rev Respir Dis 1992; 146:560–564.
21 Kips JC, Pauwels RA: Airway wall remodelling: Does it occur and what does it mean? Clin Exp Allergy 1999;29:1457–1466.
22 Tashkin DP, Altose MD, Connett JE, Kanner RE, Lee WW, Wise RA, for the Lung Health Study Research Group: Methacholine reactivity predicts changes in lung function over time in smokers with early chronic obstructive pulmonary disease. Am J Respir Crit Care Med 1996;153:1802–1811.
23 Grootendorst DC, Dahlèn S-E, van den Bos JW, Duiverman EJ, Veselic-Charvat M, Vrijlandt EJLE, Kumlin M, Sterk PJ, Roldaan AC: Benefits of high altitude allergen avoidance in atopic adolescents with severe asthma already treated with high-dose inhaled steroids. Clin Exp Allergy, in press.
24 In 't Veen JCCM, Smits HH, Hiemstra PS, Zwinderman AE, Sterk PJ, Bel EH: Lung function and sputum characteristics of patients with severe asthma during induced exacerbation by double-blind steroid withdrawal. Am J Respir Crit Care Med 1999;160:93–99.
25 Leckie MJ, ten Brinke A, Khan J, Diamant Z, Taylor DA, Walls ChM, Chung KF, Djukanovic R, Hansel TT, Holgate ST, Sterk PJ, Barnes PJ: Effects of anti-interleukin-5 on eosinophils, airway hyperresponsiveness and the late asthmatic reaction, submitted.

Prof. Peter J. Sterk
Lung Function Laboratory, C2-P
Department of Pulmonology
Leiden University Medical Centre
PO Box 9600
NL-2300 RC Leiden (The Netherlands)
Tel. +31 71 526 3578, Fax +31 71 515 4691
E-Mail p.j.sterk@lumc.nl

Airways Remodelling

Stephen T. Holgate   Donna E. Davies

RCMB Research Division, School of Medicine, University of Southampton,
Southampton General Hospital, Southampton, UK

Summary

Remodelling of the airways is a major feature of chronic persistent asthma, resulting in epithelial goblet cell metaplasia, subepithelial and mucosal fibrosis, smooth muscle hypertrophy and increased microvasculature. The epithelium is a major source of cytokines, chemokines and growth factors that control remodelling in the adjacent myofibroblasts, microvasculature and nerves. Indeed, activation of the epithelial mesenchymal trophic unit is a fundamental abnormality in chronic asthma. There are shortfalls in small animal models of relatively acute allergen-driven airway inflammatory responses, since they do not identify effects on airway remodelling.

Considering asthma as an inflammatory disorder of the airways has done much to provide a rationale for how drugs with anti-inflammatory activity, such as corticosteroids, produce their beneficial effects. Increasingly, however, patients with more severe and difficult asthma seem to respond less well to corticosteroids even at high doses [1]. Airway remodelling explains why patients with moderate to severe disease gain considerably from the addition of drugs, such as inhaled long-acting β_2-adrenoceptor agonists and cysteinyl leukotriene-1 receptor antagonists. It seems that the bronchial epithelium is especially important in orchestrating repair and proliferative responses [2]. On account of an impaired restitution response to injury, the epithelium becomes a major source of growth factors, the downstream actions of which could explain the subepithelial collagen deposition as well as wider responses including the increase in blood vessels, nerves and smooth muscle (fig. 1).

Inflammatory Cells

Most mild to moderate asthma is linked to a Th2-mediated inflammation characterized by coordinate overexpression of cytokines encoded in the IL-4 gene cluster on chromosome $5q_{31-33}$. T cells, macrophages, mast cells and eosinophils all have the capacity to generate proliferative and remodelling growth factors but, of these cells, it seems that the tissue macrophage is one of the most important sources of TGF-β, PDGF and bFGF [3]. Activated tissue macrophages are cells that are centrally involved in the pathogenesis of interstitial lung disease, although they probably do not function alone. As asthma becomes more chronic and severe, it loses its connection with atopy and adopts some of the characteristics of COPD with evidence of fixed airflow obstruction and neutrophil recruitment. This occurs in relation to expression of a second set of inflammatory cytokines involved in Th1-mediated inflammation (e.g. IFN-γ, IL-2, TNF-α) and release of neutrophil-selective chemoattractants (e.g. IL-8, GRO-α, LTB$_4$) [1]. While it has been suggested that the neutrophil response is secondary to the effect of steroids, a more likely explanation is the recruitment during a tissue-destructive phase of the disease.

Bronchial Epithelium

Structural damage to the bronchial epithelium is a feature of severe asthma that has been frequently described in post-mortem studies. Bronchial biopsy studies undertaken in asthma of differing severity have clearly shown epithelial damage, and there is now evidence to indicate that this occurs as a primary feature of asthma [2]. Char-

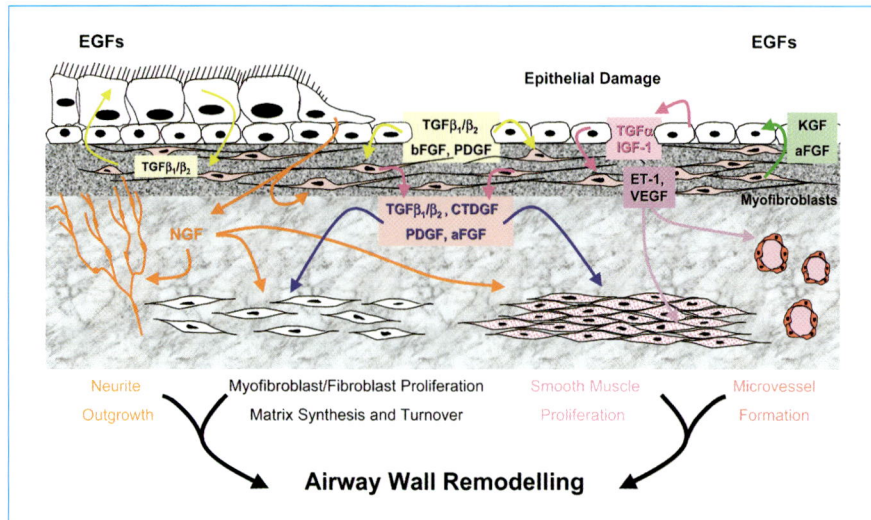

Fig. 1. Two theoretical constructs for the pathogenesis of asthma. The parallel rather than the sequential paradigm would fit the variable clinical phenotype of asthma best and also take account of a wider range of gene-environmental interactions in disease pathogenesis.

acteristically, the columnar epithelial cells detach from basal counterparts, probably as a result of premature apoptosis with loss of intercellular adhesion. The extent of epithelial damage appears to relate to both asthma severity and the level of BHR. There also occurs a characteristic thickening of the lamina reticularis component beneath the true basement membrane with the collagen deposited in this region being of the interstitial repair subtypes types I, III and V and is accompanied by the laying down of a regenerative form of laminin-β and tenascin-c [2, 4].

Loss of the protective barrier provided by the bronchial epithelium will increase the access of a wide range of environmental stimuli, including air pollutants, infectious agents and allergens to effector cells in the airway wall. For example, ICAM-1, the major receptor for the major subtypes of human rhinovirus (HRV), which is overexpressed in the basal epithelium of asthmatic airways [5], creates an easy target for lower airway involvement following the common cold.

Increased expression of mucin genes by EGFs generated by the damaged epithelium and IL-4 and IL-13 from the Th2-mediated inflammatory response explains the increased number of goblet cells within the epithelium in severe chronic asthma (fig. 2). The epithelial damage-repair cycle also initiates overexpression of a range of epithelial pro-inflammatory genes, including the inducible form of nitric oxide synthase, the cytoplasmic form of PLA_2, cyclooxygenase-2 and a number of metalloendoproteases involved in the repair response, especially MMP-9. A number of cytokines are also expressed by the activated epithelium, including GM-CSF, IL-6, TNF-α and a range of chemokines, such as eotaxin, RANTES and IL-8 [3]. The consequence of this epithelial perturbation is to enhance the airway's ability to support an inflammatory response and, at the same time, drive tissue repair processes [2, 4].

Airway Wall Fibrosis

Proliferating myofibroblasts are responsible for the 'repair' collagen deposited beneath the basement membrane in asthma, their numbers correlating with the thickness of the lamina reticularis. Myofibroblasts play an important role in chronic wound healing through their capacity to lay down matrix proteins to contract in the presence of pharmacological mediators, e.g. endothelin, and to secrete an array of growth factors (fig. 1). Growth factors derived from repairing epithelium drive the myofibroblasts to proliferate and then secrete collagen. These factors include TGF-$β_1$ and -$β_2$ (which normally inhibits proliferation of fibroblasts), bFGF, IGF-1, PDGF-BB and ET-1 [6].

Although difficult to study, there is some evidence to indicate that, in chronic severe disease, collagen deposition is increased in the submucosa and deeper reaches of the airway wall [7]. This is accompanied by other matrix proteins and proteoglycans, including decorin, versican and fibronectin. These provide important cell-surface stimuli for activating inflammatory leukocytes and prolonging their survival. They also provide a reservoir for cytokines, e.g. IL-4 (heparin), chemokines (heparan sulphate) and growth factors (TGF-β binding to decorin and bFGF factor binding to heparan sulphate). Encrypted

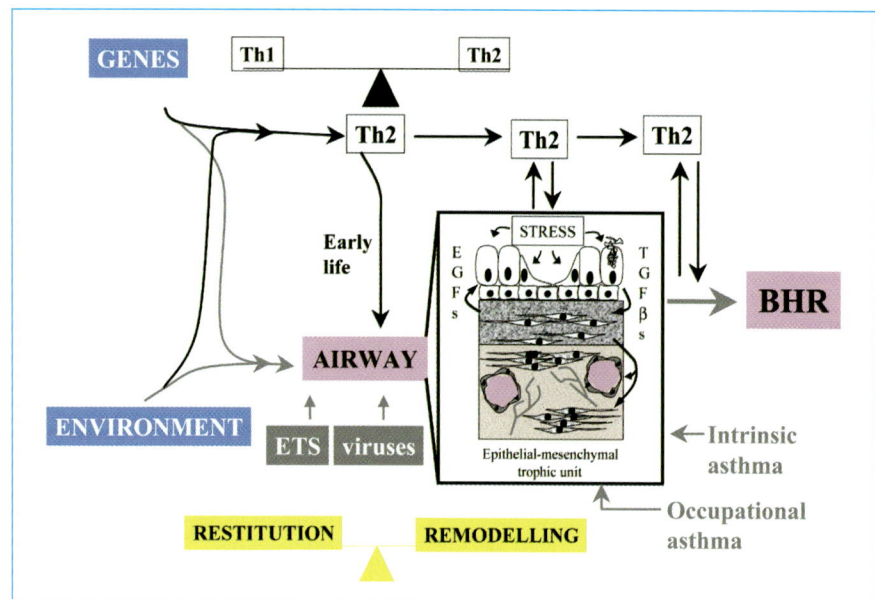

Fig. 2. Role of the abnormal damaged and stressed epithelium in airway wall remodelling in asthma.

cytokines and growth factors can be released in the presence of pro-inflammatory mediators and proteolytic enzymes, thereby providing a continuous ongoing stimulus for cell proliferation and matrix production.

An increase in thickness of the submucosa by infiltrating inflammatory cells, proteoglycans and new collagen, with water being trapped by the high molecular weight proteoglycans, will have a considerable impact on airway wall caliber with a given degree of smooth muscle shortening [8]. This alone may contribute greatly to AHR, whereas thickening of the airway wall outside the smooth muscle (which serves to spread the elastic recoil forces of the alveoli over a greater surface area) provides an explanation for the loss of the characteristic plateau response observed in normal subjects with increasing doses of a contractile agonist.

Myofibroblasts are also an important source of proinflammatory cytokines, including stem cell factor required for mast cell growth, maturation and survival and GM-CSF, a potent inhibitor of eosinophil apoptosis. Myofibroblasts are highly efficient at supporting the survival of both mast cells and eosinophils, both by the secretion of soluble products and through cell-to-cell contact [9].

Microvasculature

The small blood vessels in the submucosa play an important role in asthma, providing not only a secondary source of mediators derived from circulating plasma proteins and endothelial cells, but also a mechanisms through which effector leukocytes are recruited into the airways. In chronic severe asthma, there is ample evidence for upregulation of both endothelial selectins and adhesion molecules belonging to the immunoglobulin superclass. Of particular relevance is VCAM-1 which is under the regulation of TNF-α, IL-4 and IL-13. Through its interaction with the β_2-integrin, VLA-4, VCAM-1 is largely responsible for the selective recruitment of eosinophils, basophils and T cells into the asthmatic airway. In chronic asthma, the number of microvessels in the submucosa is increased as a consequence of enhanced secretion of vascular growth factors, including ET-1, NO and VEGF [10].

Airway Nerves

Although in mild asthma the number of sensory nerves within the asthmatic airway is unchanged, in chronic and severe disease there is increased innervation, resulting from the secretion of nerve growth factors from epithelial and inflammatory cells [3, 11]. C-fibres containing neuropeptides, such as substance P, neurokinin A and CGRP contribute to altered local vascular and smooth muscle homeostasis in asthma, although the clinical efficacy of tachykinin antagonists has been disappointing, even in patients with brittle asthma in whose airways neural pathways might be expected to be important. Another important group of sensory neurons is those bearing the rapidly adapting Aδ-receptors, which are incriminated in the production of cough. In animal models, neuropeptide receptors are under the regulation of pleiotrophic cytokines such as TNF-α.

Airway Smooth Muscle

Changes to airway smooth muscle have provided the foundations for disordered airway function in asthma [12, 13]. When airways from the lungs of asthmatic patients have been studied in vitro using a range of contractile agonists, enhanced responsiveness has only been demonstrated with adenosine and its analogues. This purine nucleoside stimulates A_{2B} receptors on primed mast cells to release contractile mediators such as histamine and cysteinyl leukotrienes [14]. Adenosine hyperresponsiveness observed in asthma probably relates to altered mast cell function rather than to any change in airway smooth muscle itself.

Morphological studies of smooth muscle in airways obtained from patients who have died from asthma reveal evidence of an increase in muscle bulk, due in large part to an increase in smooth muscle cells. Whether these cells function differently in asthma is not known [13]. However, recent electrophysiological and biochemical studies indicate that cycling of the actin and myosin cross bridges in asthmatic smooth muscle is abnormal, leading to a frozen or latched state which is difficult to relax [12]. Airway smooth muscle in asthma undergoes a process of dedifferentiation towards that of a myofibroblast cell type with more pleiotrophic cell functions, including the secretion of matrix proteins and cytokines [13]. Whether this occurs in asthmatic airways in vivo is not known, nor is it known whether the biochemical mechanisms involved in contraction of airway smooth muscle become disordered in the inflammatory milieu including ion fluxes, phosphorylation and dephosphorylation reactions and engagement of myosin with actin.

The Epithelial Mesenchymal Trophic Unit

Epithelial injury produced by inflammatory and environmental insults, such as air pollutants, environmental tobacco smoke and respiratory viruses, is usually rapidly repaired through the release and autacoid actions of EGF, amphiregulin, TGF-α and heparin-binding EGF-like growth factor [2–4]. However, in asthma it seems that epithelial proliferation and repair involving cell signalling is impaired, resulting in a change in the epithelial phenotype to one that secretes profibrogenic cytokines including TGF-β [15]. The precise biochemical site at which this block occurs is not known although it is accompanied by reduced expression of proliferating cell nuclear antigen and increased expression of the G_1 cell cycle inhibitor $p21^{waf}$.

Associated with impaired epithelial restitution is the enhanced activity of the underlying myofibroblasts which in asthma exhibit hyperresponsiveness to the TGF-β produced by the altered epithelium and a reduced capacity to degrade collagens I, III and V. The net consequence of this is the deposition of subepithelial collagen and the secretion of multifunctional growth factors by the myofibroblasts including CTGF, PDGF, NGFs, VEGF and GM-CSF with their capacity to drive fibroblast, nerve, vascular and Th2 inflammatory responses characteristic of airway wall remodelling (fig. 2). The combined involvement of the epithelial-myofibroblast unit resembles the critical involvement of the same cells in fetal branching morphogenesis (epithelial mesenchymal trophic unit) [2]. Thus, for asthma to become fully manifest, a combination of Th2-mediated inflammation and activation of the epithelial mesenchyme is required – the interaction leading to chronic inflammation and remodelling (fig. 1).

Therapeutic Targets

It is only relatively recently that the concept of an altered structure and function of the constituent elements of the conducting airways has become a recognized component of chronic asthma. While there is some evidence that the early introduction of inhaled corticosteroids are able to prevent or reverse structural changes in the airways [16, 17], there is little evidence that other therapeutic interventions can influence the natural history of asthma. Theoretical possibilities might include EGFR ligands that promote epithelial repair and increase resistance against environmental insult, inhibitors of TGF-β (e.g. blocking antibodies) that might suppress fibrogenesis and smooth muscle proliferation and similar blocking strategies against factors that lead to proliferation of nerves (e.g. NGFR antagonists) or microvessels (e.g. VEGFR antagonists). Until appropriate animal models are generated to test these agents, it will not be possible to estimate the potential usefulness of this approach.

With the clear recognition that the Th2 cytokines IL-4, IL-9 and IL-13 are involved in epithelial goblet cell metaplasia (via TGF-α) as well as epithelial production of TGF-β, the new drugs aimed at targeting these cytokine pathways, e.g. soluble IL-4R (Nuvance) and the IL-4 double mutein, look especially promising.

Clinical Trials

If novel agents are to be tested against airway remodelling in asthma, it will be important to identify clear clinical end points. One of these might include the corticosteroid-refractory component of FEV_1 or similar measure of airway calibre or a measure of BHR followed over time. To complement these physiological measures, new markers of matrix turnover and airway remodelling need to be developed to provide shorter-term surrogate indices against which to measure efficacy. Finally, in order to know whether restructuring of the airways continues in the presence of current controller therapies, long-term, natural history studies are required. Until these are available, it would be wise to treat asthma with adequate doses of controller therapies, e.g. inhaled corticosteroids as soon as it is diagnosed.

References

1 Chung KF, Godard P: Difficult Therapy Resistant Asthma: ERS Task Force Report 2000;19 (No 59):1–101.
2 Holgate ST, Davies DE, Lackie PM, Wilson SJ, Puddicombe SM, Lordan JL: Epithelial-mesenchymal interactions in the pathogenesis of asthma. J Allergy Clin Immunol 2000;105: 193–204.
3 Chung KF, Barnes PJ: Cytokines in asthma. Thorax 1999;54:825–857.
4 Elias JA: Airway wall remodelling in asthma. Unanswered questions. Am J Respir Crit Care Med 2000;161(No 3 part 2):S168–S171.
5 Wegner CD, Gundel RH, Reilly P, Haynes N, Leits LG, Rothlein R: Intercellular adhesion molecule-1 (ICAM-1) in the pathogenesis of asthma. Science 1990;247:56–459.
6 Zhang S, Howarth PH, Roche WR: Cytokine production by cell cultures from bronchial subepithelial myofibroblasts. J Pathol 1996;190: 95–101.
7 Wilson JW, Li X, Pain MCF: The measurement of reticular basement membrane and submucosal collagen in the asthmatic airway. Clin Exp Allergy 1997;27:363–371.
8 James AL, Paré PD, Hogg JC: The mechanics of airway narrowing in asthma. Am Rev Respir Dis 1989;139:242–246.
9 Zhang S, Mohammed Q, Burbridge A, Morland CM, Roche WR: Cell cultures from bronchial subepithelial myofibroblasts enhance eosinophil survival in vitro. Eur Respir J 1996;9: 1839–1846.
10 Vrugt B, Wilson S, Bron A, Holgate ST, Djukanovic R, Aalbers R: Bronchial angiogenesis in severe glucocorticoid dependent asthma. Eur Respir J 2000;15:1014–1021.
11 Ollerenshaw Sl, Jarvis D, Sullivan CE, Woolcock AJ: Substance P immunoreactive nerves in airways from asthmatics and non-asthmatics. Eur Respir J 1991;4:673–682.
12 Fredberg JJ: Airway smooth muscle: Flirting with disaster. Eur Respir J 1998;12:1252–1256.
13 John M, Hirst SJ, Jose PJ, et al: Human airway smooth muscle cells express and release RANTES in response to Th1: Regulation of Th2 cytokines and corticosteroids. J Immunol 1997;158:1841–1847.
14 Polosa R, Holgate ST: Adenosine bronchoprovocation: A promising marker of allergic inflammation in asthma? Thorax 1997;32:919–923.
15 Puddicombe SM, Polosa R, Richter A, Krishna MT, Howarth PH, Holgate ST, Davies DE: The involvement of epidermal growth factor receptor in epithelial repair in asthma. FASEB J 2000;14:1362–1374.
16 Trigg CJ, Manolitsis ND, Wang J, Calderon MA, McAulay A, Jordan SE, et al: Placebo-controlled immunopathologic study of four months of inhaled corticosteroids in asthma. Am J Respir Crit Care Med 1994;150:17–22.
17 Haahtela T: Airway remodelling takes place in asthma – what are the clinical Implications? Clin Exp Allergy 1997;27:351–353.

Stephen T. Holgate
RCMB Research Division
School of Medicine
University of Southampton
Southampton General Hospital
Southampton SO16 6YD (UK)
Tel. +44 1703 794 157, Fax +44 1703 701 771
E-Mail sth@soton.ac.uk

Exhaled Breath Analysis

Sergei A. Kharitonov   Peter J. Barnes

Department of Thoracic Medicine, National Heart and Lung Institute, Imperial College School of Medicine, London, UK

Summary

Several gases, such as NO and CO, and hydrocarbons, have been measured in exhaled air in adults and children (fig. 1). More recently, non-volatile markers and mediators (hydrogen peroxide, isoprostanes, leukotrienes, prostaglandins, cytokines, products of lipid peroxidation, nitrite/nitrate, S-nitrosothiols, nitrotyrosine) have been detected in exhaled air and condensate. There is a strong rationale to use these exhaled markers to monitor airway inflammation and oxidative stress in asthma and COPD, as well as during treatment with corticosteroids, leukotriene antagonists, antioxidants and novel therapies.

Nitric Oxide

Exhaled NO is a useful and practical non-invasive marker that is strongly related to airway inflammation [1, 2]. NO is generated by several cells in all areas of the respiratory tract by NO synthase (NOS). iNOS is activated by cytokines and is the major source of elevated NO in asthma. Exhaled NO has been standardized and validated against invasive assessment of inflammation by bronchoscopy [3] and induced sputum, and is therefore [4] reproducible and comparable between different centres.

Elevated exhaled and nasal NO levels correlate strongly with skin test scores, total IgE, and blood eosinophilia in atopic asthma, and exhaled NO may differentiate between healthy subjects with or without respiratory symptoms and patients with asthma and atopy. Addition of PC_{20} makes the NO/PC_{20} combination a very specific test for allergic asthma. Therefore, exhaled NO measurements may be used for patient selection and asthma screening.

Exhaled NO may be used to monitor the effect of anti-inflammatory treatment in stable [5] and unstable asthma [6]. Exhaled NO levels may be increased before any significant deterioration in lung function, PC_{20}, or sputum eosinophils [7] and may serve as a 'loss-of-control marker' [1]. Exhaled NO is extremely sensitive to steroid treatment, and the reduction in NO may be seen within 6 h after a single dose of nebulized steroids, or within 2–3 days following treatment with inhaled steroids [5, 6, 8, 9]. The levels of exhaled NO are higher in adults and children with severe asthma, and are related to asthma symptoms and the use of β_2-agonists in severe asthma [10], and improvement in FEV_1 also in children [11]. A correlation between exhaled NO, sputum eosinophils and eosinophil cationic protein, but not between NO and PC_{20}, is preserved in asthmatics treated with steroids [12, 13], but is lost in asthmatic smokers.

Corticosteroids have no effect on exhaled NO in normals [8], but reduce NO in asthma (table 1) and this reduction is more prominent in severe disease [11, 14]. The onset of action of inhaled budesonide on exhaled NO is short (2–3 days) and dose dependent [9] (fig. 2).

The short- and long-acting β_2-agonists have no acute effect on exhaled NO [15], as they do not have any anti-inflammatory effect on chronic inflammation in asthma.

Pranlukast inhibits the rise in exhaled NO when the dose of inhaled corticosteroids is reduced, and montelukast rapidly reduces exhaled NO by 15–30% [16] in children with asthma. This may reflect a reduced impact of inflammatory cytokines on iNOS.

NOS inhibitors by blocking NOS [17] may be important in the management of severe steroid-resistant asthma. Inhaled PGE_2 which also downregulates iNOS, decreased exhaled NO in asthma [18]. Potentially, the effect of immunosuppressants (cyclosporin and rapamycin), or cyclo-oxygenase inhibitors (ibuprofen), which are able to

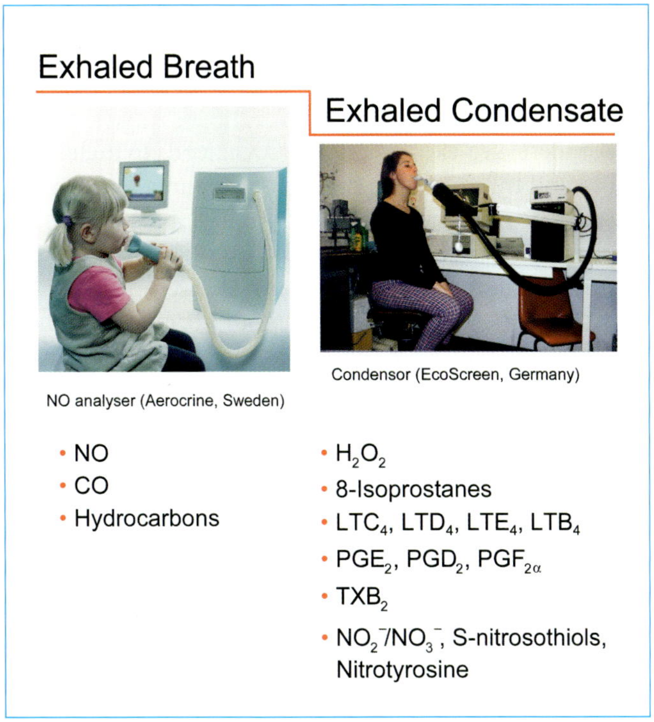

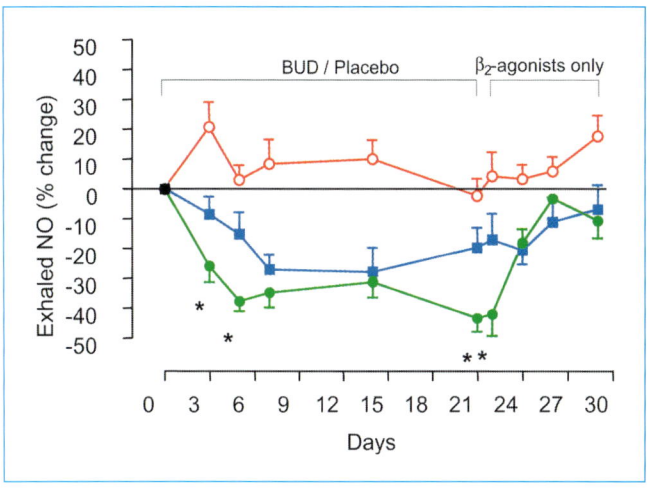

Fig. 1. Exhaled gases and condensate measurements.

Fig. 2. The effect of inhaled budesonide (BUD) on exhaled NO in patients with mild asthma. Mean values ± SEM in patients treated with 400 µg BUD (●) or 100 µg BUD (■) or placebo (○). Level of significance of difference between 400 µg BUD and 100 µg BUD: * p < 0.05.

Table 1. Effect of corticosteroids on exhaled NO

Drugs	Magnitude	Time after IS treatment	Reference
Normal subjects			
Prednisolone, 30 mg/day, 3 days[1]	no effect		8
Asthma			
Budesonide, 1,600 µg/day (mild)[1]	↓ 30%	7 days	5
Budesonide, 100 µg/day (mild)[1]	↓ 29%	28 days	28
Budesonide, 400 µg/day	↓ 50%	28 days	
Prednisolone, 30 mg/day, 3 days (mild)[1]	↓ 22%	72 h	8
Prednisolone + IS (severe)	↓ 40%	48 h	29
Prednisolone, 1 mg/kg, 5 days (severe)	↓ 46%	5 days	14
Prednisolone, 1 mg/kg, 5 days (moderate)	↓ 52%	5 days	11
Fluticasone, 1,000 µg/day, 4 weeks	↓ 76%	2 weeks	30
Budesonide, 100 µg/day (mild)	no change	3 days	9
Budesonide, 400 µg/day	↓ 26%	3 days	

IS = Inhaled steroids; ↓ = decrease; ↑ = increase.
[1] Placebo-controlled randomized trial.

inhibit both iNOS and COX-2, may be studied by monitoring exhaled NO.

Exhaled NO levels in stable COPD [19] are lower than in either smoking or non-smoking asthmatics and are not different from those in normal subjects. This is due to the effect of tobacco smoking, which downregulates NOS and reduces exhaled NO [19]. Patients with unstable COPD, however, have high NO levels [20], which may be explained by continuous neutrophilic inflammation and oxidative stress. Exhaled NO can be used to monitor COPD exacerbations.

Carbon Monoxide

CO is a product of haem degradation by haeme oxygenase, reflects oxidative stress and can be measured by electrochemical CO sensors in exhaled air of adults, children and neonates. It is affected by active or passive smoking, but a cut-off level of 6 ppm effectively separates non-smokers from smokers. Despite the early reports on elevated levels of exhaled CO in mild stable asthma, we have found significantly elevated CO levels only in patients with severe asthma. This may reflect a high level of oxidative stress and predominantly neutrophilic inflammation in these patients.

Considering the simplicity of CO measurements and portability of CO analysers, exhaled CO may be used to monitor paediatric asthma. Children with persistent asthma despite treatment with steroids have elevated exhaled CO compared with those with infrequent episodic asthma [21]. We have also found elevated CO levels in ex-smoker COPD patients, suggesting ongoing oxidative stress.

Hydrocarbons

Exhaled hydrocarbons, non-specific markers of lipid peroxidation, may help to estimate the magnitude of in vivo lipid peroxidation, and to monitor the effect of novel drugs with anti-oxidant properties. Ethane and pentane can be measured by gas chromatography from a single breath sample, in which no preconcentration is required [22], and are elevated in acute asthma [23] and in smokers [24].

Exhaled Condensate

Exhaled breath condensate is collected by cooling or freezing of exhaled air. Abnormalities in condensate chemistry and exhaled markers reflect intrinsic abnormalities of the airway lining fluid caused by inflammation and oxidative stress and may be a valuable means of monitoring of lung diseases. The collection takes 10–15 min of tidal breathing to obtain 1–3 ml of condensate and is well tolerated by patients with severe airway obstruction and children. Exhaled condensate is analysed by gas chromatography (GC), or by immunoassays (ELISA).

Hydrogen Peroxide

Activation of inflammatory cells results in increased production of H_2O_2, which is augmented in exhaled condensate in asthma and severe COPD [25].

Eicosanoids

Prostaglandins (PG), thromboxane, isoprostanes and leukotrienes are derived from arachidonic acid and have potent pro-inflammatory properties. Their non-invasive analysis provides an opportunity to assess the profile of eicosanoids in asthma and COPD directly, and may be a better predictor of clinical efficacy of leukotriene antagonists, corticosteroids, or thromboxane A_2 (TXA_2) receptor antagonist than urine, serum, or invasive BAL.

Isoprostanes

Isoprostanes, products of arachidonic acid peroxidation, can be detected in exhaled breath condensate by ELISA, which is comparable to GC analysis, and reflect cellular effects of oxidative stress. We have found that 8-isoprostane levels were doubled in subjects with mild asthma compared with normals, and increased by 3-fold in severe asthma irrespective of corticosteroids [26]. The lacking effect of corticosteroids on 8-isoprostane is most likely due to their ineffectiveness at inhibiting oxidative stress. It makes isoprostane a good marker of oxidative stress in moderate to severe asthma. We have found that the concentration of 8-isoprostane is also increased in normal cigarette smokers, but to a much greater extent in COPD patients.

Prostaglandins

An increased expression of COX-2 leads to high levels of PG and thromboxane B (TXB) in asthma and COPD. We have demonstrated that PGE_2 and $PGF_{2\alpha}$ are markedly increased in exhaled condensate of patients with COPD, but not in asthma. In contrast, TXB_2 is increased in asthma but undetectable in either normal subjects or patients with COPD. Exhaled prostaglandins and thromboxanes may be useful markers to monitor the effects of TXA_2 receptor antagonist and phosphodiesterase inhibitors in asthma and COPD.

Leukotrienes

Leukotrienes (lipid mediators derived from arachidonic acid via the 5-lipoxygenase pathway) are potent pro-inflammatory mediators in asthma and COPD. We have demonstrated further elevation of LTE_4, LTC_4, LTD_4 in exhaled condensate during the late asthmatic response to allergen challenge, and the worsening of asthma symptoms and lung function in patients with exacerbations was associated with the increase of leukotrienes and nitrotyrosine in condensate. Markedly elevated levels of exhaled LTB_4 were seen in both asthma and COPD, whereas LTE_4 was increased only in asthma [Montuschi et al., unpubl. obs.].

Oxynitrogen intermediates

Low levels of exhaled S-nitrosothiols, naturally occurring bronchodilators, have been found in asthmatic children with respiratory failure. We have shown S-nitrosothiols were reduced after 3 weeks of treatment with 400 µg, but not 100 µg of budesonide [9]. In contrast, there was a rapid and dose-dependent reduction in nitrite/nitrate (NO_2^-/NO_3^-) in the same mild asthmatics, suggesting that NO_2^-/NO_3^- are more sensitive to anti-inflammatory treatment. Increased levels of nitrotyrosine correlated with asthma symptoms during steroid withdrawal in moderate asthma, suggesting that exhaled nitrotyrosine may predict asthma deterioration caused by inflammation. Chronic oxidative stress presented to the lung by cigarette smoke may increase decomposition of nitrosothiols, explaining elevated exhaled S-nitrosothiols in healthy smokers, which were related to their smoking history.

Cytokines and Lipids

Measurement and identification of proteins in exhaled condensate is still controversial. Higher concentrations of total protein in exhaled condensate have been found in young smokers versus non-smokers, whilst the levels of IL-1β and TNF-α were not different. We have found that IL-8 levels in exhaled condensate were only mildly elevated in stable cystic fibrosis (CF), but were 2-fold higher in unstable CF patients compared with normal subjects [Balint et al., unpubl obs.]. Primary (diene conjugates) and secondary (ketodienes) products of lipid peroxidation are increased in exhaled condensate and in bronchial biopsies samples from patients with COPD and chronic bronchitis compare with normal subjects [27]. Potentially, these approaches may be of a considerable interest.

Conclusions

Accurate assessment of airway inflammation and oxidative stress is important to the clinical management of a variety of pulmonary conditions, including asthma and COPD. It may allow the clinician to monitor the progression of the disease and to assess the efficacy of anti-inflammatory or antioxidant treatment.

References

1 Kharitonov SA: Exhaled nitric oxide and carbon monoxide in asthma. Eur Respir Rev 1999;9:212–218.
2 Kharitonov SA: Exhaled nitric oxide and carbon monoxide in respiratory diseases other than asthma. Eur Respir Rev 1999;9:223–226.
3 Kharitonov SA, Chung FK, Evans DJ, O'Connor BJ, Barnes PJ: The elevated level of exhaled nitric oxide in asthmatic patients is mainly derived from the lower respiratory tract. Am J Respir Crit Care Med 1996;153:1773–1780.
4 Recommendations for standardized procedures for the online and offline measurement of exhaled lower respiratory nitric oxide and nasal nitric oxide in adults and children. Am J Respir Crit Care Med 1999;160:2104–2117.
5 Kharitonov SA, Yates DH, Barnes PJ: Inhaled glucocorticoids decrease nitric oxide in exhaled air of asthmatic patients. Am J Respir Crit Care Med 1996;153:454–457.
6 Kharitonov SA, Yates DH, Chung KF, Barnes PJ: Changes in the dose of inhaled steroid affect exhaled nitric oxide levels in asthmatic patients. Eur Respir J 1996;9:196–201.
7 Jatakanon A, Lim S, Barnes PJ: Changes in sputum eosinophils predict loss of asthma control. Am J Respir Crit Care Med 2000;161:64–72.
8 Yates DH, Kharitonov SA, Robbins RA, Thomas PS, Barnes PJ: Effect of a nitric oxide synthase inhibitor and a glucocorticosteroid on exhaled nitric oxide. Am J Respir Crit Care Med 1995;152:892–896.
9 Kharitonov SA, Donnelly LE, Corradi M, Montuschi P, Barnes PJ: Dose-dependent onset and duration of action of 100/400 mcg budesonide on exhaled nitric oxide and related changes in other potential markers of airway inflammation in mild asthma. Am J Respir Crit Care Med 2000;161:A186.
10 Stirling RG, Kharitonov SA, Campbell D, Robinson D, Durham SR, Chung KF, Barnes PJ: Exhaled NO is elevated in difficult asthma and correlates with symptoms and disease severity despite treatment with oral and inhaled corticosteroids. Thorax 1998;53:1030–1034.
11 Baraldi E, Dario C, Ongaro R, Scollo M, Azzolin NM, Panza N, Paganini N, Zacchello F: Exhaled nitric oxide concentrations during treatment of wheezing exacerbation in infants and young children. Am J Respir Crit Care Med 1999;159:1284–1288.
12 Jatakanon A, Lim S, Chung KF, Barnes PJ: An inhaled steroid improves markers of airway inflammation in patients with mild asthma. Eur Respir J 1998;12:1084–1088.
13 Jatakanon A, Lim S, Kharitonov SA, Chung KF, Barnes PJ: Correlation between exhaled nitric oxide, sputum eosinophils, and methacholine responsiveness in patients with mild asthma. Thorax 1998;53:91–95.
14 Baraldi E, Azzolin NM, Zanconato S, Dario C, Zacchello F: Corticosteroids decrease exhaled nitric oxide in children with acute asthma. J Pediatr 1997;131:381–385.
15 Yates DH, Kharitonov SA, Barnes PJ: Effect of short- and long-acting inhaled beta-2-agonists on exhaled nitric oxide in asthmatic patients. Eur Respir J 1997;10:1483–1488.
16 Bisgaard H, Loland L, Oj JA: NO in exhaled air of asthmatic children is reduced by the leukotriene receptor antagonist montelukast. Am J Respir Crit Care Med 1999;160:1227–1231.
17 Yates DH, Kharitonov SA, Thomas PS, Barnes PJ: Endogenous nitric oxide is decreased in asthmatic patients by an inhibitor of inducible nitric oxide synthase. Am J Respir Crit Care Med 1996;154:247–250.
18 Kharitonov SA, Sapienza MA, Barnes PJ, Chung KF: Prostaglandins E_2 and F_{2a} reduce exhaled nitric oxide in normal and asthmatic subjects irrespective of airway calibre changes. Am J Respir Crit Care Med 1998;158:1374–1378.
19 Kharitonov SA, Robbins RA, Yates DH, Keatings V, Barnes PJ: Acute and chronic effects of cigarette smoking on exhaled nitric oxide. Am J Respir Crit Care Med 1995;152:609–612.
20 Maziak W, Loukides S, Culpitt S, Sullivan P, Kharitonov SA, Barnes PJ: Exhaled nitric oxide in chronic obstructive pulmonary disease. Am J Respir Crit Care Med 1998;157:998–1002.
21 Uasuf CG, Jatakanon A, James A, Kharitonov SA, Wilson NM, Barnes PJ. Exhaled carbon monoxide in childhood asthma. J Pediatr 1999;135:569–574.
22 Paredi P, Kharitonov SA, Leak D, Shah PL, Cramer D, Hodson ME, Barnes PJ: Exhaled ethane is elevated in cystic fibrosis and correlates with carbon monoxide levels and airway obstruction. Am J Respir Crit Care Med 2000;161:1247–1251.
23 Olopade CO, Zakkar M, Swedler WI, Rubinstein I: Exhaled pentane levels in acute asthma. Chest 1997;111:862–865.
24 Habib MP, Clements NC, Garewal HS: Cigarette smoking and ethane exhalation in humans. Am J Respir Crit Care Med 1995;151:1368–1372.
25 Dekhuijzen PN, Aben KK, Dekker I, Aarts LP, Wielders PL, van Herwaarden CL, Bast A: Increased exhalation of hydrogen peroxide in patients with stable and unstable chronic obstructive pulmonary disease. Am J Respir Crit Care Med 1996;154:813–816.
26 Montuschi P, Corradi M, Ciabattoni G, Nightingale J, Kharitonov SA, Barnes PJ: Increased 8-isoprostane, a marker of oxidative stress, in exhaled condensate of asthma patients. Am J Respir Crit Care Med 1999;160:216–220.
27 Ignatova GL, Volchegorskii IA, Volkova EG, Kazachkov EL, Kolesnikov OL: Lipid peroxidation processes in chronic bronchitis. Ter Arkh 1998;70:36–37.
28 Jatakanon A, Kharitonov SA, Lim S, Barnes PJ: Effect of differing doses of inhaled budesonide on markers of airway inflammation in patients with mild asthma. Thorax 1999;54:108–114.
29 Massaro AF, Gaston B, Kita D, Fanta C, Stamler JS, Drazen JM: Expired nitric oxide levels during treatment of acute asthma. Am J Respir Crit Care Med 1995;152:800–803.
30 van RE, Straathof KC, Veselic-Charvat MA, Zwinderman AH, Bel EH, Sterk PJ: Effect of inhaled steroids on airway hyperresponsiveness, sputum eosinophils, and exhaled nitric oxide levels in patients with asthma. Thorax 1999;54:403–408.

Dr. Sergei A. Kharitonov
Department of Thoracic Medicine
National Heart and Lung Institute
Imperial College, Dovehouse Street
London SW3 6LY (UK)
Tel. +44 0207 8121 (ext 0025)
Fax +44 0207 351 8126
E-Mail s.kharitonov@ic.ac.uk

Clinical Studies on New Drugs

Trevor T. Hansel[a] Peter J. Barnes[b]

[a] National Heart and Lung Institute (NHLI) Clinical Studies Unit and [b] Department of Thoracic Medicine, NHLI, Imperial College, London, UK

Summary

The incidence of both asthma and COPD is increasing throughout the world, and acts as a major incentive for the development of improved therapy. For the large range of bronchodilator and anti-inflammatory therapies in current clinical development, reliable decision making is required in phase II, before entering large-scale and expensive phase III studies. With anti-inflammatory therapies for asthma, there has been a tendency to move away from the inhaled-allergen challenge as a proof of concept study, and instead test in symptomatic clinical disease in conjunction with biomarkers. Phase II studies in COPD are more difficult because inclusion criteria, monitoring parameters, comparator therapies and trial design are less well established.

Good Clinical Practice

Clinical studies within a drug development programme should be carried out under Good Clinical *Research* Practice (GCP), although GCP is not expected to be introduced into European law until 2001 at the earliest. Phase II decision making studies in asthma and COPD utilize non-invasive surrogate biomarkers, as well as pharmacokinetic and pharmacodynamic evaluation to assist in dose range finding [1].

Asthma

Asthma is generally defined on the basis of the characteristic episodic symptoms, in conjunction with assessment of lung function (table 1). It should be stressed that systemic treatments for asthmatic allergic disease have relevance to all atopic diseases, since the pharmaceutical industry has concentrated most efforts on asthma as opposed to atopic dermatitis and rhinitis [2, 3].

Table 1. Inclusion criteria and monitoring in studies on asthma and COPD

Asthma	COPD
Symptoms/history	Symptoms/history
Episodic wheeze	Smoking history
Chest tightness	Productive daily cough
Shortness of breath	Shortness of breath
Nocturnal wakening	Shuttle test, 6-min walk test
Short acting, rescue β_2-agonist usage	Health status – St. George's
Health status	
Lung function	
PEF and FEV_1	FEV_1 % predicted
Reversibility and variability	FEV_1/FVC ratio
AHR	Gas transfer, TL_{CO}
	Residual volume
	Response to inhaled SA β_2-agonists and anticholinergics
	Response to oral/inhaled steroids
Laboratory tests	
Allergy – skin prick tests	Blood gases, neutrophil CD11b,
Blood IgE, Th2 cells	Th-1 cells, oxidant/anti-oxidant
Blood and sputum eosinophils	Breath NO, eicosanoids
Exhaled NO	Sputum neutrophils, macrophages
BAL	Urine elastin/collagen degradation products
Bronchial mucosal biopsy	BAL and bronchial biopsy
X-rays and imaging	Chest X-ray
	High resolution CT scan
Concomitant therapy	
SA and LA β_2-agonists	SA and LA β_2-agonists
ICS	Anticholinergics
Oral steroids	Inhaled corticosteroids

Bronchodilation. Acute bronchodilation can be studied in patients with mild asthma who have sufficient bronchoconstriction at baseline, so that there is 'room to improve' FEV_1 following single-dose administration. In

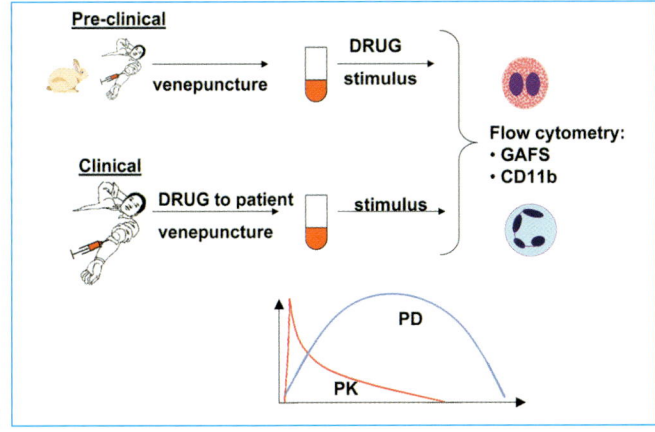

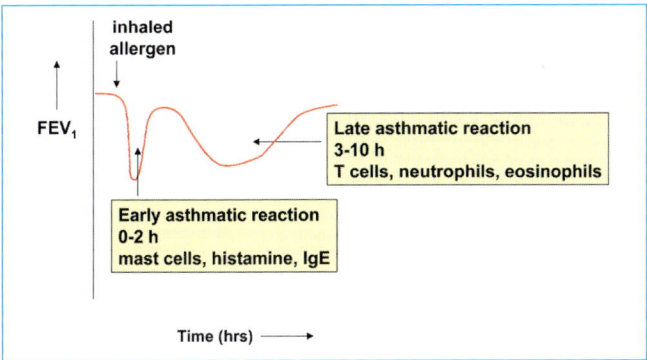

Fig. 1. Principle of using pharmacokinetic and pharmacodynamic assessments to aid dose range finding of therapies directed against eosinophils and neutrophils. Preclinically, dose-response curves are determined on volunteer or animal blood to which the novel therapeutic (drug) is added ex vivo, and then the response to a specific stimulus is determined by flow cytometry of granulocytes in whole blood. In the context of a clinical trial, the volunteer subject has received the therapeutic, and blood is taken at intervals to determine both a pharmacokinetic and pharmacodynamic profile. The graph demonstrates that the therapeutic may only be detectable pharmacokinetically for a short time, while the pharmacodynamic action may persist. GAFS = Gated autofluorescence and forward scatter; PK = pharmacokinetics; PD = pharmacodynamics.

Fig. 2. The early and late asthmatic reactions following inhalation of a nebulized relevant allergen by an allergic asthmatic that has a dual reaction. The FEV_1 is determined at intervals for up to 10 h following the inhalation.

addition bronchoprotection can be evaluated in relation to bronchoconstrictor stimuli such as histamine, methacholine, hyperventilation, adenosine and exercise.

Allergen Challenge. The inhaled-allergen challenge is the classic design for pre-clinical and clinical testing of novel anti-inflammatory drugs in asthma (fig. 2) [4]. Steroids, cromones, leukotriene antagonists, salicylates, heparin, frusemide, and cyclosporin A all cause inhibition of the late asthmatic reaction. Anti-IgE is of interest because it inhibits both the early- and late-phase response to inhaled allergen when administered by intravenous infusion [5], but not when given by inhalation [6]. In patients with allergic asthma treated with inhaled or oral steroids, anti-IgE given intravenously for 20 weeks had demonstrable efficacy and caused serum IgE to decrease by >95% [7]. However, it is relevant to therapies directed against eosinophils that agents such as anti-IL-5 and IL-12 do not affect the late asthmatic reaction, despite considerable effects on blood and sputum eosinophil numbers [8, 9].

Symptomatic Asthma. A range of recent studies have documented effects of anti-leukotrienes on patients with symptomatic mild to moderate asthma that are on inhaled β_2-agonists only [10]. These study designs provide a more clinically relevant 'wild-type' population for studying potential efficacy than utilizing an allergen challenge. However, they frequently require at least 4 weeks of anti-inflammatory therapy in conjunction with detailed monitoring to discriminate a given anti-inflammatory effect.

Steroid Add-On and Titration Studies. Theophylline and montelukast have been studied as add-on agents in asthmatics already receiving inhaled and oral steroids (fig. 3) [11, 12]. Steroid titration is a system for stepwise reduction in the dose of inhaled steroid [13, 14]. An alternative design is to abruptly discontinue ICS the day before administration of study drug; as has been performed to compare soluble IL-4 receptor (IL-4R) with placebo [15]. A whole range of important clinical studies are still being performed on ICS themselves; these address such questions as dose response finding [16–19], the possibility of once-a-day steroids, and effects on bones and growth [20].

Severe Asthma. Patients with severe asthma have more fixed airways obstruction, airways remodelling, and a tendency for neutrophilic as well as eosinophilic and IgE-mediated disease. A chimaeric monoclonal antibody against CD4 has recently been shown to be effective in chronic severe asthma [21].

Asthma Exacerbations and Emergency Asthma. Emergency asthma represents a major clinical problem with a requirement for more rapidly acting therapy, since hospitalization generally occurs for a period of at least 4 days [22]. Therapies that target TNF have the potential to cause rapid onset of anti-inflammatory effects in emergency asthma. It is important to stress that asthmatics may be vulnerable to exacerbations even when asthma is brought under apparent control.

Natural History and Disease Modification. It is a major challenge to study long-term effects of drugs on the airways in the context of structural changes in the airways that comprise airways remodelling. Current asthma therapy is palliative and neither curative nor disease modifying, and only a minority of asthmatics achieve a long-lasting remission. There are considerable ethical and clinical trial issues in studying the influence of immunomodulatory agents in the context of allergen and peptide immunotherapy. Agents such as IL-12, CpG oligodeoxynucleotides and *Mycobacterium vaccae* (SRL 172) have potential as adjuvants, but therapy may be required in childhood for genetically susceptible individuals in the context of natural allergen exposure or allergen immunotherapy [23–25]. As with disease-modifying anti-rheumatoid therapies, it is important to demonstrate disease modification in terms of prolonged efficacy following cessation of treatment.

COPD

The considerable need for effective therapy for COPD is reflected in a large range of potential therapies entering clinical development [26]. COPD is thought to involve oxidative stress, inflammation, mucus, proteases and repair mechanisms, but we do not know the relative role of these factors in clinical pathogenesis. Recently, European points to consider in clinical trials on drugs for the treatment of COPD have been issued [27].

Bronchodilators. The prolonged effects of the inhaled anticholinergic agent, tiotropium bromide, have been demonstrated in terms of bronchoprotection against methacholine-induced bronchoconstriction in asthma [28], and the dose-response relationship established in COPD [29].

Anti-Inflammatory Treatments. Ariflo is a second-generation phosphodiesterase (PDE) type 4 inhibitor that selectively inhibits the low-affinity rolipram binding form of PDE4, in an effort to minimize potential for nausea and vomiting [30]. In a 6-week study in 424 patients with COPD, Ariflo at 15 mg b.i.d. resulted in a maximum mean difference in trough clinic FEV_1 compared to placebo of 160 ml, representing an 11% improvement.

Natural History. Studies on the natural history of COPD involve monitoring post-bronchodilator FEV_1 in considerable numbers of patients over a number of years. Three major studies have recently been performed on effects of ICS on the longitudinal decline in post-bronchodilator FEV_1 over 3 years in patients with COPD [31–33]. Although effects on FEV_1 are modest, ICS are effective in preventing exacerbations and cause improvement in health status.

Exacerbations. It has already been noted that phase II studies in COPD may be poorly predictive of efficacy in

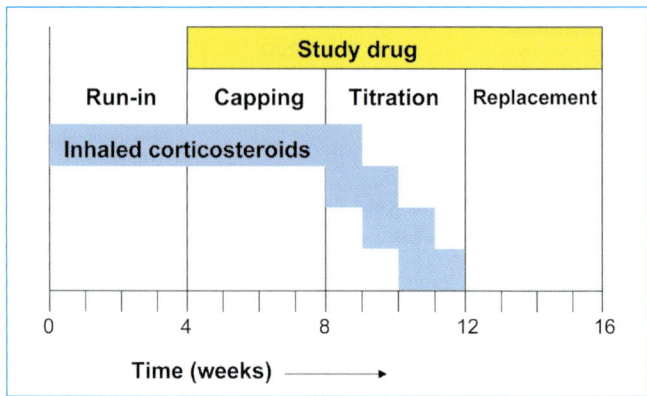

Fig. 3. The range of potential phases in a study of a novel therapeutic (study drug) in an asthmatic patient receiving inhaled corticosteroids (ICS). During the 'run in' phase, the patient maintains clinical diaries including symptoms, lung function and β-agonist usage. The 'add on' or 'capping' phase occurs when the study drug is added to a constant dose of ICS. Steroid titration is performed when the dose of ICS is gradually titrated down at intervals, although abrupt steroid withdrawal can be performed in certain circumstances, prior to steroid replacement.

larger phase III studies. Recombinant human DNAse (dornase alfa, Genentech) was evaluated in 244 patients hospitalized for acute pulmonary exacerbation of COPD, and caused a 59% reduction in mortality compared with placebo [34]. On this basis, a larger phase III study in acute exacerbations of COPD was undertaken, but when interim analysis demonstrated a negative trend in mortality data, the study was halted. Paggiaro et al. [35] have recently undertaken a study on the effects of inhaled fluticasone propionate in preventing COPD exacerbations in patients with a history of at least one exacerbation per year for 3 years. In a differing design, a recent study has documented moderate improvement in clinical outcome when using systemic glucocorticoids to treat exacerbations of COPD [36].

The Future

Based on better understanding of cellular and molecular events in asthma and COPD, we have novel rational therapies in ongoing clinical studies in asthma and COPD. Most of these new drugs inhibit components of inflammatory responses, but in the future there are real possibilities for the development of preventative and even curative treatments. We can expect clinical studies to involve assessment of genotypes and phenotypes to identify potential responders to specific therapies, as well as more sensitive monitoring of lung function, imaging methods and biomarkers of inflammation.

References

1 Bryan SA, Leckie MJ, Jenkins G, Barnes PJ, Williams TJ, Sabroe I, Hansel TT: Measurement of granulocyte pharmacodynamics in whole blood by flow cytometry; in Rogers DF, Donnelly LE (eds): Human Airway Inflammation: Sampling Techniques and Analytical Problems. Methods in Molecular Medicine. Toronto, Humana Press, in press.
2 Barnes PJ: Therapeutic strategies for allergic diseases. Nature 1999;402:B31–B38.
3 Bryan SA, Leckie MJ, Hansel TT, Barnes PJ: Novel therapy for asthma. Exp Opin Invest Drugs 2000;9:25–42.
4 Wenzel SE: Inflammation, leukotrienes and the pathogenesis of the late asthmatic response. Clin Exp Allergy 1999;29:1–3.
5 Fahy JV, Fleming HE, Wong HH, Liu JT, Su JQ, Reimann J, Fick RB, Boushey HA: The effect of an anti-IgE monoclonal antibody on the early- and late-phase responses to allergen inhalation in asthmatic subjects. Am J Respir Crit Care Med 1997;155:1828–1834.
6 Fahy JV, Cockcroft DW, Boulet L-P, Wong HH, Deschesnes F, Su JQ, Ruppel J, Su JQ, Adelman DC: Effects of aerosolized anti-IgE (E25) on airway responses to inhaled allergen in asthmatic subjects. Am J Resp Crit Care Med 1999;160:1023–1027.
07 Milgrom H, Fick RB Jr, Su JQ, Reimann JD, Bush RK, Watrous ML, Metzger WJ: Treatment of allergic asthma with monoclonal anti-IgE antibody. rhuMAb- E25 Study Group. N Engl J Med 1999;341:1966–1973.
8 Leckie MJ, ten Brinke A, Khan J, Diamant Z, O'Connor BJ, Walls CM, Mathur KA, Cowley HC, Djukanovic R, Hansel TT, Holgate ST, Sterk PJ, Barnes PJ: Effects of an interleukin-5 blocking monoclonal antibody on eosinophils, airway hyperresponsiveness, and the late asthmatic response. Lancet, in press.
9 Bryan SA, O'Connor BJ, Matti S, Leckie MJ, Kanabar V, Khan J, Warrington SJ, Renzetti L, Rames A, Bock JA, Boyce MJ, Hansel TT, Holgate S, Barnes PJ: Effects of recombinant human interleukin-12 on eosinophils, airway hyperreactivity and the late asthmatic response. Lancet, in press.
10 Adkins JC, Brogden RN: Zafirlukast: A review of its pharmacology and therapeutic potential in the management of asthma. Drugs 1998;55:121–144.
11 Evans DJ, Taylor DA, Zetterstrom O, Chung KF, O'Connor BJ, Barnes PJ: A comparison of low-dose inhaled budesonide plus theophylline and high-dose inhaled budesonide for moderate asthma (see comments). N Engl J Med 1997;337:1412–1418.
12 Laviolette M, Malmstrom K, Lu S, Chervinsky P, Pujet J-C, Peszek I, Zhang J, Reiss TF: Montelukast added to inhaled beclomethasone in treatment of asthma. Am J Respir Crit Care Med 1999;160:1862–1868.
13 Gibson PG, Wong BJO, Hepperle MJE, Kline PA, Girgis-Gabardo A, Guyatt G, Dolovich J, Denburg JA, Ramsdale EH, Hargreave FE: A research method to induce and examine a mild exacerbation of asthma by withdrawal of inhaled corticosteroid. Clin Exp Allergy 1992;22:525–532.
14 Veen JCCM, Smits HH, Hiemstra PS, Zwinderman AE, Sterk PJ, Bel EH: Lung function and sputum characteristics of patients with severe asthma during and induced exacerbation by double-blind steroid withdrawal. Am J Resp Crit Care Med 1999;160:93–99.
15 Borish LC, Nelson HS, Lanz MJ, Claussen L, Whitmore JB, Agosti JM, Garrison L: Interleukin-4 receptor in moderate atopic asthma: A phase I/II randomized, placebo-controlled trial. Am J Resp Crit Care Med 1999;160:1816–1823.
16 Taylor DA, Jensen MW, Kanabar V, Engelstatter R, Steinijans VW, Barnes PJ, O'Connor BJ: A dose-dependent effect of the novel inhaled corticosteroid ciclesonide on airway responsiveness to adenosine-5′-monophosphate in asthmatic patients. Am J Respir Crit Care Med 1999;160:237–243.
17 Jatakanon A, Kharitonov S, Lim S, Barnes PJ: Effect of differing doses of inhaled budesonide on markers of airway inflammation in patients with mild asthma. Thorax 1999;54:108–114.
18 Kelly HW: Establishing a therapeutic index for the inhaled corticosteroids. 1. Pharmacokinetic/pharmacodynamic comparison of the inhaled corticosteroids. J Allergy Clin Immunol 1998;102:S36–S51.
19 O'Byrne P, Pedersen S: Measuring efficacy and safety of different inhaled corticosteroid preparations. J Allergy Clin Immunol 1998;102:879–886.
20 Efthimiou J, Barnes PJ: Effect of inhaled corticosteroids on bones and growth (see comments). Eur Respir J 1998;11:1167–1177.
21 Kon OM, Sihra BS, Compton CH, Leonard TB, Kay AB, Barnes NC: Randomised, dose-ranging, placebo-controlled study of chimeric antibody to CD4 (keliximab) in chronic severe asthma. Lancet 1998;352:1109–1113.
22 McFadden ER, Hejal R: Asthma. Lancet 1995;345:1215–1220.
23 Huang S: Molecular modulation of allergic responses. J Allergy Clin Immunol 1998;102:887–892.
24 Van Uden J, Raz E: Immunostimulatory DNA and applications to allergic disease. J Allergy Clin Immunol 1999;104:902–910.
25 Hasko G, Szabo C: IL-12 as a therapeutic target for pharmacological modulation in immune-mediated and inflammatory diseases: Regulation of T helper 1/T helper 2 responses. Br J Pharmacol 1999;127:1295–1304.
26 Leckie MJ, Bryan SA, Hansel TT, Barnes PJ: Novel Therapy for COPD. Exp Opin Invest Drugs 2000;9:3–23.
27 Committee for Proprietary Medicinal Products (CPMP): Points to consider on clinical investigation of medicinal products in the chronic treatment of patients with chronic obstructive pulmonary disease (COPD). CPMP/EWP 562/98, 1999.
28 O'Connor BJ, Towse LJ, Barnes PJ: Prolonged effect of tiotropium bromide on methacholine-induced bronchoconstriction in asthma. Am J Respir Crit Care Med 1996;154:876–880.
29 Maesen FPV, Smeets JJ, Sledsens TJH, Wald FDM, Cornelissen PJG: Tiotropium bromide, a new long-acting antimuscarinic bronchodilator: A pharmacodynamic study in patients with chronic obstructive disease (COPD). Eur Respir J 1995;8:1506–1513.
30 Torphy TJ, Barnette MS, Underwood DC, Griswold DE, Christensen SB, Murdoch RD, Nieman RB, Compton CH: AriﬂoTM (SB 207499), a second generation phosphodiesterase 4 inhibitor for the treatment of asthma and COPD: From concept to clinic. Pulm Pharmacol Ther 1999;12:131–135.
31 Pauwels RA, Lofdahl CG, Laitinen LA, Schouten JP, Postma DS, Pride NB, Ohlsson SV: Long-term treatment with inhaled budesonide in persons with mild chronic obstructive pulmonary disease who continue smoking. European Respiratory Society Study on Chronic Obstructive Pulmonary Disease. N Engl J Med 1999;340:1948–1953.
32 Vestbo J, Sorensen T, Lange P, Brix A, Torre P, Viskum K: Long-term effect of inhaled budesonide in mild and moderate chronic obstructive pulmonary disease: A randomised controlled trial. Lancet 1999;353:1819–1823.
33 Burge PS: EUROSCOP, ISOLDE and the Copenhagen city lung study. Thorax 1999;54:287–288.
34 Hudson TJ: Dornase in treatment of chronic bronchitis. Ann Pharmacother 1996;30:674–675.
35 Paggiaro PL, Dahle R, Bakran I, Frith L, Hollingworth K, Efthimiou J: Multicentre randomised in placebo-controlled trial of inhaled fluticasone propionate in patients with chronic obstructive pulmonary disease. Lancet 1998;351:773–780.
36 Niewoehner DE, Erbland ML, Deupree RH, Collins D, Gross NJ, Light RW, Anderson P, Morgan NA: Effect of systemic glucocorticoids on exacerbations of chronic obstructive pulmonary disease. Department of Veterans Affairs Cooperative Study Group. N Engl J Med 1999;340:1941–1947.

Dr. Trevor T. Hansel
NHLI Clinical Studies Unit
Royal Brompton Hospital, Fulham Rd.
London SW3 6HP (UK)
Tel. +44 207 351 8974, Fax +44 207 351 8973
E-Mail t.hansel@ic.ac.uk

Bronchodilators

Bronchodilators: An Overview

Gary P. Anderson[a]   Klaus F. Rabe[b]

[a] Department of Pharmacology, University of Melbourne, Australia, and
[b] Pulmonology, Leiden University Center, Leiden, The Netherlands

Summary

This chapter deals with general principles in the pathophysiology and biochemistry of airflow limitation and the pharmacology of bronchodilator drugs that underlies their clinical utility. Bronchodilators are important palliative therapies for asthma and COPD because they relieve suffering and, when used appropriately, they can be life-saving. Bronchodilators work by opposing active contraction, either by blocking contractile receptors (indirectly acting) or by entraining a biochemical pathway functionally antagonistic to a contractile mediator or process (directly acting). Consequently, some bronchodilators also have other effects, such as suppression of aspects of airway inflammation, but they cannot prevent or cure disease, alone or in combination with any known agent(s). There is no convincing evidence that any clinically available or experimental bronchodilator can significantly impede disease progression in asthma or COPD.

The Nature of Airflow Limitation in Asthma and COPD

Physiological studies have demonstrated that small peripheral airways 2–3 mm in diameter are the principal site of airflow obstruction, and the site of action of most bronchodilators, in both asthma and COPD [1–3]. In vitro studies on smooth muscle from asthmatic lungs are rare and the available evidence is not uniform: there is evidence for an increased capacity to generate force, to shorten at an increased rate, to shorten excessively and there is also evidence for impaired relaxant responses to β-adrenoceptor agonists [4, 5].

In asthma, airflow limitation is at least partially reversible because it is largely due to contraction of airway smooth muscle, compounded by airway wall thickening, oedema, lumenal mucus, debris and fluid accumulation in airway intersties. Bronchodilator responses are therefore relatively easily assessed by an index of forced expiration such as FEV_1. In severe or long-standing disease, a degree of irreversible fixed airflow obstruction may develop which does not respond to bronchodilators.

Airflow limitation in COPD is more complex. Hogg et al. [1] demonstrated that the principal site of airflow limitation in smokers is in peripheral airways, including small bronchi and bronchioles <2 mm diameter. These airways are both inflamed and thickened in COPD and the surrounding alveolar walls, which normally provide elastic tethering and recoil [6], are usually disrupted, often severely, by emphysematous proteolytic destruction of elastin and collagen fibres. Airflow obstruction is further worsened by mucus secretion and loss of surfactant following transdifferentiation of Clara cells into goblet cells. The relative contributions of airway wall inflammation versus loss of elastic recoil subsequent to emphysema as causes of airflow limitation are disputed and likely to vary with severity of disease [7]. The interplay of lung parenchyma and airway wall changes in COPD compound the difficulty of assessing bronchodilator responses using FEV_1 as a response index, especially when disease is advanced and hyperinflation prominent. This may explain why some patients report great symptom relief from bronchodilators in the absence of significant changes in FEV_1. It is important to note that the perception of respiratory resistance may be very poor and breathlessness may not relate directly to measurements of impaired lung function.

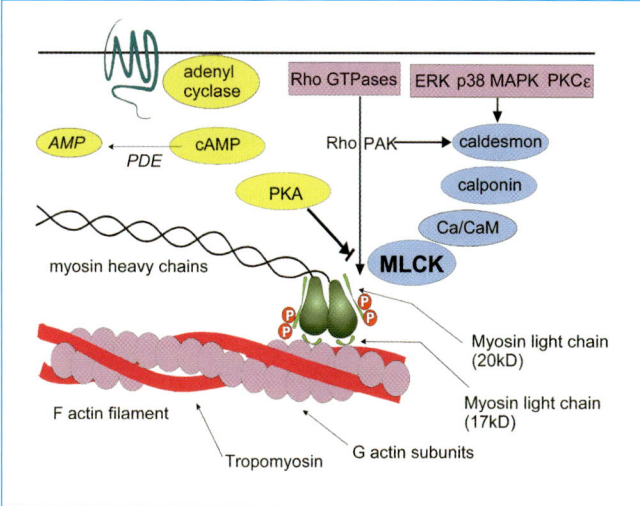

Fig. 1. Modulators of rate of contraction.

Mechanisms of Airway Smooth Muscle Contraction

Bronchodilators relax airway smooth muscle by opposing active tone and it is therefore essential to understand how airway smooth muscle contracts in order to understand bronchodilators. The contractile machinery of airway smooth muscle is shown diagrammatically in figure 1 and is composed of a myosin hexamer, comprising a pair of asymmetric heavy chains (200–204 kD) and two myosin light chains (17 and 20 kD) arranged into an active head structure and a tail. The head group contains actin attachment sites and two domains of the Ca^{2+}-stimulated Mg^{2+} dependent ATPase (myosin ATPase). The 17-kD light chain is essential for myosin ATPase activity while the 20-kD light chain is regulatory: its state of phosphorylation, which is in turn regulated by myosin light-chain kinase (MLCK), governs actin-myosin interactions by regulating myosin ATPase activity and hence contraction. The myosin head group interacts with a chain of F actin and G actin subunits interwoven with tropomysin. The number of actin-myosin cross-bridges determines the force of contraction whereas the actomyosin cycling rate determines the rate of contraction of airway smooth muscle. It has recently been suggested that perturbation of the myosin cycling in an increased rate of contraction of airway smooth muscle, particularly when disease uncouples tidal stretching forces from actually stretching airway smooth muscle, may be a princial determinant of excessive bronchoconstriction and BHR in asthma [8]. This theory is particularly important as it may help explain why BHR persists when airway inflammation has been largely resolved by inhaled glucocorticosteroids.

The actin-myosin cycling rate is influenced by (1) Ca^{2+}/calmodulin-dependent MLCK (the levels of which are believed to be upregulated in asthma); (2) Ca^{2+}/calmodulin-independent phosphorylation mechanism, and (3) p160 Rho kinase (ROCK) which phosphorylates the myosin-binding subunit of myosin light-chain phosphatase, reducing its enzymatic activity and leading to an increased duration of 20-kD light-chain phosphorylation. ROCK is also implicated in Ca^{2+} sensitization of airway smooth muscle [9].

The ease with which myosin slides over actin is also governed by actin-binding proteins, notably caldesmon and h1-calponin, which slow the rate of contraction. These proteins are phosphorylation substrates (leading to loss of actin dampening) for several kinases likely to be activated in response to inflammatory mediators and growth factors implicated in the pathogenesis of asthma, such as (1) p21-activated kinase (PAK), (2) extracellular-signal-related kinases 1 and 2 (ERK 1 and 2) and (3) protein kinase C epsilon (PKCε), but whether these phosphorylation events actually do occur in human asthma is unknown.

Bronchodilators that raise cellular cyclic adenosin monophosphate (cAMP), e.g. phophodiesterase (PDE) inhibitors and β2-adrenoceptor agonists are conventionally thought to activate protein kinase A (PKA) and possibly PKG, leading to a phosphorylation-dependent reduction in MLCK activity, together with a fall in intracellular Ca^{2+}. Similar transduction pathways converging on cyclins are thought to account for the anti-proliferative effect of β-adrenoceptor agonists on airway smooth muscle [10]. It therefore seems clear that the increasingly sophisticated understanding of the regulation of airway smooth muscle will lead to a much better understanding of how bronchodilators work, and also fail to work, in disease.

Neuro-Humoral Regulation of Airway Caliber

Some drugs cause a degree of bronchodilation indirectly by inhibiting contractile tone in the airways. Human airways are directly innervated by post-ganglionic parasympathetic neurons that increase tone by releasing acetylcholine which activates post-junctional M_3 cholinoceptors. There is almost no detectable sympathetic innervation of human airway smooth muscle at any level of the airways but noradrenalin released from sympathetic nerve varicosities may dampen cholinergic tone by inhibiting neurotransmission in ganglia via β-adrenoceptor activation. Vagal tone and vago-vagal reflexes can therefore exert strong effects on airway caliber, which are particularly evident in COPD and acute severe asthma. Both in vitro and in vivo studies suggest that excitatory non-adrenergic, non-cholinergic (NANC+) responses can be elicited in human airways, probably via neuropeptide release, although the physiological significance of this observation is not known. Humans lack physiological inhibitory NANC innervation. At least 20 known chemical mediators which have been recovered from diseased human lungs, such as histamine, endothelins, cysteinyl-leukotrienes, thromboxane, prostanoids, growth factors, kinins, some cytokine and peptides, all contract airway smooth muscle and are implicated in humoral regulation of tone. Few if any of these mediators have a physiological role in health because these antagonists produce no or trivial changes in lung function. However, in disease, antagonists of many of these mediators lessen bronchoconstriction, may also cause indirect bronchodilation and improve the maximal effect of directly acting bronchodilators notably β_2-adrenoceptor agonists: anti-cholinergic agents and leukotriene antagonists are the most prominent examples. Inflammatory mediators also promote bronchoconstriction by triggering vagal c-fibre afferents (sensory fibre) causing cholinergic reflex bronchoconstriction and facilitation of parasympathetic ganglionic neurotransmission.

Macrokinetics, Microkinetics and Biophysics of Bronchodilator Drugs

The utility of bronchodilators is governed as much by their pharmacokinetic bioavailability in the lungs as by their intrinsic pharmacological properties. Most inhaled agents are now formulated to deliver microfine particles of 0.1–10.0 μm mass median aerodynamic diameter to the lung which optimizes delivery to smaller peripheral airways. In contrast, orally administered drugs, the peak achievable plasma concentration of which must be held well within the 'therapeutic window' concentration range to prevent systemic side effects, do not reach high peak concentrations in the lung. Very small amounts of inhaled drugs actually achieve extremely high topical concentrations, sometimes as much as 1,000-fold in excess of the minimal effective concentration. This topical deposition of concentrated drug in the periciliary fluid is important because it achieves a bulk movement down local concentration gradients that forces drug to partition into the airway smooth muscle bundle but also keeps the total dose delivered to the periphery low thereby minimizing side effects. In addition to bulk partition, optimization of bio-

Table 1. Clinical useful compounds

Directly acting bronchodilators	Indirectly acting agents with bronchodilator activity

β_2-Adrenoceptor agonists
  Albuterol (salbutamol), bitolterol, fenoterol, formoterol (eformoterol), isoetharine, levalbuterol (*l* isomer of albuterol), metaproterenol, pirbuterol, salmeterol, terbutaline (bambuterol, a terbutaline pre-prodrug)
	Anticholinergic muscarinic antagonists
	  Ipratropium
	  Oxitropium
	  Tiotropium (in development)

Non-selective β-adrenoceptor agonists
  Isoprotenerol (isoprenaline)
	CysLT1 leukotriene receptor antagonists
	  Montelukast, zafirlukast,

Mixed agonists
  β_2-/dopamine $D_{2/3}$ receptor agonists
	5-Lipoxygenase inhibitors
	  Zileuton

Non-selective PDE isozyme inhibitors Theophylline, aminophylline	

physical interactions with airway smooth muscle membranes maximize retention of compound in the airways and hence duration of effect. Membrane partition coefficients (rather than simple lipophilicity alone) are reasonable predictors of duration of action, as exemplified by long-acting β-adrenoceptor agonists, such as formoterol and salmeterol, especially if the specific orientation of the drug in the lipid bilayer is also modelled [11]. Inhaled drugs which do not achieve this partitioning because of their biophysical properties, for example cromones and methylxanthines, have very short half-lives after inhalation. Most recently, drugs with discrete receptor kinetics have been discovered, such as the anticholinergic, tiotropium, which binds to all classes of muscarinic receptors with comparable affinity, but has an extremely slow dissociation from M_3 cholinoceptors on airway smooth muscle.

Effects of Disease on the Biochemistry of Bronchodilation

Most bronchodilators are functional antagonists, which means that they elicit signal transduction responses that oppose some aspect(s) of the biochemistry of airway smooth muscle contraction. The classical studies of Van Amsterdam et al. [12] established the general concept that as the intensity of contraction is increased, the pharmacological efficacy of bronchodilators is progressively diminished due to biochemical antipathy between contracting and relaxing pathways, dependent on the formation of inositol phosphates. Subsequently, the molecular nature

Table 2. Classes of experimental compounds (pre-clinical or early-phase clinical trial) awaiting demonstration of clinical utility

Directly acting bronchodilators	Indirectly acting agents with some bronchodilator activity (mostly weak or ineffective in vivo)
PDE III/IV inhibitors Selective type IV isozyme inhibitors SB 207499 Ariflo® Atrial naturetic peptide Calcium-calmodulin inhibitors Directly acting adenylyl cyclase activators Myosin light chain kinase inhibitors PAR2-activating peptides Potassium channel openers PGE$_2$ and synthetic PGE$_2$ receptor agonists ROCK inhibitors Y-27632	Prejunctional agonists suppressing cholinergic neurotransmission Opioid agonists α_2-Adrenoceptor agonists M$_2$ cholinoceptor agonists

of this cross-talk or functional antagonism has been elucidated. In the case of β-agonists, it is now clear that progressively increased tone converts agonists with high efficacy (defined as maximal extent of cAMP formation) into weak partial agonists due to impairment of cAMP generation and loss of β-adrenoceptor affinity for its agonist [13]. Moreover, it is now also understood that relaxant receptors may uncouple from their transduction pathways in very severe disease and that this uncoupling can be mimicked in vitro by exposing airway smooth muscle to inflammatory mediators such as TNF-α and especially IL-1, both of which are implicated in infectious exacerbations of asthma and COPD [14, reviewed in Anderson, 15]. Immune defects in asthma may alter airway smooth muscle function: allergic sensitization via high-affinity IgE receptors (FcεRI) has been demonstrated to promote Ca^{2+} flux into airway smooth muscle and also to increase the activity of MLCK [16]. In experimental animals, inflammatory mediators also increase the degree of electromechanical coupling between airway smooth muscle cells promoting single, rather than multi-unit, a behaviour which may favour contraction. Thus disease per se may lessen the clinical effectiveness of bronchodilators.

Compensatory Adaptations to Bronchodilation

Cellular homeostatic mechanisms tend to lessen bronchodilator responses over time although the degree to which this occurs is highly variable. Potent long-acting β$_2$-adrenoceptor-selective agonists, such as salmeterol and formoterol, cause a measurable loss of bronchoprotection against bronchoconstricition induced by inhaled methacholine, a cholinergic agonist, but no appreciable loss of bronchodilation even after years of use. G-protein-coupled receptors, such as the β$_2$-adrenoceptor undergo homologous desensitization due to receptor internalization into endosomes and possible subsequent proteolytic destruction. The fate of the receptor is dependent on phosphorylation of intracellular domains by G-protein-associated kinases and the activities of arrestins. After sustained stimulation, β-adrenoceptor mRNA may be destabilized, presumably due to ribonuclease induction, but airway smooth muscle is refractory to this process. The efficiency of signal transduction from G-coupled receptors leading to cAMP accumulation is diminished during sustained agonist exposure due to induction of PDE isoenzymes which hydrolyse cAMP [17]. In situations where endogenous bronchoconstricting agonists, e.g. acetylcholine, are tonically present, blockade of receptors by antagonists frequently causes upregulation of post-junctional effector receptors and may also downregulate prejunctional auto-inhibitory receptors. This may lead to potentiation of neurotransmitter release and enhanced bronchospasm when the antagonist is removed from the system (rebound effects) but marked changes are not usual in humans for anticholinergics, cysLT1 leukotriene blockers or antihistamines.

As the molecular regulation of vascular smooth muscle tone is broadly comparable to regulation of airway smooth muscle tone, ventilation perfusion mismatch (V/Q mismatching) is a frequent consequence of many inhaled bronchodilators especially β-adrenoceptor agonists. This may cause marked, transient falls in blood oxygen saturation. Less well known is the fact that many bronchodilators actually increase the oxygen cost of breathing, possibly via agonist activity in skeletal muscle, with unknown clinical consequences [18]. Concern has been expressed that some antagonists of some mediators, e.g. tachykinin NK1 receptor antagonist, may lessen respiratory drive as neuropeptidergic neurotransmission is important in carotid body chemoceptors. Similarly, decreased post-bronchodilator pCO$_2$ may lessen respiratory drive in hypercapnic COPD patients. A benefit of systemically bioavailable agents increasing cAMP levels, such as the non-selective PDE-blocking xanthines, is to increase respiratory muscle strength to a measurable degree.

Bronchodilator Effects on Non-Airway Smooth Muscle Tissues

Bronchodilators, especially those that increase cAMP, exert marked anti-inflammatory effects on a range of human or animal cells or tissues in vitro. Thus β-adrenoceptor agonists suppress neutrophil and eosinophil recruitment, mast cell degranulation, microvascular plasma leakage and T cell cytokine synthesis. However, these effects seem not to occur to any appreciable extent during regular use in vivo probably because inflammatory-cell β-adrenoceptors undergo rapid downregulation. A theoretical benefit of PDE inhibitors is that they may overcome this weakness; however, theophylline has no appreciable anti-inflammatory effect in biopsy studies. New type-4 PDE-selective agents strongly suppress TNF-α release from a range of cell types, a potential advantage in COPD, but whether this occurs in clinical practice is unknown. Respiratory tract infection is a frequent precipitant of acute severe asthma and some boncodilators, such as salmeterol, have been shown to protect respiratory epithelium from pathogen-mediated damage in vitro [19]. In clinical practice, β-agonists alone, however, have no effect on the rate of disease exacerbations caused by infection. Anti-leukotrienes, which bronchodilate indirectly, suppress lung eosinophilia in asthma, but the clinical significance of this finding is unknown. Very recently, it has been demonstrated that β-adrenoceptor agonists activate steroid receptors via PKA [20] – the functional significance of this discovery is currently the subject of intense research.

Genetic Variation and Polymorphisms in the Machinery of Contraction and Relaxation

Genetic studies have identified variations in dilator and contractile mechanisms that may predispose to excessive bronchoconstricition and/or impede the activity of bronchodilators:

(1) single amino acid polymorphisms in the $β_2$-adrenoceptors (4 known) and their 5′ leader cistron (1 known) [21]; (2) myosin light-chain kinase isoforms and levels of expression [22]; (3) variation in PDE isozyme expression and allosteric state [23]; (4) 5-lipoxygenase promotor mutations [24], and (5) differential protein kinase C isoform expression.

Animal and cell studies suggest that other aberrations are likely, such as genetic dysregulation of protein expression leading to aberrant signal transduction and a set of variations increasing the likelihood of airway smooth muscle proliferation and hypertrophy occurring as well as determinants of extracellular matrix deposition, particularly within the smooth muscle bundles. These changes would, in general, worsen bronchoconstriction and lessen dilator responses but they are yet to be delineated in human asthma.

With the greater insights that have recently been gained into the molecular basis of airflow obstruction and bronchodilation, it is likely that better treatment strategies with existing and new drugs will rapidly follow.

References

1 Hogg JC, Macklem PT, Thurlbeck WM: Site and nature of airway obstruction in chronic obstructive lung disease. N Engl J Med 1968; 278:1355–1360

2 Gelb AF, Gobel PH, Fairshter R, Zamel N: Predominant site of airway resistance in chronic obstructive pulmonary disease. Chest 1981;79:273–276.

3 Yanai M, Sekizawa K, Ohrui T, Sasaki H, Takishima T: Site of airway obstruction in pulmonary disease: Direct measurement of intrabronchial pressure. J Appl Physiol 1992;72: 1016–1023.

4 Opazo Saez AM, Seow CY, Pare PD: Peripheral airway smooth muscle mechanics in obstructive airways disease. Am J Respir Crit Care Med 2000;161:910–917

5 Stephens NL, Li W, Wang Y, Ma X: The contractile apparatus of airway smooth muscle. Biophysics and biochemistry. Am J Respir Crit Care Med 1998;158:S80–S94.

6 Saetta M, Ghezzo H, Kim WD, King M, Angus GE, Wang NS, Cosio MG: Loss of alveolar attachments in smokers. A morphometric correlate of lung function impairment. Am Rev Respir Dis 1985;132:894–900.

7 Di Stefano A, Capelli A, Lusuardi M, Balbo P, Vecchio C, Maestrelli P, Mapp CE, Fabbri LM, Donner CF, Saetta M: Severity of airflow limitation is associated with severity of airway inflammation in smokers. Am J Respir Crit Care Med 1998;158:1277–1285.

8 Fredberg JJ, Inouye DS, Mijailovich SM, Butler JP: Perturbed equilibrium of myosin binding in airway smooth muscle and its implications in bronchospasm. Am J Respir Crit Care Med 1999;159:959–967.

9 Yoshii A, Iizuka K, Dobashi K, Horie T, Harada T, Nakazawa T, Mori M: Relaxation of contracted rabbit tracheal and human bronchial smooth muscle by Y-27632 through inhibition of Ca^{2+} sensitization. Am J Respir Cell Mol Biol 1999;20:1190–1200.

10 Stewart AG, Harris T, Fernandes DJ, Schachte LC, Koutsoubos V, Guida E, Ravenhall CE, Vadiveloo P, Wilson JW: Beta2-adrenergic receptor agonists and cAMP arrest human cultured airway smooth muscle cells in the G(1) phase of the cell cycle: Role of proteasome degradation of cyclin D1. Mol Pharmacol 1999;56: 1079–1086.

11 Anderson GP, Linden A, Rabe KF: Why are long-acting beta-adrenoceptor agonists long-acting? Eur Respir J 1994;7:569–578.

12 Van Amsterdam RG, Meurs H, Ten Berge RE, Veninga NC, Brouwer F, Zaagsma J: Role of phosphoinositide metabolism in human bronchial smooth muscle contraction and in functional antagonism by beta-adrenoceptor agonists. Am Rev Respir Dis 1990;142:1124–1128.

13 Lemoine H, Overlack C: Highly potent beta-2 sympathomimetics convert to less potent partial agonists as relaxants of guinea pig tracheae maximally contracted by carbachol. Comparison of relaxation with receptor binding and adenylate cyclase stimulation. J Pharmacol Exp Ther 1992;261:258–270.

14 Bai TR: Abnormalities in airway smooth muscle in fatal asthma. A comparison between trachea and bronchus. Am Rev Respir Dis 1991; 143:441–443.
15 Anderson GP: Interactions between corticosteroids and beta-adrenergic agonists in asthma disease induction, progression, and exacerbation. Am J Respir Crit Care Med 2000;161: S188–S196.
16 Schmidt D, Rabe KF: Immune mechanisms of smooth muscle hyperreactivity in asthma. J Allergy Clin Immunol 2000;105:673–682.
17 Manning CD, McLaughlin MM, Livi GP, Cieslinski LB, Torphy TJ, Barnette MS: Prolonged beta adrenoceptor stimulation up-regulates cAMP phosphodiesterase activity in human monocytes by increasing mRNA and protein for phosphodiesterases 4A and 4B. J Pharmacol Exp Ther 1996;276:810–818.
18 Newth CJ, Amsler B, Anderson GP, Morley J: The ventilatory and oxygen costs in the anesthetized rhesus monkey of inhaling drugs used in the therapy and diagnosis of asthma. Am Rev Respir Dis 1991;143:766–771.
19 Dowling RB, Rayner CF, Rutman A, Jackson AD, Kanthakumar K, Dewar A, Taylor GW, Cole PJ, Johnson M, Wilson R: Effect of salmeterol on *Pseudomonas aeruginosa* infection of respiratory mucosa. Am J Respir Crit Care Med 1997;155:327–336.
20 Eickelberg O, Roth M, Lorx R, Bruce V, Rudiger J, Johnson M, Block LH: Ligand-independent activation of the glucocorticoid receptor by beta2-adrenergic receptor agonists in primary human lung fibroblasts and vascular smooth muscle cells. J Biol Chem 1999;27:1005–1010.
21 Liggett SB: Beta(2)-adrenergic receptor pharmacogenetics. Am J Respir Crit Care Med 2000;161:S197–S201.
22 Jiang H, Rao K, Halayko AJ, Liu X, Stephens NL: Ragweed sensitization-induced increase of myosin light chain kinase content in canine airway smooth muscle. Am J Respir Cell Mol Biol 1992;7:567–573.
23 Torphy TJ: Phosphodiesterase isozymes: Molecular targets for novel antiasthma agents. Am J Respir Crit Care Med 1998;157:351–370.
24 Drazen JM, Yandava CN, Dube L, Szczerback N, Hippensteel R, Pillari A, Israel E, Schork N, Silverman ES, Katz DA, Drajesk J: Pharmacogenetic association between ALOX5 promoter genotype and the response to anti-asthma treatment. Nat Genet 1999;22:168–170.

Dr. Gary P. Anderson, PhD
Senior Lecturer
Department of Pharmacology
University of Melbourne
Melbourne, Vic. 3010 (Australia)
Tel. +61 3 8344 8602, Fax +61 3 8344 0241
E-Mail g.anderson@pharmacology.unimelb.edu.au

Long-Acting β₂-Agonists

Malcolm Johnson   Gerry W.E. Hagan

GlaxoWellcome, Uxbridge, UK

Summary

The LABAs salmeterol and formoterol have both prolonged airway smooth muscle effects and non-bronchodilator activity. They have a complementary mode of action to the topical anti-inflammatory effects of corticosteroids, and inhibit mucosal oedema, increase mucociliary transport and reduce respiratory tract infection. In asthma, LABAs are currently positioned as 'add-on' therapy, where combination with inhaled steroids results in better lung function and symptom control, decreased rescue medication and fewer exacerbations. In COPD patients, LABAs such as salmeterol reduce breathlessness, decrease exacerbations and improve health-related quality of life.

Mechanism of Action

Long-acting β₂-agonists (LABAs) stimulate transmembrane β₂-adrenoceptors, leading to dissociation of the α-subunit of the associated G_s-protein and the formation, via activation of adenylate cyclase, of intracellular cAMP, which then mediates their biological and therapeutic effects [1, 2].

Formoterol is moderately lipophilic and taken up as a cell membrane depot, from where it leaches out to interact with the β₂-receptor to exert a concentration-dependent duration of action [1]. Salmeterol, which is highly lipophilic, instead diffuses laterally through the membrane to the β₂-receptor, where the side chain is anchored to an auxilliary exosite domain of hydrophobic amino acids (fig. 1) allowing the head of the molecule to repeatedly engage and disengage the active site of the receptor, resulting in an inherently long duration of action [1].

Receptor Pharmacology

Salmeterol and formoterol have high affinity for the β₂-receptor compared with salbutamol. In β₂-receptor-containing tissues, the rank order of potency is: formoterol > salmeterol > salbutamol (table 1). This activity lies predominantly in the (R)-enantiomer(s) of the molecules [3]. To date, the influence of polymorphic forms of the β₂-adrenoceptor on responses to LABAs is unclear.

Formoterol has high efficacy at the β₂-receptor (table 1), whilst salmeterol, like salbutamol, is a partial agonist [1]. This difference may influence the degree of receptor occupancy and desensitization which occurs. These pharmacological properties do not, however, affect either clinical efficacy or responsiveness of patients to short-acting β₂-agonists. Whilst both LABAs show some tolerance to protective effects against bronchostimulatory challenge (e.g. histamine, methacholine), formoterol also demonstrates reduced bronchodilator activity on chronic dosing [4]. This may be due to the full agonist properties of the molecule.

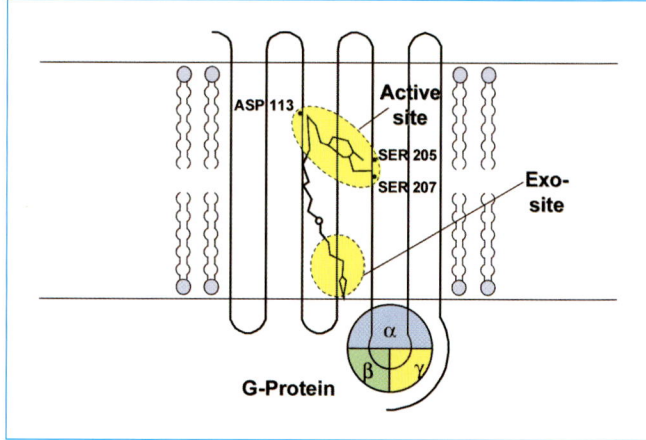

Fig. 1. The exosite mechanism of action of salmeterol.

Table 1. Comparative profile of LABAs

	Formoterol	Salmeterol
Potency	very potent	potent
Onset of action	rapid	delayed
Duration of action	– long	– long
	– dose-related	– inherent
β_2-Receptor selectivity	selective	highly selective
Efficacy	full agonist	partial agonist
Mechanism of action	membrane depot	receptor exosite
Clinical role	p.r.n./maintenance therapy?	maintenance therapy

Both formoterol and salmeterol are selective β_2-adrenoceptor agonists (table 1), but the selectivity ratio for airway β_2:cardiac β_1-receptors is higher for salmeterol [1].

Airway Smooth Muscle

In human airway tissue in vitro, the onset of bronchodilator activity is salbutamol $\leq$ formoterol $<$ salmeterol, and the duration of relaxant effect is in the rank order: salmeterol $>$ formoterol $>$ salbutamol (table 1). This profile has been confirmed clinically across the respiratory disease spectrum. Salmeterol, like salbutamol, has also been shown to inhibit smooth muscle hyperplasia induced by mitogens such as thrombin, via an action on cell cycle regulatory proteins [5], and to inhibit the release of pro-inflammatory chemokines such as eotaxin and IL-8 from smooth muscle cells [6].

Non-Smooth-Muscle Effects

The pharmacological activity of LABAs is not restricted to airway smooth muscle, possibly as a result of their ability to produce sustained elevated levels of intracellular cAMP in a range of other target cells [1].

Although LABAs inhibit mast cell mediator (histamine, PGD_2, LTC_4) release in vitro, such an effect has not been consistently demonstrated in vivo. However, after single inhaled doses in atopic asthmatic subjects, salmeterol inhibits the release of pro-inflammatory mediators (e.g., IL-4, IL-5) following segmental allergen challenge [7]. Such mediators play a role in inflammatory cell recruitment, and indeed formoterol and salmeterol have been shown to reduce submucosal eosinophils [8] and neutrophils [9], respectively, in patients with mild to moderate asthma. Clinical studies have also shown formoterol and salmeterol to inhibit plasma protein extravasation induced by histamine or allergen, thereby reducing the mucosal oedema component of the acute inflammatory response [10].

The anti-neutrophil effect of salmeterol, whereby numbers of cells, activation status and the release of mediators such as myleoperoxidase and lipocalin are reduced in tissue biopsy and BAL fluid [11], may be of relevance in COPD. In addition, LABAs have been demonstrated to increase cilial beat frequency, and at clinical doses, salmeterol has been shown to significantly increase mucociliary transport [12]. Finally, salmeterol exhibits a cytoprotective effect on the respiratory mucosa against the damaging effects of micro-organisms such as *Pseudomonas aeruginosa* and *Haemophilius influenzae* [13]. This may relate to the reduced incidence of respiratory tract infection in COPD patients treated with salmeterol [14].

Interactions with Corticosteroids

In addition to the well-documented increase in β_2-adrenoceptors induced by corticosteroids, LABAs, such as salmeterol, increase steroid-dependent translocation of the glucocorticoid receptor from the cell cytosol to the nucleus, via a possible mitogen-activated protein kinase (MAPK)-mediated phosphorylation mechanism, leading to a 'priming' of the receptor [15]. This complementary mechanism of action of the LABAs is reflected in vitro, for example, as an increase in steroid-induced eosinophil apoptosis [16], additive inhibition of cellular cytokine and chemokine release [17], and potentiation of respiratory mucosal cytoprotection [18].

In asthmatic patients, the addition of salmeterol to low-dose inhaled steroids decreases the number of eosinophils and reduces mast cells and CD4+ T cells in airway tissue [19], and significantly inhibits the degree of angiogenesis occurring as part of the remodelling process [20]. These effects were not observed with higher doses of corticosteroids, and may contribute to the increased clinical efficacy with LABA/steroid combination therapy.

Clinical Use in Bronchial Asthma

In addition to their long-acting bronchodilator activity, LABAs have been shown to produce a clinically relevant reduction in inhaled steroid dose [21], and salmeterol, unlike salbutamol, significantly decreases exacerbations in patients with moderate to severe disease [22]. However, the most important role for LABAs in asthma is as an 'add-on' combination therapy with inhaled steroids. This concept was first developed by a multi-centre study in the UK [23] in asthmatics not controlled on low-dose steroid. Treatments were divided into one group, where the dose of inhaled steroid (beclomethasone dipropionate) was increased 2.5-fold, whilst the other had salmeterol (50 μg b.d.) added to their existing steroid. In terms of lung function and symptoms, the salmeterol combination group improved more than the increased steroid group.

The FACET study [24] evaluated the risk that a LABA, although improving lung function, may be suppressing symptoms of underlying inflammation and increasing the risk of exacerbations of asthma. After stabilizing over 4 weeks on budesonide 1,600 μg daily, 800 symptomatic patients were given either low-dose (200 μg/day) or high-dose (800 μg/day) budesonide with or without formoterol (12 μg b.d.) for 1 year. The rate of exacerbations was reduced not only by increasing the inhaled steroid dose, but also by the addition of the LABA. Further evaluation [24] showed that lung function deteriorated prior to severe exacerbations after treatment with LABA or steroids, suggesting that there was no masking of inflammation in the clinical setting.

A meta-analysis (MIASMA) which compared the addition of salmeterol to at least doubling the dose of inhaled steroid has been performed [25]. The analysis on nine parallel-group trials of at least 12 weeks in 3,685 patients showed that not only did salmeterol give better lung function, symptom control and less need for rescue medication than increased inhaled steroid, but there were also fewer exacerbations (fig. 2).

Other therapeutic agents, such as theophylline and leukotriene receptor antagonists (LTRA), have been compared with LABAs as an alternative to increased doses of inhaled steroids. The addition of theophylline has also been shown to be beneficial [26], although a meta-analysis of LABAs versus theophylline by the Cochrane Airways Group [27] showed that salmeterol was more effective with less adverse events. The LTRA, montelukast added to low-dose beclomethasone dipropionate (400 μg/day) in incompletely controlled asthmatics produced an increase in morning FEV_1 from baseline in the order of 5% [28]. This modest effect was confirmed in two other comparator studies [29, 30] with zafirlukast, where the LABA, salmeterol, was at least twice as effective in increasing lung function, decreasing symptoms and reducing rescue bronchodilator use [30].

A study of salmeterol and fluticasone propionate in a single inhaler [31] showed an improvement in health status greater than fluticasone propionate alone, and significantly greater than salmeterol, which alone failed to have any benefit. The mechanism for this effect is unclear, but the simplicity and logic of the combination approach suggests that compliance with dosing would improve, but at present no data are available.

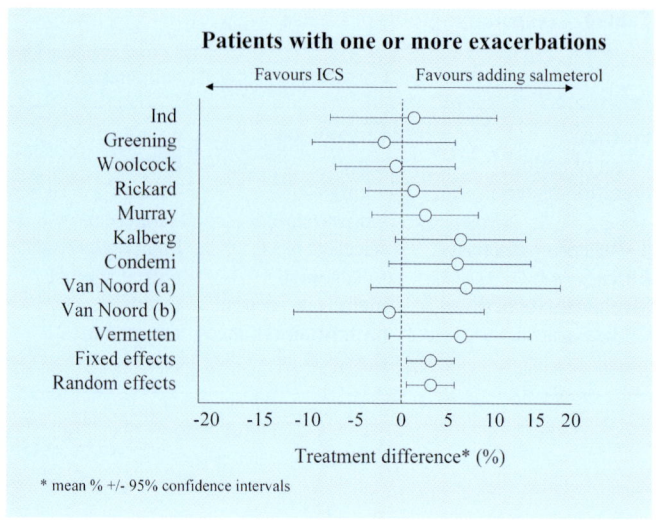

Fig. 2. Additional benefit of adding salmeterol over at least doubling the dose of ICS. From Shrewsbury et al. [25].

Clinical Use in COPD

One advantage of LABAs is their long duration of action, and as in asthma, in COPD patients both salmeterol and formoterol increase lung function for at least 12 h compared with 4–6 h for salbutamol [32, 33]. In a study of salmeterol and the shorter-acting bronchodilator, ipratropium bromide [14], the LABA also resulted in less nocturnal dyspnoea. In another study [34] of 674 COPD patients using salmeterol 50 and 100 μg b.d., whereas both groups showed a significant increase in FEV_1, only the 50 μg b.d. dose [35] resulted in a clinically significant improvement in health-related quality of life (St. George's Respiratory Questionnaire, SGRQ). Formoterol also failed to show a clinical benefit in the SGRQ score at 24 μg b.d. [36], but results at lower doses have not been reported. In the review by the Cochrane Airways Group [36] of LABAs in COPD, it was concluded that improvements in quality of life and a reduction in breathlessness can occur with only small changes in lung function.

Conclusions

LABAs have been demonstrated to be markedly effective as 'add-on' therapy in asthma, where there is increasing evidence to suggest that they have complementary actions to corticosteroids. In addition, in COPD patients, LABAs reduce breathlessness, decrease exacerbations and improve health-related quality of life. Further pharmacological and clinical studies are in progress to further understand the non-bronchodilator actions of LABAs.

References

1 Johnson M, Coleman RA: Mechanisms of action of β₂-adrenoceptor agonists; in Busse WW, Holgate ST (eds): Asthma & Rhinitis. Cambridge, Blackwell, 1995, pp 1278–1295.
2 Gilman G: G-proteins: Transducers of receptor-generated signals. Am Rev Biochem 1987; 56:615–649.
3 Johnson M, Butchers PR, Coleman RA, Nials AT, Strong P, Sumner MJ, Vardey CJ, Whelan CJ: The pharmacology of salmeterol. Life Sci 1993;52:2131–2147.
4 Pauwels RA, Löfdahl CG, Postma DS, Tattersfield AE, O'Byrne P, Barnes PJ, Ullman A: Effect of inhaled formoterol and budesonide on exacerbations of asthma. N Engl J Med 1997; 337:1405–1411.
5 Harris T, Koutsoubos V, Guida E, Stewart AG: Salmeterol modulates cell proliferation and cyclin D1 protein levels in thrombin-stimulated human cultured airway smooth muscle via an action independent of the β₂-adrenoceptor. Am J Respir Crit Care Med 1999;159:A530.
6 Pang LH, Knox A: Inhibition by β₂-adrenoceptor agonists and dexamethasone of TNFα-stimulated eotaxin release from human airway smooth muscle cells. Thorax 1999;54:A8.
7 Murray JJ, Hagaman DD, Dworski R, Keane B, Sheller JR: Inhibition by salmeterol and beclomethasone of late phase response to segmental antigen challenge in asthmatics. Am J Respir Crit Care Med 1998;157:A872.
8 Wallin A, Sandström T, Söderberg M, Howarth P, Lundbäck B, Della-Cioppa G, Wilson S, Judd M, Djukanović R, Holgate S, Lindberg A, Larsson L: The effects of regular inhaled formoterol, budesonide, and placebo on mucosal inflammation and clinical indices in mild asthma. Am J Respir Crit Care Med 1999;159:79–86.
9 Li D, Wang D, Venge P, Dahl R, Faurschou P, Jeffery P: Comparison of the anti-inflammatory effects of inhaled fluticasone propionate and salmeterol in asthma: A placebo-controlled crossover study of bronchial biopsies. Eur Respir J 1997;10:444S.
10 Proud D, Reynolds CJ, Lichtenstein LM, Kagey-Sobotka A, Togias A: Intranasal salmeterol inhibits allergen-induced vascular permeability but not mast cell activation or cellular infiltration. Clin Exp Allergy 1998;28:868–875.
11 Faurschou P, Dahl R, Jeffery P, Venge P, Egerod I: Comparison of the anti-inflammatory effects of fluticasone and salmeterol in asthma: A placebo-controlled, double-blind, crossover study with bronchoscopy, bronchial methacholine provocation and lavage. Eur Respir J 1997;10:243S.
12 Chambers CB, Corrigan BW, Newhouse MT: Salmeterol speeds mucociliary transport (MCT) in healthy subjects. Am J Respir Crit Care Med 1999;159:A636.
13 Dowling RB, Johnson M, Cole PJ, Wilson R: Effect of salmeterol on *Haemophilus influenzae* infection of respiratory mucosa in vitro. Eur Respir J 1998;11:86–90.
14 Mahler DA, Donohue JF, Barbee RA, Goldman MD, Gross NJ, Wisniewski ME, Yancey SW, Zakes BA, Rickard KA, Anderson WH: Efficacy of salmeterol xinafoate in the treatment of COPD. Chest 1999;115:957–965.
15 Eickelberg O, Roth M, Lörx R, Bruce V, Rüdiger J, Johnson M, Block L-H: Ligand-independent activation of the glucocorticoid receptor by β₂-adrenergic receptor agonists in primary human lung fibroblasts and vascular smooth muscle cells. J Biol Chem 1999;274:1005–1010.
16 Anenden V, Egemba G, Kessel B, Johnson M, Costello J, Kilfeather S: Salmeterol facilitation of fluticasone-induced apoptosis in eosinophils of asthmatics pre- and post-antigen challenge. Eur Respir J 1998;12(suppl 28):157S.
17 Korn S, Jerre A, Brattsand R: Additive inhibition of formoterol and budesonide on GM-CSF expression in cultured bronchial epithelial cells. Am J Respir Crit Care Med 1999;159: A114.
18 Dowling RB, Johnson M, Cole PJ, Wilson R: Effect of fluticasone propionate (FP) and salmeterol (SM) on *P. aeruginosa* (PA) infection of respiratory mucosa in vitro. Am J Respir Crit Care Med 1998;157:A138.
19 Sue-Chu M, Wallin A, Wilson S, Ward J, Sandström T, Djukanovic R, Holgate ST, Bjermer L: Bronchial biopsy study in asthmatics treated with low- and high-dose fluticasone propionate (FP) compared to low-dose FP combined with salmeterol. Eur Respir J 1999;14:124S.
20 Orsida BE, Ward C, Li X, Wilson JW, Thien F, Walters EH: Effect of a long-acting β₂-agonist over 3 months on airway wall vascular remodelling in asthma. Am J Respir Crit Care Med, in press.
21 Neilsen LP, Pedersen B, Faurschou P, Madsen F, Wilcke JTR, Dahl R. Salmeterol reduces the need for inhaled corticosteroid in steroid-dependent asthmatics. Respir Med 1999;93:863–868.
22 Taylor DR, Town GI, Herbison GP, Boothman-Burrell D, Glannery EM, Hancox B, Harre E, Lanbscher K, Linscott K, Ramsy CM, Richards G: Asthma control during long-term treatment with regular inhaled salbutamol and salmeterol. Thorax 1998;53:744–754.
23 Greening AP, Ind PW, Northfield M, Shaw G: Added salmeterol versus higher dose corticosteroids in asthma patients. Lancet 1994;344: 523–529.
24 Tattersfield AE, Postma DS, Barnes PJ, Svensson K, Bauer C-A, O'Byrne PM, Löfdahl C-G, Pauwels RA, Ullman A: Exacerbations of asthma: A descriptive study of 425 severe exacerbations. Am J Respir Crit Care Med 1999;160: 594–599.
25 Shrewsbury S, Pyke S, Britton M: A meta-analysis of increasing inhaled steroid or adding salmeterol in symptomatic asthma (MIASMA). BMJ 2000;320:1368–1373.
26 Evans DJ, Taylor DA, Zetterstrom O, Fan Chung K, O'Connor BJ, Barnes PJ: A comparison of low dose inhaled budesonide plus theophylline and high dose inhaled budesonide for moderate asthma. N Engl J Med 1997;337: 1412–1418.
27 Wilson AJ, Gibson PG, Coughlan J: Long-acting beta-agonists versus theophylline for maintenance treatment of asthma. Cochrane Database Syst Rev 2000;1:1–11.
28 Laviolette M, Malmstrom K, Lu S, Chervinsky P, Ppujet J-C, Peszek I, Zhang J, Reiss TF: Montelukast added to inhaled beclomethasone in treatment of asthma. Am J Respir Crit Care Med 1999;160:1862–1868.
29 Rickard KA, Yancey S, Emmett C, Kalberg CJ: Salmeterol compared to zafirlukast when added to inhaled corticosteroid therapy in patients with persistent asthma. Eur Respir J 1999;14 (suppl 30):121S.
30 Busse W, Nelson H, Wolfe J, Kalberg C, Yancey SW, Rickard KA: Comparison of inhaled salmeterol and oral zafirlukast in patients with asthma. J Allergy Clin Immunol 1999;103: 1075–1080.
31 Reese PR, Mahajan P, Woodring A: Salmeterol/fluticasone propionate combination product improves quality of life in asthmatic patients. Eur Respir J 1998;12(suppl 28):35S.
32 Matera MG, Cazzola M, Vinciguerra A, Di Perna F, Calderaro F, Caputi M, Rossi F: A comparison of the bronchodilating effects of salmeterol, salbutamol and ipratropium bromide in patients with chronic obstructive pulmonary disease. Pulm Pharmacol 1995;8:267–271.
33 Maesen BLP, Westermann CJJ, Duurkens VAM, van den Bosch JMM: Effects of formoterol in apparently poorly reversible chronic obstructive pulmonary disease. Eur Respir J 1999;13:1103–1108.
34 Boyd G, Morice AH, Pounsford JC, Siebert M, Peslis N, Crawford C: An evaluation of salmeterol in the treatment of chronic obstructive pulmonary disease. Eur Respir J 1997;10:815–821.
35 Jones PW, Bosh TK: Quality of life changes in COPD patients treated with salmeterol. Am J Respir Crit Care Med 1997;155:1283–1289.
36 Appleton S, Smith B, Veale A, Bara A: Long-acting beta-2-agonists for chronic obstructive airways disease. Cochrane Database Syst Rev 2000;2:CD001104.

Dr. Malcolm Johnson
Respiratory Therapeutic Development
GlaxoWellcome Research & Development
Building 11, Stockley Park West
Uxbridge UB11 1BT (UK)
Tel. +44 208 990 8455, Fax +44 208 990 8666
E-Mail mj0859@glaxowellcome.co.uk

Single-Isomer β-Agonists

D.A. Handley[a]   J. Morley[b]   H.S. Nelson[c]

[a]Sepracor, Marlborough, Mass., USA, [b]Haldane Research Ltd, Huntingdon, UK, and
[c]National Jewish Medical and Research Center, Denver, Colo., USA

Summary

For over a century, β-agonists have been used for the treatment of asthma and obstructive airway diseases. The drugs of this class each have a chiral carbon, thus, when synthesized, contain a 50:50 mixture of R- and S-isomers. The R-isomerisomer, being an adrenaline analog, possesses bronchodilator and bronchoprotective properties; the S-isomer has no therapeutic benefits. Studies differentiating the biological activities of R- and S-albuterol have suggested that the S-isomer has properties which are inappropriate for an asthma medication. Recently, R-albuterol (levalbuterol) has become available and seminal studies have demonstrated that the removal of S-albuterol from racemic albuterol creates a more efficacious therapeutic for mild persistent to acute asthma.

Background

β-Adrenergic agonists provide rapid and effective relief of symptoms of acute and chronic airway obstruction caused by bronchial smooth muscle contraction. This has led to extensive use of these drugs not only in asthma, but also in COPD. Currently employed β-agonists were designed to have enhanced specificity for the β_2-receptor (to avoid excessive cardiac stimulation) and structural features to achieve extended bronchodilation (prolonged pulmonary residence). Endogenous adrenaline – R-adrenaline – is a pure single isomer. In contrast, all marketed β-agonists (fenoterol, terbutaline, albuterol, salmeterol and formoterol) are racemates, composed of a 50:50 mixture of the R-isomer (an analog of adrenaline) and an S-isomer, an anti-analog of adrenaline. It is the R-isomer that provides the therapeutic benefit. While the S-isomers have been considered inert, recent evidence suggests this may be incorrect. Experimental and clinical studies reveal that the S-isomer of albuterol may cause a paradoxical intensification of airway obstruction, especially when chronic excessive doses were employed. This capacity to exacerbate asthma symptoms was seen in animal experiments [1] and provides the rationale for the development of single (homoisomer) β-agonists.

Historically, synthetic drugs containing chiral carbons have been administered as racemates containing both the isomer contributing the therapeutic benefit (eutomer) and the isomer having little or no therapeutic benefit (distomer). However, in 1992 the FDA introduced guidelines to encourage the pharmaceutical industry to switch existing marketed racemic drugs to single-isomer eutomer formulations [1]. The FDA recognized that single-isomer drugs may offer a number of advantages over existing racemic mixtures, which they considered fixed combination drugs [1]. Similar guidelines have been also been developed in Europe, Canada and Japan. From these guidelines, it would be most difficult to develop a racemate, although racemates developed outside the US before 1992 (i.e. formoterol) are still permissible.

Rationale for Single-Isomer β-Agonists

Although β-agonist drugs have been known to be composed to two isomers in equal amounts, the S-isomers have been viewed as biologically inert and hence tolerated in racemic formulations. In general, they are not inert, however, and have pharmacological properties that are singularly inappropriate for subjects with asthma or COPD [2] (table 1).

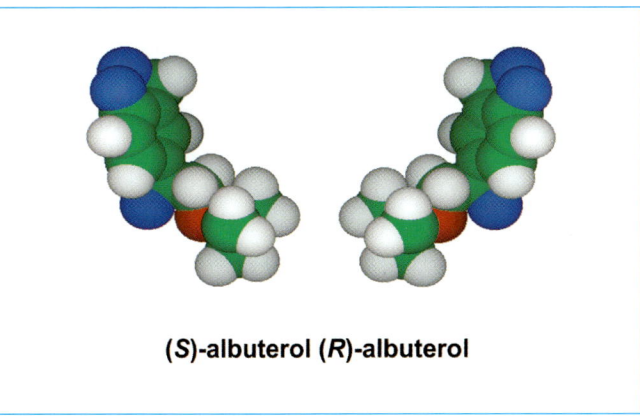

Fig. 1. 3D conformational structures of R- and S-albuterol.

Table 1. Pharmacological effects of β-agonist distomers

S-Isomer	Pharmacological effect	Differentiation from activation of β-receptors
S-Isoprenaline	potentiation of voltage-dependent influx of Ca^{2+} ions	unaffected by propranolol no elevation of cAMP
S-Albuterol	influx of Ca^{2+} ions	not mimicked by eutomer
S-Clenbuterol	stimulation of noradrenaline release	unaffected by propranolol or by desensitization
S-Albuterol	activation of human eosinophils in vitro	not mimicked by eutomer
R-Trimetoquinol	inhibition of human platelet aggrevation	not mimicked by agonists
S-Salmeterol	relaxation of guinea-pig trachea	unaffected by propranolol
S-Isoprenaline	reduced intraocular pressure	unaffected by propranolol and not accompanied by elevated cAMP
S-Albuterol	exaggerated responses to spasmogens in vitro	not mimicked by β-agonist eutomers
S-Isoprenaline, S-albuterol and S-terbutaline	exaggerated responses to spasmogens in vivo	not suppressed by β-agonist eutomers or by propranolol
S-Albuterol	acute oral and IV LD_{50} in rat	>100-fold lower than predicted by eudismic ratio[1]

[1] Eudismic ratio = potency of eutomer/potency of distomer.

When actions of the S-isomer are inappropriate for asthma and avoidable through single-isomer formulations, it could be considered clinically useful and logical to replace racemic β-agonists by single-isomer formulations, as these become available. This logic provides the basis for levalbuterol (Xopenex), the single-isomer form of racemic albuterol (fig. 1). A similar rationale may apply to R;R-formoterol and for other β-agonists which are structural analogues of adrenaline.

Mechanism of Action

Interaction between R-isomers and $β_2$-adrenoceptors activates adenyl cyclase, and reduces intracellular Ca^{2+} ions, causing smooth muscle relaxation. In general, the R-isomers are 2–3 log orders more potent than the S-isomers [3]. While this expected effect is achieved by R-albuterol (levalbuterol), S-albuterol has been shown to dose-dependently promote an influx of Ca^{2+} into isolated smooth muscle cells and will oppose, or even nullify, the dose-dependent decrease in Ca^{2+} that is produced by R-albuterol [4]. In addition, R-albuterol inhibits airway epithelial cytokine, chemokine and nitric oxide release in vitro, while S-albuterol paradoxically increased levels, suggesting a pro-inflammatory effect [5]. Studies conducted with human eosinophils stimulated with IL-5 to release superoxide [6] or ionophore-induced secretion of eosinophil peroxidase [7] showed that R-albuterol inhibited both superoxide generation and eosinophil peroxidase release, while S-albuterol augmented superoxide (statistically significantly) and eosinophil peroxidase (dose-trend) responses, indicating again a pro-inflammatory effect. Other studies demonstrated that S-albuterol augmented the contractile effect of spasmogens in vitro in human airway tissues, while R-albuterol was found to effectively inhibit a variety of direct and indirect spasmogen-induced contractions of isolated human bronchus [8], observations consistent with its known receptor binding and pharmacology. Lastly, in several toxicology models, the lethal doses (LD) for rats by intravenous or oral administration of S- and R-albuterol were nearly equivalent [9], suggesting that the S-isomer exhibits toxicology independent of $β_2$-receptor interaction. R-Albuterol has 8- to 10-fold more rapid metabolism over S-albuterol such that, depending upon the route of administration, S-albuterol accumulates in body fluids following administration of racemic albuterol. This effect is amplified during regular administration and is compounded by selective retention of S-albuterol in human airways [10, 11] as well as progressive increases and accumulation of S-albuterol in the plasma [12].

Effectiveness of Levalbuterol in Pediatrics

In pediatric patients, levalbuterol achieved dose-related improvements in FEV_1 [13]. Removal of the S-albuterol allowed for a reduction in the dose of R-albuterol so that 0.63 mg offered comparable efficacy to the bronchodilation effects of 2.50 mg racemic albuterol, resulting in a reduction in β-mediated side effects, such as nervousness, tremor and tachycardia.

Levalbuterol was evaluated in infants (3–12 months) by comparing a single nebulized dose of racemic albuterol (2.50 mg) to levalbuterol (0.63 mg) [14]. Pulmonary function was determined using crying vital capacity measurements. Levalbuterol 0.65 mg produced a similar improvement in crying vital capacity as compared to 2.5 mg racemic albuterol in these infants with reactive airway disease.

Efficacy of Levalbuterol in Exercise-Induced Bronchoconstriction

In exercise-induced asthma, a controlled study compared the efficacy of 0.63 or 1.25 mg levalbuterol to 2.50 mg racemic albuterol to prevent bronchospasm in patients with mild to moderate asthma [15]. Levalbuterol at 0.63 mg produced equal bronchoprotection to 2.50 mg racemic albuterol [15].

Efficacy of Levalbuterol in Cold Air-Induced Bronchoconstriction

A number of studies have demonstrated that 0.63 mg of levalbuterol exhibits similar bronchodilator efficacy to 2.50 mg of racemic albuterol but with fewer β-mediated side effects. In a recent controlled study [16], the bronchodilator efficacy of 0.63 mg levalbuterol was compared to 2.50 mg racemic albuterol to prevent cold-air-induced asthma. This study again showed that 0.63 mg levalbuterol produced equal bronchoprotection to 2.50 mg racemic albuterol.

Efficacy of Levalbuterol in Moderate Persistent Asthma

In a larger 4-week clinical study (n = 363), levalbuterol (0.63 mg, 1.25 mg) was compared with racemic albuterol (1.25 mg, 2.50 mg) and in patients with moderate to severe persistent asthma after 4 weeks of nebulized treatment [17]. The improvement in FEV_1 for the 0.63 mg dose of levalbuterol was comparable to 2.50 mg of racemic albuterol, but was associated with fewer β-mediated side effects and a less marked effect on serum potassium, glucose and heart rate. In subjects with a baseline $FEV_1 \leq 60\%$ and steroid naïve, the improvement in FEV_1 of levalbuterol 1.25 mg was statistically better than 2.50 mg of racemic albuterol (p = 0.0024). Relative potency, calculated by a slope ratio assay from the area under the curve, showed that in general 1 unit of levalbuterol equaled 1.6 units of racemic albuterol, suggesting enhanced potency with levalbuterol. Furthermore, 1.25 mg levalbuterol statistically improve symptom-free days (while 2.50 mg racemic albuterol did not), statistically reduced rescue metered-dose inhaler needs (as did 0.63 mg levalbuterol), while 2.50 mg racemic albuterol did not.

Efficacy of Levalbuterol in COPD and Acute Care

Levalbuterol decreased prescribed dosing and p.r.n. treatments for hospitalized patients with asthma and COPD [18]. Over 4 weeks, nebulized levalbuterol 0.63 mg was given every 6–8 h and breakthrough treatments were administered as needed [18]. Of the 60 patients who received a total of 1,252 doses of levalbuterol, only 10% breakthrough treatments were administered, a substantial reduction over historical data for racemic albuterol. Then, levalbuterol 0.63 mg administered every 6 h was initiated as the standard at this facility for hospitalized patients. After 30 days, 10% of patients required breakthrough treatments. Increasing the dose of levalbuterol to 1.25 mg (q8h) decreased the number of breakthrough treatments to approximately 6% and reduced ipratropium bromide need by 25%. The pharmacy noted a 50% decrease in the number of levalbuterol treatments compared to previous use of racemic albuterol [18].

A current study of the single-isomer β-agonist levalbuterol for effective bronchodilation in the treatment of acute asthma in the emergency department revealed significant improvements in discharge rate in comparison to the reported discharge rates of racemic albuterol [19]. Additional studies are in progress to confirm these findings.

Place in Therapy

The medical value or need to substitute single-isomer β-agonists for racemic formulations is predicted by the extent to which distomers can impair therapeutic efficacy of racemates. These results suggest that the 0.63 mg levalbuterol dose offers effective bronchodilation with an improved therapeutic index, achieved through equivalent efficacy with reduction in β-mediated side effects. The 1.25 mg dose may offer increased bronchodilator effectiveness, perhaps useful in the treatment of acute asthma exacerbations. In some patients a reduction in dosing frequency can be expected, as well as reducing or eliminating the need for concomitant medications.

Conclusions

These completed and on-going studies indicate that the levalbuterol, at 0.63 mg or 1.25 mg, offers a dosing choice and may present an improved therapeutic index. With equivalent efficacy to 2.50 mg racemic albuterol and a reduction in β-mediated side effects, 0.65 mg levalbuterol may offer benefits to patients sensitive to side effects. The on-going studies are designed to fully characterize the acute, intermediate and chronic effects of S-albuterol on pulmonary function.

References

1 FDA: Statement for the development of new stereoisomeric drugs. Chirality 1992;4:338–340.
2 Handley DA, Morley J: The pursuit of precision pharmaceuticals: Divergent effects of β-agonist isomers. Exp Opin Invest Drugs 1998; 7:1601–1616.
3 Penn RB, Frielle T, McCullough JR, Aberg G, Benovic JL: Comparison of (R)-, S-, and (R,S)-albuterol interaction with human β_1- and β_2-adrenergic receptors. Clin Rev Allergy Immunol 1996;14:37–45.
4 Mitra S, Ugur M, Ugur O, Goodman M, McCullough JR, Yamaguchi H: (S)-Albuterol increases intracellular free calcium by muscarinic receptor activation and a phospholipase C-dependent mechanism in airway smooth muscle. Mol Pharmacol 1998;53:347–354.
5 Frieri M, Pergolizz R, Milan C, Dominguez PJ: Cytokine, chemokine and nitric oxide (NO) release in stimulated small airway epithelial cells (SAEC) treated with β_2 agonist enantiomers of albuterol. J Allergy Clin Immunol 2000;105:S292.
6 Volcheck GW, Gleich GJ, Kita H: Pro- and anti-inflammatory effects of beta adrenergic agonists on eosinophil response to IL-5. J Allergy Clin Immunol 1998;101:S35.
7 Leff AR, Herrnreiter A, Naclerio RM, Baroody FM, Handley DA, Munoz NM: Effect of enantiomeric forms of albuterol on stimulated secretion of granular protein from human eosinophils. Pulm Pharmacol Ther 1997;10:97–104.
8 Templeton AGB, Chapman ID, Chilvers E, Morley J, Handley DA: Effects of (S)-albuterol on isolated human bronchus. Pulm Pharmacol 1998;11:1–6.
9 Snider ME, Rollins TE, Handley DA: Preclinical and clinical effects of (S)-albuterol. Allergy Asthma Proc 1999;20:200.
10 Gumbhir-Shah K, Kellerman D, DeGraw SS, Koch P, Jusko W: Pharmacokinetic and pharmacodynamic characteristics and safety of inhaled albuterol enantiomers in healthy volunteers. J Clin Pharmacol 1998;38:1096–1106.
11 Dhand R, Goode M, Reid R, Fink JB, Fahey PJ, Tobin MJ: Preferential pulmonary retention of (S)-albuterol after inhalation of racemic albuterol. Am J Respir Crit Care Med 1999; 160:1136–1141.
12 Schmekel B, Rydberg I, Norlander B, Sjöswärd KN, Ahlner J, Andersson RGG: Stereoselective pharmacokinetics of (S)-salbutamol after administration of the racemate in healthy volunteers. Eur Respir J 1999;13:1230–1235.
13 Gawchik SM, Saccar CL, Noonan M, Raesner DS, DeGraw SS: The safety and efficacy of nebulized levalbuterol compared with racemic albuterol and placebo in the treatment of asthma in pediatric patients. J Allergy Clin Immunol 1999;103:615–621.
14 Edell D, Perlander F, Khoshoo V: Comparative efficacy of levalbuterol (LA) and racemic albuterol (RA) in infants with reactive airway disease (RAD) using crying vital capacity (CVC) measurements. Ann Allergy Asthma Immunol, in press.
15 Busse WW, Greos L, Vaickus L: Lower doses of Xopenex are as effective as racemic albuterol in the prevention of exercise-induced asthma (EIB). J Allergy Clin Immunol 1999;103:S136.
16 Israel E, Hong C, Claus R, DeGraw SS, Rubin P: Levalbuterol is effective in the prevention of cold air induced bronchospasm and does not induce tachyphylaxis in the degree of bronchoprotection. J Allergy Clin Immunol 2000;105: S22.
17 Nelson HS, Bensch G, Pleskow WW, DiSantostefano MS, DeGraw S, Reasner DS, Rollins TE: Improved bronchodilation with levalbuterol compared with racemic albuterol in patients with asthma. J Allergy Clin Immunol 1998;102:943–952.
18 Truitt TJ, Witko J, Kotter S, Gordon I: Levalbuterol reduces total and breakthrough treatments in hospitalized patients. Am J Respir Crit Care Med 2000;137:248S.
19 Nowak R: Single isomer β agonists in the ED Department. Am Acad Allergy Asthma and Immunol, San Diego, March 2000.

Dean A. Handley, PhD, MBA
Sepracor, 111 Locke Drive
Marlborough, MA 01752 (USA)
Tel. +1 508 357 7391, Fax +1 508 357 7497
E-Mail dhandley@sepracor.com

Dual D_2 Dopamine Receptor and β_2-Adrenoceptor Agonists for the Modulation of Sensory Nerves in COPD

Paul Newbold   Dale M. Jackson   Alan Young   Iain G. Dougall   Frank Ince
Karen M.S. Rocchiccioli   Phil R. Holt

AstraZeneca R & D Charnwood, Loughborough, UK

Summary

Viozan™ is a first in class dual D_2 dopamine receptor and β_2-adrenoceptor agonist. Preclinical studies have demonstrated that activation of D_2-receptors inhibits sensory afferent driven processes including cough, mucus production and tachypnoea. Clinical studies in COPD patients have shown that Viozan significantly improves the symptoms of cough, breathlessness, sputum production and health status quality of life. The combination of D_2-receptor agonist activity to modulate sensory nerve reflexes with β_2-adrenoceptor agonist activity to provide bronchodilatation is a novel approach to the management of COPD.

COPD is a growing worldwide public health issue as exemplified by the prediction that it will become the third biggest cause of global mortality by 2020 [1]. With regard to morbidity, a treatment for the symptoms experienced by patients suffering from COPD is an unmet medical need. A therapy that reduces the symptoms of cough, breathlessness, wheeze and excess sputum production would improve patients' quality of life and may alter the course of the disease. The inhibition of sensory-nerve-driven reflex processes is a novel approach to the treatment of such symptoms as is the concept of applying dopamine D_2-receptor agonism to achieve this therapeutic effect.

Rationale for D_2 Dopamine Receptor Agonism to Modulate Airway Sensory Afferent Nerves

The symptoms of COPD can all potentially be mediated by neuronal mechanisms. Sensory afferent nerves, activated by endogenous and exogenous irritants, can generate reflexes eliciting cough, mucus production, bronchoconstriction and changes in the depth of breathing [2].

D_2 dopamine receptors are present on many neurones and their activation can modulate neuronal activity. Most studies on these receptors have focused on central nervous system effects, although D_2-receptors also have a widespread distribution in the peripheral nervous system (see review in Missale et al. [3]) including sensory ganglia [4]. In general, peripheral D_2-receptors have an inhibitory role, e.g. activation of D_2-receptors on presynaptic terminals of postganglionic sympathetic nerves inhibits release of noradrenaline thereby modulating vascular tone [5]. Additionally, we have demonstrated that dopamine inhibits histamine-induced discharge of rapidly adapting stretch receptors in the lungs of dogs, an effect that was blocked by the D_2-receptor antagonist, sulpiride [6]. Given this evidence, our working hypothesis was that stimulation of dopamine D_2-receptors on sensory nerve endings in the airways would inhibit sensory nerve activity and consequently suppress reflex-mediated cough, sputum production and dyspnoea in COPD.

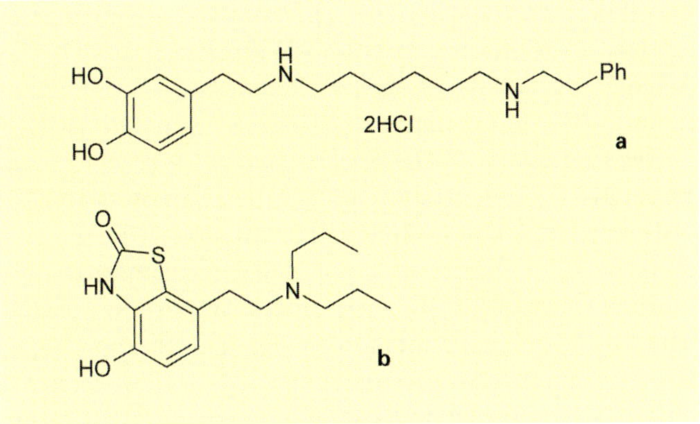

Fig. 1. Structures of Dopacard (a) and 7-hydroxy-4-[2-(di-n-propylamino)ethyl]benzothiazol-2(3H)-one (b).

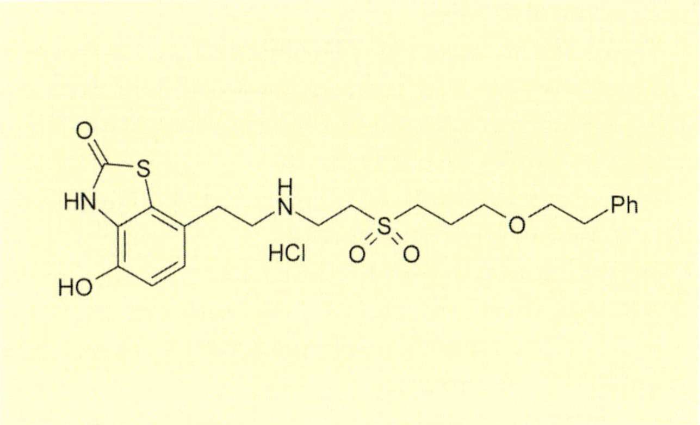

Fig. 2. Structure of Viozan (4-hydroxy-7-[2-(2-(3-(2-phenylethoxy)propylsulphonyl)ethylamino)ethyl]-1,3-benzothiazol-2(3H)-one, hydrochloride).

Chemical Rationale and Screening

Our aim was to develop potent, selective D_2 dopamine receptor agonists. In addition, β_2-agonism would provide anti-bronchoconstrictor activity and bronchodilation by a direct action on airway smooth muscle. Candidate drug selection was targeted at discovering compounds that possessed both D_2- and β_2-receptor agonist properties. These dual agonists were designed to be delivered topically to the lung.

Initial chemical leads were developed from Dopacard® (a D_1-receptor and β_2-adrenoceptor agonist, fig. 1a) [7] and the potent D_2-receptor agonist 7-hydroxy-4-[2-(di-n-propylamino)ethyl]benzothiazol-2(3H)-one (fig. 1b) [8]. These leads possessed the desired D_2-receptor and β_2-adrenoceptor agonist activity but also some α_1-adrenoceptor agonist activity, which could cause unwanted cardiovascular effects.

D_2-receptor, β_2-adrenoceptor and α_1-adrenoceptor structure activity relationships were constructed and molecules were ranked according to a potency value ($p[A]_{50}$) and intrinsic activity (maximum response relative to a standard agonist).

Molecular modelling identified parts of the molecules that were responsible for each of the receptor activities. Substituents were then added which should introduce steric and/or electronic effects to reduce the α_1-adrenoceptor potency and/or intrinsic activity whilst maintaining or enhancing D_2-receptor and β_2-adrenoceptor agonist activity.

Incorporation of an SO_2 moiety into the alkyl chain of the original lead compounds resulted in analogues with potent D_2-receptor and β_2-adrenoceptor agonist activity but with negligible α_1-adrenoceptor activity. 4-Hydroxy-7-[2-[2-[3-(2-phenylethoxy) propylsulphonyl] ethylamino] ethyl]-1,3-benzothiazol-2(3H)-one hydrochloride (Viozan™) (fig. 2) was chosen for further development and is the first in a novel class of dual D_2-receptor and β_2-adrenoceptor agonists for the treatment of COPD [9].

Viozan
- is a potent full agonist at the D_2-receptor [10];
- is a potent partial agonist at the β_2-adrenoceptor [10];
- possesses high affinity for human D_2- and D_3-receptors but low affinity for human D_1-, D_4- and D_5-receptors [10];
- exhibits no significant activity at α_2-, β_1- and β_3-adrenoceptors and low potency at α_1-receptors [10].

A summary of the D_2-receptor, β_2-adrenoceptor and α_1-adrenoceptor activities of Viozan is shown in table 1.

Table 1. Activity of Viozan at dopamine D_2-receptors and adrenoceptors [10]

Receptor	Tissue	$p[A]_{50}$	Intrinsic activity
D_2	rabbit ear artery	8.94	0.90
D_2	mouse vas deferens	8.85	–
β_2	guine pig trachea	7.95	0.69
β_2	rabbit saphenous vein	8.64	0.69
α_1	rabbit ear artery	6.08	0.08

Preclinical Studies

D_2-Mediated Properties. The ability of the D_2-receptor agonist properties of Viozan to modulate lung sensory-nerve-driven processes was examined in animal models of sensory and reflex mechanisms.

In vivo experiments demonstrated the following effects of Viozan on sensory nerves:
- Inhibition of histamine-induced discharge of rapidly adapting stretch receptors in β-blocked dogs: the activity of Viozan could be blocked with the D_2-receptor antagonist, sulpiride [6].
- Inhibition of capsaicin-induced plasma protein extravasation in rat indicating an effect on neurogenic inflammation: the activity of Viozan was again antagonised by the D_2-receptor antagonist, sulpiride [11].

Experiments in the β-blocked dog demonstrated the following effects of Viozan on reflex-mediated mechanisms:
- Inhibition of histamine-induced tachypnoea: the tachypnoea is reflex in origin as demonstrated by cooling or cutting the vagus. The activity of Viozan could be blocked with the peripherally acting D_2-receptor antagonist, domperidone [11]. Of note, in dogs that were not β-blocked, $β_2$-adrenoceptor agonists had no effect in this model.
- Inhibition of ammonia-induced mucus production: the mucus production is reflex in origin since it can be inhibited by cooling the vagus and reversed by rewarming. The activity of Viozan was again antagonised by domperidone [11]. In dogs that were not β-blocked, $β_2$-adrenoceptor agonists and ipratropium bromide had no effect on this reflex response [12].
- Inhibition of capsaicin-induced cough in conscious dogs [11]: reversal was demonstrated with domperidone.

$β_2$-Mediated Properties. In vitro, using the isolated superfused field stimulated guinea pig trachea preparation, Viozan had a rapid onset of action and a longer duration of action than formoterol and salbutamol [13].

In vivo the $β_2$-adrenoceptor activity was characterised in dogs, against a histamine-induced bronchoconstriction [14]. In this model, Viozan inhibited bronchoconstriction in a dose-dependent manner. The duration of protection of Viozan was equivalent to that of salmeterol, lasting for 10 h, and was greater than that of formoterol and salbutamol [13].

Comparison of D_2 and $β_2$ Potencies. Relative D_2- and $β_2$-receptor in vivo potencies of Viozan can be directly compared in the dog. Comparing ED_{50} values in the histamine-induced tachypnoea (D_2) and the histamine-induced bronchoconstriction ($β_2$), Viozan possesses $D_2 = β_2$ activity. In addition, compounds with $D_2 > β_2$ and $D_2 < β_2$ potency ratios have been discovered, and selected compounds are undergoing further drug development [15].

Determination of Therapeutic Index. D_2-receptor agonists have the potential to induce emesis. In order to minimise this undesirable effect, all compounds were selected on the basis of the separation of their topical pharmacodynamic D_2 activity from their emetic activity in the dog. The absorption and metabolism of Viozan show rapid first pass metabolism to a glucuronide and low bioavailability, thus minimising systemic exposure. As a result, Viozan has a therapeutic index greater than 30 in the dog [11].

Clinical Studies. The efficacy and safety of Viozan have been assessed in phase II studies in symptomatic COPD patients with a history of smoking. These studies were double blind, group comparator, placebo-controlled multinational studies in which approximately 800 patients completed treatment.

In a 6-week dose-ranging study [16], compared with placebo, Viozan dose dependently
- improved individual symptom scores for cough, sputum production, breathlessness and total symptom score;
- improved morning and evening peak flow;
- reduced the requirement for rescue medication;
- improved health status quality of life as measured by St. George's Respiratory Questionnaire on total score and the individual three quality of life domains,
- showed positive opinion of efficacy by both patient and investigator.

In a 4-week treatment period, placebo-controlled study, Viozan was compared with the standard therapies for COPD, salbutamol and ipratropium bromide. In this study, Viozan was significantly better than salbutamol and ipratropium bromide at improving the total symptom score of cough, sputum production and breathlessness in COPD patients [17].

In all studies, Viozan was well tolerated and any side effects were attributable to the $β_2$-properties of the compound. There was no evidence of a potential for nausea and vomiting compared to the control placebo groups. This confirmed the preclinical studies in the dog showing a clear separation between therapeutic effects and emesis.

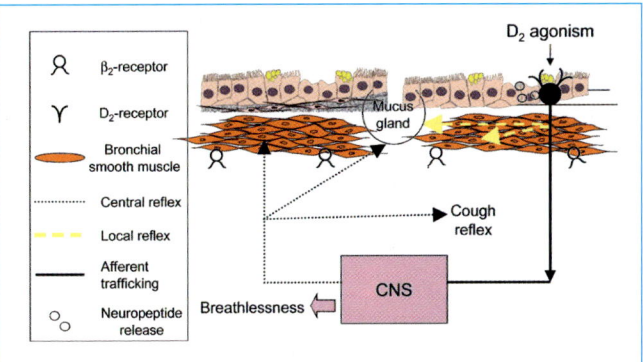

Fig. 3. Mechanism of action of Viozan. D_2-agonism modulates sensory afferent nerves, inhibiting local axon reflexes, the local release of neuropeptides and afferent trafficking to the CNS resulting in inhibition of central reflexes. β_2-Agonism relaxes airway smooth muscle, providing functional antagonism of bronchoconstrictor mechanisms.

Conclusion

We have discovered a novel class of dual D_2-receptor and β_2-adrenoceptor agonists. These molecules are able to modulate pulmonary sensory nerve activity and hence inhibit cough, mucus production and breathlessness in animal models. Preclinical data suggest that these effects are attributable to the activation of D_2-receptors on sensory nerves (fig. 3). The β_2-activity provides the added benefit of bronchodilatation. The first-in-class compound, Viozan, is currently in late clinical development for the treatment of COPD and it has been shown to have significant efficacy in improving symptoms of cough, sputum production, breathlessness and health status quality of life. D_2-receptor-mediated inhibition of sensory nerve processes in the airways is a novel approach to the management of COPD.

References

1 Murray CJL, Lopez AD: Alternative projections of mortality and disability by cause 1990–2020: Global burden of disease study. Lancet 1997;349:1498–1504.
2 Undem BJ, Riccio MM: Activation of airway afferent nerves; in Barnes PJ, Grunstein MM, Leff AR, Woolcock AJ (eds): Asthma. Philadelphia, Lippincott-Raven, 1997, pp 1009–1025.
3 Missale C, Nash SR, Robinson SW, Jaber M, Caron MG: Dopamine receptors: From structure to function. Physiol Rev 1998;78:189–225.
4 Xie G-X, Jones K, Peroutka SJ, Palmer PP: Detection of mRNAs and alternatively spliced transcripts of dopamine receptors in rat peripheral sensory and sympathetic ganglia. Brain Res 1998;785:129–135.
5 Ilhan M, Long JP: Inhibition of the sympathetic nervous system by dopamine. Arch Int Pharmacodyn Ther 1975;216:4–10.
6 Jackson DM, Simpson WT: The effect of dopamine on the rapidly adapting receptors in the dog lung. Pulmonary Pharmacol Ther 2000;13:39–42.
7 Brown RA, Dixon JD, Farmer JB, Hall C, Humphries RG, Ince F, O'Conner SE, Smith GW: Dopexamine: A novel agonist at peripheral dopamine receptors and β_2-adrenoceptors. Br J Pharmacol 1985;85:599–608.
8 Weinstock J, Gaitanopoulus DE, Stringer OD, Franz RG, Heible JP, Kinter LB, Mann WA, Flaim KE, Gessner G: Synthesis and evaluation of non-catechol D-1 and D-2 dopamine receptor agonists: Benzimidazol-2-one, benzoxazol-2-one, and the highly potent benzothiazol-2-one 7-ethylamines. J Med Chem 1987;30:1166–1176.
9 Bonnert RV, Brown RC, Chapman D, Cheshire DR, Dixon J, Ince F, Kinchin EC, Lyons AJ, Davis AM, Hallam C, Harper ST, Unitt JF, Dougall IG, Jackson DM, McKechnie K, Young A, Simpson WT: Dual D_2-receptor and β_2-adrenoceptor agonists for the treatment of airway diseases. 1. Discovery and biological evaluation of some 7-(2-aminoethyl)-4-hydroxybenzothiazol-2(3H)-one analogues. J Med Chem 1998;41:4915–4917.
10 Dougall IG, Fagura MS, Lydford SJ, Harper D, McKechnie KCW, Brown RC, Ince F: The in vitro pharmacology of AR-C68397AA, a novel dual D_2-receptor and β_2-adrenoceptor agonist. Am J Resp Crit Care Med 1999;A796.
11 Young A, Dougall IG, Blackham A, Jackson DM, Hallam C, Harper S, Ince F: AR-C68397AA: The first dual D_2-receptor and β_2-adrenoceptor agonist. Am J Resp Crit Care Med 1999;159:A522.
12 Young A, Blackham A, Taylor CV, Vendy K, Harper ST, Mistry H, Hallam C: Reflex mucus production in the anaesthetised dog. Eur Resp J 1998;12(suppl 29):66s, P509.
13 Mohammed SP, Dougall IG, Taylor CV, Ince F, Blackham A, Young A: The β_2-adrenoceptor activity and duration of action of AR-C68397AA: An in vitro and in vivo comparison. Am J Resp Crit Care Med 1999;159:A813.
14 Young A, Blackham A, Taylor CV: Activity of inhaled β_2 agonists in the anaesthetised dog. Eur Resp J 1998;12(suppl 29):68s, P521.
15 Dougall I, Fagura M, Young A, Blackham A, Taylor C, Brown R, Cheshire D, Bonnert R, Ince F: Novel dual D_2-receptor and β_2-adrenoceptor agonists with varying ratios of activity. Am J Resp Crit Care Med 2000;161:A435.
16 Wenzel S, Ind PW, Laursen LC, Deamer L, Nyström P, Rocchiccioli K: Viozan™ (AR-C68397AA) reduces breathlessness, cough and sputum production in COPD patients. Am J Resp Crit Care Med, submitted.
17 Laitinen LA, Laursen LC, Wouters E, Lloyd J, Blackshaw R, Rocchiccioli K: Efficay of Viozan™ (AR-C68397AA) versus salbutamol and ipratropium bromide in the management of COPD. Am J Resp Crit Care 2000;161:A190.

Paul Newbold
AstraZeneca R & D Charnwood
Bakewell Road
Loughborough LE 11 5RH (UK)
Tel. +44 1509 645376, Fax +44 1509 645599
E-Mail Paul.Newbold@astrazeneca.com

Anticholinergics: Tiotropium

Bernd Disse[a] Theodore J. Witek, Jr.[b]

[a]Boehringer Ingelheim Clinical Research Institute, Ingelheim/Rhein, Germany, and
[b]Boehringer Ingelheim Pharmaceuticals Inc., Ridgefield, Conn., USA

Summary

Anticholinergic bronchodilators have transformed from a fascinating ancient history of inhaling smoke from medicinal plants to the present day formulations of N-quaternary compounds such as ipratropium bromide. Ipratropium has emerged as important maintenance therapy, particularly in COPD. Recently, the new generation compound tiotropium (Spiriva®) has been shown to have unique pharmacologic properties, among the most important being its prolonged binding to muscarinic receptors. In clinical trials, this property has translated into effective once-daily bronchodilation in patients with COPD with persistent improvement before the next administration at trough (at end of dosing interval, 24 h after administration). Preliminary evaluations of health outcomes have been encouraging, including the effect of tiotropium on dyspnea and quality of life.

Mechanism of Action

There are several pathophysiologic components that contribute to the morbidity and mortality of COPD. These include mucus hypersecretion, dyscrinia and chronic productive cough (simple chronic bronchitis), airflow obstruction in the large airways, destruction of the lung periphery (emphysema) resulting in obstruction of peripheral airways and impaired gas exchange [1, 2]. In COPD, vagal tone mediated through the action of acetylcholine (ACh) at parasympathetic ganglia and neuromuscular junctions at bronchial smooth muscle may either be increased, as suggested by Gross et al. [3], and/or may provoke a higher degree of obstruction for geometric reasons if applied on top of thickened (edematous) or mucus-laden airway walls [4]. The airflow obstruction in COPD may show less reversibility to bronchodilators than in asthma and many studies have shown anticholinergics to be more effective than β_2-agonists [5–7]. Higher doses of anticholinergics may reduce the hypersecretion and expectoration, as shown following 8 weeks of treatment with 200 μg of oxitropium t.i.d. [8]. For these reasons, antagonists at muscarinic ACh receptors like ipratropium bromide are the bronchodilators of choice in COPD [1, 2, 9].

Tiotropium, like atropine and ipratropium (fig. 1), is a competitive antagonist of ACh at muscarinic receptors of the M_1 to M_5 subtype. At the receptors of airway smooth muscle or mucus glands, antagonism of ACh results in smooth muscle relaxation and inhibition of mucus secretion [10]. This competitive antagonism has been demonstrated in man using challenges with the agonist methacholine [11]. Here, tiotropium provided long-lasting protection from airway contraction, as evidenced by the increasing doses of methacholine necessary to reduce airway function as measured by FEV_1, i.e., $PC_{20}FEV_1$ (fig. 2).

The first clinical evidence of reduction of cholinergic tone with tiotropium was reported by Maesen et al. [12] who observed long-lasting increases in airflow following a single dose. These observations set the stage for development of the first once-daily-inhaled bronchodilator for treatment of COPD [13].

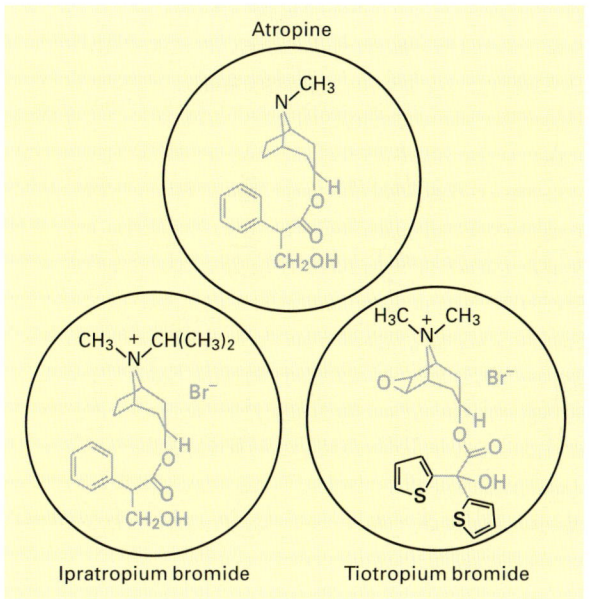

Fig. 1. The chemical structures of three generations of anticholinergic agents: atropine, ipratropium and tiotropium.

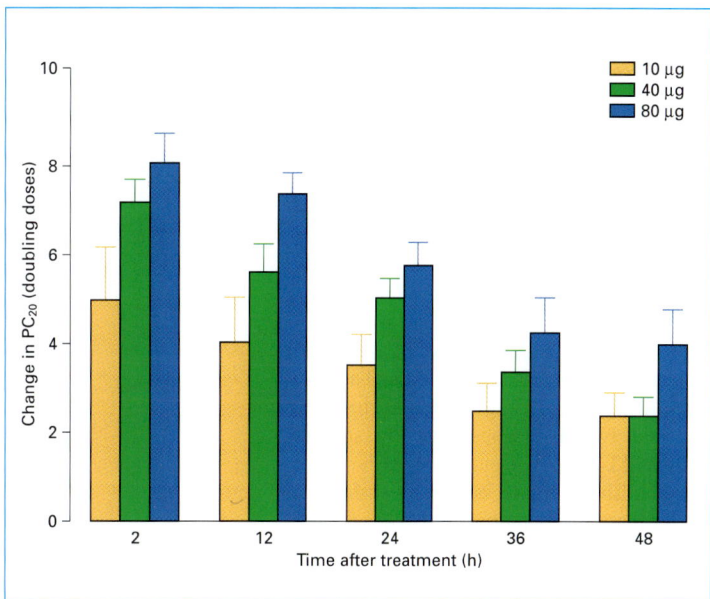

Fig. 2. Changes in PC_{20} from placebo, for each dose of tiotropium at each time point after treatment, expressed in terms of doubling dose protection (means ± SEM). From O'Connor et al. [11].

Table 1. Binding affinity of antimuscarinics and dissociation half-lives of the receptor-drug complexes

	Tiotropium		Ipratropium	
	K_D, nM	$t_{½}$, h	K_D, nM	$t_{½}$, h
M_1	0.041	14.6	0.183	0.11
M_2	0.021	3.6	0.195	0.035
M_3	0.014	34.7	0.204	0.26

Binding affinity to membrane preparations from Chinese hamster ovary K1 cells expressing human muscarinic receptors, kinetically determined at 23°C. Dissociation half-lives from 3–5 triplicate experiments [17].

Preclinical Pharmacology and Toxicology

In vitro pharmacologic studies have shown tiotropium to be a specific, highly potent antagonist at all subtypes of muscarinic receptors M_1 to M_5 showing slow dissociation with a half-life of around one day as compared to about 15 min with e.g. ipratropium (table 1) [14]. Tiotropium, similar to ipratropium, is in the classical view not subtype-selective; however, dissociation from M_2 is faster than from M_1 or M_3 (table 1) which, in functional experiments, manifested a kinetic receptor subtype selectivity of M_3 and M_1 over M_2. This feature has been demonstrated in the experiments of Takahashi et al. [15] explained in figure 3. Incubation of guinea pig tracheas in vitro with tiotropium and subsequent washout showed that inhibition of electrical field stimulation-induced contraction (M_3) persisted much longer than increased junctional ACh release (M_2). Using atropine, both effects were of short duration.

Further support for the slow dissociation of tiotropium from muscarinic receptors providing prolonged duration of functional effects was demonstrated in the test system of methacholine-stimulated ciliary beating [14]. Anticholinergics do not influence basal beat frequency. However, following near-maximal ciliary beat stimulation with methacholine, tiotropium or ipratropium can completely block this cholinergic response. Upon continuing wash of the drugs and re-introduction of methacholine, stimulation of beat frequency was reestablished at the first measurement 16 min after switching from ipratropium and not until 82 min after tiotropium.

The long duration of action was also confirmed in dogs and guinea pigs following inhalation of the drug [14]. In the latter species, a single inhalation provided protection from asphyxia induced by ACh aerosol for more than 24 h.

Toxicology studies performed with in vitro systems, or mice, rats, dogs and rabbits following inhalational, oral and parenteral administration for up to 2 years have demonstrated a wide safety margin. Systemic antimuscarinic

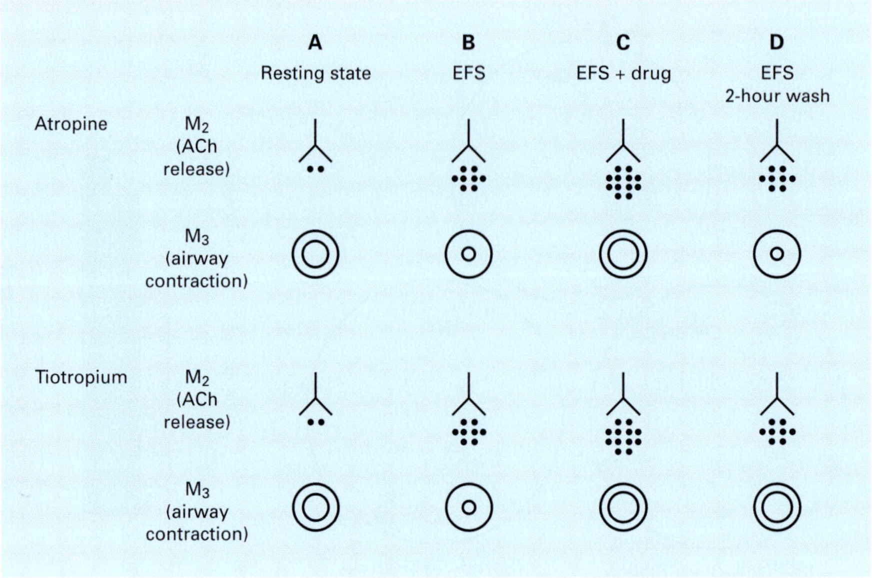

Fig. 3. The functional relevance of kinetic receptor subtype selectivity following tiotropium. Electrical-field stimulation (EFS) of guinea pig trachea leads to junctional ACh release and twitch contraction of the airway smooth muscle (A, B). Atropine and tiotropium equally enhanced the EFS-induced neuronal ACh release (prejunctional autoreceptor: M_2). Both drugs inhibited the EFS-induced twitch response (airway smooth muscle: M_3) (C). The enhanced ACh release was abolished 2 h after beginning washout of both drugs, at which time the airway smooth muscle contraction was still inhibited by tiotropium, but not after atropine (D).

effects and their sequelae were observed at higher doses and prolonged periods of exposure: inhibition of salivary and lacrimal secretion leading to dry oral mucosa or conjunctivitis, increase in heart rate, coprostasis. Substance-related mortality did not occur up to and including the high dose of about 500 μg/kg in 1-year studies in rats and dogs. Genotoxicity studies, reproduction studies and carcinogenicity studies up to 2 years did not reveal any mutagenic, teratogenic or carcinogenic potential of the drug.

The preclinical profile supports the drug to be safe and effective. The antimuscarinic responses in these preclinical test systems support the kinetic subtype selectivity of tiotropium and its long duration of action. Subtype selectivity may translate into higher efficacy (maximum effect obtainable), but this may be difficult to differentiate from higher potency (efficacious at lower doses) considering that huge parallel-group chronic dose ranging studies in patients with COPD would be required. Receptor-dissociation-mediated long duration of action is the effect that unequivocally has translated into a distinctive characteristic in clinical therapeutics.

Formulations and Device

The core clinical development of tiotropium utilizes a lactose-based powder formulation containing 18 μg of active substance. The first device with tiotropium submitted for marketing authorization will be the HandiHaler®. This device uses a single capsule which is placed in the device and is pierced when the patient presses a button. Upon inhalation, the capsule vibrates and its contents are inhaled via the inspiratory air stream. Capsule evacuation occurs at a flow rate threshold of 15–20 liters/min with patients with COPD of all severities achieving sufficient flow rates through the device [16]. Additional device developments are ongoing.

Human Pharmacology

Human pharmacology trials have demonstrated that tiotropium is well tolerated with known anticholinergic effects manifesting at doses severalfold the recommended therapeutic dose. Decreases in airway resistance, albeit of relatively small magnitude, confirmed the intended pulmonary pharmacodynamic response, even in healthy subjects. This indirectly confirms the presence of cholinergic airway tone in normal airways. The most common side effect was dry mouth explained by the fact that the next sensitive anticholinergic effect after airway smooth muscle relaxation in man is reduction in salivary secretion. In multiple-dose studies, there were no significant drug effects on heart rate or on pupillary diameter.

Pharmacokinetic evaluations of inhaled tiotropium in patients with COPD have demonstrated steady-state plasma levels after a linear accumulation period of less than 3 weeks. Beyond this time, plasma levels remain constant and the increase from single dose trough level (before next dose) to multiple-dose trough level is about a factor of two. Peak plasma tiotropium levels reach about 14 pg/ml 5 min post-dose with a subsequent rapid decline in less than 1 h to very low levels (~ 2 pg/ml range). At these low levels, plasma tiotropium was eliminated with a terminal

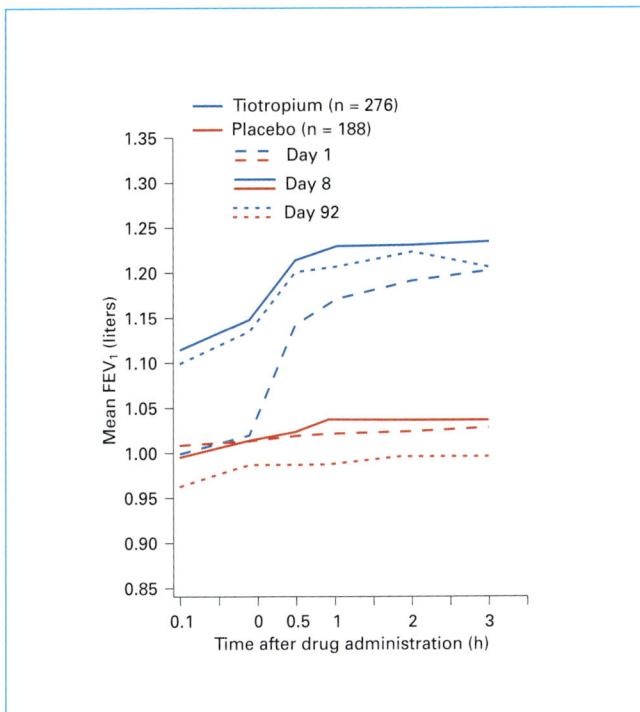

Fig. 4. The bronchodilating effects of once-daily tiotropium as evidenced by improvement in FEV_1 over 90 days. Note the improved trough response, i.e. FEV_1 improvement prior to dosing. SE for difference ranged from 0.01 to 0.02 liters. Difference is highly statistically significant ($p < 0.01$) after treatment administration. Means adjusted for the center effects and baseline. From Casaburi et al. [20].

Table 2. Improvement in airflow, dyspnea and quality of life in 1-year studies with tiotropium

Day	ΔFEV_1		TDI	SGRQ impact	SGRQ total
	trough	6-hour average			
0	–	0.15 ± 0.02			
50	0.13 ± 0.02	0.22 ± 0.02	0.9 ± 0.23	–2.1 ± 1.06	–2.3 ± 0.92
92	0.14 ± 0.02	0.20 ± 0.02	1.0 ± 0.24	–2.4 ± 1.21	–2.4 ± 1.05
176	0.16 ± 0.02	0.23 ± 0.02	1.0 ± 0.26	–4.5 ± 1.30	–4.1 ± 1.15
260	0.15 ± 0.02	0.20 ± 0.02	1.1 ± 0.27	–3.5 ± 1.30	–3.3 ± 1.19
344	0.15 ± 0.02	0.21 ± 0.02	1.1 ± 0.28	–4.6 ± 1.29	–4.1 ± 1.18

Preliminary data from 1-year clinical trial in COPD comparing tiotropium to placebo. Improvements in FEV_1 are accompanied by improvement in transitional dyspnea index (TDI) and health status as measured by St. George's Respiratory Questionnaire (SGRQ). ΔFEV_1 describes the mean difference ± SE between tiotropium and placebo in change from baseline for trough and the 6 h following inhalation of medication. TDI was measured as mean difference ± SE between tiotropium and placebo. A higher value of greater than 1 indicates clinically meaningful improvement. SGRQ impact domain and total score are reported as mean difference between tiotropium and placebo ± SE. A reduction in score by 4 points indicates a clinically significant improvement. All data are from San Pedro et al. [22], ZuWallack et al. [23] and Mahler et al. [24].

half life of 5–6 days, regardless of dose inhaled [17, 18]. At even the peak levels attainable in plasma, it can be predicted that systemic receptor occupancy would be low (e.g. 6%). At such levels, effects from systemic blockage would also be expected to be minimal [17]. These theoretical predictions, however, are being evaluated in long-term observations in man.

COPD Trials

The single-dose results in hyperreactive asthmatics [11] and patients with COPD [12] have already been reviewed as confirmatory clinical evidence in the section 'Mechanism of Action'. The first multiple-dose clinical trial in COPD was reported by Littner et al. [19] who observed significant bronchodilation over dose ranges of 4.5–36 μg. There was little dose dependency in FEV_1 among higher doses than the 4.5-μg dose. The primary endpoint in this trial was the trough FEV_1, i.e. the spirometric values measured 23–24 h after dosing. This endpoint was chosen to document the persistent efficacy just before the next dose and reflects the prolonged duration of action. After 4 weeks once-daily inhalation of 18 μg the trough FEV_1 was 0.13 liters above study baseline, not much lower than the 6-hour average (0.15 liters) immediately following the inhalation.

The core clinical development program consisted of four trials of 1 year duration. The basic design elements can be found in the reports of Casaburi et al. [20] and Van Noord et al. [21]. Bronchodilation with once-daily dosing has been established with long-term administration (fig. 4). Preliminary reports [22–24] from 1-year observations have confirmed the effectiveness of tiotropium as a once-daily bronchodilator.

Overall proportions of patients with adverse events were balanced across treatment groups as were serious events, events leading to study withdrawal, and death. The most common adverse event was dry mouth, occurring in approximately 15% of patients receiving tiotropium in the 1-year studies. Dry mouth was mild in the vast majority of cases and was associated with trial withdrawal in less than 0.5% of patients.

In addition to the ability of tiotropium to provide significant and sustained bronchodilation without evidence of tachyphylaxis, preliminary reports highlight significant improvements in dyspnea in both patient and caregiver assessments. Furthermore, significant benefits in health related quality of life were observed over both, placebo and ipratropium bromide (table 2).

Conclusion

Anticholinergic agents have emerged as important first-line therapy in patients with COPD. The sustained bronchodilation even present at trough achieved with once-daily inhalation represents a significant advance in therapeutics. More importantly, the preliminary reports of improved dyspnea and health-related quality of life can translate into meaningful impact on patients with a significant degree of chronic airflow obstruction.

References

1 ERS Consensus Statement: Optimal assessment and management of chronic obstructive pulmonary disease (COPD). Eur Respir 1995; 8:1398–1420.
2 Ferguson GT, Cherniack RM: Management of chronic obstructive pulmonary disease. N Engl J Med 1993;328:1017–1022.
3 Gross NJ, Evangeline CO, Skorodin MS: Cholinergic bronchomotor tone in COPD. Estimates of its amount in comparison with that in normal subjects. Chest 1989;96:984–987.
4 Gross NJ, Skorodin MS: State of the art, anticholinergic, antimuscarinic bronchodilators. Am Rev Respir Dis 1984;129:856–870.
5 Braun SR, McKenzie WN, Copeland C, Knight L, Ellersieck M: A comparison of the effect of ipratropium and albuterol in the treatment of chronic obstructive airway disease. Arch Intern Med 1989;149:544–547.
6 Rennard SI, Serby CW, Ghafouri Mo, Johnson PA, Friedman M: Extended therapy with ipratropium is associated with improved lung function in patients with COPD. Chest 1996;110: 62–70.
7 Calverly PMA: Symptomatic bronchodilator treatment; in Calverly PMA, Pride NB (eds): Chronic Obstructive Pulmonary Disease. London, Chapman & Hall, 1995, pp 419–446.
8 Tamaoki J, Chiyotani A, Tagaya B, Sakai N, Konno K: Effect of long term treatment with oxitropium bromide on airway secretion in chronic bronchitis and panbronchiolitis. Thorax 1994;49:545–548.
9 American Thoracic Society. Standardization of spirometry: 1994 update. Am J Respir Crit Care Med 1995;152:1107–1136.
10 Barnes PJ: Muscarinic receptor subtypes in airways. Life Sci 1993;52:521–527.
11 O'Connor BJ, Towse LJ, Barnes PJ: Prolonged effect of tiotropium bromide on methacholine-induced bronchoconstriction in asthma. Am J Respir Crit Care Med 1996;154:876–880.
12 Maesen FPV, Smeets JJ, Costongs MAL, Wald FDM, Cornelissen PJG: BA 679 BR, a new long-acting antimuscarinic bronchodilator: A pilot dose-escalation study. Eur Respir J 1993; 6:1031–1036.
13 Witek TJ, Souhrada JF, Serby CW, Disse B: Tiotropium (Ba679). Pharmacology and early clinical observations; in Spector SS (ed): Anticholinergics in the Upper and Lower Airways. New York, Dekker, 1999, pp 137–152.
14 Disse B, Reichl R, Speck G, Traunecker W, Rominger KL, Hammer R: BA 679 BR, a novel long-acting anticholinergic bronchodilator. Life Sci 1993;52:537–544.
15 Takahaski T, Belvisi MG, Patel H, Ward JK, Tadjkarimi S, Yocub MH, Barnes PJ: Effect of BA679 BR: A novel long-acting anticholinergic agent, on cholinergic neurotransmission in guinea pig and human airways. Am J Respir Crit Care Med 1994;150:1640–1645.
16 Chodosh S, Flanders J, Serby CW, Hochrainer D, Witek, TJ: Effective use of Handihaler® dry powder inhalation system over a range of COPD disease severity (abstract). Am J Respir Crit Care Med 1999;159:A524.
17 Disse B, Speck GA, Rominger KL, Witek TJ, Hammer R: Tiotropium (Spiriva): Mechanistical considerations and clinical profile in obstructive lung disease. Life Sci 1999;64:457–464.
18 Disse B, Rominger K, Serby CW, Souhrada JF, Witek TJ: The pharmacokinetic (PK) profile of tiotropium during long-term treatment in stable COPD (abstract). Am J Respir Crit Care Med 1999;159:A524.
19 Littner M, Auerbach D, Campbell S, Dunn L, Friedman M, Illowite J, Tashkin D, Taylor J, Menjoge S, Serby CW, Witek TJ: The bronchodilator effects of tiotropium in stable COPD. Am J Respir Crit Care Med 1997;155: A282.
20 Casaburi R, Briggs Jr. DD, Donohue JF, Serby CW, Menjoge SS, Witek TJ for the US Tiotropium Study Group: The spirometric efficacy of once-daily dosing with tiotropium in stable COPD: A 13-week multi-center trial, submitted.
21 Van Noord JA, Bantje ThA, Eland ME, Korducki L, Cornelissen PJG, on behalf of the Dutch Tiotropium Study Group: A randomised controlled comparison of tiotropium and ipratropium in the treatment of chronic obstructive pulmonary disease. Thorax 2000;55: 289–294.
22 San Pedro G, Elias DJ, Serby CW, Witek TJ for the American Study Group. Tiotropium (Spiriva™): One-year bronchodilator efficacy established with once-daily dosing in COPD patients. Am J Respir Crit Care Med 2000;161: A749.
23 ZuWallack R, Jones PW, Kotch A, Goodwin B, Menjoge SS, Serby CW for the American Study Group: Tiotropium (Spiriva™) improves health status in patients with COPD. Am J Respir Crit Care Med 2000;161:A892.
24 Mahler DA, Montner P, Brazinsky SA, Goodwin B, Menjoge SS, Witek TJ: Tiotropium (Spiriva™), a new long-acting anticholinergic bronchodilator, improves dyspnea in patients with COPD. Am J Respir Crit Care Med 2000; 161:A892.

Bernd Disse, MD, PhD
Boehringer Ingelheim Clinical Research
Institute, Department of Respiratory Medicine
Boehringer Ingelheim GmbH
D–55216 Ingelheim/Rhein (Germany)
Tel. +49 6132 77 3992, Fax +49 6132 77 3818
E-Mail disse@ing.boehringer-ingelheim.com

Potassium Channel Openers

Agents for the Treatment of Airway Hyperreactivity

John R. Fozard   Paul W. Manley

Preclinical Research, Novartis Pharma Ltd., Basel, Switzerland

Summary

ATP-sensitive potassium (K_{ATP}) channels link the metabolic status of the cell to the plasma membrane potential and thus play a key role in regulating cellular excitability. K_{ATP} channel openers (KCOs) may impact positively on respiratory disease by suppressing bronchoconstriction, mucus hypersecretion, cough and airway hyperreactivity (AHR). A major recent development is the emergence of KCOs which can obviate experimental AHR at doses which are devoid of cardiovascular effects. This new generation of compounds with selectivity for the airways may constitute a new class of drugs for the treatment of asthma.

ATP-sensitive potassium (K_{ATP}) channels are found in a wide variety of tissues, including skeletal and smooth muscle cells, secretory cells (such as insulin-secreting pancreatic β-cells), cardiac myocytes and neurons [1–3]. Conceptually, the presence of K_{ATP} channels in bronchiolar smooth muscle [2] and airway sensory and autonomic neurons [4] raises the possibility of their involvement in the pathophysiology of respiratory disease through the modulation of direct and reflex-induced bronchoconstriction [5], mucus secretion [6] and cough [7]. In practice, it is the phenomenon of airway hyperreactivity (AHR), whose underlying mechanisms remain ill-defined [8, 9], which is emerging as the key target with clinical relevance to respiratory disease [10]. For this reason, the emphasis in this review will be placed on the role and therapeutic significance of K_{ATP} channels in the phenomenon of AHR.

Mechanism of Action

Potassium channel openers (KCOs) act by stimulating ion flux through a distinct class of potassium channels which are inhibited by intracellular ATP and activated by intracellular nucleoside diphosphates. Such K_{ATP} channels link the metabolic status of the cells to the plasma membrane potential and in this way play a key role in regulating cellular activity [1–3]. In most excitatory cells, K_{ATP} channels are closed under normal physiological conditions and open when the tissue is metabolically compromised (e.g. when the [ATP]:[ADP] ratio falls). This promotes K^+ efflux and the cell hyperpolarizes, thereby preventing voltage-operated Ca^{2+} channels (VOCs) from opening (fig. 1). K_{ATP} channels are composed of a pore-forming tetrameric complex of inward rectifying K^+ channel (K_{ir}) subunits (either $K_{ir}6.1$ or $K_{ir}6.2$), with each subunit being associated with a regulating protein of the sulphonylurea receptor type (SUR1, SUR2A or SUR2B) [11, 12] (table 1). SUR proteins are members of the ATP-binding-cassette transporter family and their nucleotide-binding domains are believed to render the K_{ATP} channels sensitive to [ATP]/[ADP]. SURs are also the target proteins for KCOs [14]. It is likely that the various combinations of SUR and $K_{ir}6$ subunits account for the clear differences between K_{ATP} channels in various tissues, with respect to their channel properties and sensitivity to ligands which both activate and inhibit their opening (table 1).

Range of Therapies

K_{ATP} channels are activated by a diverse group of compounds which include the anti-hypertensive agents, minoxidil sulphate, diazoxide and pinacidil, as well as a variety of benzopyran derivatives such as levcromakalim (or its racemate, cromakalim), SDZ PCO 400, bimakalim, JTV 506, YM 934, KC-399, BRL 55834, rilmakalim and SDZ 217-744 (fig. 2). Only the benzopyran derivatives have been profiled as therapies for asthma [15]. K_{ATP} channels are inhibited by sulphonylurea derivatives, such as glibenclamide and tolbutamide, and the high affinity of these agents for K_{ATP} channels in pancreatic β-cells is the

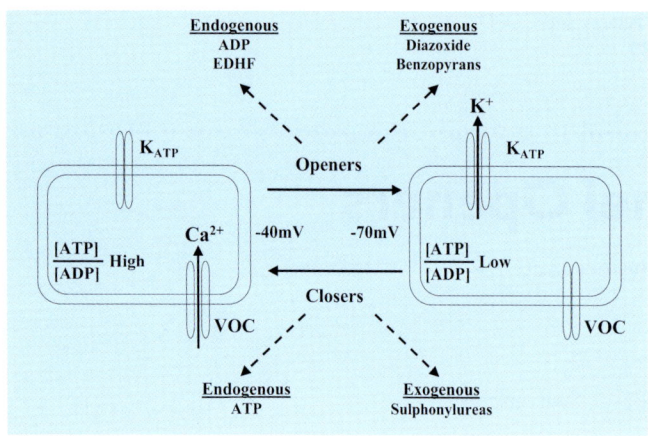

Fig. 1. Diagrammatic representation of the role of K_{ATP} channels in cell excitability. For further details see text.

Table 1. Composition and pharmacological properties of K_{ATP} channels in different tissues

Tissue	Channel composition	Inhibition by glibenclamide IC$_{50}$, µM	Activation by diazoxide EC$_{50}$, µM	Activation by levcromakalim EC$_{50}$, µM
Pancreatic β-cell	(SUR1/ K$_{ir}$6.2)$_4$	0.005–0.030	20–100	>100
Cardiac myocyte	(SUR2A/ K$_{ir}$6.2)$_4$	0.003–0.005	>500	300
Vascular myocyte	(SUR2B/ K$_{ir}$6.1)$_4$	0.025	200	0.5
Skeletal muscle	(SUR2B/ K$_{ir}$6.2)$_4$	0.01–0.2	>500	>100
Neurons	(SUR1/ K$_{ir}$6.2)$_4$[1]	2.1[2]	<200	not available

From Quast [1], Quayle et al. [2], Fujita and Kurachi [3], Babenko et al. [11] and Sakura et al. [13].
[1] A novel SUR variant, SUR1B [13].
[2] Figure refers to inhibition by the sulphonylurea, tolbutamide.

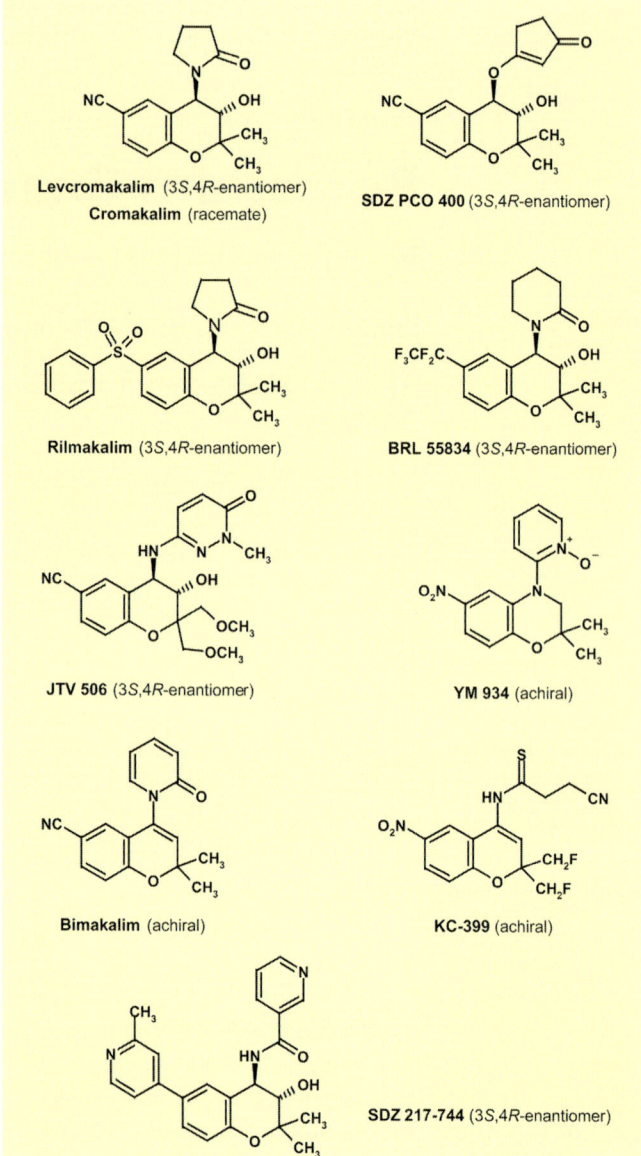

Fig. 2. KCOs profiled for asthma.

basis for their efficacy in stimulating insulin release and use in diabetes [1, 16].

Rationale for the Utility of Potassium Channel Openers in Airway Hyperreactivity

The heightened sensitivity of the airways of asthmatics to a range of bronchoconstrictor stimuli which do not usually affect normal subjects is a defining feature of asthma [17]. The phenomenon, termed bronchial (or airway) hyperreactivity (AHR), results in facilitation of bronchospasm and contributes to the airway obstruction characteristic of asthma [8, 9, 18–20]. The principal clinical symptoms of asthma, wheezing and breathlessness are a direct consequence of airway obstruction. Although the underlying mechanisms of AHR in asthma are unknown, both preclinical and clinical evidence points to an increased excitability of smooth muscle cells and/or the nervous elements of the airways as important contributory factors [18, 19]. By increasing the efflux of potassium from these cells, KCOs would induce hyperpolarization and a decrease in responsiveness to excitatory stimuli.

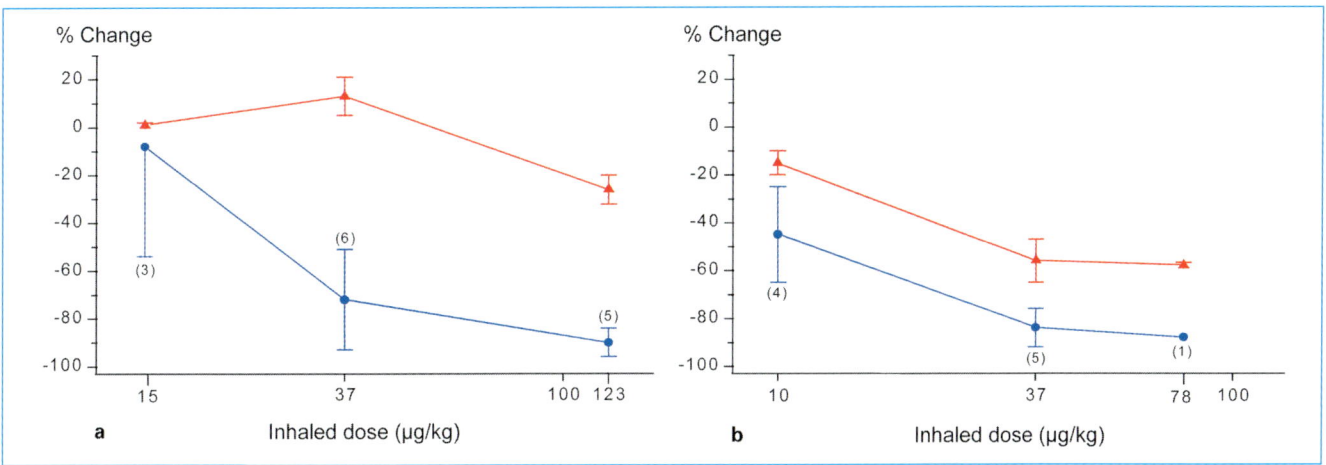

Fig. 3. Dose-response curves for the effects of SDZ 217-744 (**a**) and bimakalim (**b**) given by aerosol inhalation on the bronchoconstrictor response to inhaled methacholine (●) and diastolic blood pressure (▲) in the anaesthetized rhesus monkey. Effects were measured 5 min after the end of drug administration and are the maxima observed at each dose level. Mean values (± SEM) of the number of individual experiments shown in parentheses are presented. For further details see text.

Effects of Potassium Channel Openers in Animal Models of Airway Hyperreactivity

AHR can be induced in guinea pigs by intravenous administration of immune complexes [21, 22] or exposure to ozone [23]. Representative KCOs reverse AHR when administered locally to the airways although there are significant differences between these agents in their potencies in the two models (table 2). KCOs are significantly more potent in reversing AHR than in inducing bronchodilation in animals with normoreactive airways [20, 22]. The effects of bimakalim to suppress AHR can be blocked by pretreatment of the animals with glibenclamide, which is consistent with the involvement of K_{ATP} channels in the response [24]. The first generation KCOs, levcromakalim, bimakalim and YM 934, markedly reduce blood pressure at the doses required to inhibit AHR. In contrast, BRL 55834, JTV 506 and particularly SDZ 217-744, showed a clear separation between the two activities (table 2). Unlike salbutamol, SDZ 217-744 does not cause AHR on prolonged administration to guinea pigs; indeed, concomitant administration of SDZ 217-744 inhibits AHR induced in the same model by chronic administration of salbutamol [25]. Confirmation of the difference between first- and second-generation KCOs with respect to their therapeutic ratios for inhibiting AHR and inducing cardiovascular effects has come from experiments in rhesus monkeys (fig. 3). Thus, in animals displaying spontaneous AHR, bimakalim and SDZ 217-744 were found to be potent inhibitors of methacholine-induced bronchoconstriction.

Table 2. Comparison of potencies of benzopyran-type KCOs for their inhibition of AHR in guinea pigs induced by either immune complex (IC-AHR) or ozone (O_3-AHR) compared with their potencies in reducing mean arterial blood pressure (ΔBP)

Compound	IC-AHR ED_{50}, μg/kg	O_3-AHR ED_{50}, μg/kg	ΔBP ED_{20}, μg/kg
Levcromakalim	22	n.d.	10
Bimakalim	0.5	0.3	2
Rilmakalim	0.2	n.d.	10
JTV 506	0.5	n.d.	19
SDZ PCO 400	3.2	n.d.	30
YM 934	2.1	>100	3.4
BRL 55834	0.1	>100	10
SDZ 217-744	0.08	3	>100

From Buchheit and Hofmann [22], Yeadon et al. [23] and Buchheit [unpubl. obs.].

However, whereas bimakalim induced hypotension at similar doses, SDZ 217-744 was devoid of cardiovascular effects at doses which markedly supressed bronchoconstriction (fig. 3). Thus, a new generation of KCOs, exemplified by SDZ 217-744, is emerging with a wide therapeutic window following local administration.

Clinical Studies with Potassium Channel Openers

There have been just four clinical studies with KCOs published and all concern first generation compounds. In a study in normal volunteers, oral administration of cromakalim inhibited bronchoconstrictor responses to histamine [26]. However, in a second study with levcromakalim, the active enantiomer of cromakalim, the finding could not be confirmed and headache was reported by 19 out of the 25 patients who received the drug [27]. Nevertheless, in a study in nocturnal asthma, orally administered cromakalim attenuated the fall in the early morning FEV_1; again, though, headache was a significant side effect [28]. In a further study, bimakalim showed neither bronchodilation nor cardiovascular side effects when given by inhalation to asthma patients at cumulative doses up to 175 µg [29].

Conclusions

Major recent developments in our understanding of the structural basis of the heterogeneity of K_{ATP} channels promise to reveal opportunities for novel therapies for a variety of diseases. Nowhere is this more evident than in the area of respiratory disease where a unique approach to the treatment of AHR, one of the defining characteristics of asthma, is emerging [10] supported by a wealth of preclinical evidence. The key development has been the demonstration that certain KCOs of the benzopyran class can obviate experimentally induced AHR at doses substantially below those which produce cardiovascular side effects. Since the clinical potential of earlier, first-generation KCOs was compromised by cardiovascular side effects, the new generation of compounds with selectivity for the airways may constitute a new class of drugs for the treatment of asthma.

References

1 Quast U: ATP-Sensitive K+ channels in the kidney. Naunyn-Schmiedeberg's Arch Pharmacol 1996;354:213–225.
2 Quayle JM, Nelson MT, Standen NB: ATP-sensitive and inwardly rectifying potassium channels in smooth muscle. Physiol Rev 1997; 77:1165–1232.
3 Fujita A, Kurachi Y: Molecular aspects of ATP-sensitive K+ channels in the cardiovascular system and K+ channel openers. Pharmacol Ther 2000;85:39–53.
4 Van der Velden VHJ, Hulsmann AR: Autonomic innervation of human airways: Structure, function, and pathophysiology in asthma. NeuroImmunoModulation 1999;6:145–159.
5 Spina D, Shah S, Harrison S: Modulation of sensory nerve function in the airways. Trends Pharmacol Sci 1998;19:460–466.
6 Ramnarine SI, Liu YC, Rogers DF: Neuroregulation of mucus secretion by opioid receptors and K_{ATP} and BK_{Ca} channels in ferret trachea in vitro. Br J Pharmacol 1998;123:1631–1638.
7 Poggioli R, Benelli A, Arletti R, Cavazzutti E, Bertolini A: Antitussive effect of K+ channel openers. Eur J Pharmacol 1999;371:39–42.
8 Morley J: K+ channel openers and suppression of airway hyperreactivity. Trends Pharmacol Sci 1994;15:463–468.
9 Brusasco V, Crimi E, Pellegrino R: Airway hyperresponsiveness in asthma: Not just a matter of airway inflammation. Thorax 1998;53: 992–998.
10 Sont JB, Willems LNA, Bel EH, van Krieken HJM, Vandenbroucke JP, Sterk PJ: Clinical control and histopathologic outcome of asthma when using airway hyperresponsiveness as an additional guide to long-term treatment. Am J Respir Crit Care Med 1999;159:1043–1051.
11 Babenko AP, Aguilar-Bryan L, Bryan J: A View of $SUR/K_{ir}6.X$, K_{ATP} Channels. Ann Rev Physiol 1998;60:667–687.
12 Bryan J, Aguilar-Bryan L: Sulphonylurea receptors: ABC transporters that regulate ATP-sensitive K+ channels. Biochim Biophys Acta 1999;1461:285–303.
13 Sakura H, Trapp S, Liss B, Ashcroft FM: Altered functional properties of K_{ATP} channel conferred by a novel splice variant of SUR1. J Physiol (Lond) 1999;521:337–350.
14 Uhde I, Toman A, Gross I, Schwanstecher C, Schwanstecher M: Identification of the potassium channel opener site on sulfonylurea receptors. J Biol Chem 1999;274:28079–28082.
15 Lawson K: Potassium channel activation: A potential therapeutic approach? Pharmacol Ther 1996;70:39–63.
16 Dunne MJ, Cosgrove KE, Shepherd RM, Ammala C: Potassium channels, sulphonylurea receptors and control of insulin release. Trends Endocrinol Metab 1999;10:146–152.
17 Woolcock AJ: Definitions and clinical classification; in Barnes PJ, Grunstein MM, Leff AR, Woolcock AJ (eds): Asthma. Philadelphia, Lippincott/Raven 1997, pp 27–32.
18 O'Connor BJ, Crowther SD, Costello JF, Morley J: Selective airway responsiveness in asthma. Trends Pharmacol Sci 1999;20:9–11.
19 Cockcroft DW: Airway responsiveness; in Barnes PJ, Grunstein MM, Leff AR, Woolcock AJ (eds): Asthma. Philadelphia, Lippincott/Raven 1997, pp 1253–1266.
20 Cheung D, Sont JK, Sterk PJ: Clinical features of bronchial hyperresponsiveness. Pulm Pharmacol Ther 1999;12:91–96.
21 Chapman ID, Kristersson A, Mathelin G, Schaeublin E, Mazzoni L, Boubekeur K, Murphy N, Morley J: Effects of a potessium channel opener (SDZ PCO 400) on guinea-pig and human pulmonary airways. Br J Pharmacol 1992; 106:423–429.
22 Buchheit KH, Hofmann A: K_{ATP} channel openers reverse immune-complex-induced airways hyperreactivity independently of smooth muscle relaxation. Naunyn-Schmiedeberg's Arch Pharmacol 1996;354:355–361.
23 Yeadon M, Wilkinson D, Darley UV, O'Leary VJ, Payne AN: Mechanisms contributing to ozone-induced bronchial hyperreactivity in guinea-pigs. Pulm Pharmacol 1992;5:39–50.
24 Buchheit KH, Fozard JR: K_{ATP} channel openers for the treatment of airways hyperreactivity. Pulm Pharmacol Ther 1999;12:103–105.
25 Buchheit KH, Hofmann A, Fozard JR: Salbutamol-induced airway hyperreactivity in guinea pigs is not due to a loss of its bronchodilator effect. Eur J Pharmacol 1995;287:85–88.
26 Baird A, Hamilton TC, Richards DH, Tasker T, Williams AJ: Inhibition of histamine induced bronchoconstriction in normal healthy volunteers by a potassium channel activator, cromakalim, BRL 34915. Br J Clin Pharmacol 1988;25:1174.
27 Kidney JC, Fuller RW, Wordsell YM, Lavender EA, Chung KF, Barnes PJ: Effect of an oral potassium channel activator, BRL 38227, on airway function and responsiveness in asthmatic patients: Comparison with oral salbutamol. Thorax 1993;48:130–133.
28 Williams AJ, Lee TH, Cochrane GM, Hopkirk A, Vyse T, Chiew F, Lavender E, Richards DH, Owen S, Stone P, Church S, Woodcock AA: Attenuation of nocturnal asthma by cromakalim. Lancet 1990;336:334–336.
29 Faurschou P, Mikkelsen KL, Steffensen I, Franke B: The lack of bronchodilator effect and the short-term safety of cumulative single doses of an inhaled potassium channel opener (bimakalim) in adult patients with mild to moderate bronchial asthma. Pulm Pharmacol 1994;7: 293–297.

Dr. John R. Fozard, Dr. Paul W. Manley
Preclinical Research, Novartis Pharma Ltd.
CH–4002 Basel (Switzerland)
Tel. +41 61 6971111
E-Mail john_r.fozard@pharma.novartis.com;
paul.manley@pharma.novartis.com

Urodilatin

Kristin Forssmann[a]   Markus Meyer[a,b]   Wolf Georg Forssmann[b]

[a]CardioPep Pharma GmbH and [b]IPF PharmaCeuticals GmbH, Hannover, Germany

Summary

Urodilatin (INN: Ularitide) belongs to the family of natriuretic peptides. Results indicate that urodilatin is synthesized in kidney tubular cells and secreted luminally because this peptide is found solely in urine and not in blood plasma. In its natural function, urodilatin plays the role of a paracrine regulator for sodium and water homeostasis in the kidney. Since the discovery of urodilatin in 1988, a vast number of pharmacological and clinical investigations have been carried out. To date more than 1,000 patients have been treated with urodilatin for indications such as acute renal failure, congestive heart failure and bronchial asthma in clinical phase I and II studies.

The airway-relaxing effects of urodilatin were first shown in vitro, [1, 2] using tracheal muscle strips [3] and in in vivo experiments in rodents [4]. Urodilatin exerts bronchodilator activity by stimulation of intracellular cGMP as an alternative pathway to β_2-agonists, such as albuterol, the current first-line bronchodilator, increasing the intracellular concentration of cAMP and thereby inducing bronchodilation. In patients with mild to moderate bronchial asthma, urodilatin given intravenously exerts a bronchodilator effect on the central and peripheral airways, as shown by increasing lung function parameters such as FEV_1, PEF, and MEF_{25-75}. The best results are obtained at doses of 30 and 60 ng/kg/min. Recently, urodilatin, given as a monotherapy as well as in combination with albuterol, exerted bronchodilator effects in clinically stable asthmatic patients with severe disease [5]. The bronchorelaxant effect of urodilatin is expected to be of therapeutic benefit to patients suffering from bronchial asthma. However, due to the intravenous administration of the drug, and its rapid but short-lived action, its clinical applicability is limited to asthma exacerbation.

Molecular and Cellular Mechanisms of Action

Urodilatin is a nonglycosylated, naturally occurring human paracrine peptide [1]. Urodilatin was isolated from human urine in 1988 and belongs to the family of natriuretic peptides, namely type A, probably representing a differentially processed molecular form [2]. In contrast to the circulating atrial natriuretic peptide, ANP-99-126 urodilatin is N-terminally extended by 4 amino acids [6]. Urodilatin and ANP-99-126 are both derived from a common precursor peptide ANP-1-126 (fig. 1).

The pharmacological effect of urodilatin is based on the stimulation of intracellular guanylyl cyclase as the intracellular domain of the natriuretic peptide receptor A (NPR-A), the enzyme that catalyzes the conversion of GTP to cGMP [7]. Activation of cGMP-dependent protein kinase inhibits sodium reabsorption via an amiloride-sensitive channel and furthermore results in smooth muscle relaxation via a decrease in intracellular Ca^{2+} concentration [7–9] (fig. 2).

Urodilatin and other natriuretic peptides are inactivated by binding to the natriuretic peptide clearance receptor (NPR-C) and by enzymatic degradation through the neutral endopeptidase (NEP; EC 3.4.24.11) [10]. Urodilatin is characterized by a higher stability against enzymatic degradation by neutral endoproteases than ANP-99-126, [11], which contributes to its stronger renal effects [12].

Toxicology and Pharmacological Effects in Animal Models

Summarizing the toxicological results, no incompatibility reactions appear during or after local and systemic administration of urodilatin. The doses used in preclinical acute and long-term experiments which are 10- to 100-

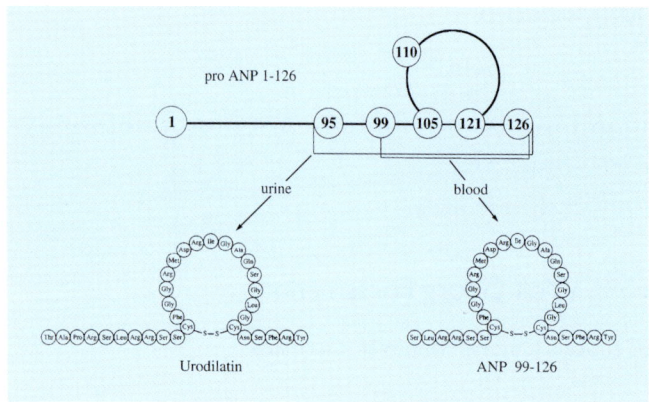
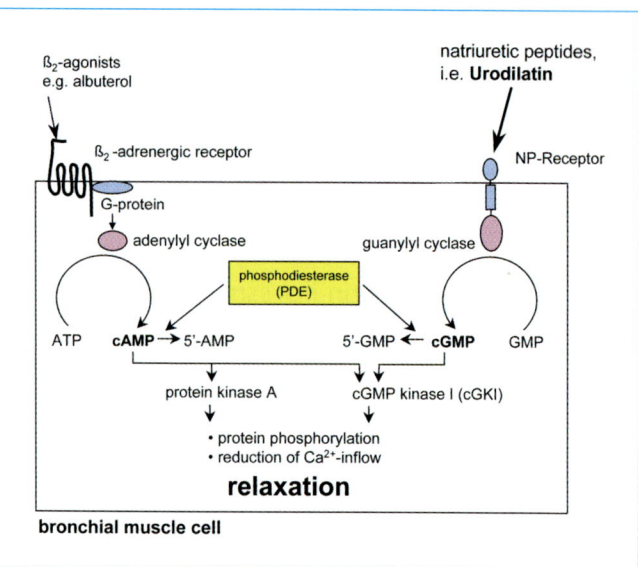

Fig. 1. Schematic exposure of the natriuretic peptides urodilatin (left), ANP-99-126 (right) and the prohormone ANP-1-126. The prohormone contains the circulating ANP-99-126 and urodilatin.

Fig. 2. Cellular and molecular mechanism of natriuretic peptides and β_2-agonists via the NP-receptor and the β_2-receptor.

fold higher than those used in clinical trials are well tolerated and do not lead to any clinical toxic effect or drug-related histopathological alterations in different species. Daily intravenous administration of urodilatin to pregnant rats during organogenesis does not result in any adverse effects on maternal performance or survival, growth, and development in utero. There are no hints of mutagenic activity or chromosomal aberrations in in vitro experiments [unpubl. Investigator's Brochure].

Intravenous administration of urodilatin to various animal species results in dose-dependent renal effects, such as natriuresis and diuresis [12, 13], and cardiovascular effects in dogs with and without heart failure [14, 15]. Urodilatin infusion causes a dose-dependent decrease in mean arterial pressure, cardiac ouput, stroke volume and right atrial pressure [12–15].

Active Ingredients, Dosage Formulation and Route of Administration

Urodilatin acetate is a basic peptide comprising 32 amino acids which represent positions 95–126 of the sequence of the naturally occurring precursor, human ANP-1-126 (fig. 1). The two L-cysteines of urodilatin acetate form an intrapeptide disulfide bridge. The peptide is manufactured synthetically in two fragments by the Merrifield solid-phase method and then condensed and highly purified. Acetate serves as the neutralizing and stabilizing counter-ion and is introduced at the final purification stage. By definition, acetate is part of the urodilatin acetate molecule and is contained in the active ingredient preparation. The finished product urodilatin acetate is provided as a sterile lyophilizate in vials for injection purposes which contain urodilatin acetate corresponding to 1.0 mg of urodilatin. The formula which will be used in clinical trials contains mannitol as the only other excipient. Urodilatin is administered by intravenous infusion after dissolution in physiological sodium chloride solution.

Therapeutic Effects (table 1)

Cardiovascular Effects – Heart Failure. Urodilatin increases cardiac index and heart rate [16]. Furthermore, it reduces mean pulmonary arterial pressure, pulmonary capillary wedge pressure, and systemic vascular resistance in healthy human volunteers [16].

In patients with congestive heart failure (NYHA III-IV), intravenously administered urodilatin increases cardiac index and decreases pulmonary artery pressure, pulmonary capillary wedge pressure, pulmonary and systemic vascular resistance [17–19]. In a randomized, double-blind, placebo-controlled study, infusion of urodilatin (15 ng/kg/min) for 10 h significantly decreases systolic blood pressure and central venous pressure. Furthermore, urine flow as well as urinary sodium excretion are significantly increased. These effects are accompanied by an increase in plasma and urinary cGMP levels. No neurohumoral activation or adverse side effects are observed [18].

The beneficial effects of urodilatin in patients suffering from cardiac failure have been confirmed by other natri-

Table 1. Major clinically relevant physiological effects of urodilatin with particular reference to acute asthma

Systemic effects of urodilatin
- Cardiovascular   vasodilation
- Renal   diuresis, natriuresis
- Endocrine   renin, angiotensin, aldosterone, endothelin, and catecholamine antagonism
- Pulmonary   bronchodilation

Effects of urodilatin relevant for pulmonary function in asthmatics
- Bronchodilation
- Decrease of pulmonary capillary wedge pressure
- Decrease of pulmonary artery pressure
- Decrease of volume load/edema
- Anti-inflammatory effects?

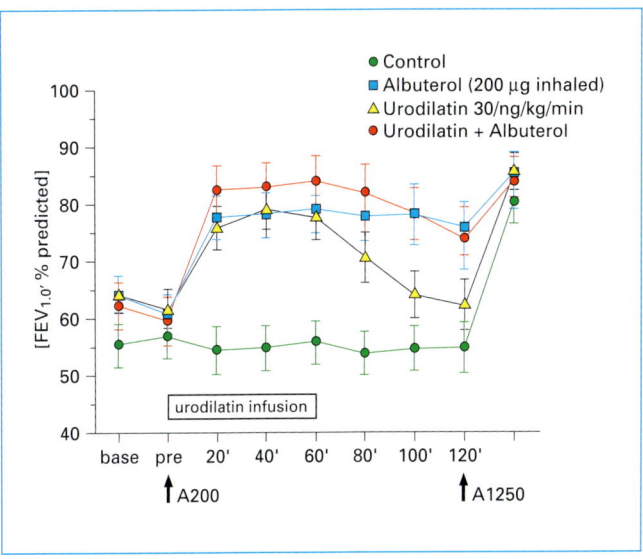

Fig. 3. Results of the clinical phase II study of urodilatin in asthmatics showing the superiority of combined urodilatin and albuterol treatment. Time course of FEV_1 in combined albuterol inhalation (200 µg, ▲ A 200) and urodilatin infusion (30 ng/kg/min), albuterol alone, urodilatin alone and control. Note that the combined application shows the strongest effects, comparable to maximum bronchodilation by 1,250 µg albuterol. base = baseline; pre = before treatment; 20′, 40′, 60′ = during treatment; 80′, 100′, 120′ = after treatment; ▲ A 1250 = following 1,250 µg albuterol. $p < 0.05$ at 20′ 40′ and 60′ vs. pre in all groups; $p < 0.05$ at 20′, 40′, 60′ and 80′ with urodilatin and albuterol monotherapy as well as with combined urodilatin-albuterol therapy vs. control. Modified from Flüge et al. [5].

uretic peptides. Infusion of ANP-99-126 or brain natriuretic peptide in patients with congestive heart failure improves left ventricular function by vasodilation and a noticeable natriuretic action [19].

Renal Effects – Renal Failure. Acute renal failure is a frequent postoperative complication after a major surgical intervention and after organ transplantation, due to cyclosporin-A induced vasoconstriction.

In initial pilot trials, the vasodilator and natriuretic peptide urodilatin showed significant and beneficial effects in preventing or treating acute renal failure [20, 21], resulting in a reduced frequency of hemodialysis or hemofiltration (HD/HF). However, these clinical studies were either noncontrolled or the number of patients was small. Therefore, a multicenter, randomized, double-blind, placebo-controlled study with urodilatin was performed in patients with oliguric acute renal failure in a pivotal phase II trial [22]. The primary objective was the avoidance of HD/HF. This study failed to show a significant difference in patient outcome in the urodilatin-treated groups versus placebo. The incidence of HD/HF was similar in all groups. These results are in contrast not only to the initial results but also to a study by Allgren et al. [23]. However, some points such as patient collective characterized by multimorbidity and high mortality rate may have contributed to the outcome of that study.

Pulmonary Effects – Bronchial Asthma. Urodilatin was shown to exert a bronchodilator activity in isolated perfused guinea pig trachea [3], in in vivo studies [4], and in patients with asthma [24, 25] by stimulation of intracellular cGMP production.

In a randomized, double-blind, placebo-controlled clinical phase II study with cross-over design, urodilatin induced beneficial effects in patients suffering from bronchial asthma. More precisely, urodilatin increased FEV_1, VC_{max}, PEF, MEF_{75}, MEF_{50} and MEF_{25} of FVC at infusion doses of 10, 30 or 60 ng/kg/min; optimal results were obtained at urodilatin doses of 30 and 60 ng/kg/min. A further approach of this study was to investigate the bronchodilatory effects of intravenously administered urodilatin compared with inhaled albuterol or a combination of both drugs. Urodilatin monotherapy resulted in a bronchodilation comparable to that induced by a standard dose of albuterol. However, when urodilatin infusion was combined with albuterol inhalation, a significantly stronger bronchodilator effect was shown compared to that obtained by monotherapy with either drug [25] (fig. 3). Urodilatin-induced effects, such as diuresis, drop in central venous pressure and pulmonary resistance, might be particularly beneficial in patients suffering from cor pulmonale. The treatment of asthma exacerbation with urodilatin combined with a β_2-agonist should therefore be of great clinical value.

Conclusion

In conclusion, urodilatin may improve pulmonary function in patients with bronchial asthma and other obstructive pulmonary diseases. Particularly in patients with a cardiovascular risk and in patients in whom the cAMP-mediated mechanism of bronchodilation is disturbed or exhausted due, for example, to receptor desensitization and downregulation, the alternative cGMP-mediated bronchodilator mechanism induced by urodilatin may be the treatment of choice.

References

1 Forssmann WG, Richter R, Meyer M: The endocrine heart and natriuretic peptides: Histochemistry, cell biology, and functional aspects of the renal urodilatin system. Histochem Cell Biol 1998;110:335–357.
2 Schulz-Knappe P, Forssmann K, Herbst F, Hock D, Pipkorn R, Forssmann WG: Isolation and structural analysis of 'urodilatin', a new peptide of the cardiodilatin (ANP)-family, extracted from human urine. Klin Wochenschr 1988;66:752–759.
3 Duft S, Marxen P, Deeb M, Kuhn M, Piepenbrock S, Forssmann WG, Frölich JC: Urodilatin and atrial natriuretic factor relax preconstricted isolated perfused guinea pig trachea and increase cyclic GMP (abstract). Naunyn-Schmiedeberg's Arch Pharmacol 1992;345 (suppl 2):R49.
4 Flüge T, Hoymann HG, Hohlfeldt J, Heinrich U, Fable H, Wagner TOF, Forssmann WG: Type A natriuretic peptides exhibit different bronchoprotective effects in rats. Eur J Pharmacol 1994;271:395–402.
5 Flüge T, Forssmann WG, Kunkel G, Schneider B, Mentz P, Forssmann K, Barnes PJ, Meyer M: Bronchodilation using combined urodilatin-albuterol administration in asthma: A randomized, double-blind, placebo-controlled trial. Eur J Med Res 1999;4:411–415.
6 Forssmann K, Hock D, Herbst F, Schulz-Knappe P, Talartschik J, Scheler F, Forssmann WG: Isolation and structural analysis of the circulating human cardiodilatin (alpha ANP). Klin Wochenschr 1986;64:1276–1280.
7 Drewett JG, Garbers DL: The family of guanylyl cyclase receptors and their ligands. Endocr Rev 1994;15:135–162.
8 Zeidel ML, Seifter JL, Lear S, Brenner BM, Silva P: Atrial peptides inhibit oxygen consumption in kidney medullary collecting duct cells. Am J Physiol 1986;251:F379–383.
9 Cornwell TL, Lincoln TM: Regulation of intracellular Ca^{2+} levels in cultured vascular smooth muscle cells. Reduction of Ca^{2+} by atriopeptin and 8-bromo-cyclic GMP is mediated by cyclic GMP-dependent protein kinase. J Biol Chem 1989;264:1146–1155.
10 Gagelmann M, Feller S, Hock D, Schulz-Knappe P, Forssmann WG: Biochemistry of the differential release, processing and degradation of cardiac and related peptide hormones; in Kaufmann W, Wambach G (eds): Endocrinology of the Heart. Berlin, Springer, 1989, pp 27–40.
11 Gagelmann M, Hock D, Forssmann WG: Urodilatin (CDD/ANP-95-126) is not biologically inactivated by a peptide from dog kidney cortex membranes in contrast to atrial natriuretic peptide/cardiodilatin (α-hANP/CDD-99-120). FEBS Lett 1988;233:249–254.
12 Shaw S, Weidmann P: Comparative therapeutic and histological effects of intravenous Urodilatin or nitroprusside combined with dopamine during established acute renal failure in rats. Kidney Int 1992;41:493–494.
13 Emmeluth C, Drummer C, Gerzer R, Bie P: Roles of cephalic Na^+ concentration and urodilatin in control of renal Na^+ excretion. Am J Physiol 1992;262:F513–F516.
14 Riegger GAJ, Elsner D, Forssmann WG, Kromer: Effects of ANP-(95-126) in dogs before and after induction of heart failure. Am J Physiol 1990;259:H1643–H1648.
15 Villarreal D, Freeman RH, Johnson RA: Renal effects of ANF (95-126), a new atrial peptide analogue, in dogs with experimental heart failure. Am J Hypertens 1991;4:508–515.
16 Kentsch M, Ludwig D, Drummer C, Gerzer R, Mueller-Esch G: Haemodynamic and renal effects of Urodilatin in healthy volunteers. Eur J Clin Invest 1992;22:319–325.
17 Kentsch M, Ludwig D, Drummer C, Gerzer R, Mueller-Esch G: Haemodynamic and renal effects of Urodilatin bolus injections in patients with congestive heart failure. Eur J Clin Invest 1992;22:662–669.
18 Elsner D, Muders F, Müntze A, Kromer EP, Forssmann WG, Riegger GAJ: Efficacy of prolonged infusion of Urodilatin [ANP-(95-126)] in patients with congestive heart failure. Am Heart J 1995;129:765–773.
19 Yasue H, Yoshimura M: Natriuretic peptides in the treatment of heart failure. J Card Fail 1996;2 (suppl 4):S277–S285.
20 Hummel M, Kuhn M, Bub A, Bittner H, Kleefeld D, Marxen P, Schneider B, Hetzer R, Forssmann WG: Urodilatin. A new peptide with beneficial effects in the postoperative therapy of cardiac transplant recipients. Clin Invest 1992;70:674–682.
21 Cedidi C, Meyer M, Kuse ER, Schulz-Knappe P, Ringe B, Frei U, Pichlmayr R, Forssmann WG: Urodilatin: A new approach for the treatment of therapy-resistant acute renal failure after liver transplantation. Eur J Clin Invest 1994;24:632–639.
22 Meyer M, Pfarr E, Schirmer G, Überbacher HJ, Schöpe K, Böhm E, Flüge T, Mentz P, Scigalla P, Forssmann WG: Therapeutic use of the natriuretic peptide Ularitide in acute renal failure. Renal Failure 1999;21:85–100.
23 Allgren RL, Marbury TC, Rahman SN, Weisberg LS, Fenves AZ, Lafayette RA, Sweet RM, Genter FC, Kurnik BRC, Conger JD, Sayegh MH, for the Auriculin Anaritide Acute Renal Failure Study Group: Anaritide in acute tubular necrosis. N Engl J Med 1997;336:828–834.
24 Flüge T, Fabel H, Wagner TOF, Schneider B, Forssmann WG: Urodilatin (ularitide, INN): A potent bronchodilator in asthmatic subjects. Eur J Clin Invest 1995;25:728–736.
25 Flüge T, Fabel H, Wagner TOF, Schneider B, Forssmann WG: Bronchodilating effects of natriuretic and vasorelaxant peptides compared to salbutamol in asthmatics. Regul Pept 1995;59:357–370.

Dr. Kristin Forssmann
CardioPep Pharma GmbH
Karl-Wiechert-Allee 76
D-30625 Hannover (Germany)
Tel. +49 511 530 4515, Fax +49 511 530 4510
E-Mail kforssmann@gmt.de

Steroids

Steroids: An Overview

Ronald Dahl[a]   Lars Peter Nielsen[b]

[a]Department of Respiratory Diseases, Aarhus University Hospital, and
[b]Department of Clinical Pharmacology, University of Aarhus, Aarhus, Denmark

Summary

Inhaled corticosteroids are the most effective drugs available to clinicians for the control inflammation in asthma, but their use in COPD remains controversial. This overview will describe the mechanism of action of corticosteroids (CS) in cellular, physiological and molecular terms. In particular, the effects of CS on symptoms, FEV_1, and AHR will be considered in relation to dose response. In an effort to minimize systemic adverse events, yet maximize local anti-inflammatory effects, a number of strategies to improve the risk-benefit of CS are available.

Immunopathology of Asthma

Bronchial asthma is characterized by an inflammatory reaction in the bronchial mucosa where an increased number of inflammatory cells and activation of resident cells give rise to a complex scenario with involvement of mediators, cytokines, chemokines, adhesion molecules and a variety of enzymes. This acute and chronic inflammation concomitantly gives rise to bronchial oedema because of increased blood volume and flow in bronchial vessels and plasma leakage. In addition changes in the airway structure develop over months and years and this airway remodelling is characterized by a thickening of the subepithelial basement membrane, proliferation of fibroblasts and smooth muscle. These bronchial abnormalities are clinically expressed as increased airway reactivity that manifests itself by acute and chronic bronchoconstriction after a variety of specific and non specific stimuli, and in symptoms of cough, wheeze and breathlessness [1].

Action on Leukocytes

CS ameliorate the inflammatory reaction in the bronchial mucosa, which can be substantiated by a decrease in cell numbers, mediators and receptors (fig. 1). There is a general reduction in markers of cell activity such as epithelial cells, lymphocytes and eosinophils [2].

Physiological Effects

The regulation by CS of the inflammatory and resident cell activity together with reduction of bronchial oedema and the inflammatory mediators result in a reduction in AHR and clinical effects on asthma (table 1). This can be quantified by challenge tests with histamine, methacholine, AMP, cold air, physical exercise or by specific allergens. This profound influence on the bronchial pathology is probably the main explanations for the substantial reduction in exacerbation rate and hospitalizations evi-

Table 1. Clinical effects of CS in asthma

Improved/normalization of lung function
Reduced/normalization of diurnal variation in lung function
Reduced/normal AHR
Reduced/no asthma symptoms (ex. cough, wheeze, dyspnoea) day and night
Reduced/no need for rescue medication
Reduced/no asthma attacks or exacerbations
Reduced/no hospitalization
Reduced/no morbidity, no mortality
Improved/normalization of quality of life

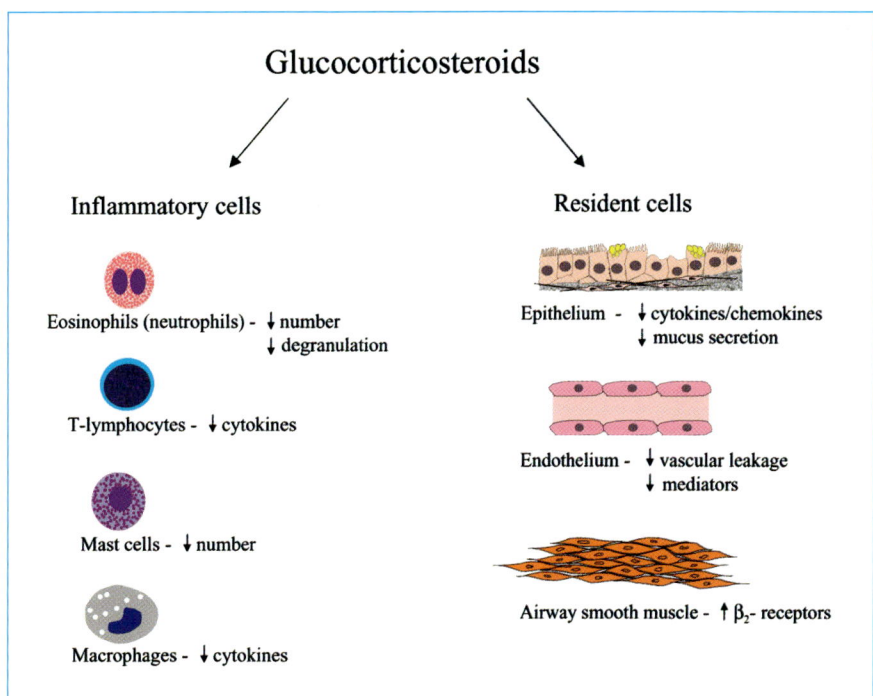

Fig. 1. Cellular actions of CS in asthma. ↓ = decrease; ↑ = increase.

dent in asthmatics treated with regular CS. After CS treatment lung function increases, symptoms during day and night as well as the need for rescue bronchodilators are reduced. These beneficial effects also result in an improved quality of life and make the treatment cost effective [3].

Time Response

The time response to the effects of CS differs between various outcome parameters, but clinical effects may be seen after a few hours (fig. 2a). Generally, symptoms and lung function improve within days or weeks, whereas a reduction in AHR may not reach its maximum before treatment has been given for several months [4].

Dose Response

The evaluation of the clinical responses to CS in asthma is in addition complicated because of the dose-response curves and slopes to the individual outcome parameters (fig. 2b). The dose-response slope to lung function is shallow, which makes it difficult to distinguish between dosages [5] (fig. 2c). The dose-response span is greater with regard to BHR which makes it possible to distinguish more clearly between dosages and more so with indirect challenges than with direct challenge procedures [6].

Adverse Events

Side effects to CS are dose dependent and of special concern are the metabolic side effects, especially, those influencing childhood growth (table 2). The profound influences of CS on protein catabolism over time result in osteoporosis, muscle weakness and skin thinning. Carbohydrate metabolism is altered in a diabetogenic direction, and changes in lipid metabolism give rise to altered fat distribution and possibly atherosclerosis. Many more side effects occur, such as mood changes, fluid retention [7]. Inhaled CS in a few instances give rise to local side effects in the mouth and pharynx (candidiasis and 'sore throat'). Voice change from husky voice to aphonia can occur. These side effects are dose dependent and totally reversible.

It is desired to separate the beneficial effects as much as possible from the undesired side effects and when evaluating various glucocorticosteroids this should be looked upon by determining a therapeutic ratio. The therapeutic ratio for glucocorticosteroids has been improved during the years for example by a diminished mineralo corticosteroid effect of the molecules, the use of inhaled drugs with topical activity and improving the topical versus the systemic effects of the inhaled drug.

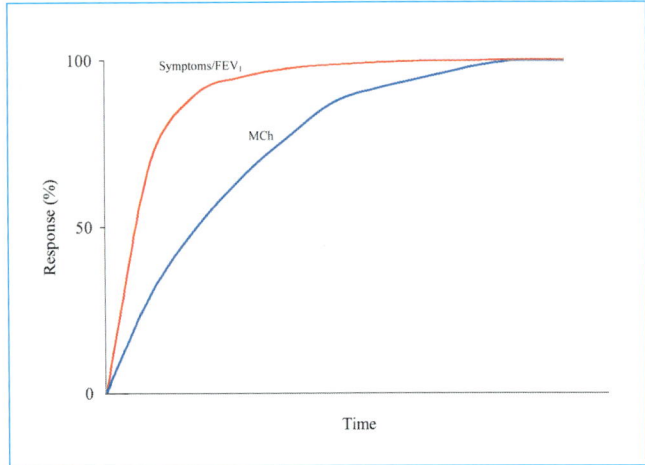

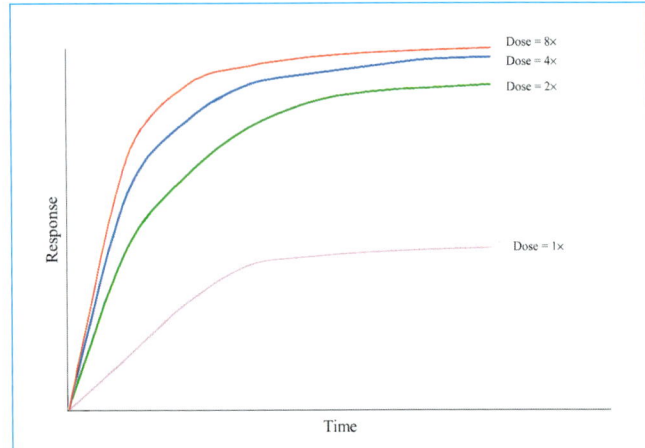

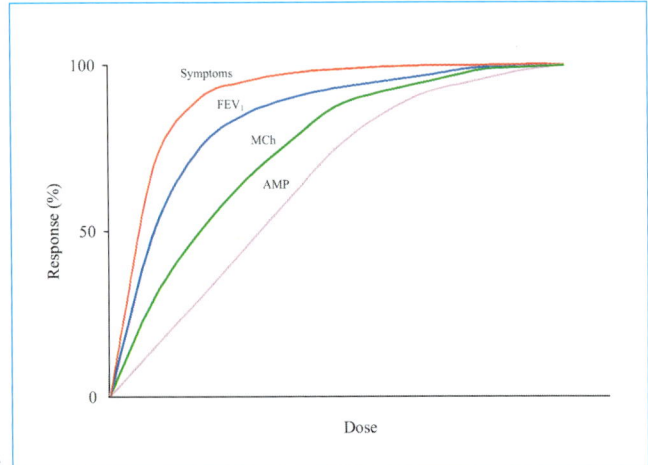

Fig. 2. Dose-response relationship of CS in bronchial asthma for different outcome parameter (**a**), time-response relationship for CS in bronchial asthma (**b**), and time-response relationship for different CS dose levels in bronchial asthma (**c**). Each dose reaches a maximum that is not influenced further over time. MCh = Bronchial reactivity to methacholine; AMP = bronchial reactivity to adenosine monophosphate.

Table 2. Unwanted effects of CS

Local side effects from inhaled CS
Sore throat
Oral/pharyngeal candidiasis
Dysphonia/aphonia
Systemic side effects
Growth retardation
Osteoporosis, skin thinning, muscle weakness
Diabetes
Weight gain and abnormal fat distribution
Adrenocortical insufficiency
Post-capsular cataract
Hyperlipidaemia
Mood changes, psychiatric disturbances
Gastric ulcer, oesophagitis
Hypertension

Table 3. Glucocorticosteroids and gene transcription

Increased transcription	
β_2-Adrenoceptor	
Inhibitory $\kappa B\alpha$	
Lipocortin	
IL-1 receptor antagonist	
IL-1 receptor II	
Secretory leukocyte inhibitor protein	
Decreased transcription	
Cytokines	IL-1, IL-2, IL-3, IL-4, IL-5, IL-6, IL-11, IL-13, TNF-α, GM-CSF, stem cell factor
Chemokines	IL-8, RANTES; MIP-1α, MCP-1, MCP-3, MCP-4, eotaxin
iNOS	
Inducible cyclooxygenase (COX-1, COX-2)	
Cytoplasmic PLA$_2$	
Adhesion molecules: ICAM-1, E selectin	
ET-1	
NK1 receptor, NK2 receptor	

Mechanism of Action of Glucocorticosteroids

The steroidal hormones, including CS, exert their action intracellularly after passive penetration of the cell membrane. In the cytoplasm, CS work by generation or suppression of mRNA production of a large number of substances of importance for the normal metabolism and homeostasis (table 3). CS exert their action by at least two different mechanisms called transactivation and transrepression [8] (fig. 3).

The intracellular CS receptor consist of 770 amino acids [9]. One area of the receptor binds CS while another

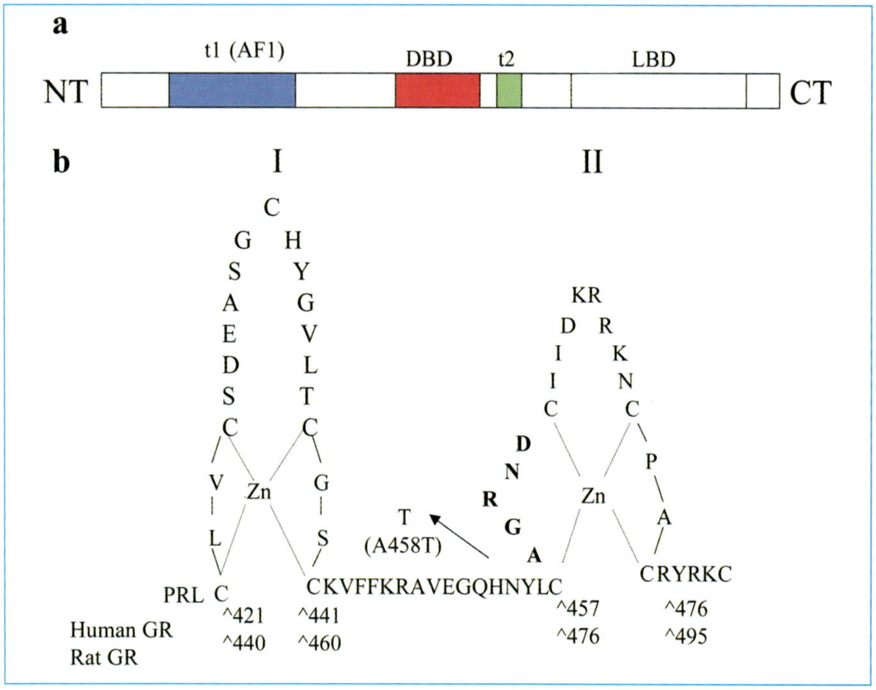

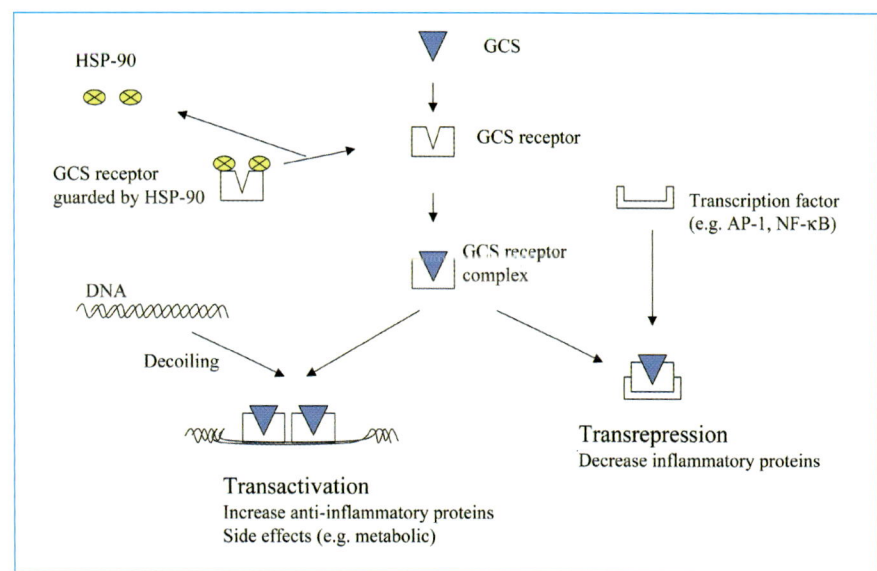

Fig. 3. Structure of the glucocorticoid receptor (GR). **a** Linear representation of the 777-amino-acid glucocorticoid receptor showing the principal domains. DBD = DNA-binding domain; LBD = ligand-binding domain; t1 and t2 = the two activation domains; NT = amino terminal; C = carboxy terminal. **b** Enlargement of part of the DNA-binding domain showing the amino acid sequence (single-letter codes) of the two zinc fingers and the dimerization loop (in bold). Numbering of both the human and rat receptors is given. The A to T mutation at position 458 that gives rise to the dimerization defective receptor is shown.

Fig. 4. Schematic representation of intracellular events of glucocorticosteroid receptor binding and resulting transactivation-transrepression of gene transcription. GCS = Glucocorticosteroid; HSP-90 = heat shock protein; AP-1 = activator protein-1; NF-κB = Nuclear factor-κB.

binds to certain DNA domains (fig. 4). In addition, activator domains are present. An area responsible for the dimerization of the receptor is situated within the DNA-binding domain. In the cytoplasm, each CS receptor is guarded by a heat shock protein which acts as a chaperone protecting the receptor from dimerization or binding to DNA or transcription-regulating proteins. The dissociation of the chaperone proteins from the receptor after CS binding makes it possible for two receptors to associate into a dimer complex. This complex has the ability to penetrate into the nucleus and to bind to specific regions on DNA. These regions are called glucocorticoid response elements and are located in the promoter region of certain genes. This binding may facilitate and initiate the corresponding gene mRNA product. Binding to non-glucocorticoid response elements inhibits mRNA translation. These mechanisms are called transactivation and include the metabolic effects of CS.

Table 4. Transactivation-transrepression

Transactivation	Transrepression
Enhanced transcription	Inhibitor of transcription
GRE	'nGRE'
Dimeric GCS receptor	Monomeric GCS receptor
Metabolic effects	Anti-inflammatory effects
Undesirable in asthma	Desirable in asthma

GRE = Glucocorticoid response elements; nGRE = non-glucocorticoid response elements; GCS = glucocorticosteroid.

Transcription of DNA to mRNA involves other complex mechanisms. First of all the promoter regions within the DNA molecules must be accessible for binding of activators. Normally, DNA is packed very densely by means of deacetylated histones. Acetylation of these glue-like proteins make the DNA unfold and expose promoter regions. CS themselves can influence both histone acetylation and deacetylation [10, 11].

Transactivation and Transrepression

The transcription of DNA to mRNA can be activated by a number of regulatory intracellular proteins such as NF-κB, activator protein 1. CS can influence transactivation by binding to these activator proteins and thereby inhibiting mRNA production (table 4). This CS mechanism is exerted through monomeric CS receptor complexes and is called transrepression.

It may be possible to reduce the unwanted systemic side effects such as metabolic effects by favouring the formation of monomeric CS receptor complexes. This will avoid the dimerization and transactivation effects on metabolism.

An increased local effect compared to a systemic effect can be achieved from inhaled CS, if they deposit on the diseased mucosa and do not access the tissue outside the bronchi. This may be achieved if deposition and retention in the lungs occur without systemic absorption. If the drug eventually reaches the systemic circulation, rapid metabolism must occur. In addition, the proportion of swallowed drug should be rapidly eliminated in the gut mucosa or, if absorbed, rapidly metabolized.

Future Directions

The pharmaceutical industry is active in the development of novel steroids and other anti-inflammatory compounds that have an improved risk-benefit ratio compared with currently available CS. Efforts to design pro-drug steroids, soft steroids and dissociated steroids all have exciting potential to achieve this aim.

References

1 Barnes PJ: Pathophysiology of asthma; in Barnes PJ, Rodger IW, Thomson NC (eds): Asthma: Basic Mechanisms and Clinical Management. London, Academic Press, 1998, pp 487–506.
2 Laitinen LA, Laitinen A, Haahtela T: A comparative study of the effects of an inhaled corticosteroid, budesonide, and of a beta-2-agonist, terbutaline, on airway inflammation in newly diagnosed asthma. J Allergy Clin Immunol 1992;90:32–42.
3 Pedersen S, O'Byrne P: A comparison of the efficacy and safety of inhaled corticosteroids in asthma. Allergy 1997;52:1–34.
4 van Essen-Zandvliet EE, Hughes MD, Waalkens HJ, Duiverman EJ, Pocock SJ, Kerrebijn KF: Effects of 22 months of treatment with inhaled corticosteroid and/or beta-2-agonists on lung function, airway responsiveness and symptoms in children with asthma. Am Rev Respir Dis 1992;146:547–554.
5 Dahl R, Lundback B, Malo JL, Mazza JA, Nieminen MM, Saarelainen P, Barnacle H: A dose-ranging study of fluticasone propionate in adult patients with moderate asthma. International Study Group. Chest 1993;104:1352–1358.
6 Taylor DA, Jensen MW, Kanabar V, Engelstatter R, Steinijans VW, Barnes PJ, O'Connor BJ: A dose-dependent effect of the novel inhaled corticosteroid ciclesonide responsiveness to adenosine-5'-monophosphate in asthmatic patients. Am J Respir Crit Care Med 1999;160:237–243.
7 WE Serafin: Drugs used in the treatment of asthma; in Hardman JG, Limbird LE (eds): The Pharmacological Basis of Therapeutics, ed 9. New York, McGraw-Hill, 1996, pp 659–682.
8 Barnes PJ: Molecular mechanisms of steroid action in asthma. J Allergy Clin Immunol 1996;97:159–168.
9 Hollenberg SM, Weinberger C, Ong ES, et al: Primary structure and expression of a functional glucocorticoid receptor cDNA. Nature 1985;318:635–641.
10 Newton R: Molecular mechanisms of glucocorticoid action: What is important? Thorax 2000;55:603–613.
11 Adcock IM, Ito K: Molecular mechanisms of corticosteorid actions. Monaldi Arch Chest Dis 2000;55:256–266.

Dr. Ronald Dahl
Department of Respiratory Diseases
Aarhus University Hospital
DK–8000 Denmark
Tel. +45 8949 2085, Fax +45 8949 2110
E-Mail akh.grp02s.rda@aaa.dk

Ciclesonide: An On-Site-Activated Steroid

K. Dietzel   R. Engelstätter   A. Keller

Byk Gulden Pharmaceuticals, Konstanz, Germany

Summary

Ciclesonide is a novel non-halogenated inhaled corticosteroid that is not directly active, but is cleaved by endogenous esterases in the lung to activated drug substance. Thus, ciclesonide is an on-site-activated drug. Because of this, it has high topical potency but essentially no oropharyngeal side effects and suppression of endogenous cortisol. In this chapter we review the encouraging preclinical and clinical data on ciclesonide.

Inhaled corticosteroids are the most effective agents currently used to treat chronic asthma in patients of all ages with differing degrees of asthma severity. However, systemic side effects limit the dose at which inhaled corticosteroids can be administered for long-term therapy. The benefits of long-term treatment with glucocorticoids must be weighed against the potential adverse effects of the treatment, such as impairment of growth [1–7], abnormalities in the metabolism of glucose [1], adrenal suppression [8–14], and the formation of cataracts [15]. Although some of the available steroids have relatively low oral bioavailability, inhaled corticosteroids are absorbed from the lung or nasal mucosa into the systemic circulation, so that they have systemic effects. Therefore, the major aim in the development of novel steroids is to design substances which have high topical potency but no or significantly reduced systemic side effects. By adopting the on-site-activation drug approach, this aim could be achieved when developing ciclesonide. This very promising novel steroid thus provides a new dimension of therapeutic benefits for the treatment of chronic asthma.

Ciclesonide is a new-generation non-halogenated glucocorticoid with high local anti-inflammatory properties. In addition, it has essentially no oral bioavailability. Most importantly, however, ciclesonide is an ester prodrug. This means that ciclesonide is not directly active. Ciclesonide has almost no binding affinity for the glucocorticoid receptor, whereas the binding affinity of the activated ciclesonide is higher by a factor of 100 (table 1). Activation of ciclesonide occurs upon cleavage by endogenous esterases, as outlined in figure 1.

The activation of ciclesonide takes place in the target organ, the lung. Pharmacokinetically, the on-site-activated drug concept leads to delayed and blunted peak serum concentrations of the active metabolite of ciclesonide. Activated ciclesonide is very rapidly metabolized to inactive breakdown products.

By virtue of its on-site-activated drug feature ciclesonide is thus expected to bring about the following clinical advantages:
- minimized systemic adverse effects,
- minimized oropharyngeal side effects.

The clinical advantages of the on-site-activated drug concept are further supported by the fact that ciclesonide is a pure epimeric substance. As a consequence there is no superfluous steroid load from the other less active epimeric form; this should also result in a beneficial safety profile and in a high topical potency already at low doses of ciclesonide.

Table 1. Binding affinities to rat lung glucocorticoid receptors [Hochhaus, unpubl. obs.]

	Relative binding affinities
Ciclesonide prodrug	12
Activated ciclesonide	1,200
Dexamethasone	100

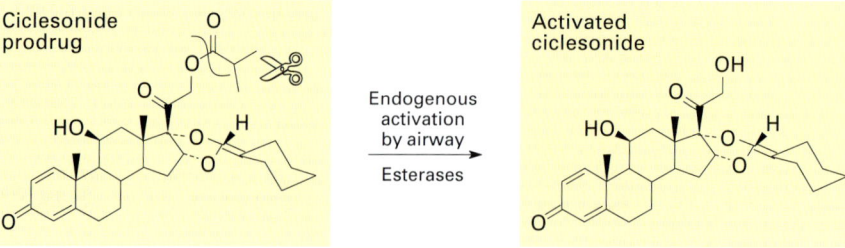

Fig. 1. The on-site-activation concept of ciclesonide.

Advantages of the on-site-activation concept
– Targeted activation in the lung
– Minimized systemic adverse effects
– Minimized oropharyngeal side effects

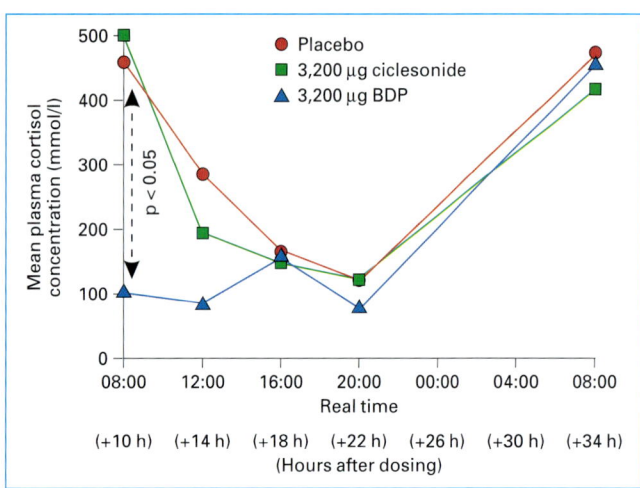

Fig. 2. Mean plasma cortisol concentrations obtained after inhalation of 3,200 μg ciclesonide, 3,200 μg beclomethasone dipropionate (BDP) and placebo (n = 6 each).

Clinical Studies

Cortisol Levels. The first clinical results obtained in healthy volunteers and in asthmatic patients confirm that the prodrug concept of ciclesonide indeed translates into a significantly improved safety profile in comparison to conventional steroids. Whereas cortisol concentrations in the serum of healthy volunteers treated with a very high dose of 3,200 μg ciclesonide behave essentially like placebo, the same dose of beclomethasone dipropionate shows a marked suppression of serum cortisol (fig. 2).

Dose Range Finding. In terms of efficacy, in vitro studies indicate that ciclesonide is at least as active as conventional steroids. In order to get early insight into how the high topical potency observed in the preclinical setting also translates into the clinical effectiveness of ciclesonide, two challenge studies were initiated.

Inhaled steroids decrease airway responsiveness in asthma by mechanisms that may involve suppressing airway inflammation and a reduction in the number of inflammatory cells in the airway. Several studies have shown that chronic treatment with inhaled steroids reduces the airway responsiveness to inhaled histamine and methacholine, however, the effect is sometimes small and thus makes it difficult to investigate the dose-effect relationship of a steroid. In a recent study [16], it was shown that budesonide reduced the response to adenosine-5-monophosphate (AMP) to a significantly higher extent compared to methacholine and sodium metabisulfite. Therefore, this model was chosen to gain first insight not only into the efficacy but also into the dose-effect relationship of ciclesonide.

The effects of 3 different ciclesonide doses (50, 200 and 800 μg, inhaled twice daily for 14 days) on airway responsiveness to AMP were assessed in 29 asthmatic patients who were hyperresponsive to AMP ($PC_{20}FEV_1 \leq 60$ mg/ml), had an $FEV_1 \geq 60\%$ predicted and were currently taking only intermittent short-acting β-agonists to treat occasional symptoms [17] (fig. 3).

Ciclesonide reduced airway responsiveness to AMP in a dose-dependent manner ($p < 0.05$). In comparison with placebo, this decrease in airway responsiveness after treatment with 100, 400, and 1,600 μg ciclesonide/day amounted to 1.6, 2.0, and 3.4 doubling doses, respectively.

Additionally, in the same study sputum induction was performed before and after treatment with ciclesonide or placebo. Although airway eosinophilia was low in all groups of patients, a statistically significant ($p < 0.05$) reduction in the percentage of eosinophils was found in induced sputum after 400 and 1,600 μg ciclesonide/day.

Allergen Challenge. In another double-blind, randomized study, 11 patients with allergic asthma underwent allergen challenge after having been treated with placebo

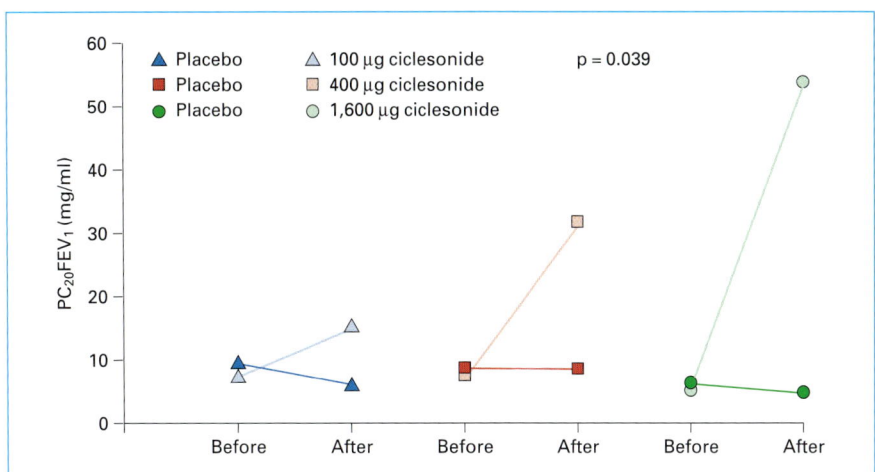

Fig. 3. Airway responsiveness to AMP (PC_{20}) before and after 2 weeks of treatment with placebo and ciclesonide. Data are geometric mean (SEM). A value of $p < 0.05$ for comparison of the post/pre PC_{20} (AMP) ratios for ciclesonide 400 and 1,600 µg daily versus respective placebo ratios.

and 800 µg b.i.d. ciclesonide for 7 days in a crossover fashion [18]. As expected ciclesonide inhibited the late-phase asthmatic reaction to allergen ($p < 0.05$). Also the early-phase reaction was significantly suppressed ($p < 0.05$) despite the short treatment period of only 1 week indicating a rapid onset of action.

Conclusion

The on-site-activated ciclesonide is the first inhaled corticosteroid having a high topical potency without causing any cortisol suppression. Cortisol suppression commonly serves as a surrogate parameter for systemic adverse effects of steroids.

References

1 Eigen H, Rosenstein BJ, FitzSimmons S, Schidlow DV: Cystic Fibrosis Foundation Prednisone Trial Group. A multicenter study of alternate-day prednisone therapy in patients with cystic fibrosis. J Pediatr 1995;126:515–523.
2 Allen DB: Growth suppression by glucocorticoid therapy. Endocrinol Metab Clin North Am 1996;25:699–717.
3 Allen DB: Influence of inhaled corticosteroids on growth: A pediatric endocrinologist's perspective. Acta Paediatr 1998;87:123–129.
4 Doull IJM, Freezer NJ, Holgate ST: Growth of prepubertal children with mild asthma treated with inhaled beclomethasone dipropionate. Am J Respir Crit Care Med 1995;151:1715–1719.
5 Allen DB, Mullen M, Mullen B: A meta-analysis of the effect of oral and inhaled corticosteroids on growth. J Allergy Clin Immunol 1994;93:967–976.
6 Todd G, Dunlop K, McNaboe J, yan MF, Carson D, Shields MD: Growth and adrenal suppression in asthmatic children treated with high-dose fluticasone propionate. Lancet 1996;337:8–14.
7 Hui-Chuan Lai RD, FitzSimmons S, Allen DB, Kosorok MR, Rosenstein BJ, Campbell PW, Farrell PM: Risk of persistent growth impairment after alternate-day prednisone treatment in children with cystic fibrosis. N Engl J Med 2000;342:851–859.
8 Clark DJ, Grove A, Cargill RI, Lipworth BJ: Comparative adrenal suppression with inhaled budesonide and fluticasone propionate in adult asthmatic patients. Thorax 1996;51: 262–266.
9 Grahnén A, Eckernäs S-A, Brundin RM, Ling-Andersson A: An assessment of the systemic activity of single doses of inhaled fluticasone propionate in healthy volunteers. Br J Clin Pharmacol 1994;38:521–525.
10 Grahnén A, Jansson B, Brundin RM, Ling-Andersson A, Lönnebo A, Johansson M, Eckernäs SA: A dose-response study comparing suppression of plasma cortisol induced by fluticasone propionate from Diskhaler and budesonide from Turbuhaler. Eur J Clin Pharmacol 1997;52:261–267.
11 Grove A, Allam C, McFarlane LC, McPhale G, Lipworth B: A comparison of the systemic bioactivity of inhaled budesonide and fluticasone propionate in normal subjects. Br J Clin Pharmacol 1994;38: 527–532.
12 Lönnebo A, Grahnén A, Jansson B, Brundin RM, Ling-Andersson A, Eckernäs S-A: An assessment of the systemic effects of single and repeated doses of inhaled fluticasone propionate and inhaled budesonide in healthy volunteers. Eur J Clin Pharmacol 1996;49:459–463.
13 Clark DJ, Lipworth BJ: Dose-response of inhaled drugs in asthma. An update. Clin Pharmacokinet 1997;32:58–74.
14 Thorsson L, Dahlström K, Edsbäcker S, Källén A, Paulson J, Wirén J-E: Pharmacokinetics and systemic effects of inhaled fluticasone propionate in healthy subjects. Br J Clin Pharmacol 1997;43:155–161.
15 Cumming RG, Mitchell P, Leeder SR: Use of inhaled corticosteroids and the risk of cataracts. N Engl J Med 1997;337:8–14.
16 O'Connor BJ, Ridge SM, Barnes PJ, Fuller RW: Greater effect of inhaled budesonide on adenosine 5-monophosphate-induced than on sodium-metabisulfite-induced broncho-constriction in asthma. Am Rev Respir Dis 1992;146:560–564.
17 Taylor DA, Jensen MW, Kanabar V, Engelstätter R, Steinijans VW, Barnes PJ, O'Connor BJ: A dose-dependent effect of the novel inhaled corticosteroid Ciclesonide on airway responsiveness to adenosine-5'-monophosphate in asthmatic patients. Am J Respir Crit Care Med 1999;160:237–243.
18 Dahl R, Nielsen LP, Christensen MB, Engelstätter R: Ciclesonide – an inhaled corticosteroid prodrug – inhibits allergen induced early and late phase reactions. Eur Respir J 1998;28: 62s.

Dr. K. Dietzel
Byk Gulden Pharmaceuticals
Byk-Gulden-Strasse 2
D-78467 Konstanz (Germany)
Tel. +49 7531 842 268, Fax +49 7531 842 402
E-Mail klaus.dietzel@byk.de

Soft Steroids

Bengt Axelsson   Ralph Brattsand

AstraZeneca R&D Lund, Lund, Sweden

Summary

Improved topical selectivity for airways and lung may be achieved if inhaled corticosteroids (ICS) were inactivated during their systemic distribution (and not just in the liver as with current ICS). Several projects have been evaluated based upon steroids inactivated by esterases. Compounds hydrolyzed by ubiquitous, nonselective esterases have failed (fluocortin butylester, itrocinonide), probably due to too rapid inactivation in the target tissue. A new approach has been attempted based upon paraoxonase-catalyzed breakdown selectivity in plasma. This may better answer the question whether soft steroids can reach the same efficacy as current ICS in the absence of systemic activity.

Pharmacokinetic Basis of Airway and Lung Selectivity of Current Inhaled Steroids

The currently used inhaled corticosteroids (ICS) are biostable at the airways and lung target, being inactivated in liver by CYP450-3A-mediated oxidative biotransformation [1]. This brings about an efficient first-pass inactivation of the swallowed part of the inhalation dose, but not of the key fraction deposited in the airways and lung (fig. 1). The latter is bioavailable and transported to the heart via the bronchial and pulmonary circulations. While one quarter of the cardiac output has the first pass to the liver for inactivation, the majority of absorbed steroid is widely distributed in the body [2]. This systemic spill-over of current ICS results in circulating plasma levels of 0.1–1 nmol/l, persisting for several hours after inhalation [3–6]. Although these levels are low, they are still in the same range as the K_D of these very potent steroids [1, 7]. While this systemic spill-over introduces a risk of adverse steroid reactions [1], it does not seem to add own anti-asthmatic efficacy [8, 9].

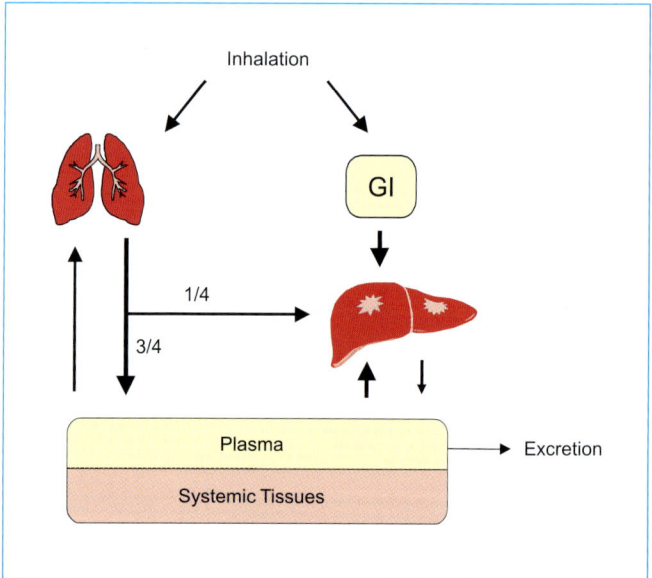

Fig. 1. Disposition of inhaled glucocorticosteroids.

Pharmacological and Chemical Aims for Soft-Drug Development

A soft drug is active by itself, has therapeutic efficacy at the site of application, and is rapidly and predictably inactivated during its systemic uptake and distribution [10]. A soft ICS should have sufficient metabolic stability for inducing the desired anti-inflammatory effect at the airways and lung target, but during its systemic uptake and distribution it has to be inactivated by further metabolic routes, in addition to hepatic CYP450.

A common approach to soft-drug design has been to start from inactive metabolites and to activate them by coupling easily hydrolyzable substituents, which can then be removed in vivo.

Glucocorticoids (GCSs) are metabolized via redox pathways. An important route of steroid metabolism is oxidation of the 17β-hydroxyacetone side chain leading to inactive 17β-keto- and 17β-carboxylic acids, and these metabolites have been the basis of soft-steroid design [10]. Carboxylesterases (EC 3.1.1.1) catalyze the hydrolysis of the active esters of GCSs to their corresponding inactive acids. The carboxylesterases have a broad and overlapping substrate specificity, and a single hydrolytic reaction is often catalyzed by several enzymes. The highest hydrolase activity occurs in the liver, but carboxylesterase activity has also been found in a number of other compartments including blood, the lung and circulating leukocytes [11]. However, their ubiquitous tissue distribution and overlapping substrate specificity make it difficult to obtain an ideal therapeutic profile for a conventional carboxylic acid ester GCS. Reduced efficacy due to rapid hydrolysis at the airway and lung target or poor selectivity because of slow inactivation during their systemic distribution have been the main obstacles. The ideal soft ICS should therefore possess the same metabolic stability and high receptor affinity at the airway and lung target as current ICS, but be rapidly inactivated by specific esterases in blood and peripheral tissue during systemic disposition.

Inactivation by Ubiquitous Esterases

Fluocortin Butylester. Fluocortin butylester (FCB) was the first soft steroid ester based on the inactive-metabolite concept (table 1). Its glucocorticoid receptor affinity and topical anti-inflammatory potency are several fold less than those of dexamethasone. When incubated with human blood in vitro, FCB is decomposed to an inactive carboxylic acid [12]. However, the in vivo relevance of this hydrolysis is questionable, since after intravenous injection the plasma $t_{1/2}$ of FCB (2.6 h) [12] is still as high as for current ICS [1]. A powder formulation was tested in a bronchial provocation test [13], with the outcome that FCB (2 mg q.d.s. for 1 week) was clearly inferior to beclomethasone dipropionate (200 μg q.d.s. for 1 week).

Itrocinonide. The aims of this Astra project, initiated in the early 1980s, were to design a soft steroid with a receptor affinity equal to the best ICS of that time, and with a faster hydrolytic rate than FCB [14]. The idea was to test whether a strong initial receptor trigger could generate a protracted functional response. Possibly, the steroid liganded within the receptor complex might be metabolically more protected than the nonliganded steroid fraction.

By introducing a carbonate ester group within the 17β-carboxylic ester moiety (table 1), it was possible to design a soft steroid candidate with a receptor affinity similar to budesonide, and with a rapid hydrolytic inactivation ($t_{1/2}$ less than 30 min in human plasma and lung tissue in vitro). In animal airway and lung models, the rapid biotransformation of itrocinonide was still compatible with topical anti-inflammatory efficacy, even though the absolute potency of the inhaled compound was rather low. However, itrocinonide exhibited a much better airway and lung selectivity than conventional ICS. Itrocinonide was administered to humans as a dry powder (Turbuhaler) formulation, and its rapid inactivation and very good tolerance were confirmed in man. After intravenous injection, the plasma $t_{1/2}$ was approximately 30 min. By inhalation, very little intact itrocinonide could be traced in plasma, and even doses up to 80 mg (nominal dose) were achieved without signs of systemic activity (cortisol depression) [14].

When itrocinonide was inhaled in daily doses of 4–8 mg, it had some efficacy in clinical asthma, in challenge-induced provocation of asthmatics, and in seasonal rhinitis [14]. However, its efficacy was much less than that of budesonide, and too low for forwarding the project. The low efficacy of itrocinonide is probably due to its rapid hydrolysis within the target tissue. Although it could initially trigger glucocorticoid receptors as strongly as current ICS, its rapid breakdown would leave insufficient compound to trigger recycled or de novo synthetized glucocorticoid receptors. Clearly, sustained local concentrations of steroid are necessary for mediating functional anti-inflammatory activity.

Loteprednol Etabonate. Loteprednol etabonate (LE) is a soft drug developed by Bodor and Buchwald [10] for local ophthalmic use, but is now tested also for respiratory indications [15]. LE has a soft-steroid profile and is broken down by plasma and tissue esterases into its inactive 17β-carboxylic acid. In the rat, LE has a $t_{1/2}$ of less than 10 min in vitro (plasma), and an in vivo terminal plasma $t_{1/2}$ of 50 min [16]. However, LE is rather stable in dog plasma, with a terminal plasma $t_{1/2}$ of 2.8 h which is similar to that of liver-inactivated ICS [17]. Its human intravenous kinetics have not been published.

Table 1.

Soft steroid projects

Drug	Structure		D-ring	Inactivation route	Inhalation project
	X	Y			
By ubiquitous esterases					
Flucocortin butyl ester (Schering AG)	H	F	COO(CH$_2$)$_3$CH$_3$, CH$_3$ (with =O)	COOH, CH$_3$ (with =O)	Cancelled
Itrocinonide (Astra)	F	F	COO(CH$_3$)CHOCOOC$_2$H$_5$, O-H, O-C$_3$H$_7$	COOH, O-H, O-C$_3$H$_7$	Cancelled
Loteprednol etabonate (N. Bodor, Asta)	H	H	COOCH$_2$Cl, OCOOC$_2$H$_5$	COOH, OH	Preclinical phase
By specific esterases					
Example from WO 9724365 (GW)	F	F	lactone with S, OCOOC$_2$H$_5$, CH$_3$	COOH, OH with S, OCOOC$_2$H$_5$, CH$_3$	See text and Note Added in Proof

Inactivation of Steroids by Esterases with Low Activity in Lung Tissue

Lactone derivatives of glucocorticosteroids are a novel class of soft GCSs that have recently been revealed by GlaxoWellcome in a series of patent applications (WO 97/24365, WO 97/24367, WO 97/24368 and WO 99/01467) and one short publication [18]. One preferred compound from application WO 97/24365 is shown in table 1. The clear aim of the project is to develop steroids with stability in their target organ (airways and lung) but high lability in blood.

The hydrolysis of the lactone ring is catalyzed by a specific esterase and gives a hydroxy carboxylic acid derivative with a very low affinity for the glucocorticoid receptor. Incubation with human plasma resulted in very rapid hydrolysis of the active compound (for example, in vitro $t_{1/2}$ in Biggadike et al. [18] is less than 1 min), whereas the lactone was stable in a human lung fraction (in vitro $t_{1/2}$ more than 480 min). The enzyme that catalyzes lactone ring hydrolysis is a paraoxonase (EC 3.1.8.1), which is present in the liver and blood, but could not be detected in brain, placenta, lung, skeletal muscle, kidney and pancreas using Northern blot analysis [19].

According to the patent applications, GCS-lactones have good topical anti-inflammatory efficacy, as documented by inhibition of croton-oil-induced ear edema and lung eosinophilia after provocation of sensitized rats. The systemic effects of lactone-GCS, measured as ACTH suppression in adrenalectomized rats, were much lower than with conventional ICS, supporting a high topical selectivity in the pharmacological models. Two compounds have subsequently been selected for clinical testing. GW 215864 (structure not revealed) has a high 'receptor potency', and a very rapid in vitro hydrolysis in human plasma ($t_{1/2}$ 1 min). This compound is now in phase II trials [data from Investext, AN 2000:724966]. The other compound, GW 250495 (structure not revealed), has a somewhat lower 'receptor potency' and a slower rate of hydrolysis, and is reported to be in phase I [data from Investext, AN 2000:724966]. According to a recent chemical presentation [Ramesh V, et al: 218th Am. Chem. Soc. Natl. Meet., New Orleans, 1999], GlaxoWellcome continues to screen for steroids with the desired combination of high receptor affinity and short plasma $t_{1/2}$.

Conclusion and Prospects

The currently used ICS-like budesonide and fluticasone propionate are both very efficacious and safe for the treatment of mild and moderate asthma. However, many asthma patients are still hesitant to use ICS, due to an unfounded steroidophobia, and cannot therefore be optimally treated. One way to reduce steroidophobia has been to develop ICS based upon the soft-drug concept, so that much less active steroid is distributed outside the target area. However, the soft steroids hitherto clinically tested have not been able to compete with conventional ICS in terms of efficacy. The earliest developed soft steroid, FCB, possessed too low receptor affinity (in the range of prednisolone). To improve the receptor affinity to the same high level as that of current ICS, the soft drug itrocinonide was developed and designed for an even faster extrahepatic metabolic rate than FCB. Also itrocinonide had too low clinical efficacy, probably due to its rapid inactivation at the target tissue, and potentially also due to its total lack of systemic activity (if there is a need for such activity).

The soft drug project at GlaxoWellcome has generated lactone-GCS conjugates with stability to conventional hydrolases, but lability to plasma paraoxonase. This affords a better opportunity to attain both topical efficacy and selectivity, since these steroids will be stable in the target tissue but susceptible to rapid inactivation during their disposition in the blood. The therapeutic outcome of these GCS may clarify the key issue for soft steroids: that is, whether it is possible to achieve anti-asthmatic efficacy comparable with that of conventional ICS in the absence of any systemic GCS distribution and activity.

Note Added in Proof

According to Adis R&D Insight 2000, Accession numbers 10129 and 10130, the development of GW 250495 and GW 215864 has been discontinued for the asthma indication. However, for GW 215864 Phase I clinical trials are in progress for the treatment of rhinitis.

References

1 Barnes PJ, Pedersen S, Busse WW: Efficacy and safety of inhaled corticosteroids: New developments. Am J Respir Crit Care Med 1998; 157:S1–S53.
2 Brattsand R: What factors determine anti-inflammatory activity and selectivity of inhaled steroids. Eur Respir Rev 1997;7:50, 356–361.
3 Thorsson L, Dahlström K, Edsbäcker S, Källén A, Paulson J, Wirén JE: Pharmacokinetics and systemic effects of inhaled fluticasone propionate in healthy subjects. Br J Clin Pharmacol 1997;43:155–161.
4 Ryrfeldt Å, Andersson PH, Edsbäcker S, Tönnesson M, Davies D, Pauwels R: Pharmacokinetics and metabolism of budesonide, a selective glucocorticoid. Eur J Respir Dis 1982; 63(suppl 122):86–95.
5 Van den Bosch JMM, Westmann CJJ, Aumann J, Edsbücker S, Tönnesson M, Selroos O: Relationship between lung tissue and blood plasma concentrations of inhaled budesonide. Biopharm Drug Dispos 1993;14:455–459.
6 Esmailpour N, Högger P, Rabe KF, Heitmann U, Nakashima M, Rohdewald P: Distribution of inhaled fluticasone propionate between human lung tissue and serum in vivo. Eur Respir J 1997;10:1496–1499.
7 Dahlberg E, Thalén A, Brattsand R, Gustafsson J-Å, Johansson U, Roempke K, Saartok T: Correlation between chemical structure, receptor binding and biological activity of some novel, highly active 16α,17α-acetal-substituted glucocorticoids. Mol Pharmacol 1984;25:70–78.

8 Toogood JRH, Frankish CW, Jennings B, Baskerville JC, Borgå O, Lefcoe NM, Johansson S-Å: A comparison of the anti-asthmatic efficacy of inhaled versus oral budesonide. J Allergy Clin Immunol 1990;85:872–880.
9 Lawrence M, Wolfe J, Webb DR, Chervinsky P, Kellerman D, Schaumberg JP, Shah T: Efficacy of inhaled fluticasone propionate in asthma results from topical and not from systemic activity. Am J Respir Crit Care Med 1997;156: 744–751.
10 Bodor N, Buchwald P: Soft drug design: General principles and recent applications. Med Res Rev 2000;20:58–101.
11 Satoh T, Hosokawa M: Mammalian carboxylesterases: From molecules to functions. Annu Rev Pharmacol Toxicol 1998;38:257–288.
12 Mützel W: Pharmacokinetics and biotransformation of fluocortin butyl ester in man. Arzneimittelforschun 1977;27:2230–2233.
13 Burge S, Efthimiou J, Turner-Warwick M, Nelmes PTJ: Double blind trial of inhaled beclomethasone dipropionate and fluocortin butyl ester in allergen-induced immediate and late asthmatic reactions. Clin Allergy 1982;12: 523–531.
14 Thalén A, Andersson PH, Andersson PT, Axelsson B, Edsbücker S, Brattsand R: Prospects for developing inhaled steroids with extrahepatic metabolism – 'soft steroids'; in Schleimer RP, O'Byrne P, Szefler S, Brattsand R (eds): Airway Activity and Selectivity of Inhaled Steroids in Asthma. New York, Dekker, in press.

15 Poppe H, Marx D, Heer S, Szelenyi I: Effects of loteprednol etabonate on TNFα and GM-CSF release in vitro and on late phase eosinophilia in guinea pigs administered intratracheally as a dry powder. Am J Respir Crit Care Med 1998; 157(suppl):A522.
16 Bodor N, Loftsson T, Wu W-M: Metabolism, distribution and transdermal permeability of a soft steroid, loteprednol etabonate. Pharm Res 1992;9:1275–1278.
17 Hochhaus G, Chen L-S, Ratka A, Druzgala P, Howes J, Bodor N, Derendorf H: Pharmacokinetic characterization and tissue distribution of the new glucocorticoid soft drug loteprednol etabonate in rats and dogs. J Pharm Sci 1992; 81:1210–1215.
18 Biggadike K, Angell RM, Burgess CM, Farrell RM, Hancock AP, Harker AJ, Irving WR, Ioannou C, Procopiou PA, Shaw RE, Solanke YE, Singh OMP, Snowden MA, Stubbs RJ, Walton S, Weston HE: Selective plasma hydrolysis of glucocorticoid γ-lactones and cyclic carbonates by the enzyme paraoxonase: An ideal plasma inactivation mechanism. J Med Chem 2000;43:19–21.
19 Kelso GJ, Stuart WD, Richter RJ, Furlong CE, Jordan-Starck TC Harmony JAK: Apolipoprotein J is associated with paraoxonase in human plasma. Biochemistry 1994;33:832–839.

Ralph Brattsand
AstraZeneca R&D Lund
SE-221 87 Lund (Sweden)
Tel. +46 46 336 209, Fax +46 46 336 624
E-Mail ralph.brattsand@astrazeneca.com

Dissociated Steroids

Thomas J. Brown   Maria G. Belvisi   Martyn L. Foster

Aventis Pharmaceuticals, Dagenham, UK

Summary

Inhaled glucocorticoids are the mainstay of asthma therapy, but their use is often limited by the associated systemic side effects. Dissociated steroids have been developed which differentiate between the two main actions of steroids (i.e. transactivation and transrepression). These compounds claim to offer the potential for a more selective anti-inflammatory profile without possessing adverse effects. The profile of one such compound is discussed below.

Glucocorticoids (GCs) remain the most effective therapy for inflammatory disorders. In terms of asthma, topical steroids are the mainstay for controlling the inflammatory component of the disease. However, topical steroid use is often limited by patient compliance issues and poor device training, particularly in the young and old. Pharmaceutical research on steroids is now focused on the discovery and development of oral drugs. However, such a strategy is limited by the constellation of adverse effects associated with chronic, oral steroid use. These include suppression of hypothalamic-pituitary axis, osteoporosis, reduced bone growth in the young, opportunistic infections, behavioural alterations, and disorders of lipid metabolism. Most of these effects may be attributed to the endocrine activity of steroids and are largely identical to the syndromes of endogenous corticosteroid excess (Cushing's syndrome). Thus the Holy Grail of steroid pharmacology is the development of agents which have a markedly better therapeutic ratio than current steroids, especially on systemic administration. This may be achieved by the identification of molecules that elicit marked anti-inflammatory effects but have a minor impact on endocrine responses. Dissociated corticosteroids are ligands for the GC receptor (GR) that may offer the potential for a more selective anti-inflammatory profile.

Transactivation by Steroids

The cellular actions of steroids are mediated by ligand diffusion across the cell membrane and its association with the GR, a member of the nuclear hormone receptor superfamily. This superfamily is characterized by a modular structure including a DNA-binding domain (DBD) comprising two zinc fingers, a ligand-binding domain (LBD) and two transactivation motifs (AF-1 and AF-2). Between the DBD and the LBD is a sequence required for dimerization of two monomers. Ligand binding of the GR results in dissociation of heat shock proteins and exposure of nuclear localization sequence, allowing nuclear transportation of the receptor homodimers. Transactivation by the GR requires binding of receptor dimers to specific palindromic sequences in the cis-regulatory region of target genes called the GC response element (GRE) [1]. GRE-bound GR homodimers induce gene expression by interacting with basic transcription machinery, co-activators and other transcription factors. It is via this mechanism that GCs regulate the expression of β_2-adrenoceptors and I-κBα, the inhibitor of the transcription factor NF-κB [2, 3]. Additionally, gene repression can be mediated by GR binding to negative GREs (nGREs) as identified in the pro-opiomelanocortin promoter. However,

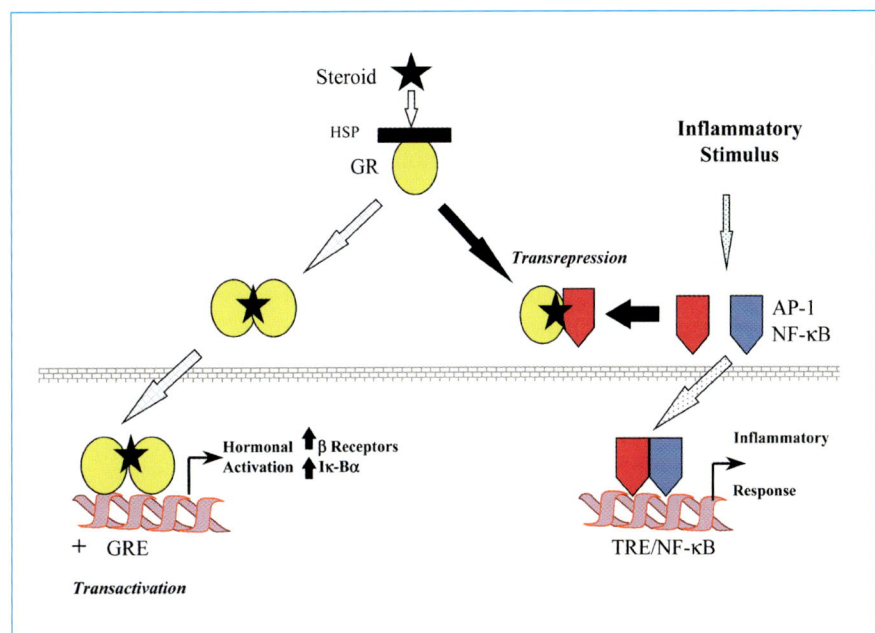

Fig. 1. Models of steroid-induced transactivation and transrepression.

many of the pro-inflammatory genes whose inhibition is central to the anti-inflammatory actions of GCs do not possess GREs or nGREs in their promoters, thus suggesting that alternative modes of regulation of these genes probably exist [1].

Transrepression by Steroids

Many of the pro-inflammatory genes whose products mediate the inflammatory process in asthma are regulated by the transcription factors activating protein-1 (AP-1) and NF-κB. In the early 1990s, a number of groups recognized that the GR can regulate gene transcription by forming protein-protein interactions with these transcription factors without the necessity for DNA binding. AP-1, which is a dimer of c-Jun and c-Fos, contributes to the regulation of cytokines and adhesion molecules. Direct protein-protein interaction between AP-1 and the liganded GR was shown to result in repression of transcriptional activity by blocking the interaction of both transcription factors with their respective response elements [4]. Mutation studies of the GR have revealed that this repressive action is most likely mediated by GR monomers rather than dimers. Heck et al. [5] illustrated, through the introduction of mutations in the DBD of the GR, that transactivation and transrepression can be dissociated. Mutations resulting in failure of the GR to dimerize and bind DNA were associated with a failure to transactivate GRE-dependent promoters in cell transfection studies. However, repression of the AP-1-dependent promoter by the mutant GR was as effective as by the wild-type receptor.

Various mechanisms have been invoked to explain the transrepressing actions of steroids. Although evidence exists for direct protein interaction through the b ZIP region of AP-1 and the DBD of the GR resulting in failure of DNA binding, this is unlikely to be the sole mechanism [6]. Nuclear footprinting studies have indicated that AP-1 DNA interactions can still occur despite transrepression by GR. In this situation, it is likely that an ineffective complex has been produced after binding of AP-1 to DNA at its cognate recognition sequence and the GR binding by protein-protein interaction to the promoter with failure to transactivate [7] (fig. 1). Further explanations of transrepression may lay in the competition for binding to shared co-activators such as CREB-binding protein (CBP) [8], whose availability is limited. Displacement of AP-1 from CBP by GR would result in failure to induce gene expression. Recently, the ability of GCs to limit the expression of JNK, a key regulator of AP-1 expression, has emerged. In cases of GC resistance, it has been reported that this regulation of JNK is impaired [9].

NF-κB is also important in the regulation of inflammatory genes. In addition to the increased expression of the inhibitory I-κBα induced by GR, GCs also have the capacity to directly interact with and repress NF-κB. The relative importance of these respective means of repressing NF-κB may be cell type dependent. The ability of steroids to transrepress the action of transcription factors probably extends beyond AP-1 and NF-κB to other transcription factors including GATA and the STATs. Furthermore, the ability to transrepress is not limited to the GR, but is also a characteristic of other members of the nuclear receptor family.

The physiological significance of the DNA binding and dimerization-independent transrepressive actions of the GR are revealed in studies in homozygous mice carrying a dimerization- and DNA-binding-defective mutant of GR (GR^{dim}). DNA binding and transcriptional regulation of genes containing GREs and nGREs were confirmed to be unresponsive to GCs, whereas repression of AP-1-mediated gene expression was shown to be intact. The GR^{dim} homozygotes appeared normal and survived to adulthood in sharp contrast to mice that were deficient in their GR. This suggests that GRE mediated gene regulation is not essential for survival or development, whereas the ability of GR to transrepress transcription factors is essential [9–11]. However, these studies do not address whether in these mutants GCs are capable of regulating the activity of other transcription factors such as NF-κB and thereby repress the expression of proinflammatory genes, e.g. cytokines. Furthermore, although GR$^{dim/dim}$ mice are resistant to GC-induced thymus involution, it is not clear whether these mice would demonstrate an anti-inflammatory effect in the lung following GC treatment.

These studies suggest that different domains of the GR are responsible for different actions, but can this be exploited pharmacologically and lead to agents with more selective, better anti-inflammatory activity compared with current drugs? The evidence is that different steroids can preferentially elicit different responses from the GR. Of considerable importance to the development of more selective steroids is the consideration as to whether different mechanisms can be triggered by different ligands following activation of the GR [13] (fig. 2).

Recently, a new compound, RU 24858, was identified, which was claimed to differentiate between the two main actions of GCs (i.e. transactivation and transrepression), while possessing potent in vivo anti-inflammatory activity [14] (fig. 3). In vitro studies have shown that this compound exhibits significant AP-1 transrepression while only weakly activating the GRE-based reporter genes. Furthermore, the in vitro anti-inflammatory activity of RU 24858 was confirmed by inhibition of IL-1β secretion from activated monocytes while the compound was unable to induce tyrosine amino transferase activity, confirming the lack of transactivating activity. However, this

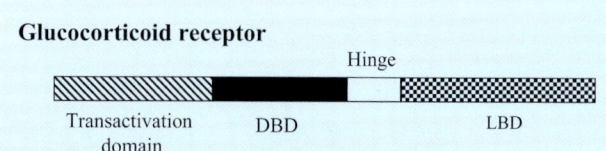

- GR represses inflammatory genes that lack GRE, but contain AP-1 sites in the promoter.
- A transactivation-defective mutant (2 amino acids deleted in the DBD) still represses AP-1.
- The GRE-binding domain and chimeric receptor still binds AP-1.
- Point mutations in the DBD reveal that transactivation and transrepression are dissociable and suggests that GRE-regulated promoters require GR dimerization whereas repression is a function of GR monomers.

Fig. 2.

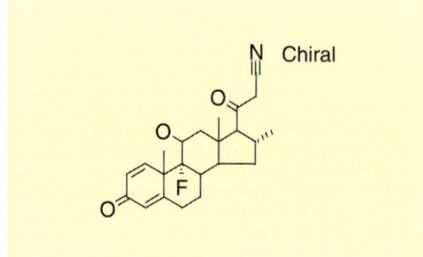

Fig. 3. Structure of RU 24858.

study did not address whether RU 24858 could exhibit the same dissociation by demonstrating anti-inflammatory properties without steroid adverse side effects in vivo. Recently, Belvisi et al. [15] have demonstrated that RU 24858 exhibits anti-inflammatory activity comparable to the standard steroids in an animal model of lung oedema. Interestingly, RU 24858 showed no differentiation, compared to standard steroids, in the ability to induce systemic changes (eg. loss in body weight, thymus involution) and in the quantitative osteopenia of the femur observed after 7 days of treatment. These results suggest that in vitro separation of transrepression from transactivation activity does not translate to an increased therapeutic ratio for GCs in vivo.

To date, the transrepression/transactivation mechanism remains an interesting approach. However, whole-animal physiological studies have failed to confirm the predicted dissociation between anti-inflammatory activity and adverse effects. Whether this indicates that homoeostatic mechanisms present in the animal models override selectivity, which argues for biochemical redundancy in the mechanism, or merely reflects limitations of the prototypical tool, RU 24858, is unknown. Alternatively, these data suggest that some of the classical hormonal actions of GCs are a consequence of transrepression rather than transactivation. It is clear that research in this area should give us fundamental insights into the molecular physiology of steroid action. Given the possible therapeutic rewards of a dissociated steroid, the contradictory data generated so far should only serve as a spur to future research.

References

1 Karin M: New twists in the gene regulation by glucocorticoid receptor: Is DNA binding dispensable? Cell 1998;93:487–490.
2 Barnes PJ: Anti-inflammatory actions of glucocorticoids: Molecular mechanisms. Clin Sci 1998;94:557–572.
3 van der Velden VHJ: Glucocorticoids: Mechanisms of action and anti-inflammatory potential in asthma. Mediators Inflamm 1998;7:229–237.
4 Gotticher M, Heck S, Herrlich P: Transcriptional cross-talk, the second mode of steroid hormone receptor action. J Mol Med 1998;76:480–489.
5 Heck S, Kullman M, Gast A, Ponta H, Rahmsdorf HJ, Herrlich P, Cato AC: A distinct modulating domain in glucocorticoid receptor monomers in the repression of activity of the transcription factor AP-1. EMBO J 1994;13:4087–4095.
6 Tuckermann JP, Reichardt HM, Arribas R, Richter KH, Schutz G Angel P: The DNA binding-independent function of the glucocorticoid receptor mediates repression of AP-1-dependent genes in skin. J Cell Biol 1999;147:1365–1370.
7 Pearce D, Matsui W, Miner JN, Yamamoto: Glucocorticoid receptor transcription activity determined by spacing of receptor and nonreceptor DNA sites. J Biol Chem 1998;273:30081–30085.
8 Sheppard KA Phelps KM, Williams AJ, Thanos D, Glass CK, Rosenfeld MG, Gerritsen ME, Collins T: Nuclear integration of glucocorticoid receptor and nuclear factor-κB signaling by CREB-binding protein and steroid coactivator-1. J Biol Chem 1998;273:29291–29294.
9 Sousa A, Lane SJ, Soh C, Lee TH: In vivo resistance to corticosteroids in bronchial asthma is associated with enhanced phosphorylation of JUN N-terminal kinase and failure of prednisolone to inhibit JUN N-terminal kinase phosphorylation. J Allergy Clin Immunol 1999;104:565–574.
10 Reichardt HM, Kaestner KH, Tuckermann J, Kretz, O, Wessely O, Bock R, Gass P, Schmid W, Herrlich P, Angel P, Schutz G: DNA binding of the glucocorticoid receptor is not essential for survival. Cell 1998;93:531–541.
11 Reichardt HM, Tronche F, Berger S, Kellendonk C, Schutz G: New insights into glucocorticoid and mineralocorticoid signaling: Lessons from gene targeting. Hormones and Signaling 2000;1–21.
12 Kellendonk C, Tronche F, Reichardt HM, Schutz G: Mutagenesis of the glucocorticoid receptor in mice. J Steroid Biochem Mol Biol 1999;69:253–259.
13 Berghe WV, Francesconi E, Bosscher KD, Resche-Rigon M, Haegman G: Dissociated glucocorticoids with anti-inflammatory potential repress IL-6 gene expression by nuclear factor-κB-dependent mechanism. Mol Pharm 1999;56:797–806.
14 Vayssière BM, Dupont S, Choquart A, Petit F, Garcia T, Marchandeau C, Gronemeyer H, Resche-Rigon M: Synthetic glucocorticoids that dissociate transactivation and AP-1 transrepression exhibit anti-inflammatory activity in vivo. Mol Endocrinol 1997;11:1245–1265.
15 Belvisi MG, Wicks S, Battram C, Bottoms S, Redford J, Webber S, Foster M: Does the synthetic glucocorticoid, RU 24858, which dissociates transactivation and transrepression in vitro possess anti-inflammatory properties without steroid adverse side effects in vivo? Am J Respir Crit Care Med 1999;153:A342.

Dr. Maria G. Belvisi
Reader in Respiratory Pharmacology
Head, Respiratory Pharmacology Group
Cardiothoracic Surgery, Imperial College
School of Medicine
National Heart and Lung Institute
Dovehouse Street
London SW3 6LY (UK)
Tel. +44 207 351 8270, +44 402 300 464 (mobile)
Fax +44 207 376 3442
E-Mail m.belvisi@ic.ac.uk

Oestradiol Metabolites

Effects on Airway Remodelling

A.G. Stewart   R. Vlahos   D.J. Fernandes   R.A. Hughes

Department of Pharmacology, University of Melbourne, Australia

Summary

Airway wall remodelling is a significant contributor to the airway hyperresponsiveness in asthma and hence to asthma symptoms. Existing anti-asthma agents (glucocorticoids) appear to have insufficient efficacy in the regulation of smooth muscle proliferation and other aspects of airway wall remodelling in severe asthma. Thus, agents that regulate airway wall remodelling will add significantly to the choice of preventative therapies available for more severe asthma. The anti-angiogenic, anti-proliferative oestradiol metabolite, 2-methoxyoestradiol, is a candidate prophylactic anti-asthma agent that may more specifically target the airway wall remodelling process.

Airway Wall Remodelling and Asthma

Asthma is characterized by chronic airways inflammation, a variable degree of reversible airway obstruction and airway wall remodelling, each of which contributes to airway hyperresponsiveness. The cellular components of airway wall remodelling include airway smooth muscle hyperplasia and hypertrophy, basement membrane thickening resulting from an increase in interstitial collagen deposited by (myo)fibroblasts, mucous cell hyperplasia, angiogenesis and infiltration of inflammatory cells [see Pare and Bai, 1, for review]. Airway wall remodelling has also been described in sudden infant death syndrome [2] and in COPD [3]. Smooth muscle hyperplasia is the most important of all of these cellular changes that contribute to airway wall thickening, and this wall thickening is now considered to explain a large part of the airway hyperresponsiveness in asthma [4].

A number of biologically diverse stimuli for proliferation of human cultured airway smooth muscle have been identified [5]. It is not clear which of the many cytokines, growth factors and other mitogens identified in the airway wall [6, 7] are the most important in causing airway wall remodelling in asthma. Furthermore, it is uncertain whether or not the remodelling process is capable of reversal, either spontaneously or after effective drug treatment. However, the results of a recent landmark study examining the effects of adjusting the dose of glucocorticoids to achieve a reduction in airway hyperresponsiveness (AHR regimen), rather than to control symptoms (reference regimen), suggest that remodelling is at least partly reversible. The AHR regimen resulted in the use of higher doses of glucocorticoids that reduced subepithelial fibrosis and the number of asthma exacerbations to a greater extent than the lower doses of glucocorticoids used in the reference treatment regimen [8]. We have proposed that development of inhibitors of airway smooth muscle growth may provide novel anti-asthma drugs that prevent/reverse airway wall thickening, reduce airway hyperresponsiveness and therefore ameliorate asthma symptoms [5, 9].

Existing Anti-Asthma Drugs and Airway Wall Remodelling

Glucocorticoids are currently the most effective drugs used to treat airway inflammation and have become the mainstay therapy for patients with asthma [10]. However, clinical studies have shown that glucocorticoids do not fully reverse airway hyperresponsiveness and that their maximal effect on this process takes several months to develop [11]. Glucocorticoids attenuate proliferation of cultured airway smooth muscle stimulated by a variety of mitogens [12, 13]. The mechanism(s) involved in these anti-mitogenic effects involve regulation of the synthesis of the key cyclin, cyclin D1, which is required for passage of cells through the restriction point of the cell cycle [13].

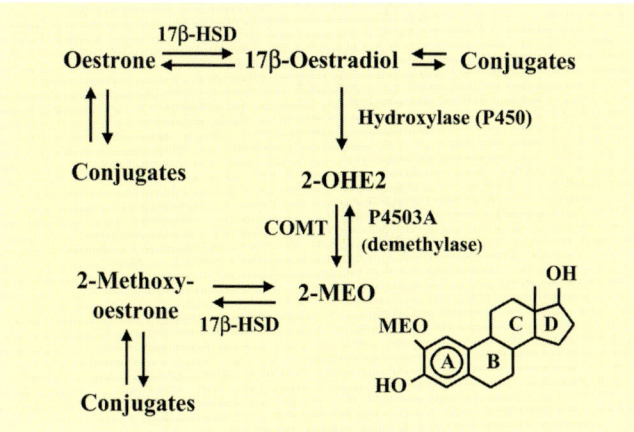

Fig. 1. Metabolic pathway of 17β-oestradiol. 17β-Oestradiol circulates in concentrations less than 10 nM. It may undergo several reversible reactions. Transformation by oestrogen sulphotransferase or glucuronyl transferase generates more polar products that are readily excreted by the kidneys. 17β-Hydroxy-steroid-dehydrogenase (17β-HSD) converts 17β-oestradiol to the oestrone that retains affinity for ER. A cytochrome P450 hydroxylase converts 17β-oestradiol into the 2OH metabolite, 2-hydroxyoestradiol (2-OHE2) that is further converted by COMT to 2-MEO. 2-MEO has less than 1/100 the affinity of 17β-oestradiol for ER. 2-MEO may itself undergo conjugation or oxidation to 2-methoxyoestrone, which has even lower affinity for ER. The activity of a number of these enzymes may be altered by phytoestrogens, the pharmacology of which resembles that of 2-MEO in some cases [19].

Even though glucocorticoids inhibit airway smooth muscle proliferation, these compounds may compromise effective negative feedback influences on remodelling, such as increased prostaglandin E$_2$ production [14]. In addition, the magnitude of the anti-proliferative effects of the glucocorticoids depends on the specific mitogen stimulating proliferation (e.g. growth factor stimulant via receptor tyrosine kinase versus stimulant of G-protein-coupled receptor) [12]. Therefore, there is a need for new agents with greater capacity to provide additional control of the remodelling that occurs in asthma and other chronic airway inflammatory conditions. In this brief review we describe the properties of 2-methoxyoestradiol (2-MEO), a metabolite of oestradiol that has potential as a novel anti-asthma agent with multiple actions on the airway wall remodelling process.

Oestradiol and Asthma

Females have a higher risk of hospital admission for asthma, possibly as a consequence of endogenous or exogenous levels of sex hormones [15]. In addition, more than 30% of asthmatic females suffer from worsening asthma symptoms around the time of menstruation [15]. Oestradiol treatment of asthmatic females results in improvement in symptoms [16], and the oral contraceptive pill attenuates cyclical change in airway reactivity [17]. Nevertheless, there are a number of studies that suggest that exogenous sex hormones exacerbate asthma [15]. In the aforementioned studies it is not apparent whether any of the actions of oestradiol were due to activation of high-affinity oestrogen receptors (ER) or due to the action of oestradiol metabolites acting through other mechanisms (fig. 1). Moreover, there is little information as to the effects of ER antagonists on airway function and disease.

2-Methoxyoestradiol

Oestradiol is metabolised by several different pathways generating metabolites that have variable degrees of oestrogenic activity/affinity for the ER (fig. 1). The conjugates (glucuronide and sulphate) may be excreted or converted back to oestradiol depending on the enzymatic profile of the organ/tissue. The hydroxylation of oestradiol to 2-hydroxyoestradiol (2-OHE2), whilst most likely to occur in the liver, may take place in many different cell types [18]. Subsequently, the widely distributed catechol-O-methyl transferase (COMT) may catalyse the conversion of 2-OHE2 to 2-MEO. The plasma concentrations of 2-MEO are not well characterized, but this compound is widely regarded as being a minor metabolite that may rise to bioactive levels in specific compartments such as the follicular fluid [18, 19].

2-MEO had been widely, though not exclusively, regarded as an inactive metabolite of oestradiol. Several studies reported some activities including inhibition of proliferation of transformed cell lines [see Zhu and Conney, 19, for references]. However, the unexpected observation of anti-angiogenic and anti-proliferative activities by Fotsis et al [20] raised interest in other actions of this catecholoestrogen metabolite. It has now been established that 2-MEO inhibits the development of various types of tumour by a combination of cytotoxic and anti-angiogenic actions [20, 21], reduces collagen-induced arthritis in the rat [22] and at the molecular level is believed to exert at least some of its anti-proliferative actions through interactions with tubulin [23]. 2-MEO has anti-proliferative effects against a variety of tumour cell types: these effects do not appear to depend on the expression of high-affinity ER by the target tumour cells [21, 23]. In addition, 2-MEO regulates the proliferation of a number of other cell types including lymphocytes [22], granulosa cells [18], smooth muscle [24, 25], endothelium and fibroblasts [20].

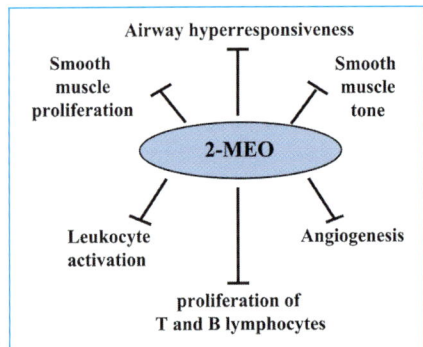

Fig. 2. Properties of 2-MEO that would make it a therapeutic agent in the treatment of asthma. 2-MEO inhibits the proliferation of airway smooth muscle and fibroblasts [24, 25], decreases lymphocyte proliferation in response to endotoxin and concanavalin A [22], has antiangiogenic actions in tumours and in the cornea [21], and reduces mast cell degranulation and macrophage prostaglandin production [24]. Collectively, these actions are likely to reduce airway hyperresponsiveness.

Fig. 3. Orthogonal views of 2-MEO showing the extra volume below the plane of the D ring occupied by electronegative substituents on compounds showing 'agonist' activity in the airway smooth muscle DNA synthesis assay.

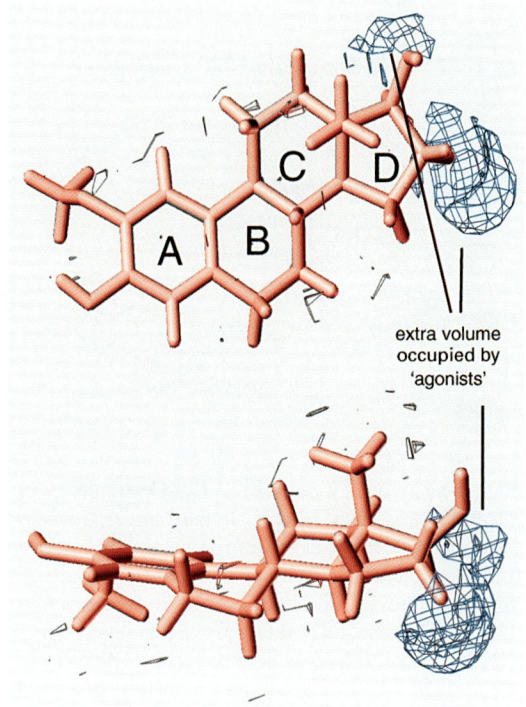

Potential Anti-Asthma Properties of 2-Methoxyoestradiol

We have demonstrated that 2-MEO has several properties desirable in the treatment of obstructive airway diseases such as asthma and COPD (fig. 2) [24, 25]. The spectrum of activities of 2-MEO make it a suitable candidate for further evaluation as an anti-asthma drug that influences several important elements of the airway wall remodelling process, including the development of new blood vessels. Angiogenesis may be critical in subserving the metabolic needs of the increased tissue mass occurring as a result of the airway wall remodelling. Our current studies are focussed on the effects of 2-MEO in models of airway wall remodelling and airway hyperresponsiveness in rats and mice. The effects of 2-MEO on proliferation of cultured airway smooth muscle proliferation are relatively well characterized.

Inhibition of Smooth Muscle Proliferation

2-MEO inhibits mitogen-stimulated DNA synthesis of human cultured airway smooth muscle (table 1). Interestingly, at a concentration of 10 μM, 2-OHE2 was as effective as 2-MEO as an inhibitor of airway smooth muscle DNA synthesis, but oestradiol itself was inactive (table 1). In contrast, 2-methoxyoestriol stimulated DNA synthesis elicited by thrombin, whereas 2-methoxyoestrone had

Table 1. Effects of oestradiol and its metabolites on human airway smooth muscle DNA synthesis and potency for displacement (IC_{50}) of 0.2 nM [^{3}H]-oestradiol binding from a preparation of rat uterine cytosol (source of high-affinity ER)

Metabolite	Thrombin-induced DNA synthesis (% control) at 10 μM metabolite mean ± SEM	Affinity for ER $-\log[IC_{50}]$ ± SEM
17β-Oestradiol	99 ± 18	9.89 ± 0.24
2-Hydroxy-17β-oestradiol	45 ± 17	9.49 ± 0.02
2-Methoxy-17β-oestradiol	40 ± 4	7.50 ± 0.15
2-Methoxyoestrone	83 ± 14	4.97 ± 0.34
2-Methoxy-3,17β-oestriol	180 ± 36	5.56 ± 0.08

no effect at 10 μM, but was stimulatory at 1 and 3 μM. Using a standard assay of affinity for the ER, namely displacement of [^{3}H]-oestradiol from a preparation of rat uterine cytosol, it was evident that there was no clear relationship between ER affinity and effects on DNA synthesis in airway smooth muscle [25]. Molecular modelling of 2-methoxyoestriol, 2-methoxyoestrone and 2-MEO showed that the former two agents, which have stimulatory effects on airway smooth muscle DNA synthesis, are characterized by extra bulk from electronegative substituents projecting below the plane of the D ring of the steroid nucleus (fig. 3).

2-MEO does not appear to act through glucocorticoid receptors because the anti-proliferative effects of 2-MEO on airway smooth muscle are not blocked by pretreatment with the glucocorticoid and progesterone receptor antagonist, RU486. Furthermore, the time-course of action of the glucocorticoid, dexamethasone and that of 2-MEO on airway smooth muscle DNA synthesis are clearly distinct. In addition, 2-MEO has no structural similarity to glucocorticoids other than the steroid nucleus and 2-MEO neither blocks nor mimics the actions of glucocorticoids [24].

A number of observations suggest that there is no role for the normal affinity states of the ER (α or β) in the effects of 2-MEO; the lack of a relationship between affinity for ER and suppression of smooth muscle DNA synthesis; the lack of activity of oestradiol; and the failure of the ER antagonist, ICI 182780, to block the actions of 2-MEO [unpubl. obs.].

Collectively, our findings provide impetus for the further development of 2-MEO as an anti-asthma agent.

Acknowledgments

We acknowledge the NHMRC (Australia) and AMRAD Operations Pty Ltd for funding of the work on 2-MEO and airway smooth muscle proliferation. We also thank Ms Trudi Harris for technical assistance with the smooth muscle DNA synthesis assessments.

References

1 Pare PD, Bai TR: The consequences of chronic allergic inflammation. Thorax 1995; 50:328–332.
2 Elliot J, Vullermin P, Carroll N, James A, Robinson P: Increased airway smooth muscle in sudden infant death syndrome. Am J Respir Crit Care Med 1999;160:313–316.
3 Kuwano K, Bosken CH, Pare PD, Bai TR, Wiggs BR, Hogg JC: Small airways dimensions in asthma and chronic airway obstructive pulmonary disease. Am Rev Respir Dis 1993;148:1220–1225.
4 James AL, Pare PD, Hogg JC: The mechanics of airway narrowing in asthma. Am Rev Respir Dis 1989;139:242–246.
5 Stewart AG, Tomlinson PR, Wilson J: Regulation of airway wall remodelling: Prospects for the development of novel anti-asthma drugs. Adv Pharmacol 1995;33:209–253.
6 Hoshino M, Nakamura Y, Sim JJ: Expression of growth factors and remodelling of the airway wall in bronchial asthma. Thorax 1998;53:21–27.
7 Vignola AM, Chanez P, Bonsignore G, Godard P, Bousquet J: Structural consequences of airway inflammation in asthma. J Allergy Clin Immunol 2000;105:514–517.
8 Sont JK, Willems LN, Bel EH, van Krieken JH, Vandenbroucke JP, Sterk PJ: Clinical control and histopathologic outcome of asthma when using airway hyperresponsiveness as an additional guide to long-term treatment. The AMPUL Study Group. Am J Respir Crit Care Med 1999;159:1043–1051.
9 Stewart AG, Tomlinson PR, Wilson J: Airway wall remodelling in asthma: A novel target for the development of anti-asthma drugs. Trends Pharmacol Sci 1993;14:275–279.
10 Barnes PJ, Pedersen S, Busse WM: Efficacy and safety of inhaled corticosteroids: New developments. Am J Respir Crit Care Med 1998; 157:S1–S53.
11 Haahtela T, Jarvinen M, Kava T, Kirivanta K, Koskinen S, Lehtonen K, Nikander K, Persson T, Selroos O, Sovijarvi A, Stenius-Aarniala B, Svahn T, Tammivara R, Laitinen L: Effects of reducing or discontinuing inhaled budesonide in patients with mild asthma. N Engl J Med 1994;331:700–705.
12 Stewart AG, Fernandes DJ, Tomlinson PR: The effect of glucocorticoids on proliferation of human cultured airway smooth muscle. Br J Pharmacol 1995;116:3219–3226.
13 Fernandes D, Guida E, Koutsoubos V, Harris T, Vadiveloo P, Wilson JW, Stewart AG: Glucocorticoids inhibit proliferation, cyclin D1 expression and retinoblastoma protein phosphorylation, but not activity of the extracellular-regulated kinases in human cultured airway smooth muscle. Am J Respir Cell Mol Biol 1999;21:77–88.
14 Vlahos R, Stewart AG: Interleukin-1alpha and tumour necrosis factor-alpha modulate airway smooth muscle DNA synthesis by induction of cyclo-oxygenase-2: Inhibition by dexamethasone and fluticasone propionate. Br J Pharmacol 1999;126:1315–1324.
15 Forbes L: Do exogenous oestrogens and progesterone influence asthma? Thorax 1999;54:265–267.
16 Chandler MHH, Schuldheisz S, Phillips BA, Muse KN: Premenstrual asthma: The effect of estrogen on symptoms, pulmonary function, and β_2-receptors. Pharmacotherapy 1997;17:224–234.
17 Tan KS, McFarlane LS, Lipworth, BJ: Modulation of airway reactivity and peak flow variability in asthmatics receiving the oral contraceptive pill. Am J Respir Crit Care Med 1997;155:1273–1277.
18 Spicer LJ, Hammond JM: Catecholestrogens inhibit proliferation and DNA synthesis of porcine granulosa cells in vitro: Comparison with estradiol, 5α-dihydrotestosterone, gonadotrophins and catecholamines. Mol Cell Endocrinol 1989;64:119–126.
19 Zhu BT, Conney AH: Is 2-methoxyestradiol an endogenous estrogen metabolite that inhibits mammary carcinogenesis? Cancer Res 1998; 58:2269–2277.
20 Fotsis T, Zhang Y, Pepper MS, Adlercreutz H, Montesano R, Nawroth PP, Schweigerer L: The endogenous oestrogen metabolite 2-methoxyoestradiol inhibits angiogenesis and suppresses tumour growth. Nature 1994;368:237–239.
21 Klauber N, Parangi S, Flynn E, Hamel E, D'Amato RJ: Inhibition of angiogenesis and breast cancer in mice by the microtubule inhibitors 2-methoxyestradiol and taxol. Cancer Res 1997;57:81–86.
22 Josefsson E, Tarkowski A: Suppression of type II collagen-induced arthritis by the endogenous estrogen metabolite 2-methoxyestradiol. Arthritis Rheum 1997;40:154–163.
23 Cushman M, He HM, Katzenellenbogen JA, Varma RK, Hamel E, Lin CM, Ram S, Sachdeva YP: Synthesis of analogs of 2-methoxyestradiol with enhanced inhibitory effects on tubulin polymerization and cancer cell growth. J Med Chem 1997;40:2323–2334.
24 Stewart AG: Treatment of asthma and airway diseases. 1999 United States Patent Number 5,962,445.
25 Stewart AG, Harris T, Guida E, Vlahos R, Koutsoubos V, Hughes RA, Robertson A: The estradiol metabolite, 2-methoxyestradiol inhibits proliferation of human cultured airway smooth muscle. Am J Respir Crit Care Med 1998;159:A530.

Alastair G. Stewart
Department of Pharmacology
University of Melbourne
Melbourne, Vic. 3010 (Australia)
Tel. +61 3 8344 5675, Fax +61 3 8344 0241
E-Mail
a.stewart@pharmacology.unimelb.edu.au

Leukotriene Inhibitors

Leukotriene Inhibitors: An Overview

Paul M. O'Byrne[a]   Jeffrey M. Drazen[b]

[a]Asthma Research Group, St. Joseph's Hospital and McMaster University, Hamilton, Canada, and
[b]Respiratory Division, Brigham and Women's Hospital and Harvard Medical School, Boston, Mass., USA

Summary

The leukotrienes (LTs) are eicosanoids derived from membrane constituent arachidonic acid. The cysteinyl LTs LTC_4, LTD_4 and LTE_4 are potent airway smooth muscle constrictors with a much longer duration of action than other smooth muscle constrictors and make up the biological activity previously known as slow reactive substance of anaphylaxis. LTB_4 has minimal bronchoconstrictor effects, but is a potent neutrophil chemoattractant. The cysteinyl LTs transduce their activity through the $CysLT_1$ receptor, while LTB_4 does so through the BLT receptor. Several potent and selective anti-LTs have been developed, which have demonstrated the critical role of cysteinyl LTs in asthma pathobiology. The anti-LTs have now been extensively evaluated in clinical trials in patients with persisting asthma, several of which are available to treat the disease.

In 1938, Kellaway and Trethewie [1] identified a biological activity, which caused slow onset, but very prolonged constriction of smooth muscle; they called this activity 'slow reacting substance' (SRS). Twenty years later, Brocklehurst [2] demonstrated SRS release from lung segments from an asthmatic subject, when exposed to allergen, and slightly modified the name to 'slow reacting substance of anaphylaxis' (SRS-A). He showed, using newly available anti-histamines, that this activity could not be attributed to histamine. His findings generated great excitement among researchers interested in asthma pathogenesis, mainly because SRS-A was a potent airway smooth muscle constrictor with a much longer duration of action than other smooth muscle constrictors, such as histamine, and therefore was conjectured to be important in causing bronchoconstriction and symptoms in asthmatics after allergen inhalation. Subsequently, Samuelsson et al. [3] identified that SRS-A consists of arachidonic acid metabolites which they called 'leukotrienes' (LTs), and the biological activity of SRS-A is now known to be caused by the cysteinyl LTs, LTC_4, LTD_4 and LTE_4. They also identified a biologically distinct noncysteinyl LT (LTB_4) that has minimal bronchoconstrictor effects, but is a potent neutrophil chemoattractant [3].

Leukotriene Biosynthesis

The LTs are derived from the ubiquitous membrane constituent arachidonic acid and are members of a larger group of 20 carbon fatty-acid-derived biomolecules known as eicosanoids. Arachidonic acid (5,8,11,14-cis-eicosatetraenoic acid), is found esterified, in the sn-2 position, to cell membrane phospholipids in a wide variety of mammalian cells [4, 5]. The synthesis of LTs is initiated by the action of phospholipase A_2, which selectively cleaves arachidonic acid from cell membranes. Arachidonic acid is converted sequentially to 5-hydroperoxy-eicosatetraenoic acid and then to LTA_4 (5,6-oxido-7,9-$trans$-11,14-cis-eicosatetraenoic acid) by a catalytic complex consisting of 5-lipoxygenase [6] and the 5-lipoxygenase-activating protein [7]. In the intracellular microenvironment, and in the presence of LTC_4 synthase [8], glutathione is adducted at the C6 position of leukotriene LTA_4 to yield the molecule known as LTC_4 [5(S)-hydroxy-6(R)-glutathionyl-7,9-$trans$-11,14-cis-eicosatetraenoic acid] [9]. The LTC_4 so formed is exported from the cytosol to the

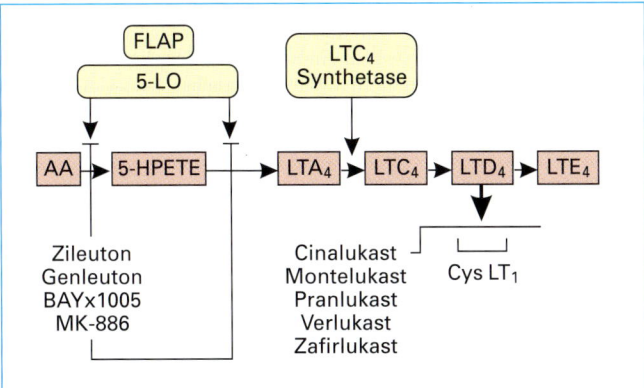

Fig. 1. The 5-lipoxygenase (5-LO) pathway of arachidonic acid (AA) metabolism, indicating the other enzymes, 5-lipoxygenase-activating protein (FLAP) and LTC$_4$ synthetase, necessary for the production of the cysteinyl LTs. Also FLAP antagonists such as BAYx1005 and MK-886, 5-lipoxygenase inhibitors such as zileuton and Cys LT$_1$ antagonists, such as zafirulast or montelukast inhibit the production or action of the cysteinyl LTs. 5-HPETE = 5-Hydroperoxyeicosatetraenoic acid. From O'Byrne PM et al. [16], with permission.

extracellular microenvironment [10] where the glutamic acid moiety is cleaved by γ-glutamyltranspeptidase to form LTD$_4$ [5(S)-hydroxy-6(R)-cysteinyl-glycyl-7,9-*trans*-11,14-*cis*-eicosatetraenoic acid] [11]. Cleavage of the glycine moiety from LTD$_4$ by a variety of dipeptidases results in the formation of LTE$_4$ [5(S)-hydroxy-6(R)-cysteinyl-7,9-*trans*-11,14-*cis*-eicosatetraenoic acid] [12]. All three cysteinyl LTs have the same range of biological effects; however, LTE$_4$ is much less potent as a bronchoconstrictor than its precursor molecules. Among the cells in the lung that possess the enzymatic activities to produce the cysteinyl LTs are mast cells [13], eosinophils [14] and alveolar macrophages [15]; eosinophils and mast cells have been strongly implicated as critical effector cells in the pathobiology of asthma.

Inhibition of Leukotriene Production or Action

It is theoretically possible to inhibit the production of the LTs by inhibition of any of the enzymes in their biosynthetic pathway (fig. 1). However, as of this time, the only enzyme that has been selectively inhibited in human studies is 5-lipoxygenase [17]. It has also been possible to interrupt LT formation by preventing the binding of arachidonic acid to the 5-lipoxygenase-activating protein [18].

The LTs transduce their effects by binding at specific receptors, which for the cysteinyl LTs is the CysLT$_1$ receptor, previously known as the LTD$_4$ receptor or LTR$_d$. This is a seven transmembrane-spanning, G-protein coupled receptor [19]; the gene which encodes this protein is located on the X-chromosome. Stimulation of the CysLT$_1$ receptor results in smooth muscle constriction, with signal transduction occurring by stimulation of phosphoinositide turnover [20]. The LTB$_4$ receptor (BLT) is also a seven-transmembrane-spanning receptor; the gene encoding this receptor is located on chromosome 14q [21]. A number of chemically distinct, specific, selective antagonists of both receptor subtypes have been identified, and CysLT$_1$ receptor antagonists have been extensively studied in human asthma.

Identifying a role for any mediator in asthma (or other inflammatory diseases) is dependent on the collection of various types of evidence. Often, when the structure of a mediator (such as the leukotrienes) is identified, and it is synthesized, the mediator is given (usually by inhalation) to humans (both nonasthmatic and asthmatic), to identify whether it can mimic some component of the asthmatic response. Then, when assays for its measurement are available, efforts are made to measure it in biological fluids, to determine whether it is released (or excreted) during asthmatic responses. This evidence is, however, indirect and can be misleading, as, for example, when very small concentrations of mediators are released locally, which cannot be measured systemically, or when a mediator is released which has its measurable biological effect hours later.

The most compelling evidence of the importance of a mediator in asthma is available when selective antagonists which block the action of the mediator on its receptor, or synthesis inhibitors which prevent its production, are available, and used to evaluate the role of the mediator in causing components of the asthmatic responses evaluated in clinical models of asthma. The final, and most difficult, hurdle is to determine whether the antagonists of the mediators' action or inhibitors of its synthesis are useful in treating asthmatic patients. These data provide the most convincing evidence available that a given mediator has an important role in the pathogenesis of asthma.

By the early 1990s, several potent and selective compounds had been developed, which were then used to demonstrate the critical role of leukotriene generation and release in the airways in causing exercise- [22], allergen- [23], cold-air- [24] and aspirin-induced [25] bronchoconstriction in asthmatics. The anti-LTs have now been extensively evaluated in clinical trials in patients with persisting asthma. The details of these studies will be reviewed in the subsequent chapters.

The studies reported since the early 1980s have not only increased the understanding of the biology of LTs, but also have provided an excellent example of the valuable interaction between the pharmaceutical industry and research efforts to understand the pathobiology of asthma. Without the tools developed by industry, the importance of the LTs in asthma would not have been clarified and, at the same time, a useful therapy for asthma has been made available to asthma patients.

References

1 Kellaway CH, Trethewie ER: The liberation of a slow-reacting smooth muscle-stimulating substance in anaphylaxis. Q J Exp Physiol 1940;30:121–145.
2 Brocklehurst WE: The release of histamine and formation of a slow reacting substance (SRS-A) during anaphylatic shock. J Physiol 1960;151: 416–435.
3 Samuelsson B, Dahlen B, Lindgren JA, Rouzer CA, Serhan CN: Leukotrienes and lipoxins: Structures, biosynthesis, and biological side effects. Science 1987;237:1171–1176.
4 Kaiser E, Chiba P, Zaky K: Phospholipases in biology and medicine. Clin Biochem 1990; 23: 340–370.
5 Ferguson JE, Hanley MR: The role of phospholipases and phospholipid-derived signals in cell activation. Curr Opin Cell Biol 1991;3:206–212.
6 Matsumoto T, Funk CD, Radmark O, Hoog JO, Jornvall H, Samuelsson B: Molecular cloning and amino acid sequence of human 5-lipoxygenase. Proc Natl Acad Sci USA 1988;85: 26–30.
7 Dixon RA, Diehl RE, Opas E, Rands E, Vickers PJ, Evans JF, et al: Requirement of a 5-lipoxygenase-activating protein for leukotriene synthesis. Nature 1990;343:282–284.
8 Lam BK, Penrose JF, Freeman GJ, Austen KF: Expression cloning of a cDNA for human leukotriene C4 synthase, an integral membrane protein conjugating reduced glutathione to leukotriene A4. Proc Natl Acad Sci USA 1994; 91: 7663–7667.
9 Lewis RA, Drazen JM, Austen KF, Clark DA, Corey EJ: Identification of the C(6)-S-conjugate of leukotriene A with cysteine as a naturally occurring slow reacting substance of anaphylaxis (SRS-A). Importance of the 11-cis-geometry for biological activity. Biochem Biophys Res Commun 1980;96:271–277.
10 Lam BK, Owen WF, Austen KF, Soberman RJ: The identification of a distinct export step following the biosynthesis of leukotriene C_4 by human eosinophils. J Biol Chem 1989;264: 12885–12889.
11 Lewis RA, Austen KF, Drazen JM, Clark DA, Marfat A, Corey EJ: Slow reacting substances of anaphylaxis: Identification of leukotrienes C-1 and D from human and rat resources. Proc Natl Acad Sci USA 1980;77:3710–3714.
12 Parker CW, Koch D, Huber MM, Falkenhein SF: Formation of the cysteinyl form of slow reacting substance (leukotriene E4) in human plasma. Biochem Biophys Res Commun 1980; 97:1038–1046.
13 Schliemer RP, MacGlashan DW, Peters SP, Pinckard RN, Adkinson NFJr, Lichtenstein LM: Characterization of inflammatory mediator release from purified human lung mast cells. Am Rev Respir Dis 1986;133:614–617.
14 Weller PF, Lee CW, Foeter DW, Corey EJ, Austen KF, Lewis RA: Generation and metabolism of 5-lipoxygenase pathway leukotrienes by human eosinophils: Predominant production of leukotriene C_4. Proc Natl Acad Sci USA 1983;80:7626–7630.
15 Rankin JA, Hitchcock M, Merrill W, Bach MK, Brashler JR, Askenase PW: IgE-dependent release of leukotriene C_4 from alveolar macrophages. Nature 1982;297:329–331.
16 O'Byrne PM, Israel E, Drazen JM: Anti-leukotrienes in the treatment of asthma. Ann Intern Med 1997;127:472–480.
17 Carter GW, Young PR, Albert DH, Bouska J, Dyer R, Bell RL, Summers JB, Brooks DW: 5-Lipoxygenase inhibitory activity of zileuton. J Pharmacol Exp Ther 1991; 256:929–937.
18 Ford-Hutchinson AW: FLAP: A novel drug target for inhibiting the synthesis of leukotrienes. Trends Pharmacol Sci 1991; 12:68–70.
19 Lynch KR, O'Neill GP, Liu Q, Im DS, Sawyer N, Metters KM, et al: Characterization of the human cysteinyl leukotriene CysLT1 receptor. Nature 1999;399:789–793.
20 Crooke ST, Mattern M, Sarau HM, Winkler JD, Balcarek J, Wong A, Bennett CF: The signal transduction system of the leukotriene D_4 receptors. Trends Pharmacol Sci 1989;10:103–107.
21 Yokomizo T, Masuda K, Kato K, Toda A, Izumi T, Shimizu T: Leukotriene B4 receptor. Cloning and intracellular signaling. Am J Respir Crit Care Med 2000;161:S51–S55.
22 Manning PJ, Watson RM, Margolskee DJ, Williams VC, Schwartz JI, O'Byrne PM: Inhibition of exercise-induced bronchoconstriction by MK-571, a potent leukotriene D4-receptor antagonist. N Engl J Med 1990;323:1736–1739.
23 Taylor IK, O'Shaughnessy KM, Fuller RW, Dollery CT: Effect of a cysteinylleukotriene receptor antagonist, ICI 204-219 on allergen-induced broncho-constriction and airway hyperactivity in atopic subjects. Lancet 1991;337: 690–694.
24 Israel E, Dermarkarian R, Rosenberg M, Sperling R, Taylor G, Rubin P, Drazen J: The effects of a 5-lipoxygenase inhibitor on asthma induced by cold, dry air. N Engl J Med 1990;323: 1740–1744.
25 Israel E, Fischer AR, Rosenburg MA, Lilly CM, Callery JC, Shapiro J, Cohn J, Rubin P, Drazen J: The pivotal role of 5-lipoxygenase products in the reaction of aspirin-sensitive asthmatics to aspirin. Am Rev Respir Dis 1993;148:1447–1451.

Paul M. O'Byrne
St Joseph's Hospital, Firestone Clinic, Rm. 113
50 Charlton Ave. East
Hamilton, Ontario L8N 4A6 (Canada)
Tel. +1 905 522 1155 (ext. 3694)
Fax +1 905 521 6125

Cysteinyl Leukotriene Antagonists

Rodger M. McMillan

Respiratory and Inflammation Research Area, AstraZeneca, Macclesfield, UK

Summary

Cysteinyl leukotrienes are products of the 5-LO pathway. They are potent mediators of allergic bronchospasm and inflammation. Considerable effort in the pharmaceutical industry has focussed on the development of agents that modulate their synthesis or actions. Recently, three selective antagonists of the cysLT1 receptor have been launched for the treatment of asthma. This review summarizes the discovery and development of this new class of asthma therapy.

Metabolism of arachidonic acid via 5-LO gives rise to two unstable intermediates, 5-hydroperoxyeicosatetraenoic acid (5-HPETE) and an epoxide intermediate leukotriene A_4 (LTA_4). Metabolic conversion of LTA_4 can occur via two pathways. The first forms a dihydroxy acid LTB_4 which is a potent chemoattractant and activator of polymorphonuclear leukocytes. An alternative pathway of (LTA_4) metabolism gives rise to the so-called cysteinyl leukotrienes which account for the biological activity previously ascribed to 'slow-reacting substance of anaphylaxis'.

The term 'slow reacting substance' (SRS) was coined in the 1930s to describe a substance released from guinea pig lungs following injection of the animals with cobra venom. The smooth-muscle-contracting property of this material was slower in onset and of longer duration than that produced by histamine. Extension of these studies revealed that a substance with similar pharmacological properties was released from guinea pig lung during anaphylactic shock. This substance was termed 'slow-reacting substance of anaphylaxis' (SRS-A) to distinguish it from the SRSs released by non-allergic stimuli [1].

Considerable research continued in this area for over 40 years and by the late 1970s a wealth of information had accrued on the properties of SRS-A. These included the presence of sulphur, a precursor role for arachidonic acid and the presence within SRS-A of a conjugated triene. At the same time, Samuelsson [2] had discovered the 5-LO pathway and he noted a number of similarities between SRS-A and the recently discovered LTB_4. Subsequent large-scale purification and physicochemical characterization revealed that SRS-A comprises a family of peptidyl leukotrienes which contain a hydroxyl substituent at position 5 and either glutathione (LTC_4), cysteinyl glycine (LTD_4), or cysteine (LTE_4).

Now that the structure of SRS-A was known, rational approaches to the design of selective antagonists were believed to be greatly enhanced. In reality, almost 20 years elapsed before the translation of this knowledge into drugs which were approved for clinical use. It is noteworthy that the launch of the first leukotriene antagonists preceded the identification and molecular cloning of the first cysteinyl leukotriene receptor.

Cysteinyl Leukotriene Antagonism

Most major pharmaceutical companies initiated programmes to search for either inhibitors of leukotriene biosynthesis or selective receptor antagonists. The absence of any information about the leukotriene receptor genes and the chemical challenges in producing synthetic leukotrienes meant that discovery programmes aimed at cysteinyl leukotriene receptors were initiated using natural SRS-A preparations and conventional bioassay.

In the mid 1980s, synthetic preparations of cysteinyl leukotrienes became widely available to academic investigators and this allowed much better characterization of their actions and receptors. In human airways, it is now

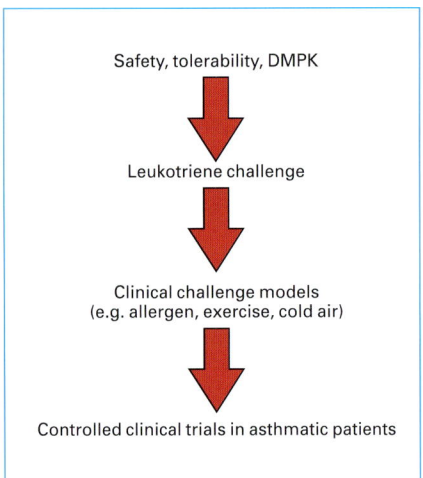

Fig. 1. Clinical evaluation of cysteinyl leukotriene antagonists.

After initial safety and tolerability studies, compounds were tested for their ability to antagonize the bronchoconstrictor activity of inhaled leukotrienes. Compounds achieving appropriate levels of blockade would then be evaluated in one or more challenge models. Only those drugs achieving target levels of efficacy in the challenge models progressed to full-blown asthma trials.

In the late 1980s, several cysteinyl leukotriene antagonists with improved potency over FPL55712 entered clinical trials. These included a Lilly compound LY171883 and several compounds from Merck Frosst, including L648051 and MK0571 [5–7]. Although none of these agents was sufficiently potent to justify progression to asthma studies, they did serve to validate the challenge models. In addition, studies with compounds increased confidence that leukotriene modulation would provide clinical benefit and also help to define the target criteria for future drugs more clearly.

Zafirlukast, Montelukast and Pranlukast

In the 1990s, the leukotriene approach moved from concept to proof. This was based on the successful development and subsequent launch of three cysteinyl leukotriene antagonists: ICI 204219 (zafirlukast; Accolate, AstraZeneca), MK0476 (montelukast; Singulair, Merck) and ONO1078 (pranlukast, ONO).

As shown in figure 2, these three drugs possess substantial structural diversity but there is now extensive clinical literature which demonstrates that their clinical effects are consistent and complementary. All three antagonists were highly effective against LTD_4 challenge models in volunteers or patients [8–10]; for example, administration of zafirlukast produced a shift of 50–100 times in the concentration response curve to inhaled LTD_4. This translated to inhibition of bronchoconstriction in a variety of challenge models, including allergen, cold air and exercise. As predicted from studies with the earlier weaker antagonists, inhibition of both early and late-phase bronchoconstriction and hyperreactivity was observed. An interesting feature was that these studies also uncovered inhibitory effects on cell recruitment; thus 1 week treatment with zafirlukast significantly reduced allergen-induced accumulation of eosinophils, lymphocytes and basophils in BAL fluid [11]. This anti-inflammatory effect is consistent with the previous report that inhalation of LTE_4 in asthmatics stimulated eosinophil influx into the bronchial mucosa [12].

clear that LTC_4, LTD_4 and LTE_4 are potent spasmogens and all seem to work through the same receptor (CysLT1) [3]. The effects of the three leukotrienes at this receptor were blocked by an SRS-A antagonist, FPL55712, which had been discovered by Fisons (now AstraZeneca) more than 5 years before the elucidation of the 5-LO pathway. Synthetic leukotrienes and the later introduction of radiolabelled versions allowed pharmaceutical scientists to move from bioassay to higher-volume assays such as radioligand binding. However, most programmes preceded the widespread use of truly high throughput screening approaches. Thus most companies employed rational design strategies based either on the structure of FPL55712 [4] or on the structures of the synthetic leukotrienes themselves. The target for most companies was a potent selective and orally active antagonist of cysteinyl leukotrienes. Oral activity was a particularly important criterion. Inhaled therapies (β-agonists and steroids) were (and are) the mainstays of asthma therapy and side effect concerns preclude their oral use. In contrast, selective antagonists of single classes of mediators were presumed to offer potential for a better efficacy:side effect ratio and therefore were ideally suited to oral therapy with its advantages in patient acceptability and compliance.

Clinical Evaluation

A common stepwise approach to clinical evaluation evolved during the testing of a number of leukotriene antagonists from several different pharmaceutical companies (fig. 1).

Asthma Efficacy Studies

Having demonstrated a favourable profile in pre-clinical and clinical challenge models, studies with leukotriene antagonists now moved into their evaluation in asthma. A common feature of trials with these antagonists is an improvement in baseline lung function in asthmatics which is observed rapidly after the first dose is administered. The magnitude of the effects vary with the treatment regime and with the extent of lung function impairment in the patients being studied. However, improvements of 10–15% in FEV_1 are commonly reported in studies with zafirlukast and montelukast [13, 14]. This improvement in lung function is additive with inhaled $β_2$-agonists and occurs in the presence or absence of inhaled corticosteroids [15, 16].

In contrast to $β_2$-agonists, cysteinyl leukotriene receptor antagonists do not improve lung function in non-asthmatics and therefore the effects cannot be attributed to direct relaxation of bronchial smooth muscle. The data imply that increased airway tone in asthmatics is maintained at least in part by synthesis of cysteinyl leukotrienes. It is not clear whether this is mediated via the direct bronchoconstrictor effects of the leukotrienes or indirectly via pro-inflammatory effects of cysteinyl leukotrienes such as the cellular effects described above. Whatever the precise mechanisms involved, the observation that improved lung function is produced by cysteinyl leukotriene antagonists, even in the presence of inhaled corticosteriods and $β_2$-agonists, indicates that these drugs will find a place in asthma therapy in addition to current treatments.

Longer-term studies of leukotriene antagonists in asthma have confirmed the acute improvement in lung function. Thus improvement in FEV_1 is maintained in trials of 6- to 13-week duration and there is no evidence for development of tolerance. These effects are associated with improvements in a variety of symptom scores (e.g. total asthma symptoms, night time awakenings and morning asthma symptoms) as well as decreased use of inhaled $β_2$-agonists. Symptom improvements have been demonstrated in 3-month studies of zafirlukast or montelukast [17, 18]. These improvements are generally in the range of 25–50%, although the magnitude of the changes depends on the symptoms which are measured as well as the severity of the asthma. Direct comparison with pranlukast is more difficult since the majority of the studies have been carried out in Japan with somewhat different protocols. However, a 4-week study in the USA with pranlukast has reported improvement in symptoms of a magnitude similar to those described above for zafirlukast and montelukast [19].

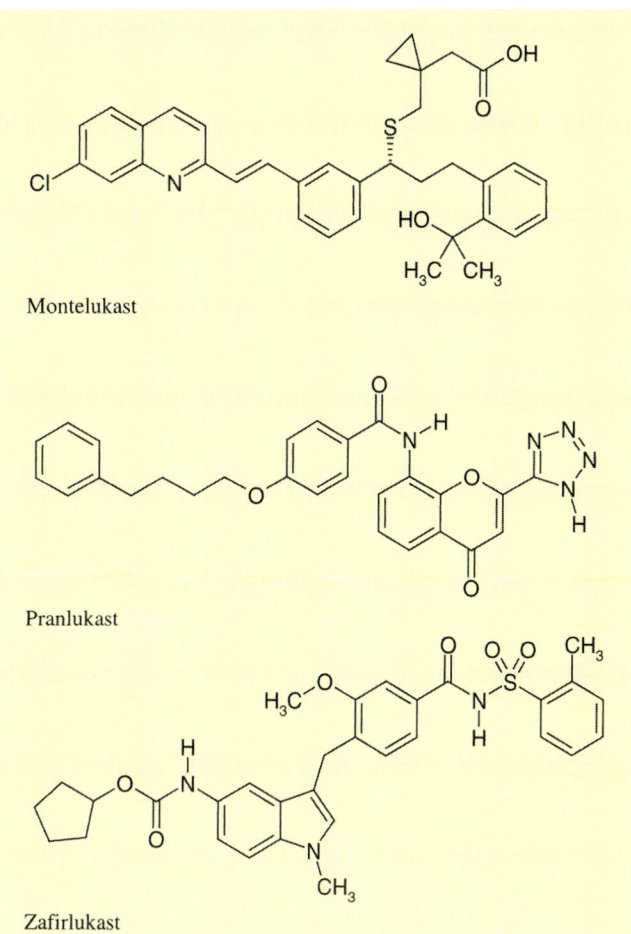

Fig. 2. Structures of cysteinyl leukotriene antagonists.

A reduction in asthma exacerbations (measured as requirement for oral steroids to treat asthma attacks) was reported in a 3-month study of montelukast in asthma [18]. This has been confirmed in a meta-analysis of five clinical trials of at least 3 months' duration with zafirlukast. Although the definition of exacerbation varied in the individual trials, the overall reduction in asthma exacerbations shown in this analysis was approximately 50% [20].

A number of studies have been carried out with combinations of cysteinyl leukotriene antagonists and inhaled corticosteroids. The effect of zafirlukast in patients who remain symptomatic on low-dose inhaled corticosteroids was compared to the effect of doubling the dose of inhaled steroid. At the end of this 13-week study, asthma symptoms and morning peak expiratory flow were improved to an equivalent extent in the zafirlukast patients and those who received the double steroid dose [21]. A different protocol has been used in studies of montelukast in combination with inhaled steriods. In that protocol a higher dose of inhaled steriods was used at the start of the study. Treatment with either montelukast or placebo resulted in a reduction in the inhaled steroid dose. The reduction in the montelukast patients was significantly greater than that seen with placebo, although the magnitude of the difference was small [22].

Conclusion

Cysteinyl leukotriene antagonists represent the first new therapeutic class to be introduced for the treatment of asthma in the last 25 years. Previously, a variety of other single mediator approaches had been unsuccessful (e.g. PAF antagonism). This led to a dogma that broader approaches were necessary in asthma. The success of cysteinyl leukotriene antagonists has exploded that myth and has demonstrated that such selective approaches provide a different balance of efficacy and side effects to drug classes with broader modes of action such as corticosteroids. An important lesson from the leukotriene area is that proof can be obtained only in the clinic since a number of the unsuccessful single-mediator approaches had shown a comparable pre-clinical profile in asthma or allergy models. The introduction of zafirlukast, montelukast and pranlukast has provided clinical proof of the leukotriene hypothesis in asthma which had evolved over almost 70 years since the discovery of SRSs. It now remains to be determined, based on extensive clinical experience, where the cysteinyl leukotriene antagonists will fit into asthma treatment guidelines.

References

1 Feldberg W, Kelloway CH: Liberation of histamine and formation of lysolecithin-like substance by cobra venom. J. Physiol (Lond) 1938; 94:187–226.
2 Samuelsson B: The discovery of the leukotrienes. Am J Respir Crit Care Med 2000; 161(suppl):2S–6S.
3 Coleman RA, Eglen RM, Jones RL, Narumiya S, Shimizu T, Smith WL, Dahlén SE, Drazen JM, Gardiner PJ, Jackson WT, Jones TR, Krell RD, Nicosia S: Prostanoid and leukotriene receptors: A progress report from the IUPHAR Working Parties on Classification and Nomenclature. Adv Prostaglandin Thromboxane Leukotriene Res 1994;23:283–285.
4 Augstein J, Farmer JB, Lee TB, Sheard P, Tattersall ML: Selective inhibitor of slow reacting substance of anaphylaxis. Nature 1973;245: 215–217.
5 Bell EH, Timmers MC, Dijkman JH, Stahl EG, Sterk PJ: The effect of an inhaled leukotriene antagonist, L-648,051 on early and late asthmatic reactions and subsequent increase in airway responsiveness in man. J Allergy Clin Immunol 1990;85:1067–1075.
6 Philips GD, Rafferty P, Robinson C, Holgate ST: Effect of the oral leukotriene D_4 induced bronchoconstriction by p.o. administration of LY-171,883 in non-asthmatic subjects. J Pharmac Exp Ther 1988;246:732–738.
7 Ramussen JB, Eriksson LO, Margolskee DJ, Tagari P, Williams VC, Andersson KE: Leukotriene D_4 receptor blockade inhibits the immediate and late bronchoconstrictor responses to inhaled antigen in patients with asthma. J Allergy Clin Immunol 1992;90:193–201.
8 Smith LJ, Geller S, Ebright L, Glass M, Thyrum PT: Inhibition of leukotriene D_4 induced bronchoconstriction in normal subjects by the oral LTD_4 receptor antagonist ICI 204-219. Am Rev Respir Dis 1990;141:988–992.
9 O'Shaughnessy TC, Georgiou P, Howland K, Dennis M, Compton CH, Barnes NC: Effect of pranlukast, an oral leukotriene receptor antagonist on leudotriene D_4 (LTD_4) challenge in normal vulunteers. Thorax 1997;52:519–522.
10 De Lepelaire I, Reiss TF, Rochette F, Botto A, Zhang J, Dundu S, Decramer M: Montelukast causes prolonged potent leukotriene D_4 receptor antagonism in the airways of patients with asthma. Clin Pharmacol Ther 1997;61:83–92.
11 Calhoun WJ, Lavins BJ, Minkwitz MC, Evans R, Gleich FJ, Cohn J: Effect of zafirlukast (Accolate) on cellular mediators of inflammation: Bronchoalveolar lavage fluid findings after segmental antigen challenge. Am J Respir Crit Care Med 1998;157:1381–1389.
12 Laitinen LA, Laitinen A, Haahtela T, Vikka V, Spur BW and Lee TH: Leukotriene E_4 and granulocytic infiltration into asthmatic airways. Lancet 1993;341:989–990.
13 Kane GC, Tillino M, Pollice M, Kim CJ, Cohn J, Murray JJ, Dworski R, Sheller J, Fish JE, Peters SP: Insights into IgE-mediated lung inflammation derived from a study employing a 5-lipoxygenase inhibitor. Prostaglandins 1995; 50:1–18.
14 Sheldon SL, Smith LJ, Glass M: Effects of 6 weeks of therapy with oral doses of ICI-204-219, a leukotriene D_4 receptor antagonist in subjects with bronchial asthma. Am J Respir Crit Care Med 1994;150:618–623.
15 Hui KP, Barnes NC: Lung function improvement in asthma with a cysteinyl leukotriene receptor antagonist. Lancet 1991;337:1062–1063.
16 Reiss TF, Sorknes CA, Strickler W, Botto A, Busse WW, Kundo S, et al: Effects of montelukast (MK-0476), a potent cysteinyl leukotriene receptor antagonist, or bronchodilation in asthmatic subjects treated with and without inhaled corticosteroids. Thorax 1997;52:45–48.
17 Fish JE, Kemp RF, Lockey M, Glass M, Hanby LA, Bonuccelli CM: Zafirlukast improves symptomatic mild to moderate asthma: A 13-week multicenter study. Clin Ther 1997;19: 675–690.
18 Reiss TF, Chervinsky P, Dockhorn RJ, Shingo S, Seidenberg B, Edwards TB: Montelukast, a once-daily leukotriene receptor antagonist in the treatment of chronic asthma: A multicenter, randomised, double-blind trial. Arch Intern Med 1998;158:1213–1220.
19 Yokoyamo A, Kohno N, Sakai K, Hirasawa Y, Knodo K, Hiwada K: Effect of pranlukast, a leukotriene receptor antagonist, in patients with severe asthma refractory to corticosteroids. J Asthma 1998;35:57–62.
20 Barnes N C, Black B, Syrett N, et al: Reduction of exacerbations of asthma in multinational trials with zafirlukast (Accolate). Allergy 1996; 51(suppl 30):84.
21 Nayak, AS, Anderson P, Kharous BL, Williams K, Simonson S: Equivalence of adding zafirlukast versus double-dose inhaled corticosteroids in asthmatic patients symptomatic on low dose inhaled corticosteroids (abstract). J Allergy Clin Immunol 1998;101:S333.
22 Lofdähl C-G, Reiss TF, Leff JA, Israel E, Noonan MJ, Finn AF, Seidersberg BC, Capizzi T, Kunda S, Godard P: Randomised, placebo controlled trial of effect of a leukotriene receptor antagonist, Montelukast, on tapering inhaled corticosteroids in asthmatic patients. BMJ 1999;319:87–90.

Rodger M. McMillan, PhD
Respiratory and Inflammation Research Area
AstraZeneca, Mereside Alderley Park
Macclesfield, SK10 4TG (UK)
Tel. +44 1625 513 221, Fax +44 1625 517 840
E-Mail rodger.mcmillan@astrazeneca.com

5-Lipoxygenase Inhibitors

Sven-Erik Dahlén

Unit for Experimental Asthma and Allergy Research, The National Institute of Environmental Medicine, Karolinska Institutet, Stockholm, Sweden

Summary

Inhibition of 5-LO will inhibit the formation of LTB_4 as well as that of the cysteinyl leukotrienes (LTC_4, LTD_4 and LTE_4). Many 5-LO inhibitors have been developed but only one drug, zileuton (Zyflo®) has been registered for treatment of asthma, and this only in the US. The market share of zileuton is very limited compared with the leukotriene receptor antagonists, due to the requirement for administration 3–4 times daily and the occurrence of a 5% incidence of liver function test abnormalities. From the clinical observations with in particular zileuton, but also from studies with other 5-LO inhibitors, it appears, however, that the anti-asthmatic effects of 5-LO inhibition and those of the selective $CysLT_1$ receptor antagonist are indistinguishable in asthmatics. Mechanistically, this suggests that LTB_4 is not involved in asthma. Inhibition of 5-LO may nevertheless be an effective strategy for oral treatment of asthma and lung diseases with a prominent neutrophilic component, such as COPD, especially as current data suggest that current 5-LO inhibitors do not completely inhibit leukotriene formation. In addition, there are receptors for cysteinyl leukotrienes that are not blocked by the current class of receptor antagonists.

Introduction

5-LO is the initial enzyme in the biosynthesis of leukotrienes and a logical target for development of anti-leukotriene drugs. In fact, an early experimental drug, U-60257, was found to be an effective inhibitor of allergen-induced leukotriene biosynthesis in lung tissue from asthmatics in vitro [1]. In addition, the compound blocked the Schultz-Dale contraction of bronchi from atopic asthmatics [1], providing further arguments in favor of the idea that leukotrienes were mediators in asthma. However, when the same compound was inhaled by asthmatics, it failed to attenuate allergen-induced bronchoconstriction [2]. This finding was, at the time, taken as evidence that leukotrienes were unimportant in vivo and contributed to the termination of anti-leukotriene development among several pharmaceutical companies. In retrospect, it is clear that the dose of U-60257 used in that particular study [2] was insufficient.

Many 5-LO inhibitors have subsequently been developed, and several have displayed efficacy in asthma models, such as allergen-induced bronchoconstriction. One drug, zileuton (Zyflo®) has been documented to have clinical efficacy, and it is registered in the US for the treatment of asthma. The market share of zileuton is however very limited compared with the leukotriene receptor antagonists. This is *not* because of inferior efficacy in the treatment of asthma. Rather, the requirement for administration 3–4 times daily and the occurrence of a 5% incidence of liver function test abnormalities have been competitive disadvantages. In the rest of the world, no 5-LO inhibitor is currently on the market.

Pharmacology

As indicated in figure 1, 5-LO inhibitors will decrease the biosynthesis of LTB_4 as well as that of the cysteinyl-containing leukotrienes (LTC_4, LTD_4 and LTE_4). This overall action on the leukotriene pathway by 5-LO inhibitors thus differs from that of the leukotriene receptor antagonists, which selectively block the effects of either LTB_4, or of the cysteinyl leukotrienes.

During the search for 5-LO inhibitors, a newly synthesized indole compound, MK-886, was found that inhibited leukotriene biosynthesis in intact cells but not when tested against the isolated 5-LO enzyme [3]. Investigations into the mechanism behind these seemingly paradoxical results discovered a cofactor in leukotriene bio-

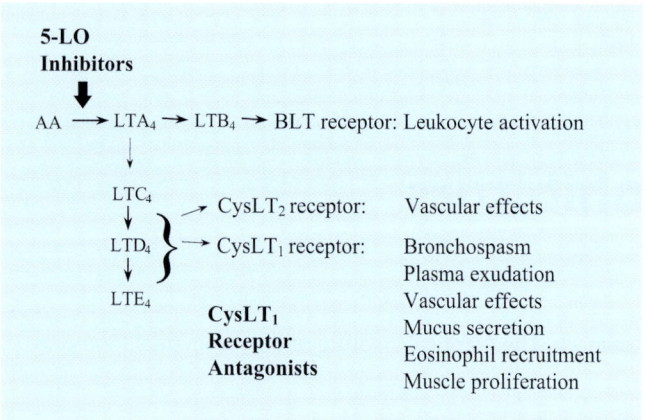

Fig. 1. The 5-LO pathway with indications of biological effects exerted by leukotrienes, their receptors and the points of attack for the anti-leukotriene drugs used to treat asthma.

synthesis, FLAP (5-LO-activating protein) [4]. It was found that this 18-kD protein was a prerequisite for efficient endogenous leukotriene biosynthesis and that MK-886 inhibited leukotriene generation because it prevented the interaction between FLAP and 5-LO [3, 5]. As a consequence, leukotriene biosynthesis inhibitors should mechanistically be divided into those that act directly on 5-LO (for example, zileuton and ABT-761) and those that are FLAP antagonists (MK-886, MK-591 and BAY x1005).

Similar to the leukotriene receptor antagonists, all 5-LO inhibitors are administered orally. Zileuton is a hydroxyurea compound that is well absorbed with peak plasma concentrations occurring within hours after an oral dose [6]. Its mean plasma half-life is about 2 h with a slightly prolonged elimination time during the night [7]. This has led to the recommendation to administer zileuton 4 times a day, but further studies have suggested that 3 times a day may be sufficient for clinical efficacy [8]. Elimination of zileuton is via first-pass excretion in the liver [6]. The FLAP antagonist MK-886 was also found to be an efficient inhibitor of leukotriene biosynthesis in humans in vivo [9], but as zileuton, it suffered from a relatively short plasma half-life. The compounds MK-591 [10] and ABT-761 [11] were therefore developed and both could be administered once or twice daily. The FLAP antagonist BAY x1005 has an intermediate position with a plasma half-life of 5–8 h [12].

It would seem straightforward to establish the effective dose of a 5-LO inhibitor by measuring the degree by which it inhibits endogenous leukotriene formation. During the development of 5-LO inhibitors, measurements of ex vivo formation of LTB_4 in ionophore-stimulated blood have generally been used to assess the degree of 5-LO inhibition [13]. This measure correlates well with plasma drug level, but there are good reasons to believe that it overestimates the degree of tissue inhibition of leukotriene formation [14]. For LTB_4, there is, however, no indicator metabolite that can be measured in urine or blood [14]. For the cysteinyl leukotrienes, measurements of urinary excretion of the end product LTE_4 is the most reliable estimate of the degree of inhibition of endogenous whole body biosynthesis [14].

It is therefore worth considering that the level of inhibition of urinary LTE_4 has consistently been less than 50% in the studies where significant effects on clinical outcome variables have been established [15–17]. This may indicate either that this level of inhibition is sufficient to obtain maximal clinical efficacy, or that the clinical efficacy can be increased further if the inhibition of leukotriene formation is increased. The latter possibility gains some support from the results of the only allergen challenge study performed with the highest dose of BAY x1005 so far tested [18]. There was more than 80% inhibition of allergen-induced urinary excretion of LTE_4 and more than 75% inhibition of the bronchoconstriction, which incidentally is the greatest degree of inhibition reported for this particular outcome variable for any anti-leukotriene drug. The phase II treatment trials with the same drug were subsequently performed at a lower dose level and the results led to the discontinuation of further development of this drug.

Effects in Patients with Asthma

Bronchoprovocation Studies. Most data on 5-LO inhibitors have been published with zileuton and it was indeed used in many of the initial studies that proved the hypothesis that leukotrienes were mediators of trigger-factor-evoked bronchoconstriction, as well as subsequently in treatment studies. Thus, zileuton was first shown to block isocapnic hyperventilation [19] and allergen-induced rhinitis [20]. Pre-treatment with zileuton for 1–4 weeks has also been documented to effectively block aspirin-induced bronchoconstriction in aspirin-intolerant asthmatics [15, 17] as well as exercise induced bronchoconstriction [21]. The follow-up compound ABT-761 was also found to inhibit exercise-induced bronchoconstriction [22, 23] and in addition, it blocked the airway response to adenosine [22].

In an early trial in allergen-induced bronchoconstriction, zileuton had no significant effect on the airway response [24], but this was hardly surprising as it was administered as a single dose and there was only marginal inhibition of leukotriene formation. Subsequently, the 5-LO inhibitors MK-886 [9], MK-591 [10] and BAY x1005 [18, 25] have all been found to inhibit both the early and the late phase of allergen-induced airway obstruction. Interestingly, in a study employing local segmental allergen challenge of atopic asthmatics [26], it was documented that zileuton inhibited local leukotriene generation and also suppressed the eosinophil infiltration that was observed in subjects treated with placebo. This was one of the first indications that anti-leukotrienes also had the potential to affect airway inflammation.

Therefore, it can be concluded that 5-LO inhibition attenuates airway obstruction induced by indirectly acting bronchoconstrictors (table 1). This supports the observation that release of leukotrienes constitutes a final common path for different trigger factors in asthma. As a corollary, 5-LO inhibitors may be used to prevent bronchospasm in response to many common environmental trigger factors such as allergen and exercise. The profile of anti-bronchoconstrictor activity appears identical to that of selective $CysLT_1$ antagonists.

Chronic Treatment. The effects of 5-LO inhibition is asthmatics is summarized in table 1. Again, the data almost exclusively derive from studies with zileuton. Regrettably, many trials with other 5-LO inhibitors have only been reported in abstract form. Thus, in placebo comparison trials, zileuton has been found to significantly improve conventional asthma outcome measures, such as FEV_1, peak flow values, day and night symptoms, and β-agonist use [16]. The effect of zileuton on pulmonary function involves an acute bronchodilating effect in patients with baseline bronchoconstriction, and a chronic effect with continued treatment. The acute effect is observed within a few hours after oral intake, and incidentally highlights the rapid turnover of leukotrienes in human airways. The chronic effect on airway function has reached its maximum after a week in some studies, whereas other studies reported progressive improvement over the observed treatment period. Presumably, the extent of improvement and the time course for the outcome much relate to the level of baseline airway obstruction and disease severity in the study population.

In trials on mild to moderate asthma, the number of asthma exacerbations requiring prednisone rescue were highly significantly reduced and not surprisingly this has coincided with improved quality of life [19]. Furthermore, in a 1-year surveillance trial with zileuton, the number of hospitalizations, emergency room visits and the

Table 1. Effects of 5-LO inhibition in asthma

Prevention of bronchoconstriction induced by allergen, adenosine, exercise and aspirin
Acute bronchodilation
Chronic improvement in pulmonary function
Reduced use of bronchodilators
Less asthma symptoms (day and night)
Fewer asthma exacerbations
Improved quality of life
Additive to inhaled glucocorticosteroids

requirement for prednisone rescue were significantly reduced among the 1,400 patients that were given zileuton [27]. It is noteworthy that zileuton was given as add-on treatment in the latter trial where 56% of the patients were on inhaled glucocorticosteroids, 30% on theophylline and 11% on cromoglycate.

One study has compared 3 months of treatment with zileuton or theophylline in US steroid naïve patients with moderate persistent asthma [28]. The results showed quite remarkable acute (18–24%) and chronic (30%) improvements in FEV_1, reduced β-agonist use and improved nocturnal asthma for both compounds, with no significant difference between theophylline and zileuton.

There are also studies supporting additive effects with inhaled steroids. For example, in a cross-over study of 40 aspirin-intolerant asthmatics, there was a global improvement over and above that provided by moderate to high doses of steroids in these patients [17]. Despite 90% of the patients being maintained since years on more than 1,000 μg of inhaled glucocorticosteroids daily, and about one third in addition also on oral prednisone, there was a 7% improvement in FEV_1 during zileuton treatment but no change during the placebo period. This suggests that patients who seemed to be controlled on conventional therapy could achieve a further improvement by addition of a 5-LO inhibitor. The findings are in line with recent observations with $CysLT_1$ receptor antagonists [29–32], and with a large body of evidence demonstrating that glucocorticosteroids do not inhibit leukotriene formation in asthmatics [e.g. 33–36]. Furthermore, in a study in 320 patients with moderate to severe asthma, it was found that addition of zileuton to 400 μg of beclomethasone had the same therapeutic effect as doubling the dose of beclomethasone to 800 μg daily [37]. In both groups, the FEV_1 increased by about 10%, concomitant with similar improvements in other asthma outcome variables. Finally in this context, the FLAP antagonist MK-591 has been reported to produce highly significant improvements in asthma outcome scores and pulmonary function in asthmatics already maintained on inhaled glucocorticosteroids [38].

In the study of the aspirin-intolerant asthmatics, there was a significant improvement in nasal function including return of smell [17]. Zileuton has also been documented to block the nasal response to oral aspirin provocation in aspirin-intolerant asthmatics [15]. A more recent open study in 36 patients with nasal rhinosinusitis supports an effect of zileuton on nasal symptoms [39].

In the study with zileuton in aspirin-intolerant asthma [17], there was also a small but significant reduction in BHR following addition of zileuton to the steroid treatment. As these patients had been treated with steroids for many years, the further improvement in BHR following a brief 6-week treatment with zileuton is worth considering. The possibility that zileuton affects BHR, and by inference, airway inflammation, is also supported by a study where the response to isocapnic hyperventilation [40] was reduced following a 2-week treatment with zileuton. The challenge was performed at a time point when zileuton treatment had been withheld for several days, and its influence on leukotriene biosynthesis thus should have been terminated.

That leukotrienes contribute to chronic airway inflammation gains further support from the findings that zileuton treatment caused a reduction in circulating eosinophils in asthmatics [41]. Such observations with zileuton were in fact among the first indications that anti-leukotriene drugs had long-term 'anti-inflammatory' effects. As discussed elsewhere, a chronic effect on eosinophils has now consistently been demonstrated with leukotriene receptor antagonists. Furthermore, in a study of nocturnal asthma, Wenzel et al. [42] showed that there was a decrease in BAL fluid cellularity and leukotriene concentrations in subjects given zileuton.

Conclusions

From the observations in particular with zileuton, but also with other 5-LO inhibitors, it appears that the antiasthmatic effects of 5-LO inhibition and selective CysLT1 receptor antagonist in asthmatics are indistinguishable. Mechanistically, this suggests that LTB_4 is not involved in asthma; this may be in line with the observation that a selective antagonist of LTB_4 had no effect on the airway physiology in allergen-induced bronchoconstriction in man [43]. This conclusion may, however, be premature as the number of studies are few and there has been no head-to-head comparison between a potent 5-LO inhibitor and a $CysLT_1$ antagonist. In fact, at closer scrutiny, it seems that zileuton may have greater effects on BHR than $CysLT_1$ antagonists which generally had no or minimal effects on this outcome variable.

Despite the approval of zileuton in the US, and the overall quite impressive efficacy profile of zileuton and other 5-LO inhibitors in asthma or asthma models, the pharmaceutical industry has been less inclined to develop 5-LO inhibitors. This is because of the currently more favorable side effect profile of $CysLT_1$ antagonists. The incidence of adverse events has been greater for zileuton (liver function test abnormalities) or MK-591 (skin rashes) than for $CysLT_1$ antagonists. There are, however, no data to support that these particular side effects are due to inhibition of 5-LO. In fact, it has been concluded that the side effects are compound-related rather than related to the specific mode of action of the drugs.

As discussed, a major uncertainty concerns the true efficacy of zileuton and other 5-LO inhibitors as inhibitor of endogenous leukotriene formation in the treatment studies performed so far. More research is needed to establish what are the best metabolites to monitor for correct assessment of endogenous leukotriene biosynthesis, and where to measure (blood? urine? exhaled air? induced sputum? BAL fluid?). It will then be important to use such measures to correlate the effective dose level of 5-LO inhibitors with both leukotriene biosynthesis and clinical outcome variables.

It may therefore, for several reasons, be rewarding to revisit 5-LO inhibition as an effective strategy for treatment of asthma and other pulmonary disorders. As LTB_4 is the major leukotriene generated in neutrophils, 5-LO inhibition may be a more logical intervention than selective antagonism of the cysteinyl leukotrienes for treatment of COPD and other lung diseases with a prominent neutrophilic component. It is also likely that 5-LO inhibition may be of interest in the treatment of rhinitis [20] as well as extrapulmonary diseases, not only because of the possibility of an involvement of LTB_4, but also because there are additional receptors for cysteinyl leukotrienes [44] that are not blocked by the current class of receptor antagonists.

Acknowledgment

The author is grateful for the support of the following Swedish organizations: The Heart Lung Foundation, The Medical Research Council (Project 9071), The Foundation for Health Care and Allergy Research (Vårdalstiftelsen) and Karolinska Institutet.

References

1 Dahlén S-E, Hansson G, Hedqvist P, Björck T, Granström E, Dahlén B: Allergen challenge of lung tissue from asthmatics elicits bronchial contraction that correlates with the release of leukotrienes C4, D4 and E4. Proc Natl Acad Sci USA 1983;80:1712–1716.

2 Mann JS, Robinson C, Sheridan AQ, Clement P, Bach MK, Holgate ST: Effect of inhaled piriprost (U-60,257), a novel leukotriene inhibitor, on allergen and exercise induced bronchoconstriction in asthma. Thorax 1986;41:746–752.

3 Rouzer CA, Ford-Hutchinson AW, Morton HE, Gillard JW: MK-886, a potent and specific leukotriene biosynthesis inhibitor blocks and reverses the membrane association of 5-lipoxygenase in ionophore-challenged leukocytes. J Biol Chem 1990;265:1436–1442.

4 Miller DK, Gillard JW, Vickers PJ, Sadowski S, Léveillé C, Mancini JA, Charleson P, Dixon RAF, Ford-Hutchinson AW, Fortin R, Gauthier JY, Rodkey J, Rosen R, Rouzer C, Sigal IS, Strader CD, Evans JF: Identification and isolation of a membrane protein necessary for leukotriene production. Nature 1990;343:278–281.

5 Dixon RAF, Diehl RE, Opas E, Rands E, Vickers PJ, Evans JF, Gillard JW, Miller DK: Requirement of a 5-lipoxygenase-activating protein for leukotriene synthesis. Nature 1990; 343:282–284.

6 Awni WM, Braeckman RA, Granneman GR, Witt G, Dubé LM: Pharmacokinetics and pharmacodynamics of zileuton after oral administration of single and multiple dose regimens in healthy volunteers. Clin Pharmacokin 1995;29(suppl 2):22–33.

7 Awni WM, Locke CS, Dube LM, Cavanaugh JH: Evaluation of the diurnal variation in the pharmacokinetics of zileuton in normal healthy volunteers. J Clin Pharmacol 1997;37: 388–394.

8 DuBuske LM, Grossman J, Swanson LJ, Dubé LM, Lancaster JF and the zileuton study group: Randomized trial of zileuton in patients with moderate asthma: Effect of reduced dosing frequency and amounts on pulmonary function an asthma symptoms. Am J Manag Care 1997; 3:633–640.

9 Friedman BS, Bel EH, Buntinx A, Tanaka W, Han YHR, Shingo S, Spector R, Sterk PJ: Oral leukotriene inhibitor (MK-886) blocks allergen-induced airway responses. Am Rev Respir Dis 1993;147:839–844.

10 Diamant Z, Timmers MC, van der Veen H, Friedman BS, De Smet M, Depré M, Hilliard D, Bel EH, Sterk PJ: The effect of MK-0591, a novel 5-lipoxygenase activating protein inhibitor, on leukotriene biosynthesis and allergen-induced airway responses in asthmatic subjects in vivo. J Allergy Clin Immunol 1995;95:42–51.

11 Wong SL, Drajesk J, Chang M, Lanni C, Witt G, Hansen R, Awni WM: Pharmacokinetic and pharmacodynamics of single and multiple oral doses of a novel 5-lipoxygenase inhibitor (ABT-761) in healthy volunteers. Clin Pharmacol Ther 1998;63:324–331.

12 Horstmann R, Beckermann B, Seitz I, Dietrich G, Böttcher M, Lemm G, Beneka M: Tolerability and pharmacokinetics of the new leukotriene synthesis inhibitor BAY x1005. Naunyn-Schmiedebergs Arch Pharmacol 1993;347: 133.

13 Wong SL, Locke C, Dubé LM, Granneman GR, Awni WM: Meta-analysis of the pharmacodynamic relationship between the ex vivo LTB_4 inhibition in whole blood and zileuton plasma concentrations from phase I studies in normal volunteers using NONMEM approach. Pharm Res 1994;11(suppl 10):S434.

14 Kumlin M: Measurements of leukotrienes in humans. Am J Resp Crit Care Med 2000;161: S102–S106.

15 Israel E, Fischer AR, Rosenberg MA, Lilly CM, Callery JC, Shapiro J, Cohn J, Rubin P, Drazen JM: The pivotal role of 5-lipoxygenase products in the reaction of aspirin-sensitive asthmatics to aspirin. Am Rev Respir Dis 1993; 148:1447–1451.

16 Israel E, Rubin P, Kemp JP, Grossman J, Pierson W, Siegel SC, Tinkelman D, Murray JJ, Busse WW, Segal AT, Fish J, Kaiser HB, Ledford D, Wenzel SE, Rosenthal R, Cohn J, Lanni C, Pearlman H, Karahalios P, Drazen JM: The effect of inhibition of 5-lipoxygenase by Zileuton in mild-to-moderate asthma. Ann Intern Med 1993;119:1059–1066.

17 Dahlén B, Nizankowska E, Szczeklik A, Zetterström O, Bochenek G, Kumlin M, Mastalerz L, Pinis G, Swanson LJ, Boodhoo TI, Wright S, Dubé LM, Dahlén S-E: Benefits from adding the 5-lipoxygenase inhibitor zileuton to conventional therapy in aspirin-intolerant asthmatics. Am J Respir Crit Care Med 1998;157: 1187–1194.

18 Dahlén B, Kumlin M, Ihré E, Zetterström O, Dahlén S-E: Inhibition of allergen-induced airway obstruction and leukotriene generation in atopic asthmatics by the leukotriene-biosynthesis inhibitor BAY x1005. Thorax 1997;52:342–347.

19 Israel E, Dermarkarian R, Rosenberg M, Sperling R, Taylor G, Drazen JM: The effects of a 5-lipoxygenase inhibitor on asthma induced by cold, dry air. N Engl J Med 1990;323:1740–1744.

20 Knapp HR: Reduced allergen-induced nasal congestion and leukotriene synthesis with an orally active 5-lipoxygenase inhibitor. N Engl J Med 1990;323:1745–1748.

21 Meltzer SS, Hasday JD, Cohn J, Bleecher ER: Inhibition of exercise-induced bronchoconstriction by zileuton, a 5-lipoxygenase inhibitor. Am J Respir Crit Care Med 1996;153:931–935.

22 Van Schoor J, Joos GF, Kips JC, Drajesk JF, Carpentier PJ, Pauwels RA: The effect of ABT-761, a novel 5-lipoxygenase inhibitor, on exercise and adenosine-induced bronchoconstriction in asthmatic subjects. Am J Respir Crit Care Med 1997;155:875–880.

23 Lehnigk B, Rabe KF, Dent G, Herst RS, Carpentier PJ, Magnussen H: Effects of a 5-lipoxygenase inhibitor, ABT-761, on exercise-induced bronchoconstriction and urinary LTE_4 in asthmatic patients. Eur Respir J 1998;11: 617–623.

24 Hui KP, Taylor IK, Taylor GW, Rubin P, Kesterson J, Barnes NC, Barnes PJ: Effect of a 5-lipoxygenase inhibitor on leukotriene generation and airway responses after allergen challenge in asthmatic patients. Thorax 1991;46: 184–189.

25 Hamilton AL, Watson RM, Wyile G, O'Byrne PM: Attenuation of early and late phase allergen-induced bronchoconstriction in asthmatic subjects by a 5-lipoxygenase activating protein antagonist, BAY x1005. Thorax 1997;52:358–354.

26 Kane GC, Pollice M, Kim C-J, Cohn J, Dworski RT, Murray JJ, Sheller JR, Fish JE, Peters SP: A controlled trial of the effect of the 5-lipoxygenase inhibitor, zileuton, on lung inflammation produced by segmental antigen challenge in human beings. J Allergy Clin Immunol 1996;97:646–654.

27 Data on file displayed for author by Abbot Laboratories, Chicago, USA.

28 Schwartz HJ, Petty T, Reed R, Dubé LM, Swanson LJ, and the zileuton study group: The comparative effects of zileuton, a 5-lipoxygenase inhibitor, vs theophylline in patients with moderate asthma: Results from a 13 week multicentre trial. Am J Respir Crit Care Med 1995; 151:A376.

29 Tamaoki J, Kondo M, Sakai N, Nakata J, Takemura H, Nagai A, Takizawa T, Konno K: Leukotriene antagonist prevents exacerbation of asthma during reduction of high-dose inhaled corticosteroid. Am J Respir Crit Care Med 1997;155:1235–1240.

30 Löfdahl C-G, Reiss TF, Leff JA, Israel E, Noonan MJ, Finn AF, Seidenberg BC, Capizzi T, Kundo S, Godard P: Randomised, placebo controlled trial of effect of a leukotriene receptor antagonist, montelukast, on tapering inhaled corticosteroids in asthmatic patients. Br Med J 1999;319:87–90.

31 Laviolette M, Malmström K, Lu S, Chervinsky P, Pujet J-C, Peszek I, Zhang J, Reiss TF: Montelukast added to inhaled beclomethaxone in treatment of asthma. Am J Respir Crit Care Med 1999;160:1862–1868.

32 Virchow JC, Prasse A, Naya I, Summerton, Harris A: Zafirlukast improves asthma control in patients receiving high-dose inhaled corticosteroids. Am J Respir Crit Care Med 2000;162: 578–585.

33 Sebaldt RJ, Sheller JR, Oates JA, Roberts LJ, FitzGerald GA: Inhibition of eicosanoid biosynthesis by glucocorticoids in humans. Proc Natl Acad Sci USA 1990;87:6974–6978.

34 Manso G, Baker AJ, Taylor IK, Fuller RW: In vivo and in vitro effects of glucocorticoids on arachidonic acid metabolism and monocyte function in humans. Eur Respir J 1992;5:712–716.

35 O'Shaughnessy KM, Wellings R, Gillies B, Fuller RW: Differential effects of fluticasone proprionate on allergen-evoked bronchoconstriction and increased urinary leukotriene E4 excretion. Am Rev Respir Dis 1993;147:1472–1476.

36 Dworski R, FitzGerald GA, Oates JA, Sheller JR: Effect of oral prednisone on airway inflammatory mediators in atopic asthma. Am J Respir Crit Care Med 1994;149:953–959.

37 O'Connor BJ, Godard P, Dubé LM, Swanson LJ, Rountree LV: The effect of zileuton, a 5-lipoxygenase inhibitor, plus low-dose inhaled beclomethasone, compared to higher dose beclomethasone alone in patients with asthma. Eur Respir J 1996;9:S273.

38 Data on file displayed to author by Merck Research Laboratories, Rahway, USA.

39 Parnes SM, Chuma AV: Acute effects of anti-leukotrienes on sinonasal polyposis and sinusitis. Ear Nose Throat J 2000;79:18–25.

40 Fischer AR, McFadden CA, Frantz R, Awni R, Cohn J, Drazen JM, Israel E: Effect of chronic 5-lipoxygenase inhibition on airway hyperresponsiveness in asthmatic subjects. Am J Respir Crit Care Med 1995;152:1203–1207.

41 Liu MC, Dubé LM, Lancaster J: Acute and chronic effects of a 5-lipoxygenase inhibitor in asthma: A 6-month randomized multicenter trial. J Allergy Clin Immunol 1996;98:859–871.

42 Wenzel SE, Trudeau JB, Kaminsky DA, Cohn J, Martin RJ, Westcott JY: Effect of 5-lipoxygenase inhibition on bronchoconstriction and airway inflammation in nocturnal asthma. Am J Respir Crit Care Med 1995;152:897–905.

43 Evans DJ, Barnes PJ, Spaethe SM, van Alstyne EL, Mitchell MI, O'Connor BJ: Effects of a leukotriene B4 receptor antagonist, LY293111, on allergen-induced responses in asthma. Thorax 1996;51:1178–1184.

44 Dahlén S-E: Pharmacological characterization of leukotriene receptors. Am J Respir Crit Care Med 2000;161:S41–S45.

Sven-Erik Dahlén
Unit for Experimental Asthma and Allergy Research
The National Institute of Environmental Medicine
Karolinska Institutet
SE–171 77 Stockholm (Sweden)
Tel. +46 8728 7203, Fax +46 8300 619
E-Mail se.dahlen@imm.ki.se

LTB$_4$ Antagonism

H.M. Jennewein R. Anderskewitz C.J. Meade M. Pairet F. Birke

Boehringer Ingelheim KG, Department of Pulmonary Research, Ingelheim, Germany

Summary

LTB$_4$ is one of the most important mediators for neutrophil granulocyte survival, trafficking and activation. A major role has been proposed in the pathophysiology of respiratory diseases characterized by a neutrophilic-type of inflammation, such as chronic bronchitis, severe asthma and cystic fibrosis. Elevated LTB$_4$ levels have been found in sputum and BAL fluid of patients with COPD, cystic fibrosis and severe asthma. This constitutes the medical rationale for testing LTB$_4$ antagonists in certain forms of asthma and in COPD. A first clinical trial has demonstrated that an LTB$_4$ antagonist could reduce the number of BAL fluid neutrophils in patients with mild asthma. Several LTB$_4$ antagonists are known, the most important ones being CP 195543, SC 53228, CGS 25019C, ONO 4057, LY 293111 Na, and BIIL 284 BS. All these compounds are specific LTB$_4$ antagonists, but they differ with respect to efficacy and pharmacokinetic properties. Their clinical evaluation is ongoing.

Mechanism of Action

In contrast to the cysteinyl leukotrienes, which primarily cause bronchoconstriction, but may also have some proinflammatory effects, LTB$_4$ acts mainly as a chemoattractant and activator of leukocytes [1, 2].

LTB$_4$ is formed by a variety of cells, primarily macrophages and neutrophils but also keratinocytes, lymphocytes or mast cells. Its most important effect is the attraction and activation of neutrophilic granulocytes and macrophages. Both cell types are major sources of LTB$_4$. Therefore even an unspecific activation of macrophages may cause a self-amplification process. This positive feedback is further supported by an LTB$_4$-induced production of cytokines, such as IL-1, IL-4, IL-6, and IL-8, by lymphocytes. Consequently, LTB$_4$ may both trigger and maintain inflammatory processes.

LTB$_4$ synthesis from arachidonic acid is mediated by the activity of 5-lipoxygenase together with a 5-LO-activating protein (FLAP). LTB$_4$ is produced from LTA$_4$ via LTA$_4$ hydrolase. 12R-HETE (formed via 12-lipoxygenase) can also activate the LTB$_4$ receptor but less effectively.

LTB$_4$ is formed near the nuclear envelope. One of its intracellular effects is on lipid catabolism through the activation of transcription factors (i.e. PPAR-α). When released into the extracellular space, LTB$_4$ binds to a specific membrane-located receptor (BLTR), which has been cloned [3]. So far there is no evidence for LTB$_4$ receptor subtypes, but LTB$_4$ receptor high- and low-affinity binding sites have been described [4]. The LTB$_4$ receptor belongs to the G-protein-coupled receptor family that spans seven membranes and uses, amongst other mediators, phospholipase C and Ca^{2+} for signal transduction. LTB$_4$ receptors are located on a variety of cells, primarily neutrophils but also macrophages, lymphocytes, eosinophils and lung epithelial cells. In polymorphonuclear leukocytes (PMNLs) LTB$_4$ causes chemoattraction, chemokinesis, oxidative burst and the upregulation or shedding of adhesion molecules as a prerequisite of adhesion [2, 5]. It also inhibits neutrophil apoptosis, thereby prolonging the inflammatory response [6]. LTB$_4$ antagonists, either competitively or noncompetitively, are able to counteract all these LTB$_4$-induced effects.

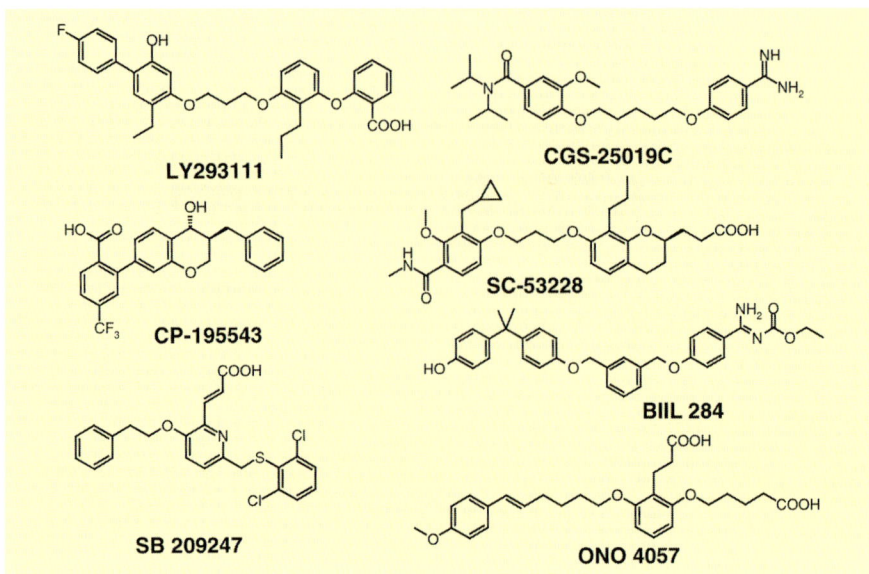

Fig. 1. Structure of LTB$_4$ antagonists.

Medical Rationale

LTB$_4$ antagonists are being considered for the treatment of diseases in which LTB$_4$ levels are elevated and in which these levels correlate with disease severity. In this sense, LTB$_4$ and neutrophilic granulocytes may play an important, probably detrimental, role in respiratory diseases, such as certain forms of asthma, COPD and cystic fibrosis.

Asthma. In asthmatics elevated LTB$_4$ levels can be detected in sputum [7] and BAL fluid [8], which corresponds to early- and late-phase reductions in FEV$_1$ [9]. Attention should be paid to cases of severe and nocturnal asthma. Both groups respond relatively poorly to glucocorticosteroids and, besides eosinophils, their lungs exhibit relatively large amounts of neutrophils [10]. In nocturnal asthma LTB$_4$ levels were increased in the BAL fluid as compared to normals at 4 a.m. but not at 4 p.m. These changes and therapeutic modulations of LTB$_4$ appear to correlate with lung eosinophilic infiltration and with decreases in FEV$_1$ values [8], suggesting that LTB$_4$ is an important mediator in nocturnal asthma.

COPD. In sputum, serum and BAL fluid of patients with chronic bronchitis, the percentage of neutrophils was higher than in healthy subjects or in asthmatics. In a 15-year follow-up study, 46 smokers and ex-smokers with airway obstruction and expectorations had higher neutrophil counts in their sputum than nonsmokers. Hereby the decline of FEV$_1$ was significantly correlated with neutrophils in the sputum [11]. In sputum from patients with bronchiectasis, LTB$_4$ comprised about one third of the chemotactic activity, as demonstrated by inhibition of LTB$_4$ using an LTB$_4$ antagonist [12]. Another interesting study investigated the effect of dietary intake of eicosapentaenoic acid (EPA) on the risk of developing COPD. EPA, the major constituent of fish oil, competes with arachidonic acid, resulting in the formation of LTB$_5$ instead of LTB$_4$. LTB$_5$ is much less effective than LTB$_4$. The EPA intake was inversely related to the risk of developing COPD [13].

Cystic Fibrosis. In addition to its putative role in COPD, LTB$_4$ may be important in cystic fibrosis (CF). Patients with CF have a persistent neutrophilic infiltration of the airways and LTB$_4$ is elevated in the bronchial epithelial lining fluid of those patients [14]. Thus large amounts of LTB$_4$ were also measured in patients with CF [15]. Treating CF patients with EPA led to an improvement [16]. In conclusion, there is some evidence that LTB$_4$ plays a role in the development of symptoms of CF patients.

Other Diseases. Besides the potential usefulness of LTB$_4$ antagonists in respiratory diseases there may be opportunities in other diseases, such as rheumatoid arthritis, inflammatory skin diseases, NSAID gastropathy and inflammatory bowel diseases.

LTB$_4$ Antagonists

In recent years, several selective LTB$_4$ antagonists have been developed [5]. The structures of the most important ones are summarized in figure 1. Little information is published about the toxicology of these compounds; however, LTB$_4$ antagonists are generally well tolerated. This is supported by the finding that 5-LO knockout mice showed no pathological phenotype [17].

LY 293111 Na (Eli Lilly)

This compound demonstrated potent in vitro LTB$_4$ antagonism [5, 18]. Studies using human PMNLs revealed inhibition of [^{3}H]LTB$_4$ binding with an IC$_{50}$ of 17 nM. LTB$_4$-induced effects of human PMNLs, such as superoxide production, were also inhibited by LY 293111 Na. LTB$_4$-induced CD11b (Mac-1) upregulation was inhibited in isolated PMNLs with an IC$_{50}$ of 3.9 nM; however, in whole blood IC$_{50}$ was found to be 362 nM, suggesting protein binding or metabolism. In vivo LY 293111 Na inhibited LTB$_4$-induced airway obstruction in guinea pigs after oral administration (ED$_{50}$ = 0.4 mg/kg) and LTB$_4$ induced pulmonary neutrophilia in conscious monkeys at a dose of 10 mg/kg p.o. Endogenous LTB$_4$ released by Ca ionophore inhalation in guinea pigs was inhibited by LY 293111 Na as well.

In two phase I studies [19, 20] LY 293111 Na was well tolerated and showed good efficacy against a surrogate parameter of ex vivo LTB$_4$ induced upregulation of Mac-1 (CD11b/CD18) on neutrophils.

An interesting phase IIa double-blind placebo-controlled crossover trial was done on 12 patients with atopic asthma [21]. LY 293111 Na was given orally at a dose of 112 mg three times a day for 7 days. Early and late asthmatic response was induced by allergen challenge. There was no change in lung function, airway hyperresponsiveness and BAL fluid eosinophils. However, neutrophils and LTB$_4$ levels as well as myeloperoxidase in BAL fluid were significantly reduced in the verum arm. Consequently, in patients with mild asthma, LTB$_4$ does not seem to play a major role, but it may be important in diseases where neutrophils are prominent. Results have been disappointing in ulcerative colitis and in psoriasis using LY 293111 Na.

CGS 25019C (Novartis)

CGS 25019C, a benzamidine-type compound, is a strong LTB$_4$ antagonist as evidenced from in vitro and in vivo studies. It inhibits [^{3}H]LTB$_4$ binding on human neutrophils with an IC$_{50}$ of 4 nM. Also LTB$_4$-induced calcium rise, chemotaxis and aggregation were inhibited with an IC$_{50}$ of 2, 2.4 and 0.1 nM, respectively.

In vivo, CGS 25019C inhibited LTB$_4$-induced neutropenia in rats (ED$_{50}$ 4 mg/kg); arachidonic acid induced ear inflammation in mice (ED$_{50}$ 1 mg/kg) and was active in a collagen-II-induced model of arthritis in mice. In this model 1, 3 and 10 mg/kg were given orally and CGS 25019C caused a dose-dependent inhibition of symptoms.

The ability of CGS 25019C to inhibit ex vivo LTB$_4$-induced Mac-1 upregulation was tested in phase I studies [21, 22]. The compound inhibited the Mac-1 upregulation with an ED$_{50}$ of 50 mg (ED$_{100}$ = 300 mg). Maximum inhibition was reached after 3 h and t$_{½}$ was 3–5 h. In a repeated-dose study, no accumulation or induction of tolerance was seen. Doses greater than 500 mg induced symptoms of gastrointestinal intolerance like diarrhea. The compound is being tested for the treatment of chronic bronchitis [5].

ONO-4057 (ONO)

ONO-4057 is a relatively weak LTB$_4$ antagonist. Although human neutrophil LTB$_4$ receptor binding was inhibited with a K$_i$ of 3.7 nM, LTB$_4$-stimulated cell function was only moderately influenced with inhibition values in the micromolar range.

ONO-4057 was effective in in vivo models of LTB$_4$-induced neutropenia and neutrophilic dermal infiltration in guinea pigs. ONO-4057 has been shown to be active in several animal models of colitis, dermatitis, pulmonary hypertension, lung anaphylaxis and transplant rejection. In a phase I study, 300 mg p.o. demonstrated efficacy using ex vivo LTB$_4$-induced calcium mobilization in human neutrophils as a pharmacodynamic measure. The compound is being tested for the treatment of psoriasis and ulcerative colitis [5], but whether development is being continued is unknown.

SB 209247 (SKB)

This drug binds selectively to the LTB$_4$ receptor with a K$_i$ of 0.78 nM [23]. LTB$_4$-induced Ca^{2+} mobilization and degranulation were also inhibited, with IC$_{50}$ values of 6.6 and 53 nM, respectively. In an arachidonic-acid-induced modal of inflammation in the mouse ear, SB 209247 demonstrated an anti-inflammatory effect with an ED$_{50}$ of 14.8 mg/kg p.o. SB 209247 has been reported to be under investigation for dermatologic indications. However, the psoriasis study was terminated.

CP 195543 (Pfizer)

CP 195543 is the follow-up compound of CP 105696, whose development was discontinued because of an extremely long terminal elimination half-life and high protein binding. From its pharmacodynamic properties, CP 195543 is largely comparable to CP 105696 [24]. In vitro, CP 195543 inhibited [^{3}H]LTB$_4$ binding to human neutro-

Table 1. Summary of biological results of BIIL 284 BS, its active metabolites BIIL 260 CL, CGS 25019C and LY 293111

	^{3}H-LTB$_4$ binding	LTB$_4$-induced transdermal chemotaxis, ED$_{50}$, mg/kg p.o.		LTB$_4$-induced neutropenia[1] ED$_{50}$, mg/kg p.o.		
	human U937 K$_i$ nmol/l	mouse (ear)	guinea pig	monkey	guinea pig	rat
BIIL 284 BS	150 (BIIL 260: 1.3)	0.01	0.02	0.05 (24)	0.3 (17)	0.05 (8)
CGS 25019C	0.9	5.3	12.0	2.5 (1)	1.4 (2)	2.5
LY 293111	24	>20	2.2	3.1 (3)	0.17 (2)	>10

[1] Figures in parentheses are half-lives in hours.

phils with an IC$_{50}$ of 6.8 nM (K$_i$ = 4.9 nM). It further inhibited LTB$_4$-mediated chemotaxis of human and mouse neutrophils with IC$_{50}$ values of 2.4 and 7.5 nM, respectively. CP 195543 was a non competitive LTB$_4$ antagonist of the high-affinity LTB$_4$ receptor (binding and chemotaxis) and a competitive antagonist of the low-affinity receptor as demonstrated in binding experiments. LTB$_4$-mediated CD11b (Mac-1) upregulation on human neutrophils was inhibited competitively with a p$_{A2}$ value of 7.66. In whole blood inhibition of Mac-1 upregulation resulted in a p$_{A2}$ value of 7.12. CP195543 was not able to antagonize Mac-1 upregulation induced by other mediators, such as IL-8 and PAF. In vivo CP 195543 inhibited LTB$_4$-induced neutrophilic infiltration in mice and guinea pigs with ED$_{50}$s of 2.8 and 0.1 mg/kg p.o., respectively. Because of its shorter half-life of ca. 1.5 h, CP 195543 was administered via osmotic minipumps in a model of collagen-II-induced arthritis in mice. The compound demonstrated good efficacy with half-maximal effects at plasma drug levels of around 0.5 µg/ml. Currently, the compound is being clinically investigated.

SC 53228 (Searle)

SC 53228 is the successor compound of SC 41930 which, due to various reasons, was discontinued. It is a potent inhibitor of [^{3}H]LTB$_4$ binding (K$_i$ = 1.3 nM) [25]. LTB$_4$-mediated chemotaxis was competitively and selectively inhibited (IC$_{50}$ = 32 nM). LTB$_4$-induced degranulation of human neutrophils was inhibited (IC$_{50}$ = 19 nM) as well in a noncompetitive fashion, however. In vivo SC 53228 inhibited LTB$_4$-induced skin inflammation in guinea pigs with an ED$_{50}$ of 0.07 mg/kg p.o. and inflammation induced by 12R-HETE was counteracted as well (ED$_{50}$ = 5.8 mg/kg). SC 53228 was active in acetic-acid-induced colitis in mice and spontaneous colitis in cotton-top tamarins. The compound was selected for clinical trials. Indications were ulcerative colitis and psoriasis.

BIIL 284 BS (Boehringer Ingelheim)

BIIL 284 BS is a prodrug, BIIL 260 being the structure obtained when the ethoxycarbonyl masking group is removed. BIIL 260 displaced [^{3}H]LTB$_4$ from the receptor of human neutrophils with a K$_i$ value of 1.7 nM. LTB$_4$-mediated degranulation of human neutrophils apparently was noncompetitively inhibited (IC$_{50}$ = 1.9 nM). LTB$_4$-induced Mac-1 upregulation in human whole blood revealed an IC$_{50}$ of 30 nM. BIIL 260 is a specific LTB$_4$ antagonist as Mac-1 upregulation stimulated by other mediators was not influenced. In vivo, LTB$_4$-induced ear inflammation in mice was antagonized quite efficiently with an ED$_{50}$ of 0.01 mg/kg p.o. and an ED$_{50}$ of 0.02 mg/kg p.o. was obtained in a model of transdermal chemotaxis in guinea pigs. LTB$_4$-induced neutropenia could be counteracted in monkeys, guinea pigs and rats (table 1). In addition, ex vivo LTB$_4$-induced Mac-1 upregulation in monkeys was dose-dependently antagonized after oral gavage, resulting in an ED$_{50}$ of 0.05 mg/kg p.o. In toxicology, no results of concern were found and the compound is currently being clinically investigated for the indication asthma/COPD.

Conclusion

LTB$_4$ is a strong chemoattractant and chemoactivator of neutrophilic granulocytes. LTB$_4$ levels together with neutrophils are elevated in COPD, some forms of asthma and other diseases. Several potent LTB$_4$ antagonists are known. Clinical investigations are still ongoing.

References

1 Bray MA: The pharmacology and pathophysiology of leukotriene B_4. Br Med Bull 1983;39: 249–254.
2 Ford-Hutchinson AW: Leukotriene B_4 in inflammation. Crit Rev Immunol 1990;10:1–12.
3 Yokomizo T, Izumi T, Chang K, Takuwa Y, Shimizu T: A G-protein-coupled receptor for leukotriene B_4 that mediates chemotaxis. Nature 1997;387:620–624.
4 Showell HJ, Pettipher ER, Cheng K, Breslow R, Conklyn MJ, Farrell CA, Hingorani GP, Salter ED, Hackman BC, Wimberly DJ: The in vitro and in vivo pharmacologic activity of the potent and selective leukotriene B_4 receptor antagonist CP-105696. J Pharmacol Exp Ther 1995;273:176–184.
5 Jackson WT: LTB_4 receptor antagonists; in Folco G, Samuelsson B, Murphy RC (eds): Novel Inhibitors of Leukotrienes. Progress in Inflammatory Research. Basel, Birkhäuser, 1999, pp 299–316.
6 Lee E, Lindo T, Jackson N, Meng Choong L, Reynolds P, Hill A, Haswell M, Jackson S, Kilfeather S: Reversal of neutrophil survival by leukotriene B(4) receptor blockade and 5-lipoxygenase and 5-lipoxygenase activating protein inhibitors. Am J Respir Crit Care Med 1999;160:2079–2085.
7 O'Driscoll BRC, Cromwell O, Kay AB: Sputum leukotrienes in obstructive airway diseases. Clin Exp Immunol 1984;55:397–404.
8 Wenzel SE: Leukotrienes in nocturnal asthma; in Folco G, Samuelsson B, Murphy RC (eds): Novel Inhibitors of Leukotrienes. Progress in Inflammatory Research. Basel, Birkhäuser, 1999, pp 177–184.
9 Seggev JS, Thornton WH, Edes TE: Serum leukotriene in obstructive pulmonary disease. Chest 1991;99:289–291.
10 Lamblin C, Gosset P, Tillie-Leblond I, Saulnier F, Marquette CH, Wallaert B, Tonnel AB: Bronchial neutrophilia in patients with noninfectious status asthmaticus. Am J Respir Crit Care Med 1998;157:394–402.
11 Stanescu D, Sanna A, Veriter C, Kostianev S, Calcagni PG, Fabbri LM, Maestrelli P: Airway obstruction, chronic expectoration, and rapid decline of FEV_1 in smokers are associated with increased levels of sputum neutrophils. Thorax 1996;51:267–271.
12 Mikami M, Llewellyn-Jones C, Bayley D, Hill S, Stockley R: The chemotactic activity of sputum from patients with bronchiectasis. Am J Respir Crit Care Med 1998;157:723–728.
13 Britton J: Dietary fish oil and airway obstruction. Thorax 1995;50:511–515.
14 Konstan MW, Walenga RW, Hilliard KA, Hilliard JB: Leukotriene B_4 markedly elevated in the epithelial lining fluid of patients with cystic fibrosis. Am Rev Resp Dis 1993;148:896–901.
15 Cromwell O, Morris HR, Hodson ME, Walport MJ, Taylor GW, Batten J, Kay AB: Identification of leukotrienes D and B in sputum from cystic fibrosis patients. Lancet 1981;ii:164–165.
16 Lawrence R, Sorrell T: Eicosapentaenoic acid in cystic fibrosis: Evidence of pathogenetic role for leukotriene B_4. Lancet 1993;342:465–469.
17 Chen XS, Sheller JR, Johnson EN, Funk CD: Role of leukotrienes revealed by targeted disruption of the 5-lipoxygenase gene. Nature 1994;372:179–182.
18 Sawyer JS: LY293111 Sodium. Drugs Future 1996;21:610–614.
19 Marder P, Spaethe SM, Froelich LL, Cerimele BJ, Petersen BH, Tanner T, Lucas RA: Inhibition of ex vivo neutrophil activation by oral LY293111, a novel leukotriene B_4 receptor antagonist. Br J Clin Pharmacol 1996;42:457–464.
20 van Pelt JPA, de Jong EMGJ, van Erp PEJ, Mitchell MI, Marder P, Spaethe SM, van Hooijdonk CAEM, Kuijpers ALA, van de Kerkhof PCM: The regulation of CD11b integrin levels on human blood leukocytes and leukotriene B4 stimulated skin by a specific leukotriene B4 receptor antagonist (LY293111). Biochem Pharmacol 1997;53:1005–1012.
21 Evans DJ, Barnes PJ, Spaethe SM, van Alstyne EL, Mitchell MJ, O'Connor BJ: The effect of a leukotriene B_4 antagonist LY293111 on allergen-induced responses in asthma. Thorax 1996;51:1178–1184.
22 Morgan J, Stevens R, Uziel Fusi S, Lau H, Hirschhorn WL, Marshall P, Palmisano M, Piraino A: Multiple dose pharmacokinetics of a mono-aryl-amidine compound (CGS-25019C) and its inhibition of dihydroxy-leukotrienes (LTB_4) induced CD11b expression. Clin Pharmacol Ther 1995;57:153.
23 Daines RA, Chambers PA, Foley JJ, Griswald DE, Kingsburg WD, Martin LD, Schmidt DB, Sham KKC, Saran HM: (E)-3-[6-[[(2,6-dichlorophenyl)thio]methyl]-3-(2-phenylethoxy)-2-pyridinyl]-2-propenoic acid: A high-affinity leukotriene B_4 receptor antagonist with oral antiinflammatory activity. J Med Chem 1996; 39:3837–3841.
24 Showell HJ, Conklyn MJ, Alpert R, Hingorani GP, Wright KF, Smith MA, Stam E, Salter ED, Scampoli DN, Meltzer S, Reiter LA, Koch K, Piscopio AD, Cortina SR, Lopez-Anaya A, Pettipher ER, Milici AJ, Griffiths RJ: The preclinical pharmacological profile of the potent and selective LTB_4 antagonist CP-195543. J Pharm Exp Ther 1998;285:946–954.
25 Yu SS, Djuric SW, Dygos JH, Tsai BS, Paulson SK, Smith PF, Fretland DJ: SC53228. Drugs Future 1994;19:1093–1097.

Prof. Dr. H.M. Jennewein
Boehringer Ingelheim KG
Department of Pulmonary Research
D-55216 Ingelheim am Rhein (Germany)
Tel +49 6132 77 21 35
Fax +49 6132 77 98 123
E-Mail
jennew@ing.boehringer-ingelheim.com

Mediator Inhibitors and Agonists

Hansel TT, Barnes PJ (eds): New Drugs for Asthma, Allergy and COPD.
Prog Respir Res. Basel, Karger, 2001, vol 31, pp 128–132

H_1-Antihistamines

C. De Vos J.P. Rihoux

UCB Pharma SA, Brussels, Belgium

Summary

The therapeutic index of an H_1-antihistamine depends on several biochemical aspects: pharmacokinetics, metabolism, tissue distribution, lack of interference with active transport systems and existence of anti-allergic activities. Although the ideal H_1-antagonist does not yet exist, new approaches will probably allow the synthesis of more potent and more specific drugs in the near future. In this paper, we are going to briefly review the present knowledge about the available H_1-antihistamines.

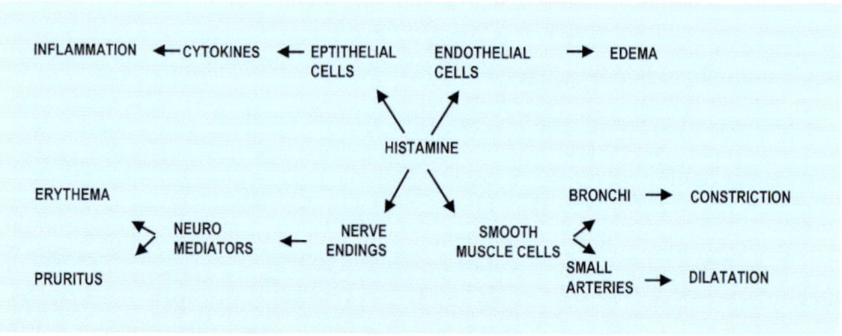

Fig. 1. Role of histamine in allergic diseases.

The H_1-Receptors

The human H_1-receptor is a protein of 487 amino acid residues (molecular weight: 55,781) showing 7-membrane-spanning hydrophobic domains like other G-protein-coupled receptors [1]. It is very similar to the bovine, rat and guinea pig H_1-receptors, and also has some similarity with the muscarinic receptor.

In allergic diseases, the main target cells for histamine via H_1-receptor-dependent activation could be the endothelial cells of the capillaries, the epithelial cells of nose, bronchial and conjunctival mucosae, the smooth muscle cells of the bronchi and small arteries, and the nerve endings (fig. 1).

Preclinical Pharmacology of H_1-Antagonists

The pharmacological screening of H_1-antihistamines is performed on particular cell lines (Chinese hamster ovary cells) expressing human H_1-receptor as well as other G-protein-coupled receptors. Using such a testing, it is possible to define the affinity and selectivity profiles of a large number of tested compounds and to establish their respective receptograms. Such studies showed that the affinity constants of second-generation H_1-receptor antagonists are very similar, the weakest affinity being found for loratadine [2]. As far as selectivity is concerned, terfenadine, loratadine and epinastine are not really H_1-selective in vitro and or in vivo in pharmacological models. They only have an apparent selectivity linked to their limited penetration into the CNS where the other receptors are mainly distributed [3–5].

H_1-Inverse Antagonism

It is well established that the binding of histamine to the H_1-receptor is rapidly followed by the activation of phospholipase C (PLC) that leads to the production of inositol-1,4,5-trisphosphate (IP_3) and 1,2-diacylglycerol (DAG). Interestingly, recent experiments carried out by the group of Timmerman [6] showed that some H_1-antihistamines not only occupy the receptor and prevent histamine from activating IP_3 formation, but also induce a decrease in IP_3, even in the absence of the agonist histamine. The relevance of this inverse agonistic effect in terms of efficacy remains to be determined (fig. 2).

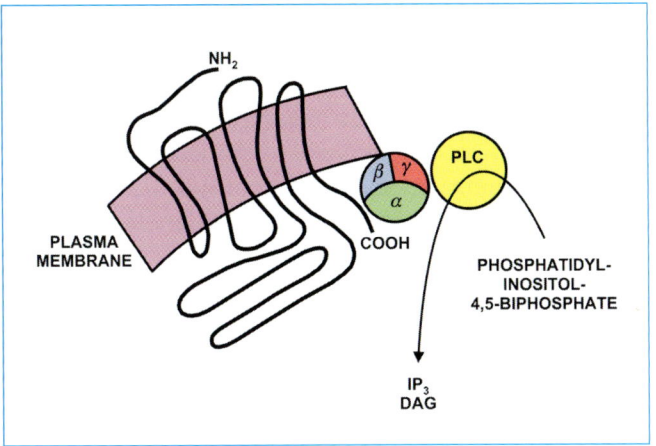

Fig. 2. H_1-receptor and signaling pathway.

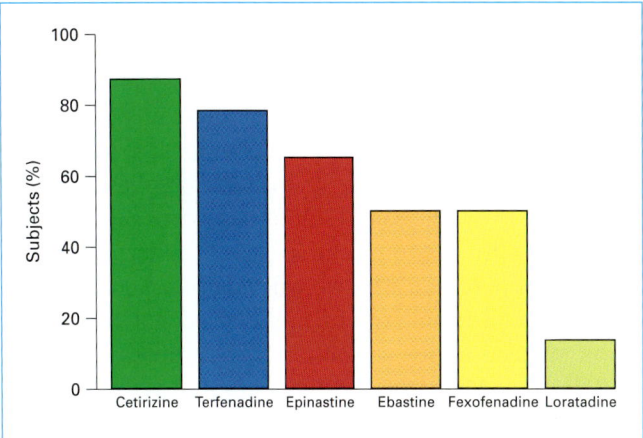

Fig. 3. Percentage of subjects with greater than 95% inhibition of flare surface areas at one time point for each treatment (n = 14 for all treatments).

Clinical Pharmacology

H_1-Receptor Antagonism. The anti-H_1-activity measured in the skin, nose and bronchi not only depends on the binding characteristics of the drugs to the peripheral H_1-receptors, but it is importantly linked to the bioavailability of the drugs at the level of the targets. In other words, it is linked to the pharmacokinetics (table 1).

Skin. Only a few double-blind crossover experiments performed in healthy volunteers compared several H_1-antagonists using the histamine-induced wheal and flare reactions [7–9]. They showed that most compounds are rapidly effective (0.5–2 h after oral intake), more or less potent and with a duration of action of at least 24 h. In other studies, no tachyphylaxis was observed (fig. 3).

Nose. The investigation of an H_1-antagonist effect in the nose is easy to perform using histamine applied locally and measuring subjective and objective induced symptoms. Very few comparative studies were performed in this area. Using double-blind and crossover conditions, Frossard et al. [10] showed that cetirizine 10 mg is more rapidly effective and longer lasting than loratadine 10 mg. By contrast, the two drugs were equally effective at their peak of action, a result that differs from skin data and shows that nose and skin are different as far as histamine and related drugs are concerned.

Bronchi. Only one clinical pharmacology study compared several H_1-antagonists at bronchial level in asthmatic subjects submitted to a bronchial provocation test with increasing concentrations of histamine given by aerosol [7]. In this study, the PC_{20} histamine (the provocation concentration of histamine required to cause a 20%

Table 1. Pharmacokinetic and pharmacodynamic characteristics of second-generation H_1-antihistamines

	Time to peak plasma level, h	Plasma half-life, h	Onset of action[1], h	Duration of action[1], h
Acrivastine	0.85 ± 1.4	1.4 ± 2.1	0.5	>7 <24
Astemizole	4	1.1 days	several hours	several days
Azelastine	5.3 ± 1.6	22 ± 1.4	2	>24
Cetirizine	1.0 ± 0.5	10.9 ± 2.2	<1	>24
Ebastine	4–6 (Carebastine)[2]	13.8→15.3	2	>24
Epinastine	1.9	11.5	0.5	24
Fexofenadine	0.83→1.33	10→12	1→2	24
Loratadine	1.0 ± 0.3	11.0 ± 9.4	1→2	12–24
Mizolastine	1.5	17 ± 4.6	1	24
Terfenadine	0.78 ± 1.1	16→23	1	24

[1] Evaluated with histamine-induced skin reaction after single oral administration.
[2] Unchanged ebastine is undetectable.

fall in the FEV_1) was measured before and after drug administration. It was shown that cetirizine 10 mg is the most potent drug, followed by terfenadine 60 mg, while the other H_1-antihistamines displayed nonsignificant shifts of PC_{20}. In other studies, loratadine 10 mg was not significantly effective while azelastine 8.8 mg was more or less similar to terfenadine 60 mg.

Anti-Allergic Activity. Unexpected pharmacological activities were recently described for histamine via H_1-

dependent mechanisms. Let us mention for instance the production of IL-6, IL-8 and GM-CSF by epithelial cells [11]. Similarly, unexpected pharmacological activities were recently described for some H_1-antagonists, drawing the attention to the possible new therapeutic interest of these drugs. Nevertheless, it must be emphasized that most of the available data result from in vitro experiments performed with very high and irrelevant concentrations.

This is the reason why we will mention here only the data collected from experiments carried out in vivo in atopic subjects taking various oral H_1-antihistamines.

Release of Mediators in vivo. Experiments carried out in atopic subjects submitted to nasal antigenic provocation showed that there was a significant decrease in histamine level in the nasal lavage fluid after treatment with terfenadine and loratadine. After cetirizine, there was no change in histamine but a decrease in LTC_4 levels [12].

Modulation of Adhesion Proteins and Cell Trafficking in vivo. In other investigations, cetirizine and loratadine were shown to significantly decrease the expression of ICAM-1 by conjunctival epithelial cells in subjects submitted to antigenic conjunctival provocation. Terfenadine given for 7 days to patients with seasonal rhinitis also reduced the expression of ICAM-1 by nasal epithelial cells. Cetirizine showed the same effect in asthmatic children treated for 2 weeks. Moreover, the same drug also decreased the expression of VCAM-1 by endothelial cells of patients with atopic dermatitis submitted to a cutaneous provocation test with DPT [13, 14]. Such a modulating effect on different adhesion molecules might explain the actions of some H_1-antihistamines on leukocyte function. Reduction of eosinophil accumulation in allergic tissues in vivo under experimental and clinical condition is repeatedly described with cetirizine [15].

Clinical Indications

Conventional Indications. H_1-antihistamines are used for the treatment of seasonal and perennial allergic rhinitis and chronic idiopathic urticaria. According to a common opinion, they are more or less equally effective in these clinical situations. This opinion is based upon a very large series of clinical double-blind studies, which were said to demonstrate equivalence between reference H_1-antihistamines.

Nevertheless, clinical trials that show no statistically significant difference between treatments do not prove that these treatments are equivalent. The demonstration of equivalence requires well-defined statistical approaches. In order to get more objective and relevant comparisons, some authors developed new experimental approaches, which deserve to be mentioned.

Quality-of-Life Approach. The aim of a quality-of-life (QOL) questionnaire is to measure the problems that patients experience in their day-to-day lives. The disease-related questionnaire may be patient specific when each patient is asked to identify activities that are important to him and in which he is limited or impaired by his allergic condition. Patients are invited to score their limitations before and during various treatments [16]. Using a generic questionnaire, Bousquet et al. [17] showed that the QOL of patients suffering from perennial allergic rhinitis is markedly affected and that it may be importantly improved by the administration of a potent H_1-antagonist.

Controlled Allergen Exposure Techniques. Some investigators developed a new objective approach of allergic rhinitis in a rigorously controlled, yet clinically relevant setting: the 'environmental exposure unit' and the 'Vienna challenge chamber' [18, 19]. Using such settings, it becomes possible to expose all the patients at the same time to the same precise relevant level of pollen, to control the intake of drugs and to establish a ranking between the different tested drugs as far as onset of action, peak, efficacy, duration of action and side effects are considered. Interestingly, such a ranking of effects in the nose correlates very well with the rankings established during objective clinical pharmacology studies performed on the skin [8].

As a conclusion, the clinical approach of any new H_1-antihistamines should combine the above-mentioned traditional and nontraditional approaches.

Nonconventional Indications. Asthma. It seems clear that some H_1-antihistamines could be of interest for the treatment of asthma, probably in addition to other drugs such as corticosteroids, leukotriene antagonists or inhibitors and β_2-agonists. Loratadine plus zafirlukast, produced an almost complete inhibition of allergen-induced early- and late-phase airway obstruction in asthmatics. Azelastine administration was accompanied by a significant corticosteroid-sparing effect. Cetirizine induced a bronchospasmolytic effect in asthmatic subjects that was additive to the bronchodilating effect of albuterol, and the same drug given at the usual dose to patients with seasonal allergic rhinitis significantly improved the symptoms of concomitant asthma [20]. Additional studies are needed in order to precisely define the role and usefulness of these drugs in this particular disease.

Safety

With the use of second-generation H_1-antihistamines, the central side effect, sedation, has become rather negligible, but other safety issues are now taken into consideration: cardiac toxicity, interferences with the hepatic enzymatic complex cytochromes P-450 (Cyt P450) and interferences with transporter proteins.

In the late eighties, rare but severe ventricular arrhythmias were described in patients taking terfenadine and astemizole. Experimental data collected since that time revealed that such toxic events usually depend on variable combinations of the following factors: overdose, hepatic failure, concomitant use of Cyt P450 inhibitors and or cardiotoxic drugs, and finally preexistence of rhythm disturbances and more especially congenital long Q-T syndrome.

Actually, several second-generation H_1-antihistamines are substrates and modulators of Cyt P450. Accordingly, their plasma and tissue levels may be increased and become toxic in case of polymedication, as well as the plasma and tissue levels of concomitantly administered drugs [21–23].

Furthermore, recent investigations showed that some H_1-antagonists may interfere with transporter proteins expressed in organs involved in drug disposition, such as intestinal P-glycoprotein: this is the case for terfenadine, fexofenadine and possibly other Cyt P450 modulators [24]. Such an interference also contributes to unpredictable increased plasma and tissue concentrations of drugs accompanied by unexpected toxicities.

Finally, the volume of distribution (V_D) of an H_1-antihistamine may also be an important factor for its therapeutic index: with a low V_D, the risk of tissue accumulation is limited as well as the risk of particular tissue toxicity [25].

Conclusions

Despite the recent discovery of numerous cytokines involved in allergic inflammation, histamine remains a pleiotropic mediator involved in different allergic conditions. Its inhibition by selective and well-tolerated drugs remains of value in the available therapeutic arsenal. Nevertheless, recent pharmacological and toxicological investigations showed that several second-generation H_1-antihistamines lack specificity since they have modulating effects on biological targets such as ion channels, Cyt P450 isoforms and transporter proteins. New H_1-antihistamines characterized by effectiveness, improved specificity and suitable pharmacokinetics and distribution are wanted: they will constitute the third-generation H_1-antihistamines.

References

1 De Backer MD, Gommeren W, Moereels H, Nobels G, Van Gompel P, Leysen JE, Luyten WHML: Genomic cloning, heterologous expression and pharmacological characterization of a human histamine H_1-receptor. Biochem Biophys Res Commun 1993;197:1601–1608.

2 Ter Laak T: Histamine H_1-Receptor Agonists and Antagonists. Modeling and Drug Design, Thesis, Amsterdam, 1995.

3 Snyder JM, Snowman AM: Receptor effects of cetirizine. Ann Allergy 1987;59/2:4–8.

4 Kreutner W, Chapman RW, Gulbenkian A, Siegel MI: Antiallergic activity of loratadine, a non-sedating antihistamine. Allergy 1987;42:57–63.

5 Fügner A, Bechtel WD, Kuhn FJ, Mierau J: In vitro and in vivo studies of the non-sedating antihistamine epinastine. Arzneimittel-Forschung 1998;38:1446–1453.

6 Bakker RA, Wieland K, Timmerman H, Leurs R: Constitutive activity of the human histamine H1 receptor reveals inverse agonism of anti-allergic H_1-antagonists. Eur J Pharmacol 2000;387:R5–R7.

7 Wood Baker R, Holgate ST: The comparative actions and adverse effect profile of single doses of H_1-receptor antihistamines in the airways and skin of subjects with asthma. J Allergy Clin Immunol 1993;91:1005–1014.

8 Grant JA, Danielson L, Rihoux JP and De Vos C: A comparison of cetirizine, ebastine, epinastine, fexofenadine, terfenadine, and loratadine versus placebo in suppressing the cutaneous response to histamine. Int Arch Allergy Immunol 1999;118:339–340.

9 Simons FER, McMillan JL, Simons KJ: A double-blind, single-dose, crossover comparison of cetirizine, terfenadine, loratadine, astemizole, and chlorpheniramine versus placebo: Suppressive effects on histamine-induced wheals and flares during 24 hours in normal subjects. J Allergy Clin Immunol 1990;86:540–547.

10 Frossard N, Benabdesselam O, Melac M, Glasser N, Lacronique J, Pauli G: Nasal effect of cetirizine and loratadine at 24 hours in patients with allergic rhinitis. Am J Ther 1998;5:307–311.

11 Weimer LK, Gamache DA, Yanni JM: Histamine-stimulated cytokine secretion from human conjunctival epithelial cells: inhibition by the histamine H_1-antagonist emedastine. Int Arch Allergy Immunol 1998;115:288–293.

12 Naclerio RM, Proud D, Kagey-Sobotka A, Freidhoff L, Norman PS, Lichtenstein LM: The effect of cetirizine on early allergic response. Laryngoscope 1989;99:596–599.

13 Ciprandi G, Catrullo A, Cerqueti P, Tosca M, Fiorino N, Canonica GW: Loratadine reduces the expression of ICAM-1. Allergy 1998;53:545–546.

14 Fasce L, Ciprandi G, Pronzato C, Cozzani S, Tosca MA, Grimaldi I, Canonica GW: Cetirizine reduces ICAM-1 on epithelial cells during nasal minimal persistent inflammation in asymptomatic children with mite-allergic asthma. Int Arch Allergy Immunol 1996;109:272–276.

15 De Vos C: H1-receptor antagonists: effects on leukocytes, myth or reality? Clin Exp Allergy, 1999;29/3:60–63.

16 Juniper EF, Thompson AK, Ferrie PJ, Roberts JN: Validation of the standardized version of the rhinoconjunctivitis quality of life questionnaire. J Allergy Clin Immunol 1999;104:364–369.

17 Bousquet J, Duchateau J, Pignat JC, Fayol C, Marquis P, Mariz S, Ware JE, Valentin B, Burtin B: Improvement of quality of life by treatment with cetirizine in patients with perennial allergic rhinitis as determined by a French version of the SF-36 questionnaire. J Allergy Clin Immunol 1996;98:309–316.
18 Day JH, Briscoe MP, Clark RH, Ellis AK, Gervais P: Onset of action and efficacy of terfenadine, astemizole, cetirizine, and loratadine for the relief of symptoms of allergic rhinitis. Ann Allergy Asthma Immunol 1997;79:163–172.
19 Horak F, Stübner P, De Vos C, Burtin B, Donnelly F: Comparison of the efficacy and safety of cetirizine 10 mg O.D. (oral tablets) and fexofenadine 120 mg O.D. (oral tablets) in reducing symptoms of seasonal allergic rhinitis. Eur Respir J 1999;14(suppl):478s.
20 Grant JA, Nicodemus CF, Findlay SR, Glovsky M, Grossman J, Kaiser H, Meltzer EO, Mitchell DQ, Pearlman D, Selner J, Settipane G, Silvers W: Cetirizine in patients with seasonal rhinitis and concomitant asthma: Prospective, randomized, placebo-controlled trial. J Allergy Clin Immunol 1995;95:923–932.
21 Renwick AG: The metabolism of antihistamines and drug interactions: The role of cytochrome P450 enzymes. Clin Exp Allergy 1999; 29:116–124.
22 Hamelin BA, Bouayad A, Drolet B, Gravel A, Turgeon J: In vitro characterization of cytochrome P450 2D6 inhibition by classic histamine H_1-receptor antagonists. Drug Metab Dispos 1998;23:536–539.
23 Nicolas JM, Whomsley R, Collart P, Roba J: In vitro inhibition of human liver drug metabolizing enzymes by second generation antihistamines. Chem Biol Interact 1999;123:63–79.
24 Cvetkovic M, Leake B, Fromm MF, Wilkinson GR, Kim RB: OATP and P-glycoprotein transporters mediate the cellular uptake and excretion of fexofenadine. Drug Metab Dispos 1999; 27:866–871.
25 Tillement JP: A low distribution volume as a determinant of efficacy and safety for histamine (H_1) antagonists. Allergy 1995;50:12–16.

Christine De Vos, UCB Pharma SA
Allée de la Recherche 60
B–1070 Brussels (Belgium)
Tel. +32 2 559 9389, Fax +32 2 559 9016
E-Mail christine.devos@ucb-group.com

Histamine H₃ Antagonists

Robbie L. McLeod[a]   Robert W. Egan[a]   Francis M. Cuss[a]   Donald C. Bolser[b]
John A. Hey[a]

[a]Allergy, Schering-Plough Research Institute, Kenilworth, N.J., and [b]Department of Physiological Sciences, University of Gainesville, Fla., USA

Summary

Treatment of allergic rhinitis often involves the use of H_1 antihistamines which block histamine, a primary mediator in allergic responses. Antihistamines alone do not provide significant benefit against the congestion associated with allergic rhinitis and are commonly given in combination with α-adrenergic decongestants. Whereas these decongestants are effective in reducing the congestion associated with allergic nasal disease, they may produce undesirable side effects, such as hypertension, agitation and insomnia. Presently, we discuss preclinical findings showing that combination histamine H_1 and H_3 receptor blockade produces decongestant activity without the hypertensive liability characteristic of α-adrenoceptor agonists.

Allergic rhinitis is an inflammation of the nasal mucosa characterized by nasal congestion and rhinorrhea. This allergic nasal disease has been estimated to occur in up to 22% of the US population [1]. Untreated rhinitis often leads to sinusitis, otitis media, nasal polyps and aggravation of bronchial asthma [2]. In the nose, mast cell histamine mediates the immediate hypersensitivity reactions that occur secondary to antigen exposure in sensitized individuals [3]. Histamine is a primary mediator responsible for the increases in nasal mucus secretion, rhinorrhea, sneezing and pruritus found in allergic rhinitis [4]. Although antihistamines are the primary treatment for allergic rhinitis, present findings indicate that the antiallergy efficacy of antihistamines against mast-cell-mediated nasal congestion may be expanded by cotreatment with a histamine H_3 receptor antagonist [5].

Antihistamines and α-Adrenergic Nasal Decongestants

Many of the allergic effects of histamine are attenuated by first- and second-generation H_1 blockers [6]. However, antihistamines are often used in combination with α-adrenergic agonist decongestants because the congestion associated with allergic rhinitis is refractory to H_1 antihistamines [7]. The use of α-agonists is limited, however, due to their potential to produce hypertensive and CNS-stimulant effects.

Modulation of Autonomic Responses by Histamine H₃ Receptors

The discovery by Arrang et al. [8] of a unique histamine H_3 receptor has rekindled interest in exploring the role of histamine and the potential for a new class of therapeutic agents that act at this receptor. Histamine H_3 receptors are widely distributed on peripheral autonomic nerves, and are found presynaptically on postganglionic nerve terminals. Activation of these receptors inhibits neurally induced cholinergic contraction in guinea pig trachea [9], human bronchus [10] and guinea pig ileum [11, 12]. They are also found presynaptically on postganglionic sympathetic nerves, and activation attenuates a variety of effector responses [13, 14]. Specifically, H_3 receptors modulate vascular responses by inhibition of norepinephrine release from sympathetic nerve terminals [15–17].

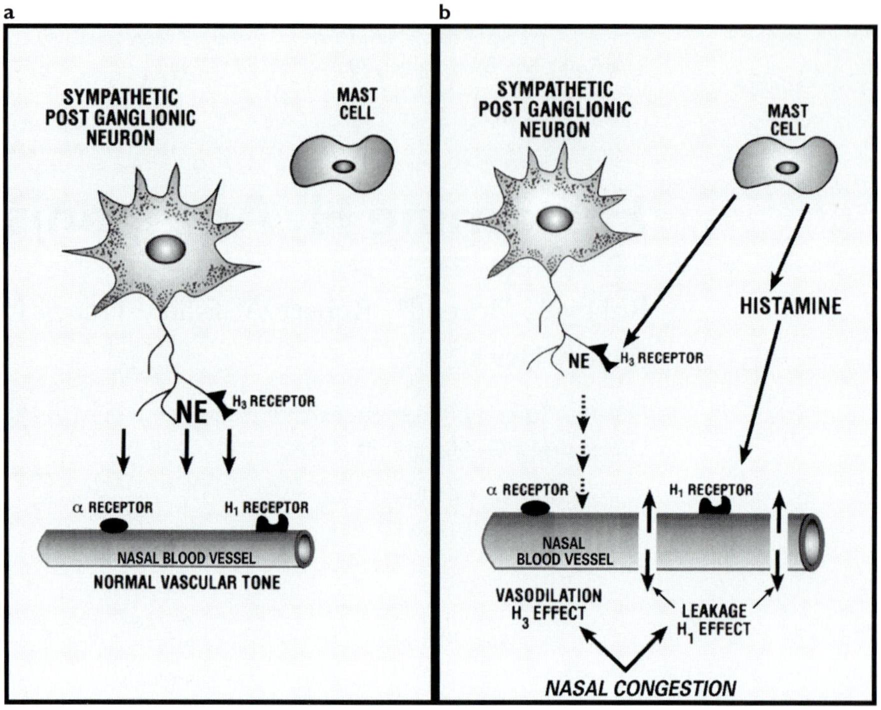

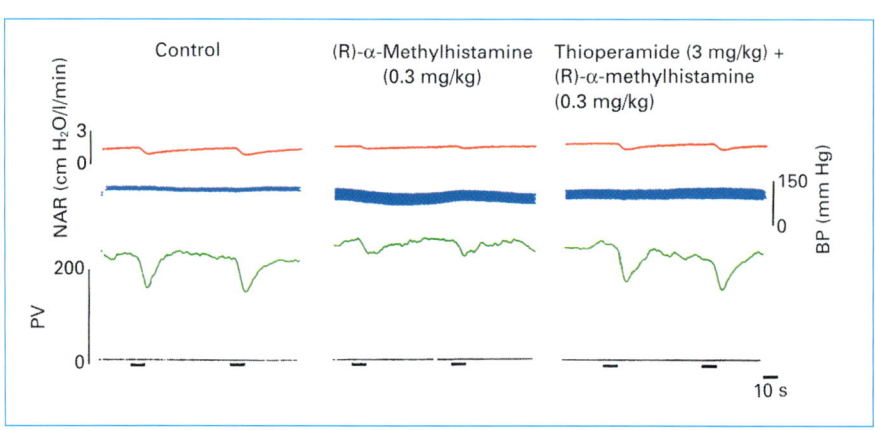

Fig. 1. Proposed mechanism for the nasal decongestant effect of combined histamine receptor H_1/H_3 blockade. **a** Nasal vascular tone is under autonomic sympathetic control mediated by tonic release of norepinephrine (NE) from postganglionic sympathetic neurons. **b** During an allergic reaction, combined H_1/H_3 treatment blocks both the direct vascular effects (plasma extravasation) of mast cell histamine and the vasodilation that occurs secondary to inhibition of sympathetic tone mediated by histamine-induced activation of presynaptic H_3 receptors.

Fig. 2. Effect of histamine H_3 receptor activation on sympathetic modulation of nasal blood flow (PV = perfusion value, an index of blood flow measured by laser Doppler) and nasal resistance (NAR). Shown on the chart recordings are the effects of (R)-α-methylhistamine on sympathetic-mediated decreases in nasal resistance and nasal blood flow. BP = Blood pressure.

Rationale for Combined Histamine H_1/H_3 Treatment for Allergic Rhinitis

In the nose, sympathetic modulation of nasal blood flow is a regulator of nasal patency. Because antihistamines do not block all the nasal effects of histamine, we studied the nasal effects of combined histamine H_1/H_3 blockade in an experimental model of nasal congestion. Under quiescent conditions, nasal vascular tone is maintained by continuous sympathetic regulation of nasal blood vessel patency (fig. 1a). After mast cell degranulation produced by an allergic reaction or by compound 48/80 as in our studies, released histamine acts on postsynaptic H_1 receptors to cause H_1-mediated plasma extravasation, vasodilation and mucus secretion. In addition, histamine produces vasodilation by activating presynaptic H_3 receptors located on postganglionic sympathetic neurons producing a decrease in norepinephrine release (fig. 1b). Combined dual H_1/H_3 treatment blocks both H_1- and H_3-mediated consequences of mast cell histamine liberation.

Histamine H_3 Modulation of Nasal Blood Flow and Nasal Resistance

Recent studies have shown a physiological role for peripheral sympathetic presynaptic H_3 receptors on regulation of nasal vascular tone. Bolser et al. [18] found that activation of histamine H_3 receptors inhibits the decrease in nasal blood flow and nasal resistance elicited by electrical stimulation of the cervical sympathetic trunk in cats. Figure 2 displays a typical effect of (R)-α-methylhis-

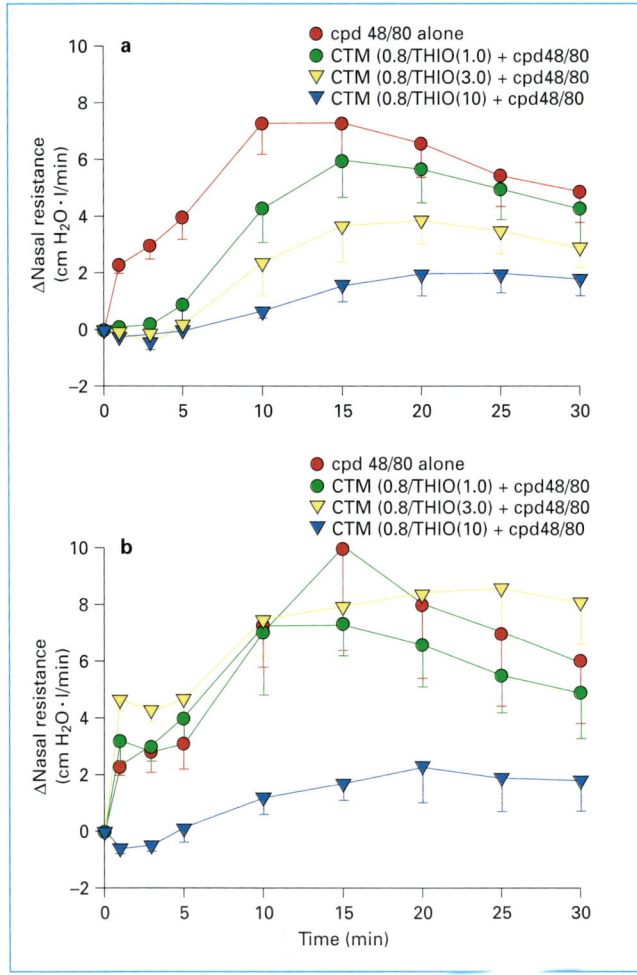

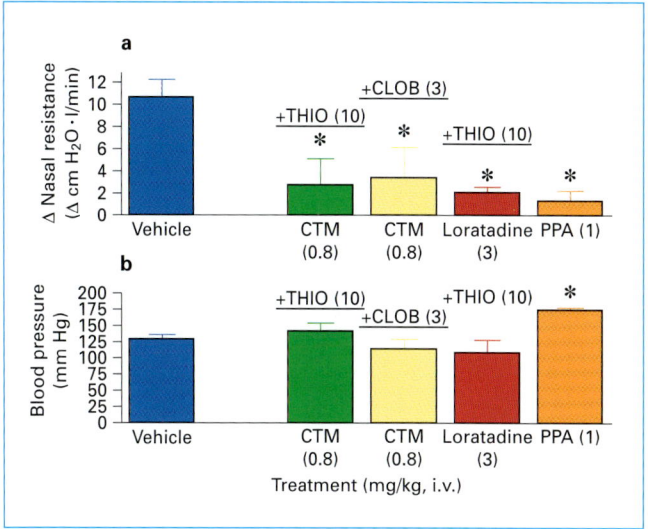

Fig. 3. Effect of combined histamine H_1/H_3 treatment with chlorpheniramine (CTM, 0.8 mg/kg, i.v.) and thioperamide (THIO 1.0–10 mg/kg, i.v.) on aerosolized compound 48/80 (1%)-induced increase in nasal resistance. Each point represents the mean ± SEM of 4–7 animals (* $p < 0.05$ compared to compound 48/80 alone).

Fig. 4. Effect of combined histamine H_1/H_3 treatment on nasal resistance and blood pressure. **a** Effect of chlorpheniramine (CTM; 0.8 mg/kg, i.v.) plus thioperamide (THIO; 10 mg/kg, i.v.); CTM (0.8 mg/kg, i.v.) plus clobenpropit (CLOB; 3 mg/kg, i.v.); loratadine (3 mg/kg, i.v.) plus THIO (10 mg/kg, i.v.) and phenylpropanolamine (PPA; 1 mg/kg, i.v.) on the increase in nasal resistance produced by aerosolized compound 48/80 (1%). **b** Effect of various H_1/H_3 combinations on blood pressure. Each point represents the mean ± SEM of 4–7 animals (* $p < 0.05$ compared to vehicle).

tamine (0.3 mg/kg, i.v.), an H_3 agonist, on nasal blood flow and resistance. In these studies, (R)-α-methylhistamine inhibited the sympathetic-mediated decrease in blood flow and nasal resistance by 49 ± 11 and 34 ± 11%, respectively. The activity of (R)-α-methylhistamine was blocked by the H_3 antagonist thioperamide (3.0 mg/kg, i.v.).

Evaluation of the Nasal Decongestant Activity of Combined H_1/H_3 Blockade

We evaluated the effect of combined H_1 and H_3 receptor blockade on the increases in nasal resistance produced by nasal provocation with aerosolized compound 48/80 in the cat [5, 19]. Figure 3 illustrates the decongestant effect of dual histamine H_1/H_3 receptor blockade on compound 48/80 (1%)-induced nasal responses. Chlorpheniramine (0.8 mg/kg, i.v.) plus thioperamide (0.1–10 mg/kg, i.v.) given before nasal exposure to compound 48/80 produced a dose-dependent inhibition of nasal resistance. Similar results were obtained with clobenpropit, an H_3 antagonist that is structurally different from thioperamide. The combination of clobenpropit (3.0 mg/kg, i.v.) and chlorpheniramine (0.8 mg/kg, i.v.) also produced nasal decongestion (fig. 4). Moreover, the nonsedating antihistamine, loratadine (3.0 mg/kg, i.v.) plus thioperamide (10 mg/kg, i.v.) inhibited the nasal congestion due to compound 48/80 (fig. 4). When evaluated separately, the H_3 antagonists thioperamide (10 mg/kg, i.v.) and clobenpropit (3.0) or the H_1 antagonists chlorpheniramine (3.0 mg/kg, i.v.) or loratadine (3.0 mg/kg, i.v.) did not produce decongestion (fig. 3b; clobenpropit and loratadine data not shown). Run as a positive standard, the α-agonist phenylpropanolamine (1.0 mg/kg, i.v.) also blocked the congestive actions of compound 48/80 while significantly increasing blood pressure (fig. 4). In contrast to the hypertension produced by phenylpropanolamine, dual histamine H_1/

Table 1. Effect of oral histamine H_1/H_3 blockade on nasal cavity geometry and blood pressure

Treatment, mg/kg, p.o.	n	Decrease in nasal cavity volume, %	Systolic BP mm Hg
Compound 48/80 alone	8	68 ± 8	89 ± 8
CTM (10)/THIO (30) + cpd 48/80	6	19 ± 12*	81 ± 8
PPA (10) + cpd 48/80	6	18 ± 9*	138 ± 8*
CTM (10) + cpd 48/80	7	64 ± 14	81 ± 6
THIO (30) + cpd 48/80	5	40 ± 10	89 ± 7

* $p < 0.05$, statistically different from control animals given compound 48/80 (cpd 48/80) alone.

H_3 blockade with chlorpheniramine plus thioperamide, chlorpheniramine plus clobenpropit, or loratadine plus thioperamide did not affect blood pressure (fig. 4).

Combined oral H_1/H_3 treatment was also found to attenuate the decrease in nasal cavity volume produced by topical exposure to compound 48/80 (1%, 50 µl). Using acoustic rhinometry, we evaluated the nasal decongestant activity of chlorpheniramine (10 mg/kg, p.o.) administered in combination with thioperamide (30 mg/kg, p.o.) on nasal cavity geometry (table 1). The nasal volume data are expressed as the percent decrease in nasal cavity volume from a naive group of animals (no compound 48/80 exposure) 3 h after oral treatments. Phenylpropanolamine (10 mg/kg, p.o.) also produced nasal decongestion. Treatment with chlorpheniramine (10 mg/kg, p.o.) or thioperamide (30 mg/kg, p.o.) alone or together had no effects on systolic blood pressure, while phenylpropanolamine (10 mg/kg, p.o.) produced an increase in blood pressure.

Conclusions

Our results suggest that combined H_1/H_3 blockade may provide a novel approach for the treatment of allergic nasal congestion without the hypertensive liability of current α-adrenergic agonist decongestant therapies. In allergic nasal disease, mast-cell-derived histamine in addition to producing H_1-receptor-mediated effects, such as plasma extravasation, sneezing and mucus secretion, may also inhibit sympathetic outflow producing nasal vasodilation by a prejunctional H_3 receptor mechanism. In conclusion, the addition of an H_3 antagonist to an H_1 antagonist confers decongestant activity upon the H_1 blocker by attenuating autonomic effects of histamine not blocked by antihistamines.

References

1 Naclerio R: Allergic rhinitis [Review]. New Eng J Med 1991;325:860–869.
2 Engler DB, Grant AJ: Allergic rhinitis: A practical approach. Hosp Pract 1991;1:105–108.
3 Baraniuk JN: Mechanisms in rhinitis. Allergy Asthma Proc 1998;19:343–346.
4 Naclerio R: Clinical manifestations of the release of histamine and other inflammatory mediators. J Allergy Clin Immunol 1999;103:S382–S3825.
5 McLeod RL, Mingo GG, Herczku C, DeGennaro-Culver F, Kreutner W, Egan RW, Hey JA: Combined histamine H_1 and H_3 receptor blockade produces nasal decongestion in an experimental model of nasal congestion. Am J Rhinol 1999;13:391–399.
6 Babe KS, Serafin WE: Histamine bradykinin and their antagonists; in Hardman G, Limbind LE (eds): Goodman and Gilman, The Pharmacological Basis of Therapeutics, ed 9. New York, McGrawHill, 1996, pp 581–600.
7 Spector S: Ideal pharmacotherapy for allergic rhinitis. J Aller Clin Immunol 1999;103:S386–S387.
8 Arrang J-M, Garbarg M, Schwartz JC: Autoinhibition of brain histamine release mediated by a novel class (H_3) of histamine receptor. Nature 1983;302:832–837.
9 Ichinose M, Stretton C, Schwartz J, Barnes P: Histamine H_3-receptors inhibit cholinergic neurotransmission in guinea-pig airways. Br J Pharmacol 1989;97:21–25.
10 Ichinose M, Barnes P: Histamine H_3-receptors modulate nonadrenergic noncholinergic neural bronchoconstriction in guinea-pig in vivo. Eur J Pharmacol 1989;174:383–386.
11 Trzeciakowski JP: Inhibition of guinea pig ileum contractions mediated by a class of histamine receptors resembling the H_3 subtype. J Pharmacol Exp Ther 1987;243:874–880.
12 Coruzzi G, Poli E, Bertaccini G: Histamine receptors in isolated guinea pig duodenal muscle: H_3 receptors inhibit cholinergic neurotransmission. J Pharmacol Exp Ther 1991;258:325–331.
13 Malinowska B, Schlicker E: H_3 receptor-mediated inhibition of neurogenic vasopressor responses in pithed rats. Eur J Pharmacol 1991;205:307–310.
14 Koss MC, Hey JA: Activation of histamine H_3 receptors produces presynaptic inhibition of neurally evoked cat nictitating membrane responses in vivo. Naunyn-Schmiedeberg's Arch Pharmac 1992;346:208–212.
15 Hey JA, del Prado M, Egan RW, Kreutner W, Chapman RW: Inhibition of sympathetic hypertensive responses in the guinea-pig by prejunctional histamine H_3-receptors. Br J Pharmacol 1992;107:347–351.
16 Hutchison RW, Hey JA: Pharmacological characterization of the inhibitory effect of (R)-α-methylhistamine on sympathetic cardiopressor responses in the pithed guinea pig. J Auton Pharmacol 1994;14:393–402.
17 McLeod RL, Gertner SB, Hey JA: Hemodynamic profile of activation of histamine H_3 receptors by R-α-methylhistamine in a guinea pig. Gen Pharmacol 1996;27:1001–1007.
18 Bolser DC, DeGennaro FC, Chapman RW, Hey JA: Histamine H_3 modulation of nasal airway blood flow and resistance in the cat. Am J Res Crit Care Med 1994;149:A909.
19 McLeod RL, Mingo G, Herczku C, Corboz MR, Ramos SI, DeGennaro-Culver F, Pedersen OF, Hey JA: Changes in nasal resistance and nasal geometry using pressure and acoustic rhinometry in a feline model of nasal congestion. Am J Rhinol 1999;13:375–383.

Robbie L. McLeod, PhD
Allergy, Schering-Plough Research Institute
2015 Galloping Hill Road
Kenilworth, NJ 07033-0539 (USA)
Tel. +1 908 740 3286, Fax +1 908 740 7175
E-Mail robbie.mcleod@spcorp.com

Kinin Receptor Antagonists

Stefania Meini   Carlo Alberto Maggi

Pharmacology Department, Menarini Ricerche SpA, Florence, Italy

Summary

Kinins are small peptides which are produced in the blood or tissues during inflammation. They act by stimulating distinct receptors, B_1 and B_2. The B_1 receptor is induced during inflammation whereas the B_2 receptor is constitutively expressed. Kinins produce a number of effects which are relevant for airway pathophysiology (bronchoconstriction, plasma protein extravasation, mucus secretion, stimulation of inflammatory cells). It is currently proposed that kinin receptor antagonists could represent a novel class of drugs useful for the treatment of chronic airway diseases, including asthma.

Kinins and Kinin Receptors

Kinins are a family of small peptides which are produced by proteolytic cleavage from inactive precursors (kininogens): bradykinin (Arg-Pro-Pro-Gly-Phe-Ser-Pro-Phe-Arg; BK) and kallidin (Lys-BK) are the two main mammalian kinins formed from circulating and tissue kininogens, respectively [1]. Alternative pathways for kinins production by lysosomal enzymes (tryptases and elastases) released from mast cells and neutrophils at the site of inflammation have also been documented [2]. Under the action of carboxypeptidases, which remove their C-terminal Arg residue, BK and Lys-BK yield the respective des-Arg metabolites [1] which are biologically active as well (see below).

Kinins produce their biological effects by activating two distinct receptors, B_1 and B_2 [3], which both belong to the family of G-protein-coupled receptors [4, 5]. BK and Lys-BK are high-affinity ligands for B_2 receptors, whereas their des-Arg derivatives are inactive at B_2 receptors and possess high affinity for B_1 receptors.

The two kinin receptors, besides having low sequence homology (36%), differ in their expression: the B_2 receptor is constitutively expressed by a number of cell types throughout the body, whereas the B_1 receptor has a very low, if any, level of expression in normal tissues and is upregulated or de novo expressed during inflammation or tissue injury [3, 6]. An upregulation of B_2 receptors in human bronchial smooth muscle cells following exposure to inflammatory mediators has been reported as well [7].

Actions of Kinins Relevant for Airway Pathophysiology

Since their discovery, kinins have been characterized as autacoids endowed with powerful inflammatory actions, chiefly produced during pathological processes. The concept that kinins may have a role in the airway pathophysiology was raised from the observation that inhaled BK induces bronchoconstriction in asthmatics but not in healthy subjects [8], and that kinin peptides can be detected in the BAL fluid of asthmatics [9].

In experimental animals kinins induce a number of responses which are in keeping with a proposed role as mediators in airway pathophysiology (fig. 1). In this respect, the bulk of available data is related to B_2 receptors. In fact, for reasons which are presently not understood, it has not yet been possible to conclusively demonstrate the expression of B_1 receptors in guinea pigs, the species most commonly used for studies on airway pathophysiology.

The effects of kinins at airway level are both direct and indirect: the latter involve the release of other mediators of inflammation/autacoids, including prostanoids [10],

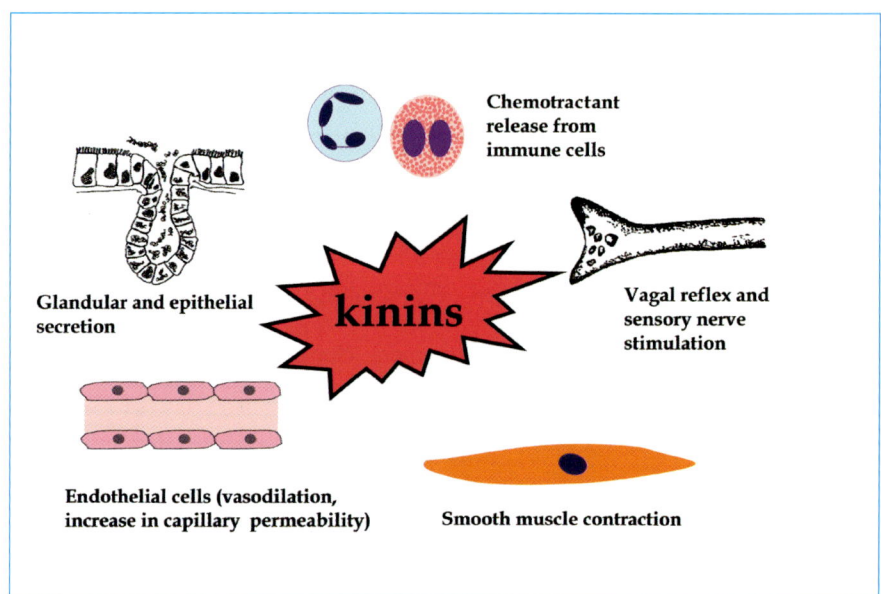

Fig. 1. Scheme depicting the main actions of kinins on different target cells which at airway level are relevant for supporting a role of kinins in airway pathophysiology. These are as follows: epithelial and glandular cells, through which kinins stimulate airway secretion; immune cells which are activated and/or primed by kinins to contribute the cellular component of airway inflammation and release cytokines which further amplify the inflammatory process; nerve endings through which kinins stimulate afferent discharge inducing cough and reflex bronchoconstriction and modulate local release of neurotransmitters; smooth muscle cells through which kinins can directly affect bronchomotor tone, and endothelial cells through which kinins can induce vasodilation (at arterial level) and increase in permeability to plasma protein and induce edema (at the level of postcapillary venules).

nitric oxide [11] and release of mediators following degranulation of mast cells [12].

Kinins, via B_2 receptors, induce powerful bronchoconstriction in the guinea pig following systemic or topical administration. This may involve both a direct effect on airway smooth muscle and also an indirect effect through afferent nerve stimulation and reflex (parasympathetic) bronchoconstriction [10, 13]. The mechanisms of BK-induced bronchoconstriction also depend upon its route of administration: intravenously administered BK caused bronchoconstriction in anesthetized guinea pigs mainly via the release of cyclooxygenase products and also by activating acetylcholine release [10]. The release of sensory neuropeptides does not appear to play a role, since their depletion by capsaicin pretreatment was without effect [10]. In contrast, when BK was administered directly into the airway lumen, the evoked bronchoconstriction was mediated *via* cholinergic mechanisms and through the release of sensory neuropeptides, without a contribution of cyclooxygenase products [10]. The latter result is similar to what has been observed in asthmatic patients since the bronchoconstrictor response to inhaled BK was not affected by aspirin [8].

Besides inducing bronchoconstriction, kinins also exert a number of inflammatory and proinflammatory effects at airway level: these include the induction of tissue edema, linked to an increase in plasma protein exudation at the level of postcapillary venules [14, 15], stimulation of mucus secretion [16], recruitment and priming of inflammatory cells and fibroblasts [17, 18]. Besides the above-mentioned indirect effects, kinins also induce the release of cytokines from inflammatory cells, which may further amplify their proinflammatory effects and also contribute to overexpression of the B_2 kinin receptors [19].

Airway microvascular leakage, induction of cell infiltration, and subsequent airway-wall edema, all contribute to the development of AHR [20], a hallmark in the pathophysiology of asthma.

As mentioned above only few data are available with regard to B_1 receptors in the airways: Huang et al. [21] reported an up-regulation of B_1 receptor in rat airways after exposure to allergen and presented evidence for their involvement of AHR to acetylcholine. Perron et al. [22] presented evidence suggesting a role of both B_1 and B_2 in pulmonary eosinophil accumulation in a model of Sephadex-induced lung inflammation in guinea pigs.

Preclinical Studies with B_2 Kinin Receptor Antagonists

The development of potent and selective antagonists for the B_2 kinin receptor, of both peptide and nonpeptide nature [23], has enabled the use of these pharmacological tools to probe a possible involvement of kinins in animal models of airway diseases. The major part of relevant data on this topic have been obtained with the peptide antagonist Icatibant [24] and the nonpeptide antagonist FR173657 [25].

Both compounds antagonize BK-induced bronchoconstriction and airway microvascular leakage in guinea pigs [24–26], FR173657 being also active after oral administration.

Kinins are generated during allergic reactions and this event can be detected by measuring an increase of kinin and kallikrein-like activity e.g. in the BAL fluid of sensitized guinea pigs after exposure to the allergen. Icatibant inhibits the increase in lung resistance provoked by antigen exposure in sensitized guinea pigs by about 50% [27], and concomitantly reduces plasma protein extravasation at airway level to about the same extent [28]. Watanabe et al. [26] showed that FR173657 inhibits the microvascular leakage induced by antigen (aerosolized ovalbumin) in guinea pig airways by about 80%. Both antagonists were equieffective in the same study in inhibiting the BK-induced plasma protein extravasation [26].

An involvement of endogenous kinins in airway inflammation has also been demonstrated in an experimental model of pleurisy induced by allergen challenge in sensitized guinea pigs, an inflammatory response characterized by mast cell degranulation, plasma leakage and neutrophil accumulation (4 h after the challenge), and a later eosinophil accumulation (24 h after the challenge) [29]. In this study, both Icatibant and FR173657 blocked the allergen- and BK-induced mast cell degranulation and the other mentioned parameters of inflammation [29] without affecting plasma leakage and eosinophil infiltration triggered by compound 48/80 and PAF, respectively.

Icatibant has also been shown to inhibit the bronchoconstriction evoked by citric acid inhalation in guinea pigs, a model which mimicks airway dysfunction caused by gastroesophageal acid reflux: in asthmatic patients, this event causes bronchoconstriction by activating a vagal reflex. Icatibant inhibits the increase in lung resistance due to citric acid aerosol [30] by about 50%, likely by preventing tachykinin release from sensory nerves.

By using kinin B_1 receptor antagonists evidence has been presented suggesting a participation of this receptor in allergen-induced AHR in rats [21] and Sephadex-induced pulmonary leukocyte accumulation in guinea pigs [22].

Summarizing this section, the data collected in various animal models of airway disease indicate that kinins are generated in the lungs during allergy/inflammation and that these autacoids, by activating both B_1 and B_2 receptors, contribute to the pathogenesis of airway inflammation. The data also advocate a possible use of kinin receptor antagonists for treatment of human airway diseases including asthma.

Clinical Studies

Inhalation of BK induces cough and retrosternal discomfort in both healthy volunteers and asthmatics, and bronchoconstriction in asthmatics only [8]. In asthmatics the BK-induced bronchoconstriction is partly reduced by ipratropium, suggesting that it is partly indirect and linked to activation of a vagal reflex. Moreover, the presence of kinins has been detected in the BAL fluid from asthmatic patients [9].

To date, only one study has reported the efficacy of a B_2 receptor antagonist in asthmatic patients: in this clinical trial [31] Icatibant was administered by aerosol (900 or 3,000 μg), compared to placebo: after 2 weeks single-blind placebo, patients were treated three times daily with nebulized Icatibant. The study indicated that 4 weeks of treatment with Icatibant led to a dose-dependent improvement in terms of respiratory parameters (FEV_1 and PEFR), although no clinically relevant improvement in subjective parameters was found. It has to be noted that no indication was provided about the efficacy and duration of action of Icatibant, at the dosages selected for the study in effectively blocking B_2 receptors at airway level, i.e. the observed improvement in airway function may have been produced by suboptimal doses of the drug, in terms of efficacy/duration of action of Icatibant.

Conclusions

In conclusion, the available data indicate that kinins are generated at airway level during allergy and inflammation and may contribute to induce various effects which are relevant to the pathophysiology of human airway diseases (bronchoconstriction, cough, inflammation, mucus secretion). Kinin receptor antagonists are effective in animals model of pulmonary allergy/inflammation. A preliminary clinical study with Icatibant demonstrated in principle that this class of drugs could be effective in ameliorating airway functions in asthmatics. It appears a challenge for future research, especially at clinical level, to demonstrate whether kinin receptor antagonists have sufficient efficacy and tolerability to be proposed as a novel class of drugs to be used in human therapy.

References

1 Bhoola KD, Figueroa CD, Worthy K: Bioregulation of kinins: Kallikreins, kininogens, and kininases. Pharmacol Rev 1992;44:1–80.
2 Kozik A, Moore RB, Potempa J, Imamura T, Rapala-Kozik M, Travis J: A novel mechanism for bradykinin production at inflammatory sites. J Biol Chem 1998;273:33224–33229.
3 Regoli D, Barabé J: Pharmacology of bradykinin and related kinins. Pharmacol Rev 1980; 32:1–46.
4 Hess JF, Borkowski JA, Young GS, Strader CD, Ransom RW: Cloning and pharmacological characterization of a human bradykinin (BK-2) receptor. Biochem Biophys Res Commun 1992;184:260–268.
5 Menke JG, Borkowski JA, Bierilo KK, Macneil T, Derrick AW, Schneck KA, Ransom RW, Strader CD, Linemeyer DL, Hess JF: Expression cloning of a human B_1 bradykinin receptor. J Biochem Chem 1994;269:21583–21586.
6 Marceau F, Hess FJ, Bachvarov DR: The B_1 receptors for kinins. Pharmacol Rev 1998;50: 357–386.
7 Schmidlin F, Scherrer D, Daeffler L, Bertrand C, Landry Y, Gies J-P: Interleukin-1β induces bradykinin B_2 receptor gene expression through a prostanoid cyclic AMP-dependent pathway in human bronchial smooth muscle cells. Mol Pharmacol 1998;53:1009–1015.
8 Fuller RW, Dixon CMS, Cuss FMC, Barnes PJ: Bradykinin-induced bronchoconstriction in humans: Mode of action. Am Rev Respir Dis 1987;135:176–180.
9 Christiansen SC, Proud D, Cochrane CG: Detection of tissue kallikrein in the bronchoalveolar lavage fluid of asthmatic subjects. J Clin Inves 1987;79:188–197.
10 Ichinose M, Belvisi MG, Barnes PJ: Bradykinin-induced bronchoconstriction in guinea pig in vivo: Role of neural mechanisms. J Pharmacol Exp Ther 1990;253:594–599.
11 Ricciardolo FLM, Nadel JA, Yoishihara S, Geppetti P: Evidence for reduction of bradykinin-induced bronchoconstriction in guineapigs by release of nitric oxide. Br J Pharmacol 1994;113:1147–1152.
12 Vietinghoff G, Paegelow I, Reissmann S: Induction of histamine release from rat mast cells by bradykinin analogues. Peptides 1996;17: 1467–1470.
13 Fox AJ, Banrnes PJ, Urban L, Dray A: An in vitro study of the properties of single vagal afferents innervating guinea-pig airways. J Physiol (Lond) ;469:21–35.
14 Nakajima N, Ichinose M, Takahashi T, Yamauchi H, Igarashi A, Miura M, Inoue H, Takishima T, Shirato K: Bradykinin-induced airway inflammation: Contribution of sensory neuropeptides differs according to airway site. Am J Respir Crit Care Med 1994;149:694–698.
15 Ortiz JL, Cortijo J, Vallés JM, Bou J, Morcillo EJ: Rolipram inhibits airway microvascular leakage induced by platelet-activating factor, histamine and bradykinin in guinea-pigs. J Pharm Pharmacol 1993;45:1090–1092.
16 Nagaki M, Shimura S, Irokawa T, Sasaki T, Oshiro T, Nara M, Kakuta Y, Shirato K: Bradykinin regulation of airway submucosal gland secretion: Role of bradykinin receptor subtype. Am J Physiol 1996;270:L907–L913.
17 Sato E, Koyama S, Nomura H, Kubo N, Sekiguchi M: Bradykinin stimulates alveolar macrophages to release neutrophil, monocyte, and eosinophil chemotactic activity. J Immunol 1996;157:3122–3129.
18 Koyama S, Sato E, Numanami H, Kubo K, Nagai S, Izumi T: Bradykinin stimulates lung fibroblasts to release neutrophil and monocyte chemotactic activity. Am J Respir Cell Mol Biol 2000;22:75–84.
19 Schmidlin F, Loeffler S, Bertrand C, Landry Y, Gies J-P: PLA_2 phosphorylation and cyclyoxygenase-2 induction, through p38 MAP kinase pathway, is involved in the IL-1β- induced bradykinin B_2 receptor gene transcription. Naunyn-Schmiedebergs Arch Pharmacol 2000;361: 247–254.
20 Kimura K, Hiroshi I, Ichinose M, Miura M, Katsumata U, Takahashi U, Takahashi T, Takishima T: Bradykinin causes airway hyperresponsiveness and enhances maximal airway narrowing. Am Rev Respir Dis 1992;146: 1301–1305.
21 Huang T-J, Haddad E-B, Fox AJ, Salmon M, Jones C, Burgess G, Chung KF: Contribution of bradykinin B_1 and B_2 receptors in allergen-induced bronchial hyperresponsiveness. Am J Respir Crit Care Med 1999;160:1717–1723.
22 Perron M-S, Gobeil FJR, Pelletier S, Regoli D, Sirois P: Involvement of bradykinin B_1 and B_2 receptors in pulmonary leukocytes accumulation induced by Sephadex beads in guinea pigs. Eur J Pharmacol 1999;376:83–89.
23 Altamura M, Meini S, Quartara L, Maggi CA: Nonpeptide antagonists for kinin receptors. Regul Pept 1999;80:13–26.
24 Wirth K, Hock FJ, Albus U, Linz W, Alpermann HG, Anagnostopoulos H, Henke St, Breipohl G, König W, Knolle J, Schölkens BA: Hoe 140 a new potent and long acting bradykinin-antagonist: In vivo studies. Br J Pharmacol 1991;102:774–777.
25 Asano M, Inamura N, Hatori C, Sawai H, Fujiwara T, Katayama A, Kayakiri H, Satoh S, Abe Y, Inoue T, Sawada Y, Nakahara K, Oku T, Okuhara M: The identification of an orally active, nonpeptide bradykinin B2 receptor antagonist, FR173657. Br J Pharmacol 1997;120: 617–624.
26 Watanabe M, Yoshihara S, Abe T, Oyama M, Arisaka O: Effects of the orally active nonpeptide bradykinin B_2 receptor antagonist, FR173657, on plasma extravasation in guinea pig airways. Eur J Pharmacol 1999;367:373–378.
27 Featherstone RL, Parry JE, Church MK: The effects of a kinin antagonist on changes in lung function and plasma extravasation into the airways following challenge of sensitized guineapigs. Clin Exp Allergy 1996;26:235–240.
28 Bertrand C, Nadel JA, Yamawaki I, Geppetti P: Role of kinins in the vascular extravasation evoked by antigen and mediated by tachykinins in guinea pig trachea. J Immunol 1993;151: 4902–4907.
29 Bandeira-Melo C, Calheiros AS, Silva PMR, Cordeiro RSB, Teixeira MM, Martins MA: Suppressive effect of distinct bradykinin B_2 receptor antagonist on allergen-evoked exudation and leukocyte infiltration in sensitized rats. Br J Pharmacol 1999;127:315–320.
30 Ricciardolo FLM, Rado V, Fabbri LM, Sterk PJ, Di Maria GU, Geppetti P: Bronchoconstriction induced by citric acid inhalation in guinea pigs. Am J Respir Crit Care Med 1999; 159:557–562.
31 Akbary AM, Wirth KJ, Schölkens BA: Efficacy and tolerability of Icatibant (Hoe 140) in patients with moderately severe chronic bronchial asthma. Immunopharmacology 1996;33: 238–242.

Carlo Alberto Maggi
Menarini Ricerche SpA
Pharmacology Department
via Rismondo 12A, I–50131 Florence (Italy)
Tel. +39 055 5680360, Fax +39 055 5680419
E-Mail camaggi@menarini-ricerche.it

Endothelin Antagonists

Douglas W.P. Hay[a]   Christopher H. Compton[b]

[a]Department of Pulmonary Biology, SmithKline Beecham Pharmaceuticals, King of Prussia, Pa., USA, and [b]Department of Clinical Investigation, SmithKline Beecham Pharmaceuticals, Harlow, UK

Summary

Endothelin-1 (ET-1), a 21-amino acid peptide discovered in 1988, and its receptors (ET_A and ET_B), are abundant in human lung. ET-1 fits several of the standard criteria for a pathophysiologically relevant substance in lung disease, including mimicry of features of asthma, COPD, pulmonary hypertension and allergic rhinitis. Furthermore, increased levels and/or expression of ET-1 are detected in patients with many pulmonary disorders, including asthma and COPD. However, clarification of the mediator role of ET-1 in pulmonary disorders awaits the clinical evaluation of ET receptor antagonists or ET synthesis inhibitors.

In 1988 a pioneer publication described the isolation and characterization of a novel peptide, endothelin-1 (ET-1), which possessed potent vasoconstrictor activity. ET-1 is a member of a family of 21-amino acid peptides, which are related to a group of snake venom toxins, the sarafotoxins; the other ETs are ET-2 and ET-3 [1]. Since the discovery of ET-1 there has been an incredible amount of research on this peptide family, reflected by the thousands of publications, including several hundred in the pulmonary system.

Synthesis, Release, Distribution and Metabolism of Endothelin-1 in the Lung

ET-1 is produced via a two-stage proteolytic process, initially involving the formation of a 39-amino-acid intermediate, called 'big endothelin', from a 212 (human)-residue preproendothelin polypeptide, followed by cleavage of the Try^{73} and Val^{74} linkage of big ET-1 by an endothelin-converting enzyme (ECE) to produce the bioactive ET-1 (fig. 1). The machinery for the synthesis, release and metabolism of ET-1 is present in mammalian lung [2, 3], with enhanced ECE expression in patients with chronic rhinitis [4].

ET-1 is found in various lung cells including the endothelium, epithelium, submucosal glands and some inflammatory cells, such as macrophages [3, 5]. The ETs, including ET-1, are metabolized in the lung predominantly via the activity of epithelium-derived, phosphoramidon-sensitive neutral endopeptidase [6]. ET-1 is also cleared in the lung, via a mechanism involving the ET_B receptor subtype [3].

ET Receptors in the Lung

The biological actions of ET-1 are produced via receptors which belong to the superfamily of G-protein-coupled, seven-transmembrane-spanning receptors. Two subtypes of ET receptor, termed ET_A and ET_B, have been cloned, sequenced and characterized [1]. Both receptor populations are located in mammalian airways [3]. High-affinity binding of $[^{125}I]$-ET-1 (nonselective ligand) occurs in human lung, predominantly to airway and vascular smooth muscle, with some associated with nerves and ganglia [3]. The percentages of ET_A and ET_B receptors in airway smooth muscle (about 85% ET_B and 15% ET_A) and peripheral lung (about 70% ET_B and 30% ET_A) are not altered in asthmatic tissues [7, 8]. However, an alteration in the ratio of ET_A and ET_B receptor mRNA – with an increase in ET_B receptor message – in patients with asthma and COPD has been described [9]. In normal human pulmonary artery the percentages are 10% ET_B and 90% ET_A [3]. Stimulation of ET_A and ET_B receptors produces many effects in mammalian lung, including airway smooth muscle and pulmonary vascular smooth muscle contraction (ET_A and ET_B), airway and vascular smooth muscle proliferation (ET_A), mediator release (ET_A), inflammatory cell recruitment (ET_A) and enhancement of nerve-induced responses (ET_A and ET_B) [3].

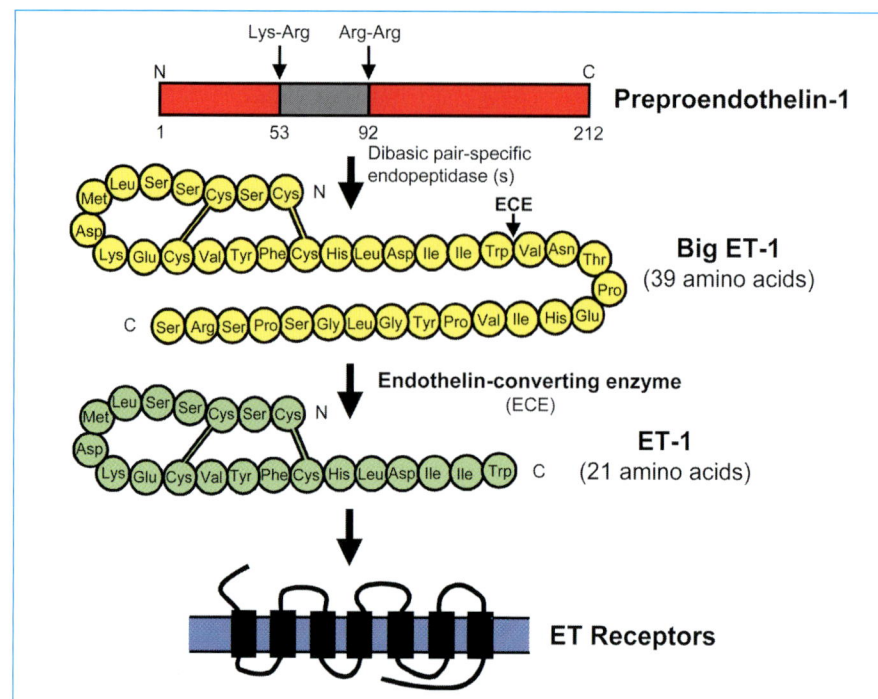

Fig. 1. Synthetic pathway for ET-1.

Table 1. ET and the pathophysiology of asthma

	Features of asthma	ET
1	Increased bronchial tone	+++
2	Airway smooth muscle hyperplasia/airways remodeling	+
3	Mucus hypersecretion	+, –
4	Airway hyperresponsiveness	+, –
5	Bronchial edema	+, –
6	Inflammatory cell influx	+, –
7	Inflammatory cell activation	+, –
8	Epithelial damage	–
9	Associated with increased i-ET levels/ET expression	++, –

+ = Stimulatory effect; – = no effect or inhibitory influence; equivocal information.
Adapted from Hay et al. [10].

Table 2. ET and the pathophysiology of COPD

	Features of COPD	ET
1	Mucus hypersecretion	+, –
2	Mucus gland hypertrophy	?
3	Cough	?
4	Airway smooth muscle hyperplasia/airways remodeling	+
5	Pulmonary vasoconstriction	+++
6	Pulmonary vascular remodeling	++
7	Inflammatory cell influx	+, –
8	Inflammatory cell activation	+, –
9	Increased bronchial tone	+++
10	Associated with increased i-ET levels/ET expression	+, –

+ = Stimulatory effect; – = no effect or inhibitory influence; equivocal information; ? = no information.

Mimicry of Features of Lung Diseases by Endothelin-1

ET-1 mimics several of the features of asthma, COPD, pulmonary hypertension and allergic rhinitis. However, some of the reported results are conflicting and/or high concentrations are required (tables 1, 2).

Asthma. ET-1 is one of the most potent contractile agonists in human isolated airway smooth muscle [3, 7, 11], producing contraction predominantly via stimulation of ET_B receptors [7], with a possible contribution from ET_A receptors [12]. Isolated bronchial smooth muscle from asthmatics had a lower sensitivity to ET-1 than tissues from nonasthmatics; it has been postulated that this may reflect chronic exposure to enhanced ET-1 release [7]. Aerosol administration of ET-1 produced bronchoconstriction in asthmatics, with minimal influence in nonasthmatic subjects, suggesting that asthmatic airways have an increased sensitivity to ET-1 in vivo [13].

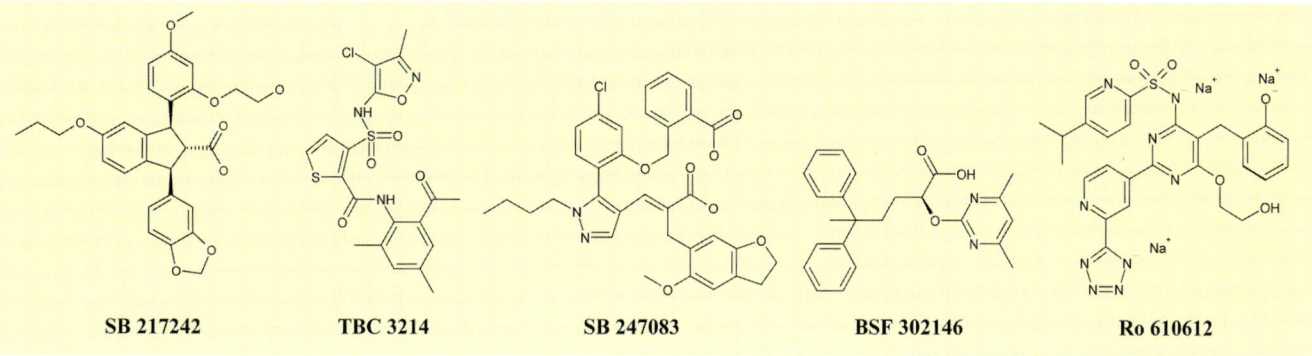

Fig. 2. Structures of ET receptor antagonists.

ET-1 potently potentiates the effects of a mitogen, epidermal growth factor, on proliferation in cultured human tracheal smooth muscle cells [14]. ET also induces proliferation of rat pulmonary artery fibroblasts, human alveolar fibroblasts and porcine tracheal epithelial cells [3].

There is conflicting evidence that ET-1 recruits and activates inflammatory cells proposed to play key roles in pulmonary disease [3]. In a mouse model of lung inflammation ET_A receptor antagonists inhibited antigen-induced influx of airway eosinophils and neutrophils [15].

ET ligands potentiated cholinergic nerve-induced responses in human bronchus, by prejunctional activation of ET_A and ET_B receptors [16]. There is equivocal evidence in animal models that ET-1 mimics other features of asthma including edema/microvascular permeability, mucus hypersecretion and AHR [3].

COPD and Pulmonary Hypertension. Pulmonary hypertension is a common potentially serious complication of COPD. ET-1 mimics the two classical features of pulmonary hypertension, namely pulmonary vasoconstriction and vascular remodeling, in human pulmonary vessels in vitro: the constriction of blood vessels occurs via ET_A and ET_B receptors [3, 10, 17], and mitogenesis of human pulmonary artery smooth muscle cells via activation of ET_A receptors [18]. Other effects of ET-1 of potential relevance to COPD include neutrophil and alveolar macrophage influx and activation, and enhancement of mucous secretion [3, 19].

Allergic Rhinitis. Immunoreactive ET (ir-ET) is present in the human nasal mucosa, including the vascular endothelium and submucosal glands [19]. ET-1 increased secretions from serous and mucous cells, and prostanoid release from human cultured nasal mucosa [4, 19]. Intranasal exposure to ET-1 increased nasal secretion weights, lysozyme secretion and symptoms of rhinorrhea, itch and sneezing in allergic and nonallergic volunteers [20]. The responses to ET-1 were greater in allergic subjects, suggesting enhanced sensitivity of the upper airways to ET-1 in allergic inflammation.

Levels of Endothelin-1 in Lung Disorders

Asthma. Increased expression and/or release of the ETs in subjects with asthma compared with asymptomatic asthmatic or nonasthmatic individuals has been demonstrated in several studies [3, 21]. The major source of ET-1 is probably the airway epithelium [21]. However, other studies revealed similar concentrations of ET-1 in peripheral blood, or in induced sputum samples of asthmatics and control individuals [22]. There is conflicting information about a correlation between the amounts of ET and disease severity. Therapies for asthma attenuate elevated airway ET levels, concomitant with improvements in lung function [3].

COPD and Pulmonary Hypertension. There is equivocal information regarding elevations in ET levels in COPD patients, although an increase in sputum samples has been reported [23], particularly in association with COPD exacerbation [24]. Enhanced plasma ET levels in patients with pulmonary hypertension have been described in many reports [3].

Allergic Rhinitis. An increase in expression of ir-ET, and also ir-ECE-1, in patients with chronic rhinitis was reported [4].

Therapeutic Benefit in Lung Diseases of Drugs Which Block the Release or Effects of Endothelins

A number of endothelin antagonists are presently in development for several indications, including cardiovascular, cerebrovascular and renal diseases. Clinical studies in man have confirmed a role for endothelin in maintaining vascular tone and demonstrated progressive vasodilation in forearm blood flow [25]. Furthermore, bosentan, a mixed ET_A/ET_B receptor antagonist, lowered pulmonary artery pressure and vascular resistance and increased cardiac index in patients with cardiac failure [26]. ET receptor antagonists have efficacy in animal models of asthma, airway inflammation and pulmonary hypertension [3, 14]. However, there is no published information on the clinical effects of ET receptor antagonists, or ECE inhibitors, in lung disease. Several potent and selective ET receptor antagonists have been identified and hopefully some will be evaluated clinically in pulmonary disease. A key question relates to what is the optimal pharmacological profile with respect to the receptor subtype, and whether this depends upon the specific disease: ET_A receptor-selective, ET_B receptor-selective or a mixed ET_A/ET_B receptor antagonist?

Conclusions

There is accumulating scientific rationale that ET-1 is a pathophysiologically relevant mediator in lung diseases, with several of the criteria required for a relevant mediator in asthma, pulmonary hypertension and allergic rhinitis being fulfilled for ET-1. Thus, ET-1 and its receptors are present in abundance in human lung, ET-1 mimics several of the features of asthma, COPD, pulmonary hypertension and allergic rhinitis, and enhanced levels or expression of ET are detected in these diseases. A significant caveat is that some of the information is preliminary, and, with respect to some parameters, equivocal. Clarification of the true pathophysiological influence of ET-1 in the lung awaits the results of clinical trials with potent and selective ET receptor antagonists in various pulmonary diseases.

References

1 Masaki T, Yanagisawa M, Goto K: Physiology and pharmacology of endothelins. Med Res Rev 1992;12:391–421.
2 Pons F, Touvay C, Lagente V, Mencia-Huerta JM, Braquet P: Involvement of a phosphoramidon-sensitive endopeptidase in the processing of big endothelin-1 in the guinea-pig. Eur J Pharmacol 1992;217:65–70.
3 Goldie RG, Knott PG, Carr MJ, Hay DWP, Henry PJ: The endothelins in the pulmonary system. Pulm Pharmacol 1996;9:69–93.
4 Furukawa K, Saleh D, Bayan F, Emoto N, Kaw S, Yanagiswaw M, Giaid A: Co-expression of endothelin-1 and endothelin-converting enzyme-1 in patients with chronic rhinitis. Am J Respir Cell Mol Biol 1996;14:248–253.
5 Giaid A, Polak JM, Gaitonde V, Hamid QA, Moscoso G, Legon S, Uwanogho D, Roncalli M, Shinmi O, Sawamura T, Kimura S, Yanagisawa M, Masaki T, Springall DR: Distribution of endothelin-like immmunoreactivity and mRNA in the developing and adult human lung. Am J Respir Cell Mol Biol 1991;4:50–58.
6 Hay DWP: Guinea-pig tracheal epithelium and endothelin. Eur J Pharmacol 1989;171:241–245.
7 Goldie RG, Henry PJ, Knott PG, Self GJ, Luttmann MA, Hay DWP: Endothelin-1 receptor density, distribution and function in human isolated asthmatic airways. Am J Respir Crit Care Med 1995;152:1653–1658.
8 Knott PG, D'Aprile AC, Henry PJ, Hay DWP, Goldie RG: Receptors for endothelin-1 in asthmatic human peripheral lung. Br J Pharmacol 1995;114:1–3.
9 Möller S, Uddman R, Granström B, Edvinsson L: Altered ratio of endothelin ET_A- and ET_B receptor mRNA in bronchial biopsies from patients with asthma and chronic airway obstruction. Eur J Pharmacol 1999;365:R1–R3.
10 Hay DWP, Henry P, Goldie RG: Endothelin and the respiratory system. Trends Pharmacol Sci 1993;14:29–32.
11 Brink C, Gillard V, Roubert P, Mencia-Huerta JM, Chabrier PE, Braquet P, Verley J: Effects and specific binding sites of endothelin in human lung preparations. Pulm Pharmacol 1991; 4:54–59.
12 Fukuroda T, Ozaki S, Ihara M, Ishikawa K, Yano M, Miyauchi T, Ishikawa S, Onizuka M, Goto K, Nishikibe M: Necessity of dual blockade of endothelin ET_A and ET_B receptor subtypes for antagonism of endothelin-1-induced contraction in human bronchus. Br J Pharmacol 1996;117:995–999.
13 Chalmers GW, Little SA, Patel KR, Thompson NC: Endothelin-1-induced bronchoconstriction in asthma. Am J Respir Crit Care Med 1997;156:382–388.
14 Panettieri RA, Jr, Goldie RG, Rigby PJ, Eszterhas AJ, Hay DWP: Endothelin-1-induced potentiation: an ET_A receptor-mediated phenomenon. Br J Pharmacol 1996;118:191–197.
15 Fujitani Y, Trifilieff A, Tsuyuki S, Coyle AJ, Bertrand C: Endothelin receptor antagonists inhibit antigen-induced lung inflammation in mice. Am J Respir Crit Care Med 1997;155: 1890–1894.
16 Fernandes LB, Henry PJ, Rigby PJ, Goldie RG: Endothelin$_B$ (ET_B) receptor-activated potentiation of cholinergic nerve-mediated contraction in human bronchus. Br J Pharmacol 1996;118:1873–1874.
17 McCulloch KM, Docherty CC, Morecroft I, MacLean MR: Endothelin$_B$ receptor-mediated contraction in human pulmonary resistance arteries. Br J Pharmacol 1996;119:1125–1130.
18 Zamora MA, Dempsey EC, Walchak SJ, Stelzner TJ: BQ213, an ET_A receptor antagonist, inhibits endothelin-1-mediated proliferation of human pulmonary artery smooth muscle cells. Am J Respir Cell Mol Biol 1993;9: 429–433.
19 Mullol J, Chowdhury BA, White MV, Ohkubo K, Rieves RD, Baraniuk J, Hausfeld JN, Shelhamer JH, Kaliner MA: Endothelin in human nasal mucosa. Am J Respir Cell Mol Biol 1993; 8:393–402.
20 Riccio MA, Reynolds CJ, Hay DWP, Proud D: Effects of intranasal administration of endothelin-1 to allergic and nonallergic individuals. Am J Respir Crit Care Med 1995;152:1757–1764.
21 Springall DR, Howarth PH, Counihan H, Djukanovic R, Holgate ST, Polak JM: Endothelin immunoreactivity of airway epithelium in asthmatic patients. Lancet 1991;337:697–701.
22 Chalmers GW, Thomson L, Macleod KJ, Dagg KD, McGinn BJ, McCharry C, Patel KR, Thomson NC: Endothelin-1 levels in induced sputum samples from asthmatic and normal subjects. Thorax 1997;52:625–627.
23 Chalmers GW, Macleod KJ, Sriram S, Thomson LJ, McSharry C, Stack BHR, Thomson NC: Sputum endothelin-1 is increased in cystic fibrosis and chronic obstructive pulmonary disease. Eur Respir J 1999;13:1288–1292.
24 Roland MA, Bhowmik A, Sapford RJ, Seemungal T, Warner T, Wedzicha JA: Endothelin-1 at COPD exacerbation. Am J Respir Crit Care Med 2000;161:A245.
25 Haynes WG, Webb DJ: Contribution of endogenous generation of endothelin-1 to basal vascular tone. Lancet 1994;344:852–854
26 Kiowski W, Sutch G, Huniziker P, Muller P, Kim J, Oechslin E, Schmitt R, Jones R, Bertel O: Evidence for endothelin-1 mediated vasoconstriction in severe chronic heart failure. Lancet 1995;346:732–736.

Douglas W.P. Hay, PhD, Group Director
Department of Pulmonary Biology, UW2532
SmithKline Beecham Pharmaceuticals
709 Swedeland Road
King of Prussia, PA 19406 (USA)
Tel. +1 610 270 6839, Fax +1 610 270 5381
E-Mail douglas_w_hay@sbphrd.com

Tachykinin Antagonists

Douglas W.P. Hay

Department of Pulmonary Biology, SmithKline Beecham Pharmaceuticals, King of Prussia, Pa., USA

Summary

The tachykinins are a family of small neurotransmitter peptides – main members are substance P (SP), neurokinin A (NKA) and neurokinin B (NKB) – found in the central and peripheral nervous systems. The major location of the tachykinins in the periphery are the unmyelinated sensory C fibres, although non-neuronal sites exist. The biological effects of the tachykinins are mediated via three receptors, NK-1, NK-2 and NK-3, which belong to the superfamily of G-protein-coupled, seven-transmembrane-spanning receptors. The tachykinins, SP and NKA, and the three tachykinin receptors are found in human lung; levels of the tachykinins are elevated in asthma and COPD. The tachykinins produce multiple effects in the lung which may be relevant to pathophysiological influences, and they play a pivotal role in neurogenic inflammation. Potent and selective antagonists of the three tachykinin receptors have been identified and comprehensive investigation of the clinical effects of some of these compounds will clarify the roles of the tachykinins and the individual tachykinin receptors in pulmonary disease.

Table 1. Some milestones in tachykinin research

Year	Milestone
1931	SP discovered [1]
1971	Purification and chemical characterization of SP [2]
1983	NKA and NKB isolated [3]
1987	Bovine NK-2R cloned [4]
1990	Human NK-2R cloned [5]
1991	Human NK-1R cloned [7]
	First potent and selective non-peptide antagonist (NK-1R antagonist) identified (CP-96,345) [7]
1992	First potent and selective non-peptide NK-2R antagonist identified, SR 48,968 [8]
	Human NK-3R cloned [9]
1995	First potent and selective non-peptide NK-3R antagonist identified, SR 142,801 [10]

Tachykinin research began in 1931 with the pioneer work by Von Euler and Gaddum [1], who extracted from equine brain and intestine a novel substance, named substance P (from 'Preparation'; SP), which produced hypotension and contraction of smooth muscle tissues. The peptide nature of SP was demonstrated 5 years later, but it was not until 1971 that it was purified and characterized chemically [2]. This key finding led to an explosion in research on SP and related peptides; some milestones are highlighted in table 1. SP was shown subsequently to be a member of a family of peptides which share the common C-terminal sequence, Phe-X-Gly-Leu-Met-NH$_2$; the other main mammalian tachykinins are NKA and NKB [11, 12] (fig. 1). Despite extensive research and significant evidence for potential pathophysiological roles of tachykinins in many diseases, including lung disorders, concomitant with the identification of numerous potent and selective tachykinin research antagonists, the first tachykinin-based therapeutic has yet to be introduced.

Synthesis, Distribution and Metabolism of Tachykinins in the Lung

SP and NKA, on the one hand, and NKB, on the other, are produced from distinct precursor genes: preprotachykinin-I (PPT-I or PPT-A) and preprotachykinin-II (PPT-II or PPT-B), respectively [11, 12] (fig. 1). Alternative RNA splicing produces four precursors, α-PPT-I, β-PPT-I, γ-PPT-I and δ-PPT-I, from PPT-I, and two from PPT-

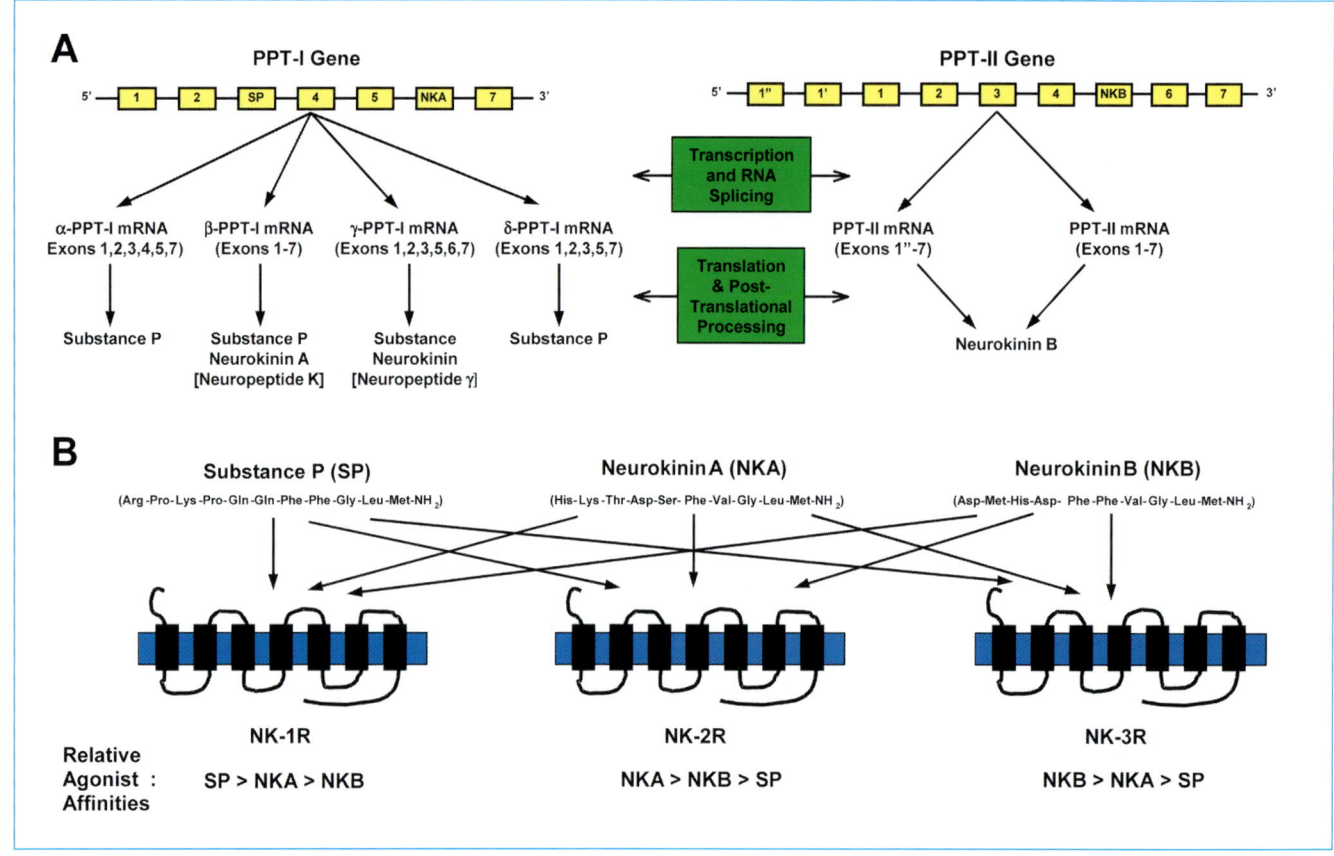

Fig. 1. Synthetic pathway for the tachykinins (**A**) and tachykinin interactions with the tachykinin receptors (**B**).

II. The major distribution of the tachykinins in the peripheral nervous system is in capsaicin-sensitive, primary afferent neurons (unmyelinated sensory C fibres) that are found extensively in several sites, including the lung [11, 12]. The tachykinins play a critical role in the classical neurogenic inflammation. Non-neuronal sites for the tachykinins include the endothelium, dendritic cells and some inflammatory cells (e.g., eosinophils, lymphocytes, neutrophils and macrophages) which are thought to play a role in asthma and/or COPD [11, 12]. In mammalian lung, including human, SP-containing nerves are located below and within epithelium, associated with submucosal glands, bronchial blood vessels, airway smooth muscle and ganglion cells [11, 12]. SP and NKA, but not NKB, are detected in significant quantities in mammalian lung; in human lung, the number of tachykinin-containing neurones is significantly sparser than in other species, e.g., the guinea pig. The tachykinins are metabolized predominantly via the membrane-bound neutral endopeptidase (EC 3.4.24.11) [11, 12].

Tachykinin Receptors in the Lung

The biological effects of the tachykinins are mediated via three receptors, NK-1R, NK-2R and NK-3R, which belong to the superfamily of G-protein-coupled, seven transmembrane spanning receptors (fig. 1) [13]. There are differences in the affinities of the natural ligands for the three tachykinin receptors: SP has the highest affinity for NK-1R (SP > NKA > NKB), NKA has highest affinity for the NK-2R (NKA > NKB > SP) and NKB has the highest affinity for the NK-3R (NKB > NKA > SP) [13]. However, a critical point is that SP, NKA and NKB interact potently with and are full agonists at all three receptors (fig. 1). The NK-1, NK-2 and NK-3 receptors are present in mammalian lung. The bovine NK-2R was the first tachykinin receptor cloned (in 1987) and subsequently all three human receptors have been cloned and expressed (table 1), and utilized for the identification of antagonists [13]. Since the report of the first non-peptide tachykinin receptor, CP-96,345 – an NK-1R antagonist – in 1991 [6], many potent and selective antagonists for the NK-1,

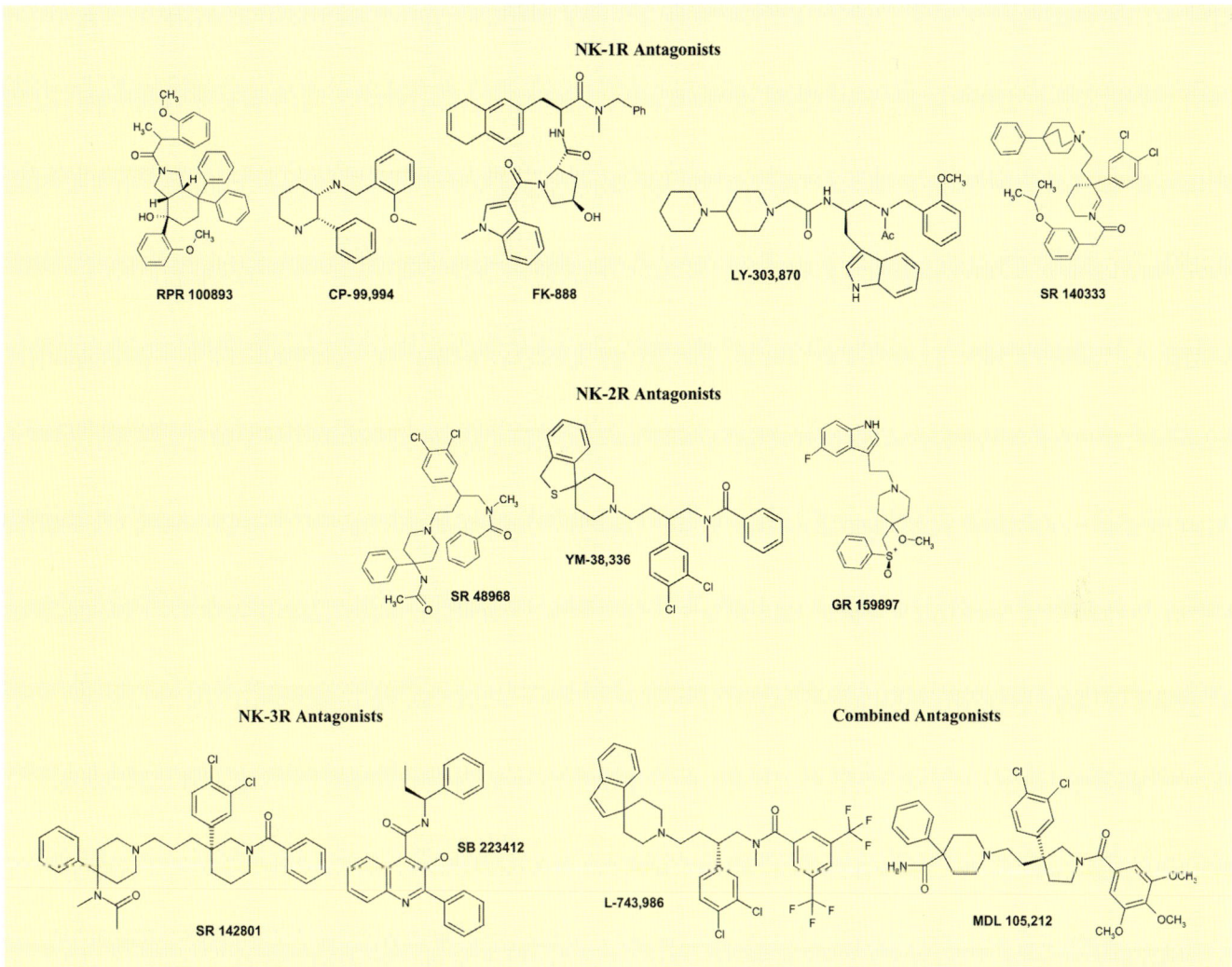

Fig. 2. Structures of representative tachykinin receptor antagonists [5–8].

NK-2 and NK-3 receptors, in addition to compounds which potently interact with more than one receptor, have been identified [13–15] (fig. 2).

Mimicry of Features of Lung Diseases by Tachykinins

The biological effects of the tachykinins and their receptors in the lung have been examined in many in vitro and in vivo systems using the natural ligands, SP, NKA and NKB, and selective antagonists and agonists for the three tachykinin receptors (tables 2, 3).

NK-1R. There is considerable evidence that NK-1R activation mediates enhanced microvascular permeability and associated plasma leakage in the lung, and pulmonary vascular vasodilatation [11, 12, 16]. SP, and selective NK-1R agonists, stimulate mucus secretion in human and animal airways; however, the effects of NK-1R antagonists have not been explored [12, 17]. Although selective NK-1R agonists have been demonstrated to potentiate cholinergic neurotransmission in rabbit and guinea pig airways, this phenomenon has not been demonstrated in human bronchus [18]. Several studies have reported that SP activates, via receptor-dependent and receptor-independent mechanisms, many inflammatory cells thought to be important in the pathophysiology of pulmonary diseases, including macrophages, T cells and leukocytes; for several of these effects, the specific tachykinin receptor responsible remains to be determined

Table 2. Tachykinins and their receptors and the pathophysiology of asthma

	Features of asthma	Influence of tachykinins	Receptor(s) involved
1	Increased bronchial tone	+++	NK-2 and NK-1
2	Airway smooth muscle hyperplasia/ airway remodelling	+	NK-1?
3	Mucus hypersecretion	++	NK-1?
4	Airway hyperresponsiveness	+, –	NK-2 and NK-3
5	Bronchial oedema and microvascular permeability	+, –	NK-1 and NK-2
6	Inflammatory cell influx	++	NK-1
7	Inflammatory cell activation	+, –	NK-1 and NK-2
8	Neuronal dysfunction	++	NK-3 and NK-2
9	Associated with increased tachykinin levels/expression	+, –	NA

+ = Stimulatory effect; – = no effect, inhibitory influence or equivocal information; NA = not applicable.

Table 3. Tachykinins and their receptors and the pathophysiology of COPD

	Features of COPD	Influence of tachykinins	Receptor(s) involved
1	Mucus hypersecretion	++	NK-1?
2	Mucus gland hypertrophy	?	?
3	Cough	++	NK-2, NK-3 and NK-1
4	Airway smooth muscle hyperplasia/ airways remodelling	+	NK-1?
5	Pulmonary vasoconstriction	–	NK-1 a
6	Pulmonary vascular remodelling	?	?
7	Inflammatory cell influx	++	NK-1
8	Inflammatory cell activation	+, –	NK-1 and NK-2
9	Increased bronchial tone	++	NK-2 and NK-1
10	Neuronal dysfunction	++	NK-3 and NK-2
11	Associated with increased tachykinin levels/tachykinin expression	+, –	NA

+ = Stimulatory effect; – = no effect, inhibitory influence or equivocal information; ? = unknown. NA = not applicable.
a Vasodilatation produced.

[11, 12, 19]. The NK-1R mediates, in part, tachykinin-induced contraction in human small airways in vitro [20] and may contribute to citric acid-induced cough in guinea pigs [21] (tables 2, 3).

NK-2R. The most recognized effect of the NK-2R is mediation of tachykinin-induced contraction of mammalian airways, including humans [20]. NKA-induced bronchoconstriction in humans in vivo is blocked by the NK-2R antagonist, SR 48948 [22]. Although, SR 48968 inhibited AHR in guinea pigs, suggesting a role for NK-2Rs in this feature of lung disease, aerosol administration of NKA did not produce AHR to methacholine in non-asthmatic or asthmatic individuals [23]. The NK-2R potentiates cholinergic neurotransmission in isolated airways of some species, but not humans [18]. This receptor is also involved in citric acid-induced cough in guinea pigs [21]. Other reported effects of NK-2R activation include NO release from airway epithelium, histamine release, activation of immune and inflammatory cells and enhanced plasma leakage [12, 13, 19] (tables 2, 3).

NK-3R. Molecular biological studies have provided conflicting information regarding the presence of the NK-3R in human lung. Electrophysiological and pharmacological analysis has provided compelling evidence that this receptor is present in guinea pig bronchial parasympathetic ganglia [24]. At this strategic location, the NK-3R has the potential to modulate neuronal inputs to several end-organs, and thus to exert a significant effect on pulmonary function. NKB- and NK-3R-selective agonists induce, whereas NK-3R antagonists inhibit, AHR in the guinea pig [25]. Furthermore, the NK-3R antagonist, SR 142,801, is effective in the citric-acid-induced cough model in guinea pigs [26]. To date, there is no evidence for effects of NK-3R activation in the lung other than modulation of neuronal inputs. Confirmation of the neuromodulatory role of the NK-3R in human airways will be important (tables 2, 3).

Levels of Tachykinins and Tachykinin Receptor Expression in Lung Disorders

Asthma. There is conflicting information on whether there is an increase in SP-containing nerves in the lungs of asthmatics versus non-asthmatics [27, 28]. The amount of immunoreactive SP and NK-1R expression was reported to be the same in lung samples of asthmatic and non-asthmatic individuals [27, 29]. In contrast, there was a 4-fold increase in NK-2R mRNA expression airways of in asthmatics versus non-smoking controls [29]. In another study treatment with corticosteroids attenuated the marked increase in NK-1R mRNA observed in the submucosa and epithelium of asthmatic individuals compared to controls [30]. In addition, elevated amounts of SP have been reported in the sputum and BAL fluid of asthmatic versus control individuals [27, 31].

COPD. In contrast to asthma, there was a decrease in NK-1R mRNA in human lung samples from patients with COPD compared to those from smokers with normal lung function; in the latter group there was a two-fold increase in NK-1R message levels compared to non-smoking con-

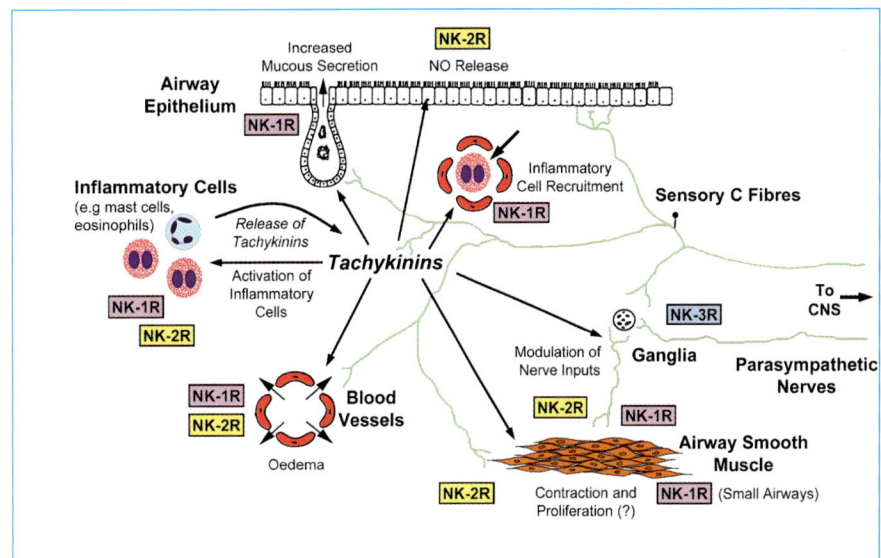

Fig. 3. Cartoon of the effects of the tachykinins and their receptors in the lung.

trols [29]. SP levels were about 20-fold higher in patients with chronic bronchitis than control subjects [31], although the number of tachykinin-containing nerves – assessed from endobronchial biopsies – was reported to be the same in these groups [28].

Therapeutic Benefit of Tachykinin Receptor Antagonists in Lung Diseases

There is minimal information on the clinical effects of tachykinin receptor antagonists in the pulmonary system, and additional studies, especially in the native disease populations, are required. SR 48,968, the NK-2R antagonist, attenuates NKA-induced bronchoconstriction in humans [22]. In a small study, FK244, a cyclic peptide NK-1R/NK-2R antagonist, given via metered-dose inhaler (4 mg), attenuated bradykinin-induced bronchoconstriction and cough in 9 asthmatics [20, 27]. However, in other studies in asthmatics, the compound was without effect on baseline pulmonary function, did not inhibit NKA-induced bronchoconstriction, and when given for 4 weeks (4 mg, q.i.d., by metered-dose inhaler) was without effect on asthma symptoms or pulmonary function [20, 27]. The NK-1R antagonist, CP-99,994 did not inhibit hypertonic-saline-induced bronchoconstriction in patients with mild asthma [20, 27]. Extensive work has been performed preclinically evaluating the effects of antagonists in different animal models of lung disease. Efficacy has been demonstrated in many systems – including animal models of bronchoconstriction (mediated via NK-2R with lesser contribution from NK-1R in some models), including that induced by antigen, sulphur dioxide, cold air and hyperpnea (a model of exercise-induced asthma), microvascular leakage (NK-1R and NK-2R), airway hyperresponsiveness (NK-2R and NK-3R), inflammatory cell recruitment (NK-1R) and cough (NK-1R, NK-2R and NK-3R) [5, 13, 20, 25].

Conclusions

Since the discovery of SP by Von Euler and Gaddum in 1931, many significant advances have been made in the tachykinin research area, including the demonstration of additional members of the tachykinin family, the identification of the NK-1, NK-2 and NK-3 receptors, which mediate the diverse biological actions of the tachykinins, and the discovery of potent and selective antagonists for the three tachykinin receptors. Using the latter tool compounds, in addition to tachykinin agonists (non-selective and selective), a wealth of preclinical information regarding the potential involvement of the NK-1R and NK-2R, and to a lesser extent the NK-3R, in the pathophysiology of asthma and COPD has been obtained (fig. 3). Overall, based upon the multiple effects of activation of the NK-1R, NK-2R and NK-3R, an optimally effective therapeutic strategy for pulmonary disease may require the utilization of antagonists which block more than one tachykinin receptor, rather than a selective NK-1R, NK-2R or NK-3R antagonist. Clarification of this key issue and whether the tachykinins play an important role in the pathophysiology of lung disease, including asthma or COPD awaits extensive clinical evaluation with appropriate compounds.

References

1 Von Euler US T, Gaddum JH: An unidentified depressor substance in certain tissue extracts. J Physiol (Lond) 1931;12:391–421.
2 Chang, MM, Leeman SE, Niall HD: Aminoacid sequence of substance P. Nature New Biol 1971;232:86–87.
3 Kimura S, Okada M, Sugita Y, Kanazawa I, Munekata E: Novel neuropeptides, neurokinin α and β, isolated from porcine spinal cord. Proc Jap Acad 1983;59B:101–104.
4 Masu Y, Nakayama K, Tamaki H, Harada Y, Kuno M, and Nakanishi S: cDNA cloning of bovine substance-K receptor through oocyte expression system. Nature 1987;329:836–838.
5 Gerard NP, Eddy RL Jr, Shows TB, Gerard C: The human neurokinin A (substance K) receptor: Molecular cloning of the gene, chromosome localization, and isolation of cDNA from tracheal and gastric tissues. J Biol Chem 1990;265:20455–20462.
6 Hopkins B, Powell S, Danks P, Briggs I, Graham A: Isolation and characterisation of the human lung NK-1 receptor cDNA. Biochem Biophys Res Commun 1991;180:1110–1117.
7 Snider RM, Constantine JW, Lowe III JA, Longo KP, Lebel WS, Woody HA, Drozda SE, Desai MC, Vinick FJ, Spencer RW, Hess HJ: A potent nonpeptide antagonist of the substance P (NK1) receptor. Science 1991;251:435–437.
8 Emonds-Alt X, Vilain P, Goulaouic P, Proietto V, Van Broeck D, Advenier C, Naline E, Neliat G, Le Fur G, Brelier JC: A potent and selective non-peptide antagonist of the neurokinin A (NK2) receptor. Life Sci 1992;50:101–106.
9 Buell G, Schulz MF, Arkinstall SJ, Maury K, Missotten M, Adami N, Talabot F, Kawashima E: Molecular characterisation, expression and localisation of human neurokinin-3 receptor. FEBS Lett 1992;299:90–95.
10 Emonds-Alt X, Bichon D, Ducoux JP, Heaulme M, Miloux B, Poncelet M, Proietto V, Van Broeck D, Vilain P, Neliat G, Soubrie P, Le Fur G, Brelier JC: SR 142801, the first potent non-peptide antagonist of the tackykinin NK3 receptor. Life Sci 1995;56:27–32.
11 Otsuka M, Yoshioka K: Neurotransmitter functions of mammalian tachykinins. Physiol Rev 1993;73:229–308.
12 Maggi CA, Giachetti A, Dey RD, Said SI: Neuropeptides as regulators of airway function: Vasoactive intestinal peptide and the tachykinins. Physiol Rev 1995;75:277–322.
13 Maggi CA: The mammalian tachykinin receptors. Gen Pharmacol 1995;25:911–944.
14 Giardina GAM, Raveglia LF, Grugni M, Sarau HM, Farina C, Medhurst AD, Graziani D, Schmidt DB, Rigolio R, Luttmann M, Cavagnera S, Foley JJ, Vecchietti V, Hay DWP: Discovery of a novel class of selective non-peptide antagonists for the human neurokinin-3 receptor. I. Identification of (S-N-(1-phenylpropyl)-3-hydroxy-2-phenylquinoline-carboxamide (SB 223412). J Med Chem 1998;42:1053–1065.
15 Leroy V, Mauser P, Gao Z, Peet NP: Neurokinin receptor antagonists. Exp Opinion Invest Drugs 2000;9:735–746.
16 Pedersen KE, Buckner CK, Meeker SN, Undem BJ: Pharmacological examination of the neurokinin-1 receptor mediating relaxation of human intralobar pulmonary artery. J Pharmacol Exp Ther 2000;292:319–325.
17 Meini S, Mak JCW, Rohde JAL, Rogers DF: Tachykinin control of ferret airways: Mucus secretion, bronchoconstriction and receptor mapping. Neuropeptides 1993;24:81–89.
18 Belvisi MG, Patacchini R, Barnes PJ, Maggi CA: Facilitatory effects of selective agonists for tachykinin receptors on cholinergic neurotransmission: Evidence for species differences. Br J Pharmacol 1994;111:103–110.
19 Maggi CA: The effects of tachykinins on inflammatory and immune cells. Regul Peptides 1997;70:75–90.
20 Advenier C, Joos G, Molimard M, Lagente V, Pauwels R: Role of tachykinins as contractile agonists of human airways in asthma. Clin Exp Allergy 1999;29:579–584.
21 Girard V, Naline E, Vilain P, Emonds-Alt X, Advenier C: Effect of the two tachykinin antagonists, SR 48968 and SR 140333, on cough induced by citric acid in the unanaesthetized guinea pig. Eur Respir J 1995;8:1110–1114.
22 Van Schoor J, Joos GF, Chasson BL, Brouard RJ, Pauwels RA: The effect of the NK2 tachykinin receptor antagonist SR 48968 (saredutant) on neurokinin A-induced bronchoconstriction in asthmatics. Eur Respir J 1998;12:17–23.
23 Cheung D, Timmers MC, Zwinderman AH, den Hartigh J, Dijkman JH, Sterk PJ: Neutral endopeptidase activity and airway hyperresponsiveness to neurokinin A in asthmatic subjects in vivo. Am Rev Respir Dis 1993;148:1467–1473.
24 Myers A, Undem B, Kummer W: Anatomical and electrophysiological comparison of the sensory innervation of bronchial and tracheal parasympathetic ganglion neurons. J Auton Nervous System 1996;61:162–168.
25 Daoui S, Naline E, Lagente V, Emonds-Alt X, Advenier C: Neurokinin B- and specific tachykinin NK_3 receptor agonists-induced airway hyperresponsiveness in guinea-pig. Br J Pharmacol 2000;130:49–56.
26 Daoui S, Cognon C, Naline E, Emonds-Alt X, Advenier C: Involvement of tachykinin NK3 receptors in citric acid-induced cough and responses in guinea pigs. Am J Respir Crit Care Med 1998;158:42–48.
27 Joos GF, Germonpré PR, Pauwels RA: Role of tachykinins in asthma Allergy 2000;55:321–337.
28 Chanez P, Springall D, Vignola AM, Moradoghi-Hattvani A, Polak JM, Godard P, Bousquet J: Bronchial mocosal immunoreactivity of sensory neuropeptides in severe airway diseases. Am J Respir Crit Care Med 1998;158:985–990.
29 Bai TR, Zhou D, Weir T, Walker B, Hegele R, Hayashi S, McKay K, Bondy GP, Fong T: Substance P (NK1)- and neurokinin A (NK2)- receptor gene expression in inflammatory airway diseases. Am J Physiol 1995;269:L309–L317.
30 Adcock IM: Increased tachykinin receptor gene expression in asthmatic lung and its modulation by steroids. J Mol Endocrinol 1993;11:1–7.
31 Tomaki M, Ichinose M, Miura M, Hirayama Y, Yamauchi H, Nakajima N, Shirato K: Elevated substance P content in induced sputum from patients with asthma and patients with chronic bronchitis. Am J Respir Crit Care Med 1995;151:613–617.
32 Wu Z-X, Lee L-Y: Airway hyperresponsiveness induced by chronic exposure to cigarette smoke in guinea pigs; role of tachykinins. J Appl Physiol 1999;87:1621–1628.

Douglas W.P. Hay, PhD, Group Director
Department of Pulmonary Biology, UW2532
SmithKline Beecham Pharmaceuticals
709 Swedeland Road
King of Prussia, PA 19406 (USA)
Tel. +1 610 270 6839, Fax +1 610 270 5381
E-Mail douglas_w_hay@sbphrd.com

Antioxidants

William MacNee

ELEGI Colt Research Laboratories, University of Edinburgh Medical School, Edinburgh, UK

Summary

The pathogenesis of COPD is closely linked to the effects of cigarette smoke. It has been proposed that an increased oxidant burden occurs in smokers and patients with COPD which produces an imbalance between oxidants and antioxidants. The oxidative stress so created in the lungs, is thought to have a role in the pathogenesis of COPD, both by direct injurious effects on lung cells and by enhancing lung inflammation. Antioxidant therapy may not only protect the lung against the injurious effects of oxidative stress but may have anti-inflammatory properties in COPD.

Oxidative Stress in the Airspaces

Since the lung epithelium is in direct contact with the environment, the airspace epithelial surface of the lung is particularly vulnerable to the effects of oxidative stress [1]. The respiratory tract lining fluids form an interface between the epithelial cells and the external environment and thus constitute the 'first line of defence' against inhaled oxidants [2].

Injury to the epithelium appears to be an important early event following exposure to cigarette smoke.

Increased epithelial permeability is present in chronic smokers compared with non-smokers and a further increase in epithelial permeability occurs following acute smoking, associated with changes in airspace antioxidants, specifically glutathione [3]. Thus cigarette smoke has a direct detrimental effect on airspace epithelial cell function.

The oxidant burden in lungs is further enhanced in smokers by the increased numbers of neutrophils (by 10-fold) and macrophages (by 2- to 4-fold) [4] in the alveolar space. Ex vitro studies have shown that the spontaneous release of reactive oxygen species from alveolar leukocytes in cigarette smokers is increased, compared to those from non-smokers [5, 6].

Oxidative Stress and Proteinase/Antiproteinase Imbalance

A 'functional α_1-AT deficiency' is thought to occur in smokers, as part of the pathogenesis of emphysema, due to inactivation of the α_1-AT by oxidation of the methionine residue at its active site [7] by oxidants in cigarette smoke and those released by leukocytes. However, there are conflicting data on whether α_1-AT lavage function lavage is decreased in cigarette smokers [8, 9].

Antioxidants in BAL Fluid

The major antioxidants in respiratory tract lining fluids include mucin, reduced glutathione, uric acid, protein (largely albumin) and ascorbic acid [10]. There is limited information on the respiratory epithelial antioxidant defences in smokers, and less in COPD. Studies have shown that GSH is elevated in BAL fluid in the airways of chronic but not acute smokers [3]. Despite the 2-fold increase in BAL fluid GSH in chronic smokers, GSH may not be present in sufficient quantities to deal with the

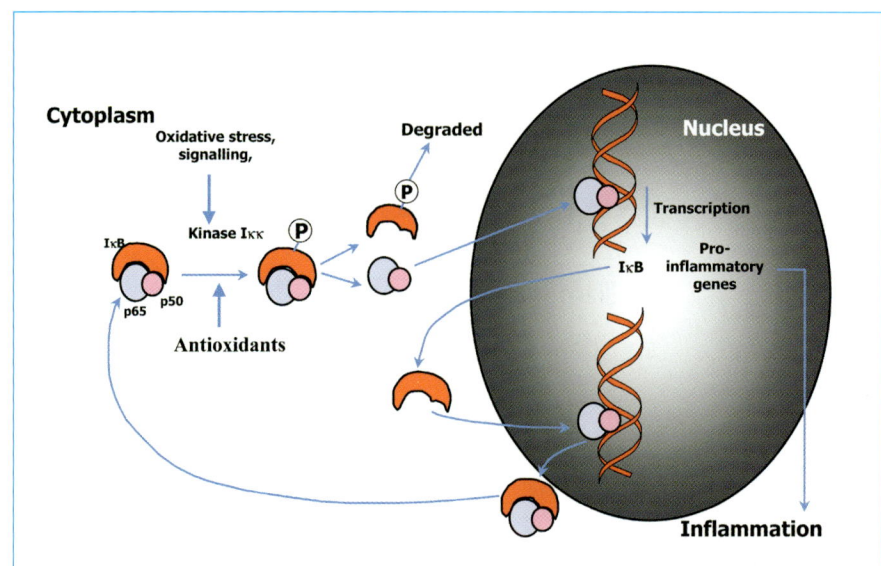

Fig. 1. Regulation of NF-κB-stimulated transcription. Iκκ = Iκ-β kinase.

excessive oxidant burden during acute smoking when acute depletion of GSH may occur.

Reduced levels of vitamin E are found in the BAL fluid of smokers compared with non-smokers [11]. By contrast, a marginal increase in vitamin C is present in BAL fluid of smokers, compared to non-smokers [12]. The apparent discrepancies between these studies of the levels of the different antioxidants in BAL fluid may be due to different smoking histories in chronic smokers, particularly the time of the last cigarette in relation to the sampling of BAL fluid.

Evidence of Systemic Oxidative Stress

There has recently been considerable interest in the systemic effects of COPD. One manifestation of such effects is the presence of markers of oxidative stress in the blood in patients with COPD.

Increased production of superoxide anion occurs from peripheral blood neutrophils obtained from patients with acute exacerbations of COPD, which returns to normal when the patients are clinically stable [13]. Polyunsaturated fats and fatty acids in cell membranes are a major target of free-radical attack, resulting in lipid peroxidation, a process that may continue as a chain reaction to generate peroxides and aldehydes. Products of lipid peroxidation reactions can be measured in body fluids as thiobarbituric acid reactive substances (TBARS). The levels of TBARS in plasma or in BAL fluid are significantly increased in healthy smokers and patients with acute exacerbations of COPD, compared with healthy non-smokers [13, 14].

Urine and plasma isoprostane $F_2\alpha$-III, which is an isomer of prostaglandin, formed by free-radical peroxidation of arachidonic acid, has been shown to be elevated in patients with COPD, compared with healthy controls, and to be even more elevated in exacerbations of this condition [15, 16]. A further manifestation of systemic oxidative stress is the decreased plasma antioxidant capacity which occurs during smoking and in exacerbations of COPD [17].

Oxidative Stress and Gene Expression

There is overwhelming evidence that COPD is associated with airway and airspace inflammation, as shown by recent bronchial biopsy studies [18]. Numerous mediators of inflammation have been shown to be elevated in the sputum of patients with COPD, including IL-8 and TNF-α [19].

Genes for many inflammatory mediators, such as the cytokines, IL-8, TNF-α, and NO are regulated by transcription factors such as NF-κB. NF-κB is present in the cytosol in an inactive form linked to its inhibitory protein IκB. Many stimuli, including cytokines and oxidants, activate NF-κB, resulting in ubiquination cleaving of IκB from NF-κB and the destruction of IκB in the proteozome [20]. This critical event in the inflammatory response is redox sensitive (fig. 1).

Thiol antioxidants, such as N-acetylcysteine and nacystelin, which have potential as therapies in COPD, have been shown in in vitro experiments to block the release of these inflammatory mediators from epithelial cells and macrophages, by a mechanism involving increasing intracellular glutathione and decreasing NF-κB.

Therapeutic Options for Redressing the Oxidant/Antioxidant Imbalance in COPD

Having demonstrated the presence of an oxidant/antioxidant imbalance in smokers and its proposed role in the pathogenesis of COPD do we have any therapeutic options?

Anti-Inflammatories. One approach would be to target the inflammatory response by reducing the sequestration or migration of leukocytes from the pulmonary circulation into the airspaces. Possible therapeutic options for this are drugs that alter cell deformability, so preventing the initial sequestration of neutrophils or the migration of neutrophils into the lungs, either by interfering with adhesion molecules necessary for migration, or preventing the release of inflammatory cytokines, such as IL-8 or LTB_4 which result in increased neutrophil chemotaxis and migration. It should also be possible to use anti-inflammatory agents to prevent the release of oxygen radicals from activated leukocytes or to quench those oxidants once they are formed, by enhancing the antioxidant screen in the lungs. Downregulating neutrophil function including the release of reactive oxygen species may be part of the anti-inflammatory effect of PDE_4 inhibitors [21].

Enhancing Lung Antioxidants. There are various options to enhance the lung antioxidant screen. One approach is the molecular manipulation of antioxidant genes, such as glutathione peroxidase or genes involved in the synthesis of glutathione, such as γ-glutamylcysteine synthetase.

Another approach would simply be to administer antioxidant therapy or by developing molecules with activity similar to those of antioxidant enzymes, such as catalase and superoxide dismutase. This has been attempted in cigarette smokers using various antioxidants. The results have been rather disappointing, although vitamin E has been shown to reduce oxidative stress in patients with COPD [22]. Attempts to supplement lung glutathione have been tried using glutathione or its precursors [23]. Glutathione itself is not efficiently transported into most animal cells and an excess of glutathione may be a source of the thiyl radical under conditions of oxidative stress. Nebulized glutathione has also been used therapeutically but this has been shown to induce bronchial hyperreactivity [24]. Cysteine is a thiol that is the rate-limiting amino acid in GSH synthesis. Cysteine administration is not possible since it is oxidized to cystine that is neurotoxic. The cysteine-donating compound N-acetylcysteine (NAC) acts as a cellular precursor of GSH and becomes de-acetylated in the gut to cysteine following oral administration. It reduces disulphide bonds and has the potential to interact directly with oxidants. The use of NAC in an attempt to enhance GSH in patients with COPD has met with varying success [25, 26]. NAC given orally in low doses of 600 mg per day to normal subjects results in very low levels of NAC in the plasma for up to 2 h after administration [25]. Bridgeman et al. [26] showed after 5 days of NAC 600 mg 3 times daily, that there was a significant increase in plasma GSH levels. However, there was no associated significant rise in BAL fluid GSH or in lung tissue. These data seem to imply that producing a sustained increase in lung GSH is difficult using NAC in subjects who are not already depleted of glutathione. In spite of this, continental European studies have shown that NAC reduces the number of exacerbation days in patients with COPD [27]. This was not confirmed in a British Thoracic Society study of NAC [28]. The contradictory results of these studies may result from several reasons: firstly, the positive studies of NAC were in patients who had relatively mild COPD, whereas in the British Study the patients had more severe COPD. Secondly, a relatively small dose of NAC was given in both studies. However, a recent meta-analysis of studies of NAC in exacerbations of COPD suggests in general favourable effects on exacerbation rates and symptoms [29].

Nacystelyn (NAL) is a lysine salt of NAC. It is also a mucolytic and oxidant thiol compound which, in contrast to NAC which is acid, has a neutral pH. NAL can be aerosolized into the lung without causing significant side effects. Studies comparing the effects of NAL and NAC found that both drugs enhanced intracellular glutathione in alveolar epithelial cells and inhibited hydrogen peroxide and superoxide anion release from neutrophils harvested from peripheral blood from smokers and patients with COPD [30]. There are no studies, as yet, of NAL in COPD.

Oxidative stress is thought to be a fundamental process in inflammation through the activation of transcription factors for genes for many pro-inflammatory mediators. Antioxidant treatment, by downregulating these processes, may have an anti-inflammatory effect in addition to a direct protective effect against oxidant-mediated injury. Support for this hypothesis comes from studies in smoke-exposed animals, a relevant model for COPD [31]. In these studies, the administration of the potent antioxidant recombinant superoxide dismutase to the airspaces was shown to abolish the influx of neutrophils into the airspaces, prevent smoke-induced IL-8 gene expression and release in the lungs and affect the fundamental inflammatory events by decreasing smoke-induced NF-

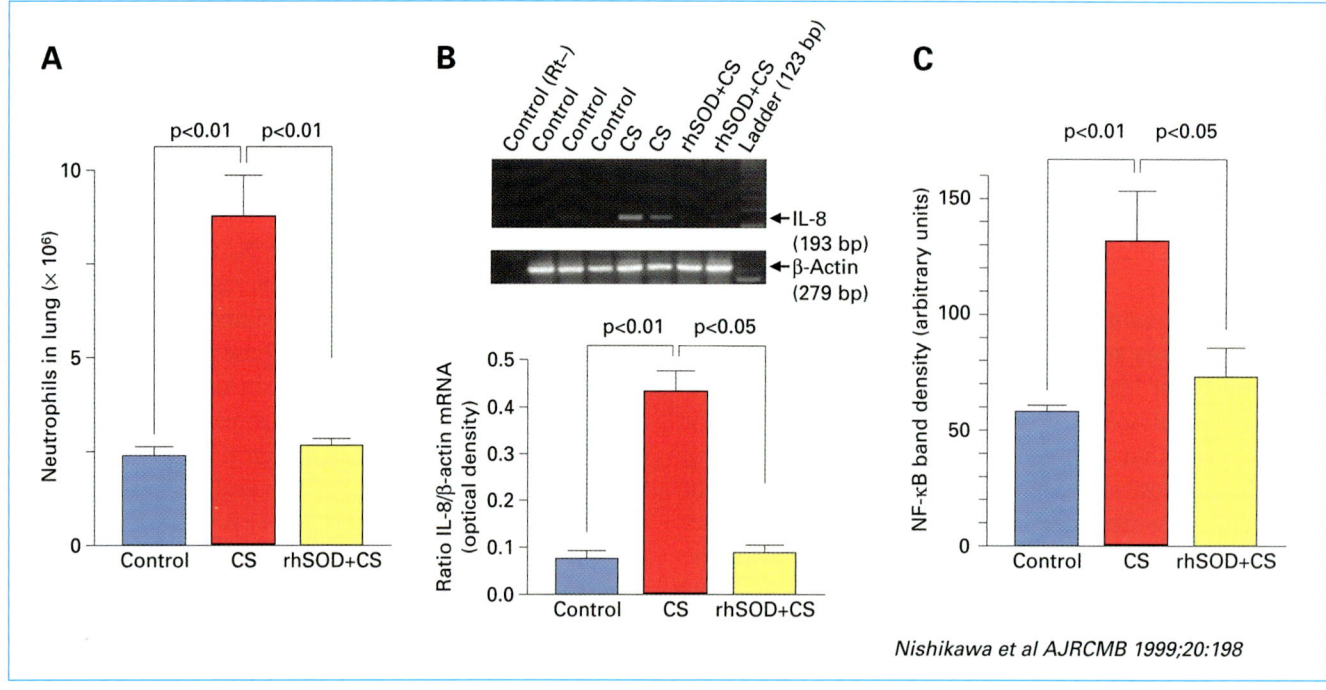

Fig. 2. Effect of recombinant superoxide dismutase (rhSOD) on cigarette-induced neutrophil influx into the lungs (**A**), IL-8 gene expression in lungs (**B**) and NF-κB nuclear binding (**C**) in guinea pig lungs. CS = Cigarette smoke. From Nishikawa et al. [31].

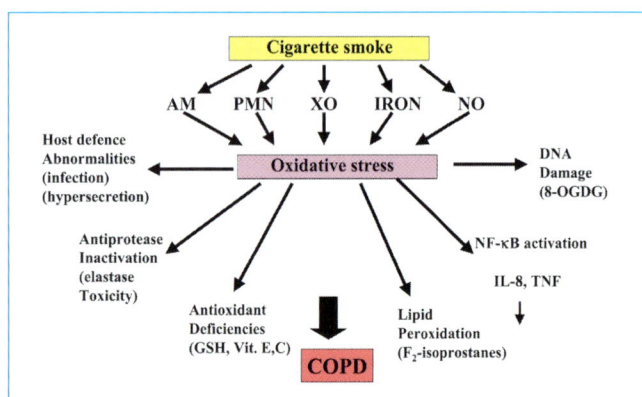

Fig. 3. Causes of cigarette-smoke-induced oxidative stress and its consequences in relation to the pathogenesis of COPD. AM = Alveolar macrophage; XO = xanthine oxidase; 8-OGDG = 8-oxyguanidine-deoxy-guanidine.

κB nuclear binding in the lungs (fig. 2). Molecules with potent antioxidant enzyme properties are being produced and if they have good bioavailability may allow proof of the cept that antioxidant therapy may have important anti-inflammatory effects in COPD.

In conclusion, there is now very good evidence for an oxidant/antioxidant imbalance in COPD and increasing evidence that this imbalance is important in the pathogenesis of this condition. There are a number of important effects of oxidative stress in smokers that are relevant to the development of COPD, which could be prevented by antioxidant therapy (fig. 3). Oxidative stress may also be critical to the inflammatory response to cigarette smoke, through the upregulation of redox-sensitive transcription factors and hence pro-inflammatory gene expression; but is also involved in the protective mechanisms against the effects of cigarette smoke by the induction of antioxidant genes. Inflammation itself induces oxidative stress in the lungs, and polymorphisms on genes for inflammatory mediators or antioxidant genes may have a role in the susceptibility to the effects of cigarette smoke. Knowledge of the mechanisms of the effects of oxidative stress should in future allow the development of potent antioxidant therapies which test the hypothesis that oxidative stress is involved in the pathogenesis of COPD, not only by direct injury to cells, but also as a fundamental factor in the lung inflammation in smoking-related lung disease.

References

1 Rahman I, MacNee W: Role of oxidants/antioxidants in smoking-induced lung diseases. Free Radic Biol Med 1996;21:669–681.
2 Cantin AM, Fells GA, Hubbard RC, Crystal RG: Antioxidant macromolecules in the epithelial lining fluid of the normal human lower respiratory tract. J Clin Invest 1990;86:962–971.
3 Morrison D, Rahman I, Lannan S, MacNee W: Epithelial permeability, inflammation and oxidant stress in the air spaces of smokers. Am J Respir Crit Care Med 1999;159:473–479.
4 Hunninghake GW, Crystal RG: Cigarette smoking and lung destruction: Accumulation of neutrophils in the lungs of cigarette smokers. Am Rev Respir Dis 1983;128:833–838.
5 Schaberg T, Haller H, Rau M, Kaiser D, Fassbender M, Lode H: Superoxide anion release induced by platelet-activating factor is increased in human alveolar macrophages from smokers. Eur Respir J 1992;5:387–393.
6 Richards GA, Theron JA, van der Merwe CA, Anderson R: Spirometric abnormalities in young smokers correlate with increased chemiluminescence responses of activated blood phagocytes. Am Rev Respir Dis 1989;139:181–187.
7 Hubbard RC, Ogushi F, Fels GA, Cantin AM, Courtney M, Crystal RG: Oxidants spontaneously released by alveolar macrophages of cigarette smokers can inactivate the active site of alpha-1-antitrypsin, rendering it ineffective as an inhibitor of neutrophil elastase. J Clin Invest 1987;80:1289–1295.
8 Morrison HM: The proteinase-antiproteinase theory of the pathogenesis of emphysema: Time for a re appraisal? Clin Sci 1987;72:151 158.
9 Abboud RT, Fera T, Richter A, Tobona MZ, Johal S: Acute effect of smoking on the functional ativity of alpha-1-protease inhibitor in bronchoalveolar lavage fluid. Am Rev Respir Dis 1985;131:79–85.
10 Cross CE, Van der Vliet A, O'Neil CA, Louie S, Halliwell B: Oxidants, antioxidants and respiratory tract lining fluid. Envion Health Perspect 1994;102(suppl 10):185–191.
11 Pacht, ER, Kaseki H, Mohammed JR, Cornwell DG, Davis WR: Deficiency of vitamin E in the alveolar fluid of cigarette smokers. Influence on alveolar macrophage cytotoxicity. J Clin Invest 1988;77:789–796.
12 Bui MH, Sauty A, Collet F, Leuenberger P: Dietary vitamin C intake and concentrations in the body fluids and cells of male smokers and nonsmokers. J Nutr 1992;122:312–336.
13 Rahman I, Morrison D, Donaldson K, MacNee W: Systemic oxidative stress in asthma, COPD, and smokers. Am J Respir Crit Care Med 1996;154:1055–1060.
14 Rahman I, Skwarska E, MacNee W: Attenuation of oxidant/antioxidant imbalance during treatment of exacerbations of chronic obstructive pulmonary disease. Thorax 1997;52:565–568.
15 Pratico D, Basili S, Vieri M, Cordova C, Violi F, Fitzgerald GA: Chronic obstructive pulmonary disease associated with an increase in urinary levels of isoprostane $F_2\alpha$-III, an index of oxidant stress. Am J Respir Crit Care Med 1997;158:1709–1714.
16 Morrow JD, Frei B, Longmire AW, Gaziano JM, Lynch M, Shyr Y, Strauss WE, Oates JA, Roberts LJ II: Increase in circulating products of lipid peroxidation (F_2-isoprostanes) in smokers. N Engl J Med 1995;332:1198–1203.
17 Cross CE, O'Neill CA, Reznick AZ, Hu ML, Marcocci L, Packer L, Frei B: Cigarette smoke oxidation of human plasma constitutents. Ann NY Acad Sci USA 1993;686:72–90.
18 Jeffery PK: Structural and inflammatory changes in COPD: A comparison with asthma. Thorax 1998;53:129–136.
19 Keating SVM, Collins PD, Scott DM, Barnes PJ: Differences in interleukin-8 and tumour necrosis factor-induced sputum from patients with chronic obstructive pulmonary disease or asthma. Am J Respir Crit Care Med 1996;153: 530 534.
20 Rahman I, MacNee W: Role of transcription factors in inflammatory lung diseases. Thorax 1998;53:601–612.
21 Torphy TJ: Phosphodiesterase isozymes. Am J Respir Crit Care Med 1998;157:351–370.
22 Hoshino E, Shariff R, Van Gossum A, et al: Vitamin E suppresses increased lipid peroxidation in cigarette smokers. J Parenter Enter Nutr 1990;40: 300–30.
23 MacNee W, Bridgeman MME, Marsden M, Drost E, Lannan S, Selby C, Donaldson K: The effects of N-acetylcysteine and glutathione on smoke-induced changes in lung phagocytes and epithelial cells. Am J Med 1991;90:60s–66s.
24 Marrades RM, Roca J, Barbera J, de Jover L, MacNee W, Rodriguez-Roisin R: Nebulized glutathione induces bronchoconstriction in patients with mild asthma. Am J Respir Crit Care Med 1997;156:425–430.
25 Bridgeman MME, Marsden M, MacNee W, Flenley DC, Ryle AO: Cysteine and glutathione concentrations in plasma and bronchoalveolar lavage fluid after treatment with N-acetylcysteine. Thorax 1991;46:39–42.
26 Bridgemen MME, Marsden M, Selby C, Morrison D, MacNee W: Effect of N-acetyl cysteine on the concentrations of thiols in plasma, bronchoalveolar lavage fluid and lining tissue. Thorax 1994;49:670–675.
27 Bowman G, Backer U, Larsson S, Melander B, Wahlander L: Oral acetylcysteine reduces exaceration rate in chronic bronchitis. Eur J Respir Dis 1983;64:405–415.
28 British Thoracic Society Research Committee: Oral N-acetylcysteine and exacerbation rates in patients with chronic bronchitis and severe airways obstruction. Thorax 1985;40:823–835.
29 Grandjean EM, Berthet P, Ruffmann R, Leuenberger P: Efficacy of oral long-term N-acetylcysteine in chronic bronchopulmonary disease: A meta-analysis of published double-blind, placebo-controlled clinical trials. Clin Ther 2000;22:209–221.
30 Nagy AM, Vanderbist F, Parij N, Maes P, Fondu P, Neve J: Effect of the mucoactive drug Nacystelyn on the respiratory burst of human blood polymorphonuclear neutrophils. Pulm Pharmacol Ther 1997;10:287–292.
31 Nishikawa M, Kakemizu N, Ito T, Kudo M, Kaneko T, Suzuki M, Udaka N, Ikeda H, Okubo T: Superoxide mediates cigarette smoke-induced infiltration of neutrophils into the airways through nuclear factor-κB activation and IL-8 mRNA expression in guinea pigs in vivo. Am J Respir Cell Mol Biol 1999;20:189–198.

Prof. W. MacNee
Respiratory Medicine
ELEGI Colt Research Laboratories
Wilkie Building, Medical School, Teviot Place
Edinburgh EH8 9AG (UK)
Tel. +44 131 651 1435, Fax +44 131 651 1558
E-Mail w.macnee@ed.ac.uk

Selective iNOS Inhibitors

Pamela T. Manning[a]   Janice M. Thompson[b]   Mark G. Currie[c]

Searle Research and Development, [a]St. Louis, Mo., and [b]Skokie, Ill., and
[c]Sepracor Inc., Marlborough, Mass., USA

Summary

Our understanding of the role of nitric oxide (NO) produced by the inducible form of nitric oxide synthase (iNOS) in the pathophysiology of pulmonary diseases, including asthma, is at an early stage. At low levels, NO acts as a bronchodilator and a stimulator of ciliary activity. However, recent evidence suggests that the sustained production of high levels of NO generated by iNOS results in the disruption of the airway epithelium, diminished ciliary function, a shift in the balance from a Th1- to a Th2-dominated response, and in addition, that it is a chemoattractant for eosinophils. For these reasons, it is likely that the selective inhibition of iNOS in asthma will result in decreased pulmonary inflammation and improved airway function. To date, no clinical study testing the efficacy of a selective iNOS inhibitor in asthma has been performed, but increasing evidence in various animal models of asthma with either selective iNOS inhibitors or iNOS gene disruption supports this concept.

Background

NO is involved in the regulation of many physiological processes, as well as in the pathophysiology of a number of diseases. It is synthesized enzymatically from L-arginine in numerous tissues and cell types by three distinct isoforms of the enzyme, NO synthase (NOS). Two of these isoforms are expressed in a constitutive manner, predominantly in the vascular endothelium (eNOS, type III NOS) and in the nervous system (nNOS, type I NOS). Under normal physiological conditions, these constitutive forms of NOS generate low, transient levels of NO (picomolar to nanomolar concentrations) in response to increases in intracellular calcium concentrations. These low levels of NO act to regulate blood pressure, platelet adhesion, gastrointestinal motility, bronchomotor tone and neurotransmission [1]. The expression of the third isoform (iNOS, type II NOS) is induced by endotoxin and/or cytokines and generates high, sustained levels of NO (up to micromolar concentrations). This excessive production of NO and resulting NO-derived metabolites (e.g., peroxynitrite) elicit cellular cytotoxicity and tissue damage which may contribute to the pathophysiology of a number of human diseases, including asthma [2].

Beneficial Actions of NO in the Lung

In a number of experimental and clinical paradigms, NO has been found to have beneficial actions in the lung with most of the emphasis placed on the actions of this agent on bronchial and vascular smooth muscle. When administered exogenously to the lung, NO acts as a bronchodilator and a vasorelaxant [3, 4]. In addition, NO decreases leukocyte activation, mobility, and adhesion to the endothelium [4]. These actions appear to represent the normal physiologic role of NO produced by the constitutive isoforms of NOS. Specifically, NO produced by nNOS in the nonadrenergic, noncholinergic (NANC) nerves is thought to modulate airway tone by serving as an endogenous bronchodilator and as a stimulator of mucociliary transport [5, 6], whereas the NO produced by eNOS appears to increase local blood flow by acting as a vasodilator and by regulating the endothelial barrier.

NO produced by iNOS may also provide a beneficial role in certain conditions. The most critical role of iNOS in many sites, including the lung, is to contribute to the host defense response to pathogens [2]. The induction of iNOS by pollutants and infectious agents may, in fact, be one cause of the increase in the incidence of asthma and may also contribute to the exacerbation of the disease by these agents.

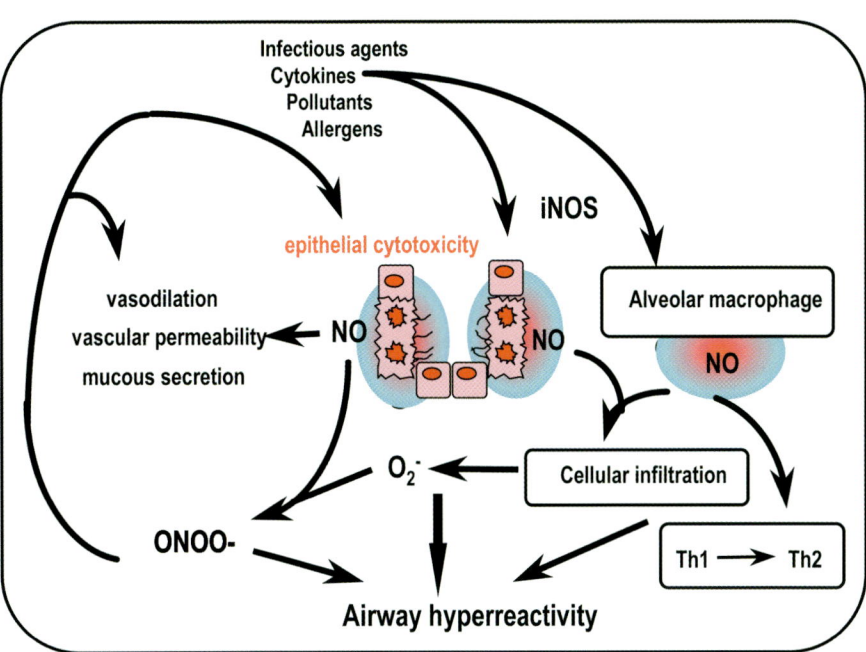

Fig. 1. Potentially deleterious actions of sustained elevated levels of NO in the lung. The sustained production of NO generated by iNOS in asthma and other inflammatory conditions in the lung may lead to cellular damage and altered lung function by a number of potential mechanisms. The expression of iNOS in the epithelium and/or inflammatory cells induced by cytokines, pollutants, allergens or infectious agents leads to the elevated production of NO. NO or its metabolites (i.e., peroxynitrite; ONOO–) produce epithelial cytotoxicity leading to cell death as well as vasodilation, increased vascular permeability, increased mucous secretion, increased cellular infiltration including eosinophils, airway hyperreactivity and stimulation of a Th2 inflammatory response.

Potential Deleterious Actions of Sustained Elevated Levels of NO Produced by iNOS

As with many inflammatory mediators, it appears that the early response of the induction of iNOS and increased levels of NO are beneficial, providing protection against pathogens. However, in many cases, these responses are either inappropriate in magnitude or fail to resolve following the disappearance of the initial insult. Subsequently, the sustained elevation of NO production causes cellular damage and alters the normal physiological functions of the lung.

A clear demonstration of the pulmonary epithelial toxicity of NO generated by iNOS occurs during *Bordetella pertussis* infection [7]. Tracheal cytotoxin released by this infectious agent results in the induction of iNOS in the pulmonary epithelial cells. The induction of iNOS appears to be mediated by interleukin-1β and results in the sustained production of NO which causes disruption of the epithelium and a marked depletion of the ciliated cells. The importance of either NO or perhaps other reactive nitrogen species in producing this damage has been demonstrated in vitro using human and hamster respiratory epithelial cells. The selective iNOS inhibitor, aminoguanidine, was found to prevent the tracheal cytotoxin-induced damage to the epithelium and ciliated cell death [7]. A similar pathology consisting of disruption of the respiratory epithelium and damage to the ciliated cells occurs in asthma [8]. In addition, 3-nitrotyrosine immunoreactivity has been localized to the epithelium in asthmatics, suggesting that the damaging radical, peroxynitrite, may contribute to this cellular cytotoxicity [9, 10]. Importantly, this staining can be eliminated following treatment with steroids which reduces both iNOS expression in the epithelium as well as cellular damage. However, it still remains to be determined whether NO or its metabolites are, in fact, the causative agent(s) of the epithelial airway damage in asthma.

Elevated levels of NO likely cause several other significant changes in the lungs of asthmatics including a shift in the balance between Th1 and Th2 lymphocyte responses, pulmonary edema, increased mucous secretion, and eosinophil accumulation [2]. These pathophysiological actions of NO may be critical in sustaining airway inflammation and ultimately in mediating the increased airway hyperresponsiveness in asthma, as summarized in figure 1.

Effect of iNOS Inhibition in Animal Models of Asthma

Following the observation that iNOS expression was elevated in the lungs of asthmatics, studies were initiated in numerous laboratories to determine whether iNOS expression was also induced in animal models of pulmonary inflammation and asthma. Early results demonstrated that iNOS expression was increased in several animal models of pulmonary inflammation, including in-

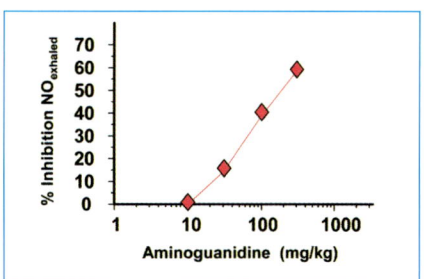

Fig. 2. Therapeutic effect of aminoguanidine on exhaled NO following endotoxin challenge. Male Lewis rats were treated with an intraperitoneal injection of 1 mg/kg of *Escherichia coli* (0111:B4) endotoxin to induce the expression of iNOS and inflammation in the lung. Following the administration of endotoxin, there was a time-dependent increase in the amount of exhaled NO ($NO_{exhaled}$). Peak increases occurred between 5 and 8 h and were elevated greater than 10-fold compared to basal levels. Aminoguanidine was administered orally 5 h following LPS administration and the amount of $NO_{exhaled}$ was measured 1.5 h later. The amount of $NO_{exhaled}$ was reduced in a dose-dependent manner by aminoguanidine. The ED_{50} was approximately 200 mg/kg.

flammation following allergen challenge [11, 12]. The cellular sources of increased iNOS expression are the pulmonary epithelium and inflammatory cells, including alveolar macrophages and eosinophils. In addition to the elevated iNOS expression, it is also feasible to measure elevated levels of exhaled NO in several of these models. We have found that the amount of exhaled NO is elevated approximately 10-fold in rats 5 h following the administration of endotoxin. This elevated level of NO can subsequently be reduced in a dose-dependent manner, 90 min following the oral administration of the selective iNOS inhibitor, aminoguanidine (fig. 2). Similar studies are in progress using rodent models of asthma. These studies demonstrate that iNOS expression and exhaled NO are elevated in animal models of pulmonary inflammation and asthma and that the production of NO can be reduced by the selective inhibition of iNOS in a manner similar to that observed following their acute administration in asthmatic patients.

There is a growing amount of data from animal models suggesting that the increased expression of iNOS plays a critical role in propagating the pulmonary inflammation associated with these models. NOS inhibitors have been shown to reverse the vascular extravasation associated with pulmonary inflammation induced by endotoxin treatment and to block the bronchial hyperresponsiveness in an air pollution model of asthma [13, 14]. In both of these models, the pulmonary expression of iNOS was elevated. However, a selective iNOS inhibitor was not utilized to demonstrate definitively the role of this NOS isoform in mediating the associated changes. In a subsequent study in the air-pollution-induced model, treatment with the modestly selective iNOS inhibitor, aminoguanidine, prevented the increase in neutrophils, eosinophils, epithelial goblet cells, and overall pulmonary inflammation, providing more convincing evidence for the role of iNOS in mediating these pathological changes [15]. The role of iNOS has also been evaluated using mice genetically engineered to lack iNOS (iNOS−/−) [16]. Following repeated allergen challenge, these iNOS−/− mice exhibited markedly reduced inflammation in the lung including decreased eosinophil infiltration, epithelial damage, microvascular leakage, pulmonary edema and airway occlusion. The suppression of the pulmonary inflammatory response appeared to result from increased levels of interferon-γ which occurred in the iNOS−/− mice (previous studies have demonstrated that NO generated from iNOS inhibits the production interferon-γ by T cells). However, the iNOS−/− mice exhibited an increase in the hyperreactivity of the bronchial airways upon challenge with methacholine, suggesting that iNOS, at least in this particular animal model of asthma, plays both a pathological role in the progression of pulmonary inflammation and a protective, bronchodilator role [16].

Challenges and Future Directions

The remarkable diversity of the biological actions of NO presents a unique pharmacological challenge. Many of these actions of NO are important to the maintenance of normal physiological functions. The strategy to discover and develop selective inhibitors of iNOS reduces some of these potential problems, but additional hurdles remain. Developing a more thorough understanding of the beneficial role that iNOS plays in host-defense and perhaps during pathological states, as well as developing clinical candidates with suitable selectivity for iNOS (to avoid compromising both normal lung function and systemic blood pressure) remain. Inhaled delivery of iNOS inhibitors for the treatment of asthma may provide an approach to reduce and/or eliminate potential systemic effects. The long-term goal, however, should be to develop an orally administered iNOS inhibitor which would be useful for the treatment of numerous conditions, including asthma and other pulmonary inflammatory disorders.

References

1 Mayer B, Hemmes B: Biosynthesis and action of nitric oxide in mammalian cells. Trends Biochem Sci 1997;22:477–481.
2 Hobbs AJ, Higgs A, Moncada S: Inhibition of nitric oxide synthase as a potential therapeutic target. Annu Rev Pharmacol Toxicol 1999;39:191–220.
3 Kacmarek RM, Ripple R, Cockrill BA, Bloch KJ, Zapol WM, Johnson DC: Inhaled nitric oxide: A bronchodilator in mild asthmatics with methacholine-induced bronchospasm. Am J Respir Crit Care Med 1996;153:128–135.
4 Weinberger B, Heck DE, Laskin DL, Laskin JD: NO in the lung: Therapeutic and cellular mechanisms of action. Pharmacol Ther 1999;84:401–411.
5 Gaston B, Drazen JM, Loscalzo J, Stamler JS: The biology of nitrogen oxide in airways. Am J Respir Crit Care Med 1994;149:538–551.
6 Runer T, Lindberg S: Ciliostimulatory effects mediated by nitric oxide. Acta Otolaryngol (Stockh) 1999;119:821–825.
7 Heiss LN, Lancaster JR Jr, Corbett JA, Goldman WE: Epithelial autotoxicity of nitric oxide: Role in the respiratory cytopathology of pertussis. Proc Natl Acad Sci USA 1994;91:267–270.
8 Holgate ST, Davies DE, Lackie PM, Wilson SJ, Puddicombe SM, Lordan JL: Epithelial-mesenchymal interactions in the pathogenesis of asthma. J Allergy Clin Immunol 2000;105:193–204.
9 Saleh D, Ernst P, Lim S, Barnes PJ, Giaid A: Increased formation of the potent oxidant peroxynitrite in the airways of asthmatic patients is associated with induction of nitric oxide synthase: Effect of inhaled glucocorticoid. FASEB J 1998;12:929–937.
10 Kaminsky DA, Mitchell J, Carroll N, James A, Soultanakis R, Janssen Y: Nitrotyrosine formation in the airways and lung parenchyma of patients with asthma. J Allergy Clin Immunol 1999;104:747–754.
11 Yeadon M, Price R: Induction of calcium-independent nitric oxide synthase by allergen challenge in sensitized rat lung in vivo. Br J Pharmacol 1995;116:2545–2546.
12 Renzi PM, Sebastiao N, al Assaad AS, Giaid A, Hamid Q: Inducible nitric oxide synthase mRNA and immunoreactivity in the lungs of rats eight hours after antigen challenge. Am J Respir Cell Mol Biol 1997;17:36–40.
13 Ohuchi Y, Ichinose M, Miura M, Kageyama N, Tomaki M, Endoh N, Mashito Y, Sugiura H, Shirato K: Induction of nitric oxide synthase by lipopolysaccharide inhalation enhances substance P-induced microvascular leakage in guinea-pigs. Eur Respir J 1998;12:831–836.
14 Lim HB, Ichinose T, Miyabara Y, Takano H, Kumagai Y, Shimojyo N, Devalia JL, Sagai M: Involvement of superoxide and nitric oxide on airway inflammation and hyperresponsiveness induced by diesel exhaust particles in mice. Free Radic Biol Med 1998;25:635–644.
15 Takano H, Lim HB Miyabara Y, Ichinose T, Yoshikawa T, Sagai M: Manipulation of the *L*-arginine-nitric oxide pathway in airway inflammation induced by diesel exhaust particles in mice. Toxicology 1999;139:19–26.
16 Xiong Y, Karupiah G, Hogan SP, Foster PS, Ramsay AJ: Inhibition of allergic airway inflammation in mice lacking nitric oxide synthase 2. J Immunol 1999;162:445–452.

Pamela T. Manning, PhD
Searle Research and Development
700 Chesterfield Village
Parkway South
Chesterfield, MO 43198 (USA)
Tel. +1 636 737 4248, Fax +1 636 737 7388
E-Mail pamela.t.manning@monsanto.com

Mucus Regulation

Duncan F. Rogers

Thoracic Medicine, National Heart and Lung Institute, Imperial College, London, UK

Summary

Patients with asthma and COPD exhibit characteristics of airway mucus hypersecretion, namely sputum production, luminal mucus, submucosal gland hypertrophy and goblet cell hyperplasia. Recent epidemiological studies show associations between sputum production and decline in lung function, morbidity and mortality. Many drugs will potentially inhibit airway mucus hypersecretion. However, more data on the similarities and differences between mucus in healthy subjects and patients with asthma or COPD are required to facilitate rational drug design.

Excessive mucus production in the airways characterises asthma and chronic bronchitis. Chronic bronchitis (hypersecretion), chronic bronchiolitis (small airway disease) and emphysema (alveolar destruction) comprise COPD. The contribution of each component to pathophysiology in any one patient is difficult to determine. The present chapter considers drug treatment of mucus hypersecretion in asthma and the 'bronchitic' component of COPD.

Mucus Hypersecretion in Asthma and COPD

Mucus hypersecretion in asthma and COPD has been considered in detail recently [1, 2]. Patients with asthma or COPD usually produce sputum at some stage of their condition, and there is excess mucus in the airway lumens of patients dying of asthma and COPD. The increased mucus is associated with submucosal gland hypertrophy and goblet cell hyperplasia. However, not all patients exhibit all characteristics of mucus hypersecretion, and there are differences between asthma or COPD (table 1). The three main differences are:

- The mucus in asthma appears more viscous than in COPD.
- Mucin gene product (MUC)5AC is a minor component of the secretions in COPD [3].
- Tethering of mucus to goblet cells in asthma but not in COPD [4].

With these differences, different drugs may be required for effective treatment of hypersecretion in asthma and COPD.

The contribution of mucus to pathophysiology and clinical symptoms is better delineated for asthma [1] than for COPD [2]. However, recent epidemiological studies in COPD find positive associations between sputum production and decline in lung function, risk of hospitalisation and death. The relationship between sputum and mucus in small airways is not clear. Mucus hypersecretion is perceived to contribute to morbidity and mortality in patients with asthma and COPD.

Drug Treatment of Mucus Hypersecretion

Drugs with the potential for inhibiting mucus hypersecretion are either currently available or are in development (fig. 1). Conventional therapy for airway inflammation should have beneficial effects on airway mucus hypersecretion. Glucocorticosteroids inhibit mucus secretion, goblet cell hyperplasia and MUC gene expression [5]. However, although glucocorticoids are effective in asthma, possibly in part due to an anti-hypersecretory action, they are not effective in stable COPD, which indicates that effective anti-hypersecretory drugs may need to be disease specific.

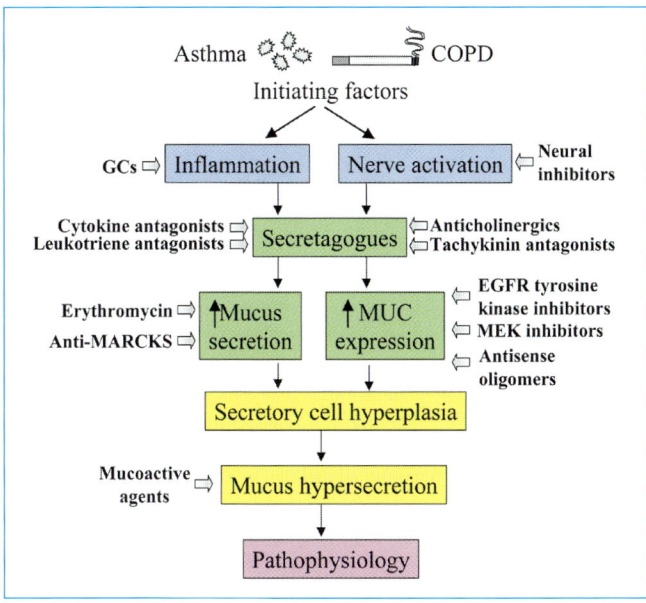

Fig. 1. Pathophysiology of mucus hypersecretion in asthma and COPD and sites of action of 'anti-hypersecretory' drugs (some compounds act at more than one site). GCs = Glucocorticosteroids.

Neural mechanisms and numerous inflammatory mediators have effects on mucus (table 2). Selective receptor antagonists might be of benefit in the treatment of airway mucus hypersecretion. For example, cysteinyl leukotriene receptor antagonists inhibit mucus output induced by ovalbumin challenge of tracheae from sensitised guinea pigs [6], an activity that may contribute to their efficacy in asthma. However, the multiplicity of mediators involved in the pathophysiology of asthma and COPD suggests that no single receptor antagonist will markedly affect mucus hypersecretion.

Mucoactive Drugs. Fifteen compounds with potentially beneficial actions on mucus are listed in pharmacopoeias worldwide [7] (table 3). However, 'mucolytic' therapy is not generally recommended in international guidelines on the management of asthma or COPD. The discrepancy between the abundance of mucoactive drugs and the caution in recommending them in treatment is related to imprecision in the design of clinical trials.

Erythromycin. Erythromycin is a macrolide antibiotic that inhibits mucin secretion in experimental prepara-

Table 1. Comparison of indices of mucus hypersecretion in asthma and COPD

Index	Asthma	COPD
Clinical definition	mucus hypersecretion not part of definition	mucus hypersecretion only in 'older' definitions
Sputum production	yes; associated with attacks	yes; recurrent and long-standing
Sputum viscosity	variable, but greater than in COPD	variable
Mucus 'markers' in sputum	yes	yes
Mucin analysis	nine-fold more mucins in plug than in COPD sputum	less mucins in sputum than in asthma
Mucus in airway lumen (gross pathology)	yes; adherent viscous 'mucus' plugs comprising mucus and exudate	yes; mucoid or mucopurulent; little evidence of asthma-like 'plugs'
Mucus in airway lumen (histology)	yes	yes
Mucus 'tethering'	yes	no
Goblet cell hyperplasia	yes (more pronounced in acute severe asthma than in chronic asthma?)	yes (except for a group of Japanese patients)
Submucosal gland hypertrophy	yes	usually, although there are exceptions
Submucosal gland mucin histochemistry	increase in mucous cells (i.e. acidic mucin)	morphologically normal, more serous glands
MUC5AC	major constituent of mucus pug	minor constituent of sputum
MUC5B	present in two glycoforms	greater proportion than in asthma
Epidemiology	mucus hypersecretion linked with decline in lung function	mucus hypersecretion and lung function decline, hospitalisation and mortality a significant risk factor in many studies, particularly as patients age

Table 2. Neural and humoral inducers of mucus secretion, goblet cell hyperplasia and MUC gene expression/synthesis in the airways

Stimulation	Secretion	Hyperplasia	MUC
Adrenergic nerves	0/+	NP	NP
α-Adrenoceptor agonists	+	NP	NP
β-Adrenoceptor agonists	+	yes	NP
Bacterial exoproducts (in culture broth)	+	yes	yes
Bradykinin	+	NP	NP
Cholinergic nerves	++	NP	NP
Cholinoceptor agonists	++	yes	NP
EGF (+ TNF-α)	NP	yes	yes
Endothelin	0/+	NP	NP
Endotoxin	+	yes	yes
Histamine	0/+	NP	NP
IL-1β	+	NP	NP
IL-4	+	yes	yes
IL-6	+	NP	yes
IL-9	NP	NP	yes
Irritant gases (e.g. cigarette smoke)	++	yes	yes
Leukotrienes	0/+	NP	NP
MMS	+	NP	NP
Neurokinin A	+	NP	NP
Nicotine	++	yes	NP
Nitric oxide	-ve/+	NP	NP
Phosphodiesterase IV inhibitors	+	NP	NP
PAF	0/+	yes[1]	yes[1]
Prostaglandins	0/+	NP	NP
Proteinases	+++	yes	NP
Purine nucleotides	+	NP	NP
Reactive oxygen species	0/+	NP	NP
Sensitisation followed by challenge	+	yes	yes
SP	++	NP	NP
Tachykininergic nerves	0/++	NP	NP
TNF-α	++	yes[1]	yes[1]

Scoring: +++ = highly potent; ++ = marked effect; + = lesser effect; 0 = minimal effect; NP = effect not published.
[1] Effect only observed with platelet-activating factor (PAF) and TNF-α in combination. MMS = Monocyte/macrophage-derived mucus secretagogue.

Table 3. 'Popular' mucoactive drugs

Mucolytic
  N-Acetylcysteine, L-ethylcysteine, sodium 2-mercaptoethane sulphonate (MESNA), methylcysteine hydrochloride, stepronine, thiopronine
Mucoregulatory
  Carbocysteine, eprazinon hydrochloride, erdosteine, letosteine
Expectorant
  Ambroxol, bromhexine, guaifenesin, sobrerol
DNAse (degrades DNA)
  Recombinant human DNase I (Dornase-α)

The 15 most frequently listed drugs in pharmacopoeias worldwide [7]. Definitions: 'mucolytic', thins mucus; 'mucoregulatory', does not thin mucus (precise mechanism of action, if any, unknown); 'expectorant', increases cough and expectoration (may induce mucus secretion).

tions. Erythromycin reduced excessive mucus secretion in a child [8] and an elderly man [9]. The mechanism of action of erythromycin is unclear, but may involve anti-inflammatory and mucoactive effects [10].

Proteinase Inhibitors. Proteinases (e.g. neutrophil elastase) have potent effects on airway mucus (table 2) [11], and proteinase inhibitors may inhibit airway mucus hypersecretion. Trifluoromethyl ketone human neutrophil elastase inhibitors (e.g. ICI 200355) inhibit elastase-mediated secretory responses. Although human trials have been alluded to [12], clinical data have not yet appeared in the literature.

Cytokine Antagonists. Interleukin-1β (IL-1β), IL-4, IL-6, IL-9 and TNF-α induce aspects of mucus hypersecretion in experimental systems (table 2). IL-4 has been suggested as a central signalling mechanism for development of a hypersecretory epithelium [13], whilst IL-9 accounts for 50–60% of the mucin-stimulating activity of lung fluids from allergic dogs [14]. Current small molecule inhibitors of IL-4 look unlikely to be effective, and biologic agents (e.g. soluble IL-4 receptors) have potential cost, administration and compliance problems.

Epidermal Growth Factor Receptor Tyrosine Kinase Inhibitors. Airway epidermal growth factor receptor (EGF-R) expression is induced by tumor necrosis factor-α (TNF-α), allergy, agarose plugs and oxidative stress, and is associated with goblet cell hyperplasia and increased expression of MUC5AC [15, 16]. Inhibitors of EGF-R tyrosine kinase, for example AG1478 and BIBX1522, block these responses. The hypersecretory response to oxidative stress is blocked by a selective mitogen-activated protein kinase (MAPK) kinase (MEK)-p44/42 MAPK (p44/42^{mapk}) inhibitor, PD98059 [16].

Myristoylated Alanine-Rich C Kinase Substrate. Myristoylated alanine-rich kinase C substrate (MARCKS) protein is a key intracellular molecule involved in intracellular movement and exocytosis of mucin granules [17]. Blockade of MARCKS by a synthetic peptide to its N-terminal region inhibited mucin secretion.

Anticholinergics. Cholinergic activation of airway mucus output is via muscarinic M_3 receptors on the secretory cells [18]. The autoinhibitory M_2 receptor regulates the magnitude of secretion. The non-selective muscarinic antagonist ipratropium bromide reduces sputum production, although without changes in viscosity or dry weight. Anticholinergics with selectivity for the M_3 receptor over the M_2 receptor may have therapeutic benefit over non-selective compounds, for example tiotropium or J-104129 [19].

Tachykinin Receptor Antagonists. Stimulation of capsaicin-sensitive tachykininergic nerves induces airway mucus secretion in experimental animals, but is less easily demonstrated in human airways. Tachykininergic nervous pathways may be upregulated with inflammation [20]. In asthma, substance P (SP)-like immunoreactivity is elevated in plasma, induced sputum and nasal lavage. SP-containing nerves and tachykinin receptor mRNA are increased. In COPD, SP is increased in induced sputum. However, the distribution of tachykinin receptors is not different between smokers and controls [21]. Tachykinin NK_1 antagonists inhibit neurogenic secretion in ferret trachea [22]. Clinical data on the effects of tachykinin receptor antagonists in asthma and COPD are equivocal, and effects on mucus secretion have not been specifically studied [20].

Neural Inhibitors. Neurally mediated mucus secretion can be attenuated by inhibition of nerve activity. Opioids and vasoactive intestinal peptide inhibit neurogenic airway mucus secretion via inhibition of neurotransmitter release [23, 24]. Inhibition is via activation of large conductance, calcium-activated K^+ (BK_{Ca}) channels [23, 24]. The BK_{Ca} channel activator NS 1619 inhibits mucus secretion in ferret trachea [23].

Antisense Oligonucleotides. An antisense oligonucleotide to MARCKS down-regulated both mRNA and protein levels and also attenuated mucin secretion [17]. An 18-mer MUC antisense oligomer suppressed mucin gene expression and wood smoke-induced epithelial metaplasia in rabbit airways [25].

Conclusions and Future Directions

Mucus hypersecretion contributes to morbidity and mortality in asthma and COPD. This suggests that it is important to develop drugs that inhibit mucus hypersecretion, although without affecting normal secretion and mucociliary clearance. Considerably more needs to be known about the identity of airway mucins in normal healthy subjects and whether or not there is an intrinsic and disease-specific abnormality in mucus in asthma and COPD. These data can be used to determine therapeutic targets for rational design of anti-hypersecretory drugs for asthma and COPD.

References

1 Liu YC, Khawaja AM, Rogers DF: Pathophysiology of airway mucus secretion in asthma; in Barnes PJ, Rodger IW, Thomson NC (eds): Asthma: Basic Mechanisms and Clinical Management, ed 3. London, Academic Press, 1998, pp 205–227.

2 Rogers DF: Mucus hypersecretion in COPD; in McNee W (ed): Chronic Obstructive Pulmonary Disease: Pathogenesis to Treatment. Novartis Found Symp. Chichester, Wiley, in press, vol 234.

3 Thornton DJ, Carlstedt I, Howard M, Devine PL, Price MR, Sheehan JK: Respiratory mucins: Identification of core proteins and glycoforms. Biochem J 1996;316:967–975.

4 Shimura S, Andoh Y, Haraguchi M, Shirato K: Continuity of airway goblet cells and intraluminal mucus in the airways of patients with bronchial asthma. Eur Respir J 1996;9:1395–1401.

5 Rogers DF: Airway goblet cells: Responsive and adaptable front-line defenders. Eur Respir J 1994;7:1690–1706.

6 Liu Y-C, Khawaja AM, Rogers DF: Effects of the cysteinyl leukotriene receptor antagonists pranlukast and zafirlukast on tracheal mucus secretion in ovalbumin-sensitized guinea pigs in vitro. Br J Pharmacol 1998;124:563–571.

7 Nightingale JA, Rogers DF: Should drugs affecting mucus properties be used in COPD? Clinical evidence; in Similowski T, Whitelaw W, Derenne J-P (eds): Clinical Management of Stable COPD. New York, Marcel Dekker, in press.

8 Suez D, Szefler SJ: Excessive accumulation of mucus in children with asthma: A potential role for erythromycin? A case discussion. J Allergy Clin Immunol 1986;77:330–334.

9 Marom ZM, Goswami SK: Respiratory mucus hypersecretion (bronchorrhea): A case discussion – possible mechanism(s) and treatment. J Allergy Clin Immunol 1991;87:1050–1055.

10 Wales D, Woodhead M: The antiinflammatory effects of macrolides. Thorax 1999;54 (suppl 2):558–562.

11 Nadel JA, Takeyama K: Mechanisms of hypersecretion in acute asthma, proposed cause of death, and novel therapy. Pediatr Pulmonol Suppl 1999;18:54–55.

12 Veale CA, Bernstein PR, Bohnert CM, Brown FJ, Damewood JR Jr, Earley R, et al: Orally active trifluoromethyl ketone inhibitors of human leukocyte elastase. J Med Chem 1997;40:3173–3181.

13 Dabbagh K, Takeyama K, Lee HM, Ueki IF, Lausier JA, Nadel JA: IL-4 induces mucin gene expression and goblet cell metaplasia in vitro and in vivo. J Immunol 1999;162:6233–6237.

14 Longphre M, Li D, Gallup M, Drori E, Ordonez CL, Redman T, Wenzel S, Bice DE, Fahy JV, Basbaum C: Allergen-induced IL-9 directly stimulates mucin transcription in respiratory epithelial cells. J Clin Invest 1999;104:1375–1382.

15 Takeyama K, Dabbagh K, Lee H-M, Agustí C, Lausier JA, Ueki IF, Grattan KM, Nadel JA: Epidermal growth factor system regulates mucin production in airways. Proc Natl Acad Sci USA 1999;96:3081–3086.

16 Takeyama K, Dabbagh K, Shim JJ, Dao-Pick T, Ueki IF, Nadel JA: Oxidative stress causes mucin synthesis via transactivation of epidermal growth factor receptor: Role of neutrophils. J Immunol 2000;164:1546–1552.

17 Li Y, Martin LD, Adler KB: MARCKS protein: A key intracellular molecule controlling mucin secretion by human airway goblet cells. Am J Respir Crit Care Med 2000;161:A259.

18 Ramnarine SI, Haddad E-B, Khawaja AM, Mak JCW, Rogers DF: On muscarinic control of neurogenic mucus secretion in ferret trachea. J Physiol 1996;494:577–586.

19 Mitsuya M, Mase T, Tsuchiya Y, Kawakami K, Hattori H, Kobayashi K, Ogino Y, Fujikawa T, Satoh A, Kimura T, Noguchi K, Ohtake N, Tomimoto K: J-104129, a novel uscarinic M_3 receptor antagonist with high selectivity for M_3 over M_2 receptors. Bioorg Med Chem 1999;7:2555–2567.

20 Rogers DF: Neurogenic inflammation in lung disease: Burnt out? Inflammopharmacology 1997;5:319–329.

21 Mapp CE, Miotto D, Braccioni F, Saetta M, Turato G, Maestrelli P, Krause JE, Karpitskiy V, Boyd N, Geppetti P, Fabbri LM: The distribution of neurokinin-1 and neurokinin-2 receptors in human central airways. Am J Respir Crit Care Med 2000;161:207–215.

22 Khawaja AM, Liu Y-C, Rogers DF: Effect of non-peptide tachykinin NK_1 receptor antagonists on non-adrenergic, non-cholinergic neurogenic mucus secretion in ferret trachea. Eur J Pharmacol 1999;384:173–181.

23 Ramnarine SI, Liu Y-C, Rogers DF: Neuroregulation of mucus secretion by opioid receptors and K_{ATP} and BK_{Ca} channels in ferret trachea in vitro. Br J Pharmacol 1998;123:1631–1638.

24 Liu Y-C, Patel HJ, Khawaja AM, Belvisi MG, Rogers DF: Neuroregulation by vasoactive intestinal peptide (VIP) of mucus secretion in ferret trachea: Activation of BK_{Ca} channels and inhibition of neurotransmitter release. Br J Pharmacol 1999;126:147–158.

25 Bhattacharyya SN, Manna B, Smiley R, Ashbaugh, Coutinho R, Kaufman B: Smoke-induced inhalation injury: Effects of retinoic acid and antisense oligodeoxynucleotide on stability and differentiated state of the mucociliary epithelium. Inflammation 1998;22:203–214.

Dr. D.F. Rogers
Thoracic Medicine
National Heart and Lung Institute
Imperial College
Dovehouse Street
London SW3 6LY (UK)
Tel. +44 171 352 8121 (ext. 3051)
Fax +44 171 351 8126
E-Mail duncan.rogers@ic.ac.uk

P2Y Receptor Agonists

Role in Mucosal Hydration and Mucociliary Clearance

William Pendergast   Richard Evans

Inspire Pharmaceuticals, Inc., Durham, N.C., USA

Summary

Binding of $P2Y_2$ purinergic agonists to their target receptor has been shown to stimulate the natural processes of mucosal hydration and mucociliary clearance in the airways. The uridine nucleotide UTP is the first aerosolized $P2Y_2$ receptor agonist in clinical studies, and is being evaluated in phase II clinical trials as an acute-use agent to stimulate the expectoration of a deep-lung sputum sample via a mucociliary clearance mechanism for use in a variety of diagnostic procedures. A next-generation $P2Y_2$ agonist, INS365, will move into phase II clinical development as a chronic treatment for obstructive respiratory disorders, such as chronic bronchitis. These compounds represent a unique approach to disorders with a high unmet medical need, and are expected to provide significant medical benefit and improvement in the patient's quality of life.

Mechanism of Action

Mucosal hydration and mucociliary clearance are the body's natural mechanisms for cleansing and/or protecting epithelial surfaces, such as those found in the lung and sinuses. Mucosal hydration requires a coordinated balance of salt, water and mucus, and is necessary to maintain the proper function of such epithelial surfaces. In addition, the process of mucociliary clearance is important in those target organs, such as the lungs and sinuses, containing ciliated epithelial cells [1]. It has been demonstrated that $P2Y_2$ receptors stimulate various components of the process of mucociliary clearance in the lung [2, 3]. At the molecular level, the cascade of events on binding of a $P2Y_2$ agonist to its receptor is illustrated in figure 1. The agonist binds to the $P2Y_2$ receptor, initiating a series of biochemical responses that result in an increase in inositol trisphosphate (IP_3) and a consequent release of calcium from the endoplasmic reticulum into the cytoplasm [4–7]. Activation of $P2Y_2$ receptors in respiratory epithelia has been associated with increased mucociliary clearance [8], presumably through the combination of the following cellular actions: increased chloride (and hence water) transport across the luminal surface via the cystic fibrosis transmembrane regulator and the 'alternate' chloride channel [9–12], the elevation of ciliary beat frequency [1], the release of mucin from goblet cells [13], and the release of surfactant from type II alveolar cells [14] (fig. 2).

Toxicology and Animal Models

UTP is well tolerated when given to rats and dogs by daily inhalation for up to 1 month. UTP has been shown to be nonmutagenic in four mutagenicity assays that have been conducted; Ames test (with or without S9 metabolic activation), mouse micronuclear cytogenetic assay, CHO cell cytogenetic test (with or without S9 activation) and the mouse lymphoma mutagenesis assay. Results from intravenous teratology studies in rats and rabbits, and a report from the literature [15] also indicate that UTP is nonteratogenic.

Although maternal toxicity and mortality were observed in the early phase of the intravenous study in rabbits, this appeared to be a species-specific effect and in several instances was related to the rate of intravenous dosing. These latter findings are not considered to be relevant to the inhalational route of administration used in clinical studies. The dose levels achieved in the 28-day inhalation toxicity studies and the intravenous studies were at least several-fold above the proposed maximum daily clinical dose on a mg/kg basis.

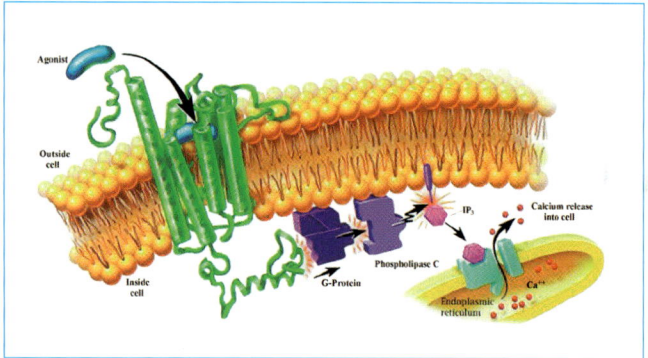
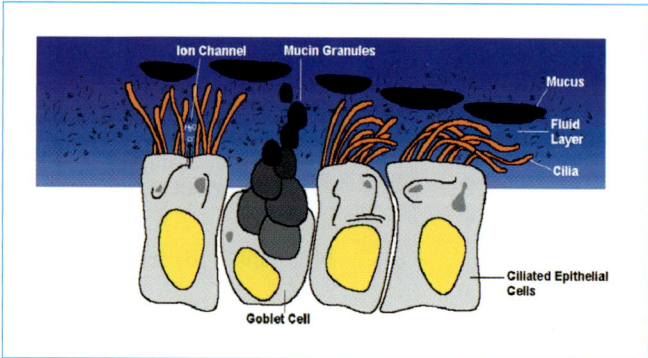

Fig. 1. Cartoon showing the agonist binding to the P2Y$_2$ receptor, initiating a series of biochemical responses that result in an increase of IP$_3$. IP$_3$ triggers the release of calcium from the endoplasmic reticulum into the cytoplasm.

Fig. 2. Cartoon showing mucin release from a goblet cell in conjunction with cilium beat in ciliated human airway epithelial cells.

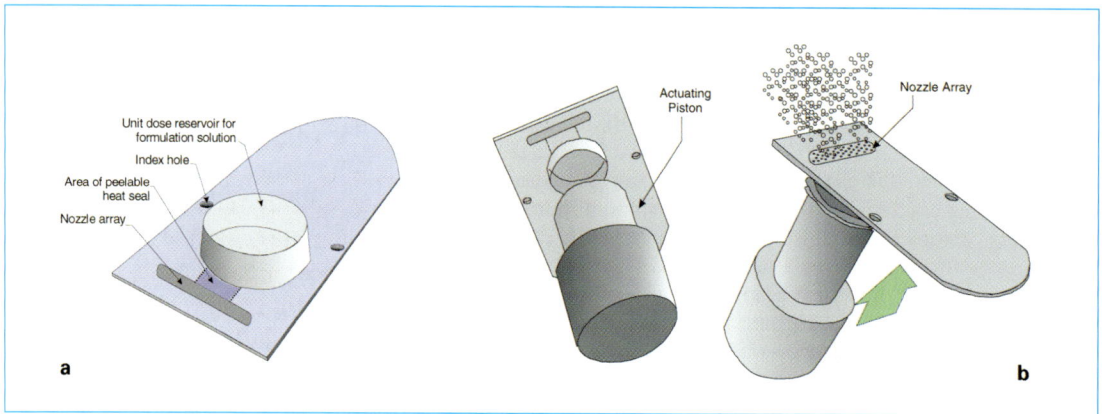

Fig. 3. Component elements of the unit-dose reservoir and the piston from the AERx® Pulmonary Delivery System. **a** The aqueous formulation is contained in a unit dose reservoir (blister) that is drawn into a polymer laminate film. During production, the liquid formulation is filled into the reservoir and a multilayer nozzle/lid assembly is heat-sealed to the top, thereby hermetically enclosing the formulation in the dosage form. To deliver the drug, the blister is placed into a reusable hand-held unit containing a piston and control electronics for administration. **b** The nozzle consists of a micromachined array of holes. At the trigger point, pressurization of the reservoir, achieved via a mechanical piston, peels open the seal in a controlled region. The liquid formulation is then forced through the nozzle array and into the inhalation air path, where it forms a gentle aerosol that is breathed into the lungs.

General acute toxicology of INS365 also demonstrated that the material was generally well tolerated by laboratory species. INS365 was found to have no clear clinical or pathological effects when given in large doses (intravenously or by inhalation) for 28 days, or acutely in dogs and rats. INS365 was without mutagenic effects in the systems described above. The exposures were greater than those proposed in the clinical protocol.

The efficacy of UTP and INS365 has been assessed in tracheal mucus velocity and whole lung mucociliary clearance studies in the sheep. These studies have been particularly useful in confirming that an increased biological stability of the nucleotides, as measured by in vitro techniques, such as metabolism on airway epithelial cells, will translate into a prolonged duration of action in vivo [16].

Route of Administration and Pulmonary Delivery Systems

The target P2Y$_2$ receptors are located on the apical surface of epithelial cells within the respiratory tract and, therefore, local delivery via inhalation of a fine respirable aerosol was chosen for the administration of both UTP

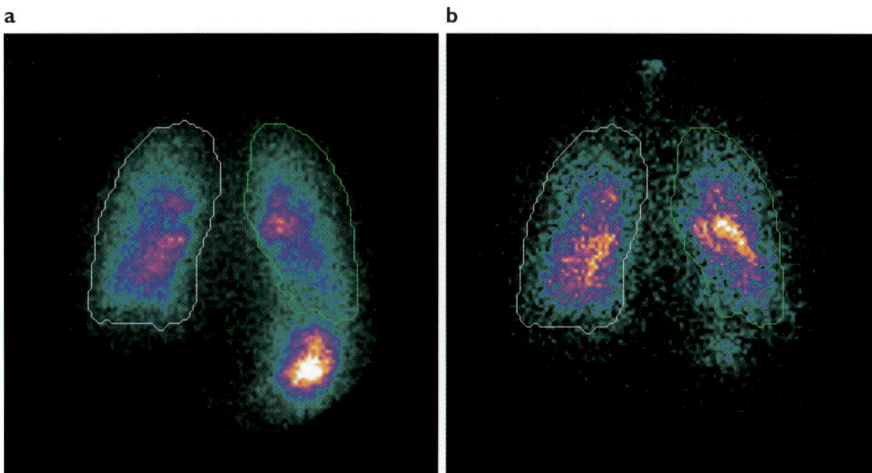

Fig. 4. Anterior lung deposition profile images obtained following the inhalation of a ^{99m}Tc DTPA-labelled INS365 solution from either the Pari LC Star nebulizer (**a**) or the AERx Pulmonary Delivery System (**b**).

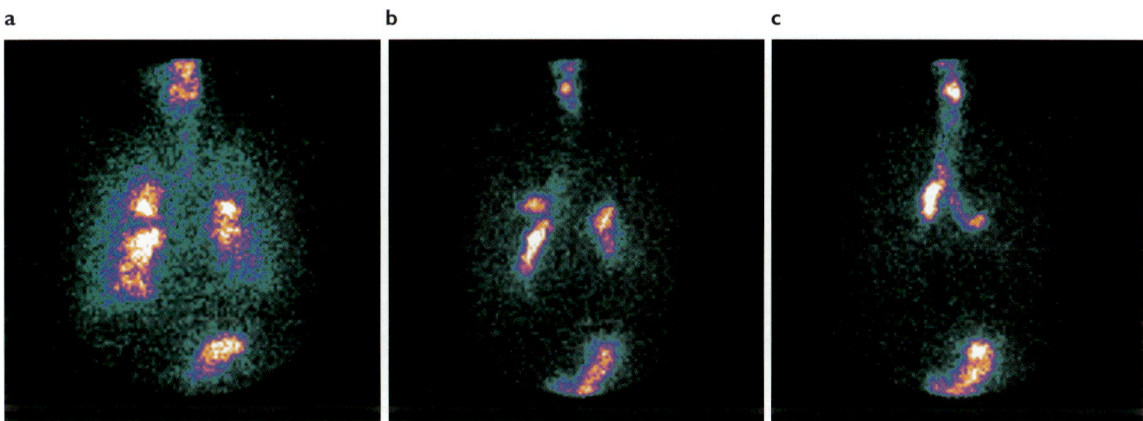

Fig. 5. Sequential images obtained 1 (**a**), 7 (**b**) and 15 min (**c**) after administration of 20 mg of INS365 solution showing clearance of the ^{99m}Tc DTPA label.

and INS365. Since both compounds are readily soluble in aqueous solution, standard air-jet nebulizers (Pari LC Plus and Star for UTP and INS365, respectively) were chosen for the initial clinical studies. Although these nebulizers (Pari Respiratory Equipment, Midlothian, Va., USA) have proven to be very effective in early studies, the administration typically takes between 12 and 15 min. Therefore, we have also evaluated a novel system that could have the potential to deliver a therapeutic amount of compound in one or two discrete inhalations. The AERx® Pulmonary Delivery System (Aradigm Corporation, Hayward, Calif., USA) uses an electro-mechanical mechanism to compress a small-volume blister (45 µl), generating and delivering a discrete bolus of fine monodispersed aerosol droplets at the optimal moment during inhalation (fig. 3).

Clinical Experience in Production of Deep-Lung Sputum Samples for Diagnosis

UTP has been studied in over 300 patients through a series of clinical trials in which it has been shown to be safe and well tolerated. Several well-controlled studies have demonstrated that UTP enhances sputum expectoration by several fold in a dose-related manner. Samples are highly enriched in lung cells of interest.

Clinical Experience in Respiratory Diseases

INS365 for the treatment of respiratory diseases, such as chronic bronchitis, has been studied in several phase I clinical trials in the UK and US. These studies have demonstrated that the compound is safe, well tolerated and that single inhaled doses significantly enhance sputum expectoration in smokers. The compound is moving into phase II in 2000.

Examples of deposition profiles, obtained immediately following dosing with either the Pari LC Star or the AERx system, taken from a gamma scintigraphy study conducted at Scintigraphics (Cardiff, UK) are shown in figure 4.

An interesting result of discrete bolus delivery of INS365 to the lungs using the AERx system appears to be a more rapid upregulation of mucociliary clearance compared to that seen for the nebulizer. Additional images taken from a second gamma scintigraphy study also conducted at Scintigraphics in 'healthy smokers' shows the clearance of the technetium label following dosing (fig. 5).

Conclusions

The outcome of enhanced mucociliary clearance, predicted from various in vitro and animal model test results, following stimulation of P2Y$_2$ receptors by novel agonists, UTP and INS365, have been demonstrated in several clinical studies. Further clinical studies are planned to confirm the utility of these molecules in anticipation of formal regulatory filings.

References

1 Drutz D, Shaffer C, LaCroix K, Jacobus K, Knowles MR, Bennett W, Regnis J, Hohneker K, Noone P, Davis W, Geary C, Boucher R: Uridine 5′-triphosphate (UTP) regulates mucociliary clearance via purinergic receptor activation. Drug Dev Res 1996;37:185.

2 Bennett WD, Olivier KN, Hohneker KW, Zeman KL, Edwards LJ, Boucher RC, Knowles MR: Effect of uridine 5′-triphosphate plus amiloride on mucociliary clearance in adult cystic fibrosis. Am J Resp Crit Care Med 1996;153: 1796–1801.

3 Knowles MR, Clarke LL, Boucher RC: Activation by extracellular nucleotides of chloride secretion in the airway epithelia of patients with cystic fibrosis N Engl J Med 1991;325: 533–538.

4 Dubyak GR, Cowen D, Mueller LM: Activation of inositol phospholipid breakdown in HL60 cells by P2-purinergic receptors for extracellular ATP. Evidence for mediation by both pertussis toxin-sensitive and pertussis toxin-insensitive mechanisms. J Biol Chem 1988; 263:18108–18117.

5 Fine J, Cole P, Davidson S: Extracellular nucleotides stimulate receptor-mediated calcium mobilization and inositol phosphate production in human fibroblasts. Biochem J 1989; 263:371–376.

6 Stutchfield J, Cockcroft S: Undifferentiated HL-60 cells respond to extracellular ATP and UTP by stimulating phospholipase C activation and exocytosis. FEBS Lett 1990;262:256–258.

7 Brown HA, Lazarowski ER, Boucher RC, Harden TK: Evidence that UTP and ATP regulate phospholipase C through a common extracellular 5′ nucleotide receptor in human airway epithelial cells. Mol Pharmacol 1991;40:648–655.

8 Olivier KN, Bennett WD, Hohneker KW, Zeman KL, Edwards LJ, Boucher RC, Knowles MR: Acute safety and effects on mucociliary clearance of aerosolised uridine 5′-triphosphate +/– amiloride in normal human adults. Am J Respir Crit Care Med 1996;154:217–223.

9 Knowles MR, Clarke LL, Boucher RC: Activation by extracellular nucleotides of chloride secretion in the airway epithelia of patients with cystic fibrosis. N Engl J Med 1991;325: 533–538.

10 Mason SJ, Paradiso AM, Boucher RC: Regulation of transepithelial ion transport and extracellular ATP in human normal and cystic fibrosis airway epithelium. Br J Pharmacol 1991; 103:1649–1656.

11 Jiang C, Finkbeiner WE, Widdecombe JA, McCray PB Jr, Miller SS: Altered fluid transport across airway epithelium in cystic fibrosis. Science 1993;262:424–427.

12 Benali R, Pierrot D, Zahm JM, de Bentzmann S, Puchelle E: Effect of extracellular ATP and UTP on fluid transport by human nasal epithelial cells in culture. J Respir Cell Mol Biol 1994; 10:363–368.

13 Lethem M, Dowell M, van Scott M, Yankaskas J, Egan T, Boucher RC, Davis C: Nucleotide regulation of goblet cells in human airway epithelial explants: Normal exocytosis in cystic fibrosis. Am J Respir Cell Mol Biol 1993;9: 315–322.

14 Gobran L, Xu Z, Lu Z, Rooney S: P2u Purinoceptor stimulation of surfactant secretion coupled to phosphatidylcholine hydrolysis in type II cells. Am J Physiol 1994;267;L625–L636.

15 Chaube S, Murphy ML: Protective effect of deoxycytidylic acid (CdMP) on hydroxyurea-induced malformations in rats. Teratology 1973;7:79–87.

16 Dougherty RW, Pendergast, W, Yerxa BR, Evans RM, Sabater JR, Lopez JA, Abraham WM, Picher M, Boucher RC: INS542 and INS37217: Novel P2Y$_2$ receptor agonists with enhanced biological stability induce prolonged stimulation of tracheal mucus velocity in vivo. Mucus and Cilia Satellite Symposium, 12th International Congress of the International Society for Aerosols in Medicine, Vienna, Austria, June 12–16, 1999.

Dr. Richard Evans
Inspire Pharmaceuticals Inc.
4222 Emperor Boulevard, Suite 470
Durham, NC 27703 (USA)
Tel. +1 919 941 9777 (ext. 280)
Fax +1 919 941 9797
E-Mail revans@inspirepharm.com

Protease Inhibitors

Tryptase Inhibition

James M. Clark   Robert E. Van Dyke   Matthias C. Kurth

Axys Pharmaceuticals, Inc., South San Francisco, Calif., USA

Summary

Tryptase, a mast-cell-specific serine protease, has been used for a number of years as a marker of mast cell activation. Elevated levels of the enzyme have been detected in allergic diseases including asthma, conjunctivitis and rhinitis, and in some diseases in which mast cell mediators have been hypothesized to play a role, such as rheumatoid arthritis, inflammatory bowel disease and interstitial cystitis. In the case of asthma, numerous studies suggested a role for tryptase in the underlying pathology of the disease. APC 366, a small molecule inhibitor of tryptase, has shown efficacy in vivo, thus confirming a causal role for tryptase in experimental models of allergic asthma. In recent phase II clinical trials, APC 366 has demonstrated efficacy in patients with mild to moderate asthma. Together, these data provide a compelling rationale for the development of tryptase inhibitors with greater potency and selectivity for the treatment of asthma and other allergic diseases.

Mechanism of Action

Tryptase is similar to trypsin in its ability to hydrolyze peptide substrates at sites C-terminal to basic amino acid residues. However, tryptase is unique among the serine proteases in having a tetrameric subunit structure stabilized by heparin [1], and in its resistance to inhibition by endogenous serine proteinase inhibitors [2]. The mechanistic basis for tryptase involvement in the pathology of asthma is not well understood. However, in vitro and ex vivo studies suggest a number of pathways through which tryptase may exert pathological effects in the airways. These include hydrolytic inactivation of endogenous bronchodilating peptides [3, 4], potentiation of histamine-induced bronchial smooth muscle contraction [5, 6], stimulation of inflammatory mediator release [7], recruitment of inflammatory cells [8, 9], stimulation of collagen synthesis [10, 11], enhanced mast cell degranulation [12], and mitogenic stimulation of lung fibroblasts [13], bronchial epithelial cells [7], or airway smooth muscle cells [14]. The ability of tryptase to inactivate vasoactive intestinal peptide and other bronchodilating peptides led to the proposal that this enzyme contributes to increased bronchoconstriction in asthma [3]. Consistent with this hypothesis, inhaled tryptase causes bronchoconstriction in allergic sheep [15]. Tryptase-induced IL-8 secretion [7] and inflammatory cell recruitment [8, 9] may contribute to the underlying airway inflammation associated with asthma (fig. 1). The mitogenic effects of tryptase on airway cells are largely blocked by active site-directed inhibitors of the enzyme, suggesting that unregulated or excessive tryptase activity may contribute to fibrotic changes in the airways. Recent reports that tryptase activates protease-activated receptor 2 (PAR2) are consistent with the requirement for catalytic activity in cell studies, and suggest a link between tryptase and intracellular signaling pathways activated by this novel class of receptors [16–18].

Preclinical Studies

APC 366, a first-generation peptidic inhibitor of tryptase (fig. 2), demonstrated efficacy in a sheep model of allergic asthma. Administered by inhalation, the compound blocked allergen-induced bronchoconstriction and reversed airway hyperresponsiveness to carbachol challenge [19]. APC 366 also reduced the allergen-induced influx of eosinophils into bronchial tissue, suggesting that tryptase inhibition promoted anti-inflammatory responses in allergen-challenged animals. Similar efficacy was noted with BABIM, a nonpeptidic inhibitor whose potency against tryptase is mediated by a unique, zinc-dependent mechanism [20]. Based on these studies, APC 366 was selected for evaluation in clinical trials to confirm the hypothesis that tryptase inhibition would indeed be a useful new therapeutic approach to treating asthma.

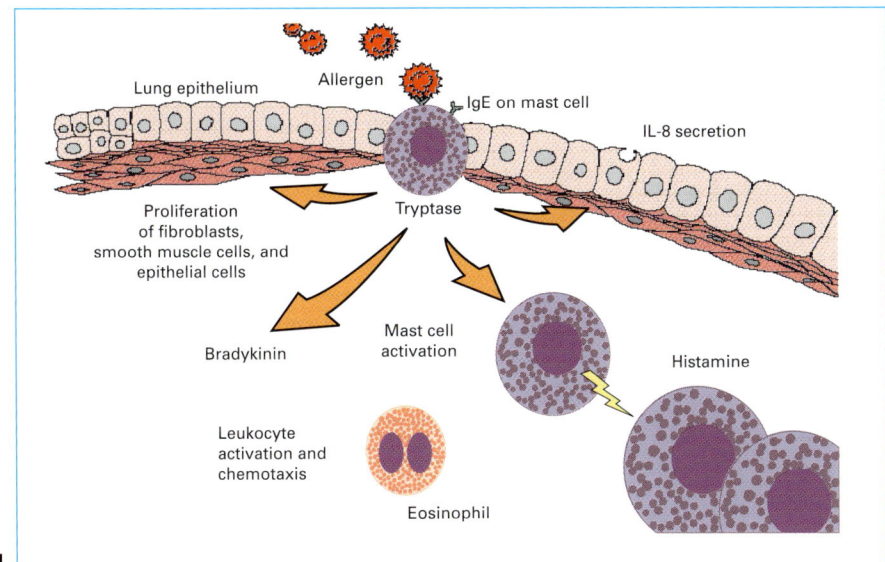
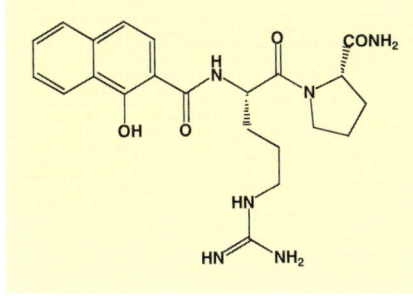

Fig. 1. Tryptase actions in asthma.
Fig. 2. Structure of APC 366.

Clinical Studies

A randomized double-blind placebo-controlled two-period cross-over study tested the hypothesis that mast cell tryptase contributes to allergen-provoked airway response in human asthmatics [unpubl. data]. The effect of APC 366 on allergen-provoked early airway response (EAR), late airway response (LAR) and the associated increase in bronchial hyperreactivity (BHR) was evaluated. Sixteen mild, atopic, nonsmoking subjects with asthma, controlled without the use of systemic or inhaled corticosteroids, participated in this study. All subjects underwent skin prick testing to aeroallergens and only those with at least one positive test were included. Subjects with significant illnesses, including respiratory infection, significant abnormalities in routine hematological and biochemical blood and urine examinations were excluded. All subjects demonstrated EAR with an FEV_1 decrease of at least 25% within 15 min of allergen challenge compared to postsaline baseline and LAR decrease of at least 15% compared to baseline occurring between 3 and 9 h after allergen inhalation. Furthermore, all subjects had ≥2-fold reduction in histamine PD_{20} compared to the pre-allergen challenge. Concomitant medications were discontinued before subjects entered the Clinical Study Unit.

In random sequence, either APC 366 (5 mg) or placebo was administered by aerosol inhalation three times daily at 6-hour intervals for 4 days and once on day 5 for a total of 13 treatments followed by another treatment period with either placebo or APC 366. Subjects underwent allergen challenge on day 4 after the 10th dose of medication followed by repeated spirometry to determine EAR and LAR. Determination of BHR via histamine challenge was performed on day 5 after the 13th dose of medication. Area under the time-response curve (AUC) was calculated for each subject for the EAR (0–2 h after allergen challenge) and LAR (3–9 h after allergen challenge). Allergen challenge resulted in both early- and late-phase reduction in FEV_1 after both active and placebo treatments (fig. 3). APC 366 treatment resulted in a slightly lower maximum FEV_1 fall compared to placebo for the EAR, but did not reach statistical significance (1.052 ± 0.209 vs. 1.183 ± 0.157). Similarly, AUC_{EAR} after APC 366 was somewhat lower than that determined after placebo treatment, but did not reach statistical significance. However, the maximum fall in FEV_1 during LAR was attenuated 21% by APC 366 treatment, a difference that was significant (0.786 ± 0.122 for APC 366 vs. 0.989 ± 0.124 for placebo, p = 0.007). Similarly, the LAR response when measured as AUC was significantly less (33%) after APC 366 treatment than after placebo treatment (–3897.2 ± 717.94 for APC 366 vs. –5856 ± 957.86 for placebo, p = 0.012). No significant differences were observed in allergen-induced BHR to histamine between the two treatment periods.

Subjects treated with APC 366 showed no drug-specific systemic adverse events. However, both active and placebo treatments resulted in some subjects experiencing transient bronchospasm after completing their inhalations. This was initially attributed to the solvent system used to administer APC 366 or placebo. However, in oth-

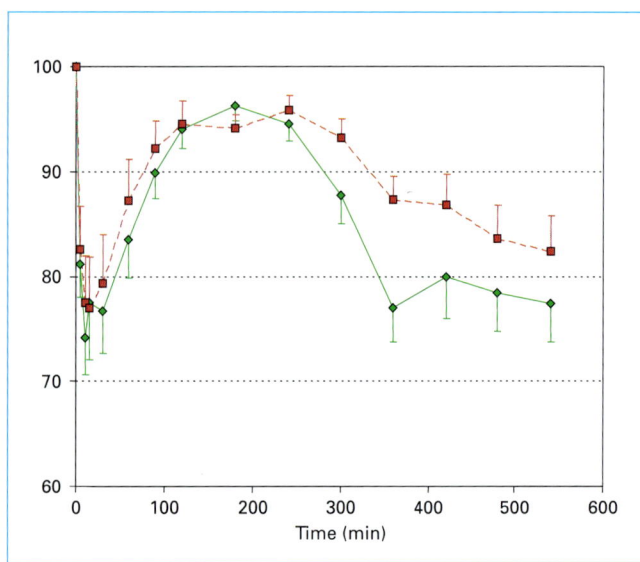

Fig. 3. Changes in FEV$_1$ in patients as a function of time after allergen challenge. —— = Placebo; - - - = APC 366.

er studies, similar results were observed with APC 366 delivered via a dry powder inhaler. While this adverse effect precluded continued clinical development of APC 366, second- and third-generation agents that are more selective, specific, and better tolerated are in development [21].

Conclusions

Initial phase II clinical studies with APC 366 strongly support the concept that mast cell tryptase contributes to the allergen-provoked airway response in human asthmatics and provide a compelling rationale for the continued development of more specific and selective tryptase inhibitors as novel treatments for asthma. The apparent link between tryptase and fibrotic responses also suggests the intriguing possibility that tryptase inhibitors may afford an advantage over existing therapeutics by mitigating the progressive fibrotic changes in the airway associated with severe, chronic asthma.

References

1 Schwartz LB, Lewis RA, Seldin D, Austen KF: Acid hydrolases and tryptase from secretory granules of dispersed human lung mast cells. J Immunol 1981;126:1290–1294.
2 Alter SC, Kramps JA, Janoff AA, Schwartz LB: Interactions of human mast cell tryptase with biological protease inhibitors. Arch Biochem Biophys 1990;276:26–31.
3 Tam EK, Caughey GH: Degradation of airway neuropeptides by human lung tryptase. Am J Respir Cell Mol Biol 1990;3:27–32.
4 Lilly CM, Martins MA, Drazen JM: Peptidase modulation of vasoactive intestinal peptide pulmonary relaxation in tracheal superfused guinea pig lungs. J Clin Invest 1993;91:235–243.
5 Sekizawa K, Caughey GH, Lazarus SC, Gold WM, Nadel JA: Mast cell tryptase causes airway smooth muscle hyperresponsiveness in dogs. J Clin Invest 1989;83:175–179.
6 Johnson PR, Ammit AJ, Carlin SM, Armour CL, Caughey GH, Black JL: Mast cell tryptase potentiates histamine-induced contraction in human sensitized bronchus. Eur Respir J 1997;10:38–43.
7 Cairns JA, Walls AF: Mast cell tryptase is a mitogen for epithelial cells. Stimulation of IL-8 production and intercellular adhesion molecule-1 expression. J Immunol 1996;156:275–283.
8 He S, Peng Q, Walls AF: Potent induction of a neutrophil and eosinophil-rich infiltrate in vivo by human mast cell tryptase: Selective enhancement of eosinophil recruitment by histamine. J Immunol 1997;159:6216–6225.
9 Huang C, Friend DS, Qiu WT, Wong GW, Morales G, Hunt J, Stevens RL: Induction of a selective and persistent extravasation of neutrophils into the peritoneal cavity cavity by tryptase mouse mast cell protease 6. J Immunol 1998;160:1910–1919.
10 Cairns JA, Walls AF: Mast cell tryptase stimulates the synthesis of type I collagen in human lung fibroblasts. J Clin Invest 1997;99:1313–1321.
11 Gruber BL, Kew RR, Jelaska A, Marchese MJ, Garlick J, Ren S, Schwartz LB, Korn JH: Human mast cells activate fibroblasts: Tryptase is a fibrogenic factor stimulating collagen messenger ribonucleic acid synthesis and fibroblast chemotaxis. J Immunol 1997;158:2310–2317.
12 He S, Gaca MD, Walls AF: A role for tryptase in the activation of human mast cells: Modulation of histamine release by tryptase and inhibitors of tryptase. J Pharmacol Exp Ther 1998;286:289–297.
13 Ruoss SJ, Hartmann T, Caughey, GH: Mast cell tryptase is a mitogen for cultured fibroblasts. J Clin Invest 1991;88:493–499.
14 Brown JK, Tyler CL, Jones CA, Ruoss SJ, Hartmann T, Caughey GH: Tryptase, the dominant secretory granule protein in human mast cells, is a potent mitogen for cultured dog tracheal smooth muscle cells. Am J Respir Cell Mol Biol 1995;13:227–236.
15 Molinari JF, Scuri M, Moore WR, Clark J, Tanaka R, Abraham WM: Inhaled tryptase causes bronchoconstriction in sheep via histamine release. Am J Respir Crit Care Med 1996;154:649–653.
16 Molino M, Barnathan ES, Numerof R, Clark J, Dreyer M, Cumashi A, Hoxie JA, Schechter N, Woolkalis M, Brass LF: Interactions of mast cell tryptase with thrombin receptors and PAR-2. J Biol Chem 1997;272:4043–4049.
17 Corvera CU, Dery O, McConalogue K, Bohm SK, Khitin LM, Caughey GH, Payan DG, Bunnett NW: Mast cell tryptase regulates rat colonic myocytes through proteinase-activated receptor 2. J Clin Invest 1997;100:1383–1393.
18 Schechter NM, Brass LF, Lavker RM, Jensen PJ: Reaction of mast cell proteases tryptase and chymase with protease activated receptors (PARS) on keratinocytes and fibroblasts. J Cell Physiol 1998;176:365–373.
19 Clark JM, Abraham WM, Fishman CE, Forteza R, Ahmed A, Cortes A, Warne RL, Moore WR, Tanaka RD: Tryptase inhibitors block allergen-induced airway and inflammatory responses in allergic sheep. Am J Respir Crit Care Med 995;152:2076–2083.
20 Katz BA, Clark JM, Finer-Moore JS, Jenkins TE, Johnson CR, Ross MJ, Luong C, Moore WR, Stroud RM: Design of potent selective zinc-mediated serine protease inhibitors. Nature 1998;391:608–612.
21 Rice KD, Tanaka RD, Katz BA, Numerof RP, Moore WR: Inhibitors of tryptase for the treatment of mast cell-mediated diseases. Curr Pharm Design 1998;4:381–396.

James M. Clark, Axys Pharmaceuticals, Inc.
180 Kimball Way
S. San Francisco, CA 94080 (USA)
Tel. +1 650 829 1003, Fax +1 650 829 1350
E-Mail clark@axyspharm.com

Neutrophil Elastase Inhibitors

Robin A. Smith[a]   Robert A. Stockley[b]   Simon T. Hodgson[a]

[a]GlaxoWellcome R&D, Stevenage, and [b]Department of Medicine, Queen Elizabeth Hospital, Birmingham, UK

Summary

Neutrophil elastase has been implicated in COPD for many years. The enzyme has a variety of effects that can contribute to the disease process, particularly in lung degradation and mucus secretion. Several approaches have been taken to the design and delivery of elastase inhibitors to the lung. The pros and cons of each are discussed in this review.

The first direct studies demonstrating that a proteolytic enzyme has the ability to induce emphysema were carried out by Gross et al. [1] in 1964. These authors induced changes similar to emphysema using the plant proteinase papain. Subsequent animal studies suggested that only enzymes able to degrade elastin could induce these changes. Instillation of elastase into the airway led to a rapid loss of lung elastin [2]. This was gradually replaced, but there was disruption of the normal alveolar architecture. The central role of elastin in maintaining alveolar structure is also indicated by the tendency of patients with cutis laxa (a genetic defect of elastin formation) to develop emphysema spontaneously [3]. Additionally, prevention of normal elastin repair leads to the development of more severe emphysema [4].

Enzymes Responsible

Animal models show that the serine proteases human neutrophil elastase (NE) and human proteinase 3 can produce emphysema [5, 6]. Cathepsin B also has this capability [7] after activation of its pro-enzyme by NE [8]. The central role of NE and proteinase 3 is also consistent with the increased tendency of subjects with α_1-AT deficiency to develop rapid early onset emphysema [9], since α_1-AT is their major inhibitor.

Interest in MMPs in emphysema has increased recently. For example, human collagenase [10] and macrophage metalloelastase [11], have been implicated. However, classic studies by Damiano et al. [12] suggest that NE is the key enzyme involved by clearly correlating the amount of immunoreactive NE in the lung tissue with the degree of emphysema. There is much interplay between MMPs, serine proteases and their respective inhibitors, and it is probable that emphysema results from the concentrated actions of both classes of protease. Inhibition of elastase alone may well prove critical, however.

Hypersecretory Diseases

Early evidence implicated NE in emphysema, but the enzyme has several other potential roles in lung disease (fig. 1). It may play a major part in airway mucus production in chronic bronchitis and other bronchial diseases such as bronchiectasis, cystic fibrosis and asthma [13, 14]. NE has been shown to promote both mucin gene transcription [15] and release from airway cells [16]. Since patients often exhibit elements of both emphysema and of mucus production, NE inhibition might prove to be a very effective therapy for COPD.

Mechanism Involved in Emphysema

Both NE and proteinase 3 are stored fully formed and as active enzymes bound to chondritin and heparan sulphates within the azurophil granules of the mature neutrophil. Activation of adherent neutrophils indicates that the degradation of connective tissue is largely dependent

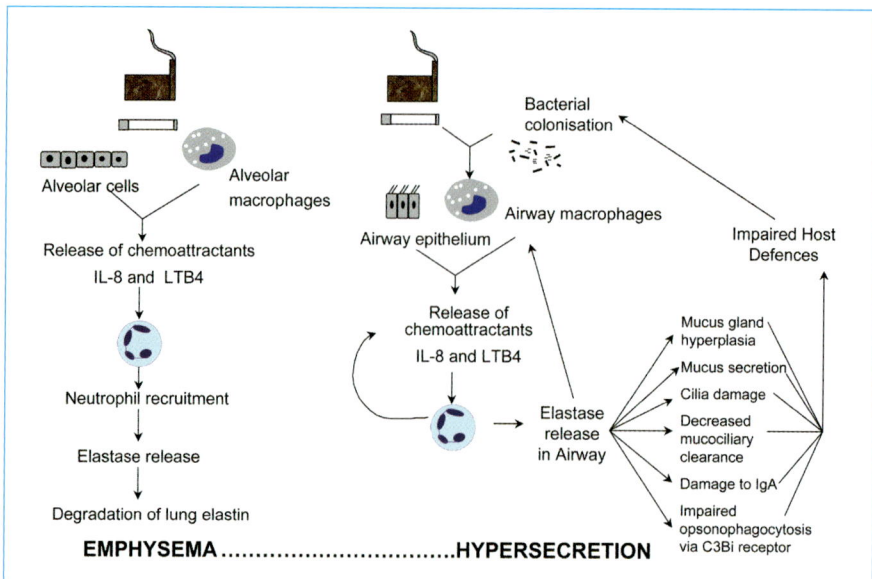

Fig. 1. Effects of NE in lung disease.

on NE [17]. Surprisingly, this process cannot be completely inhibited even by supernormal concentrations of α_1-AT. Several factors combine to decrease this inhibition: (1) exclusion of the protein from the very narrow interface between the adherent neutrophil and the connective tissue [18]; (2) some NE is released as the azurophil granule is exocytosed and spreads along the cell surface [19] where it retains its proteolytic activity, but is more resistant to inactivation by α_1-AT; (3) the concentration of NE in the azurophil granule is approximately 5 mM, which is at least 2 orders of magnitude above the normal physiological concentration of α_1-AT. As NE diffuses away from the granule, its concentration rapidly drops and it is inactivated; (4) elastase released from the azurophil can become bound to elastin. Here it is poorly inhibited by α_1-AT [20]. By contrast, secretory leukoproteinase inhibitor (SLPI) can inhibit NE while still bound to elastin, preventing further degradation [20].

Therapeutic Approach

In emphysema, pathogenic processes take place in the lung interstitium so that an effective inhibitor would need to:
1. achieve prolonged and possibly irreversible, inhibition of the enzyme
2. inhibit enzyme bound to elastin
3. maintain a sufficient concentration in the interstitium
4. inhibit cell surface elastase

The ideal inhibitor would be administered orally and be of small molecular weight. Very few clinical studies of such compounds have been published. However, MR 889, a relatively weak, reversible elastase inhibitor reduced urinary desmosine levels (a marker of elastin breakdown) in a subset of COPD patients after 4 weeks of oral dosing [21]. This result suggests that a more potent inhibitor might prove therapeutically useful long-term.

Alternatively, the agent could be administered as an aerosol into the airway. To treat emphysema, however, it would need to penetrate the tight epithelial cell junctions to reach the interstitium. This barrier creates a major therapeutic problem, unlike the more easily penetrated endothelial barrier from the systemic circulation [22]. It is now believed, however, that NE may also play a major role in bronchial diseases [13, 14], in which elastase in the airway would be an important target. Here inhalation might be appropriate. The potential effectiveness of topically dosed NE inhibitors in vivo is shown for GR 243214, a prototype inhibitor that could be administered by aerosol (fig. 2a).

Finally, perhaps the most attractive approach would be to target the neutrophil itself. Intracellular elastase inhibitors have been designed which penetrate neutrophils and inactivate the enzyme within the azurophil granule. This limits the area of damage produced during cell migration and degranulation. Such compounds should avoid many of the pitfalls mentioned above. Very effective and long-lasting inhibition of intracellular elastase has been achieved with this approach. Figure 2b shows the effect in dogs given a single dose of GW 311616 (a prototype intracellular elastase inhibitor). Importantly, effective inhibi-

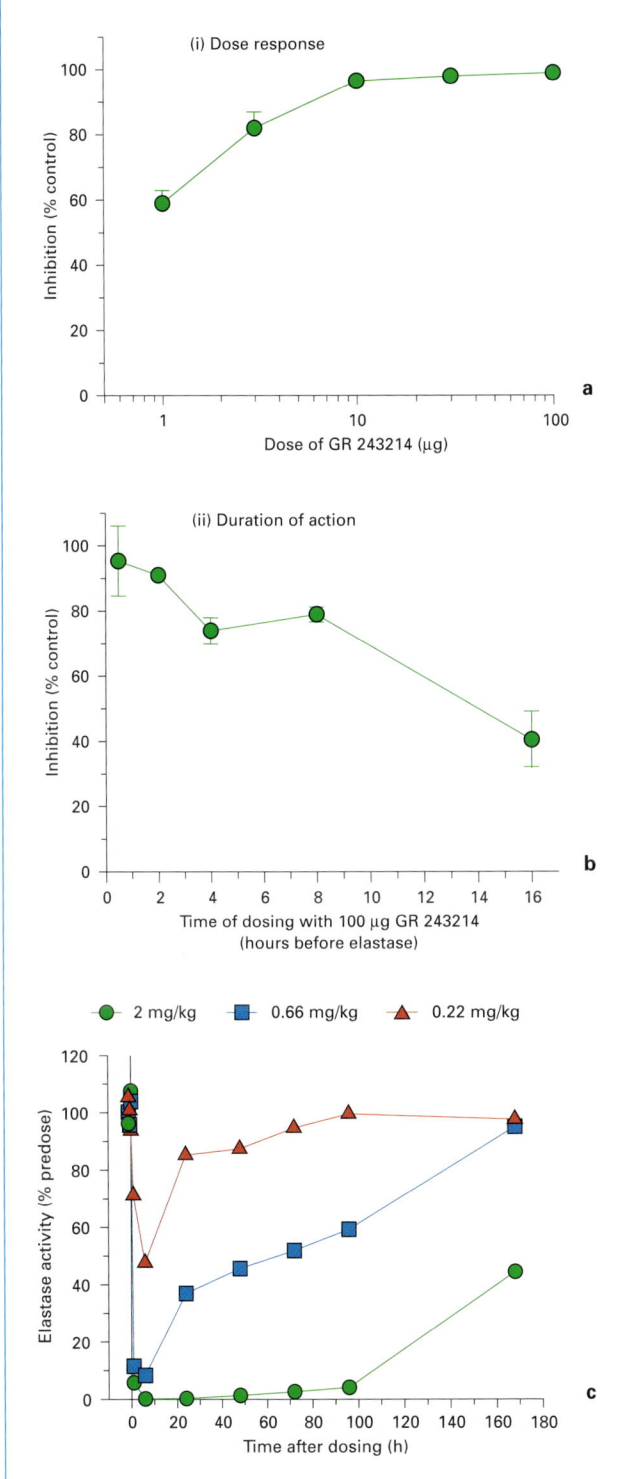

Table 1. Examples of elastase inhibitors

	Chemical class	Properties	Status
Endogenous inhibitors			
α_1-AT, SLPI, elafin	natural products	several approaches taken: purified, oxidation resistant recombinant, genetic transfer	some in phase II
Synthetic compounds			
Sivelestat (ONO-5046)	ester	extracellular, injectable	registered for acute lung injury associated with SIRS; in phase III for IPF
Midesteine MR889	ester	oral, reversible	phase III
ZD 8321	peptidyl-trifluormethyl ketone	extracellular, oral, slowly reversible	in phase II
DMP 777	β-lactam	intracellular, oral pseudo-irreversible	in phase II
ZD 0892	peptidyl-trifluormethyl ketone	extracellular, oral, reversible	in phase I
GW243214	translactam	extracellular, inhaled pseudo-irreversible	
GW311616	translactam	intracellular, oral, pseudo-irreversible	

SIRS = Systemic inflammatory response syndrome; IPF = idiopathic pulmonary fibrosis.

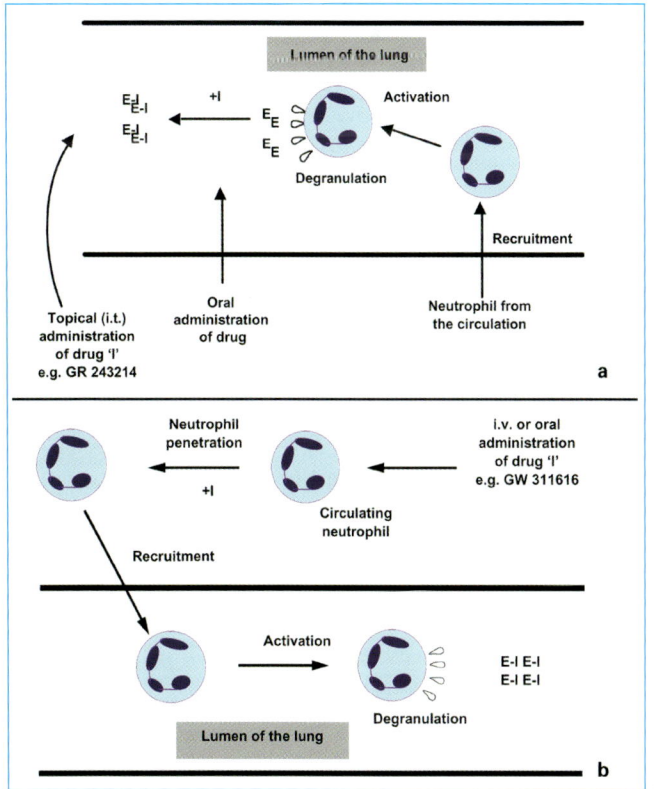

Fig. 2. Methods of inhibition of elastase. **a**, **b** Inhibition of extracellular elastase in vivo. Hamsters were dosed intratracheally with GR243214 for either 30 min (**a**) or for variable times (**b**) before elastase. **c** Inhibition of intracellular elastase in peripheral blood neutrophils in vivo. Dogs were dosed orally with GW311616.

Fig. 3. Elastase inhibition in vivo. **a** Extracellular. **b** Intracellular.

tion of elastase in the lung has been demonstrated in man with DMP 777, a compound of this type [23]. (A cartoon illustrating the different mechanisms of action of extra- and intracellular inhibitors is shown in fig. 3.)

Table 1 shows some NE inhibitors considered for development.

Safety

The major physiological role of NE is believed to be in host defence. Knockout mice lacking the enzyme are more vulnerable to overwhelming infections by 2 strains of gram-negative bacteria. Conversely, they are less susceptible to the strains of gram-positive bacteria tested [24]. The mice grow and develop normally, and are not at increased risk of spontaneous infection. Limited data have been published on the toxicology of synthetic elastase inhibitors. Minor effects only were reported for ONO 5046 (a competitive elastase inhibitor, registered for use in patients with acute lung injury associated with systemic inflammatory response syndrome) in animals [25]. Other compounds (e.g. DMP 777 and ZD 8321) are in phase II, suggesting that toxicity is not a problem. MR 889 was last reported to be in phase III and is known to be well tolerated [21].

Conclusion

NE has many detrimental effects relevant to COPD. Industrial and academic groups have sought inhibitors of the enzyme for many years, but identification of molecules with the appropriate profiles for use in the disease has proved difficult and few clinical data with inhibitors have been published. The true worth of NE inhibition in COPD will only be demonstrated once well-designed trials with effective inhibitors have been conducted. Results with the new elastase inhibitors are keenly anticipated.

References

1 Gross P, Pfitzer EA, Tolker E et al: Experimental emphysema, its production with papain in normal and silicotic rats. Arch Environ Health 1964;11:50–58.
2 Kuhn C, Slodkowska J, Smith T, Starcher B: The tissue response to exogenous elastase. Bull Europ Physiopath Resp 1980;16 (suppl) 127–137.
3 Harris RB, Heaphy MR, Perry HO: Generalized elastolysis (cutis laxa). Am J Med 1978;65: 815–822.
4 Kuhn C, Starcher BC: The effect of lathyrogens on the evaluation of elastase-induced emphysema. Am Rev Respir Dis 1980;122:453–460.
5 Janoff A, Sloan B, Weinbaum G et al: Experimental emphysema induced with purified human neutrophil elastase: Tissue localization of the instilled protease. Am Rev Respir Dis 1977;115:461–478.
6 Kao RC, Wehner NG, Skubitz KM et al: Proteinase 3 – a distinct human polymorphonuclear leukocyte proteinase that produces emphysema in hamsters. J Clin Invest 1988;82: 1963–1973.
7 Lesser M, Padilla ML, Cardozo C: Induction of emphysema in hamsters by intra-tracheal instillation of cathepsin B. Am Rev Respir Dis 1992;145:661–668.
8 Buttle DJ, Abrahamson M, Burnett D, et al: Human sputum cathepsin B degrades proteoglycan, is inhibited by α_2-macroglobulin and is modulated by neutrophil elastase cleavage of cathepsin B precursor and cystatin C. Biochem J 1991;276:325–331.
9 Larsson C: Natural history and life expectancy in severe α_1 antitrypsin deficiency, Pi Z. Acta Med Scand 1978;204:345–351.
10 D'Armiento J, Dalal SS, Okaela Y, et al: Collagenase expression in the lungs of transgenic mice causes pulmonary emphysema. Cell 1992; 71:955–961.
11 Hautamaki RD, Kobayashi DK, Senior RM, Shapiro SD: Requirement for macrophage elastase for cigarette smoking-induced emphysema in mice. Science 1997;277:2002–2004.
12 Damiano VV, Tsang A, Kucich U, et al: Immunolocalization of elastase in human emphysematous lungs. J Clin Invest 1986;78:482–493.
13 Stockley RA: Bronchiectasis – new therapeutic approaches based on pathogenesis. Clin Chest Med 1987;8:481–494.
14 Nadel JA, Takeyama K, Agusti: Role of neutrophil elastase in hypersecretion in asthma. Eur Respir J 1999;13:190–196.
15 Voynow JA, Young LR, Wang Y, Horger T, Rose MC, Fischer BM: Neutrophil elastase increases MUC5AC mRNA and protein expression in respiratory epithelial cells. Am J Physiol 1999;276:L835–L843.
16 Sommerhoff CP, Nadel JA, Basbaum CB, Caughey GH: Neutrophil elastase and to a lesser extent, cathepsin G stimulate secretion from cultured bovine airway serous cell. J Clin Invest 1990;85:682–689.
17 Chamba A, Afford SC, Stockley RA, Burnett D: Extracellular proteolysis of fibronectin by neutrophils: Characterization and the effects of recombinant cytokines. Am J Respir Cell Mol Biol 1991;4:330–337.
18 Campbell EJ, Senior RM, McDonald JA, Cox DW: Proteolysis by neutrophils. Relative importance of cell-substrate contact and oxidative inactivation of proteinase inhibitors in vitro. J Clin Invest 1982;70:845–852.
19 Owen CA, Campbell MA, Sannes PL, Boukedes SS, Campbell EJ: Cell-surface-bound elastase and cathepsin G on human neutrophils: A novel, non-oxidative mechanism by which neutrophils focus and preserve catalytic activity of serine proteinases. J Cell Biol 1995; 131:775.
20 Morrison HM, Welgus HG, Stockley RA, et al: Inhibition of human leukocyte elastase bound to elastin: Relative ineffectiveness and two mechanisms of inhibitory activity. Am J Respir Cell Mol Biol 1990;2:263–269.
21 Luisetti M, Sturani C, Sella D, Madonini E, Galavotti V, Bruno G, Peona V, Kucich U, Dagnino G, Rosenbloom J, Starcher B, Grassi C: MR889, a neutrophil elastase inhibitor, in patients with chronic obstructive pulmonary disease: A double-blind, randomised, placebo-controlled clinical trial. Eur Respir J 1996;9: 1482–1486.
22 Gorin AB, Stewart PA: Differential permeability of endothelial and epithelial barriers to albumin flux. J Appl Physiol 1979;47:1315–1324.
23 Vender RL, Burcham DL, Quon CY: DMP 777: A synthetic human neutrophil-elastase inhibitor as therapy for cystic fibrosis. Ped Pulmonol 1998;17S:136–137.
24 Belaaouaj A, McCarthy R, Baumann M, Gao ZM, Ley TJ, Abraham SN, Shapiro AD: Mice lacking neutrophil elastase reveal impaired host defense against gram-negative bacterial sepsis. Nat Med 1998;4:615–618.
25 J Toxicol Sci 1998;23(suppl III):409–538.

Dr. Robin A. Smith
Enzyme Pharmacology, GlaxoWellcome R&D
Gunnelswoods Road
Stevenage, Herts SG1 2NY (UK)
Tel. +44 1438 764 070, Fax +44 1438 763 363
E-Mail ras0782@glaxowellcome.co.uk

Macrophage Metalloelastase Inhibitors

Robert L. Martin[a]   Steven D. Shapiro[b]   Sandra E. Tong[a]   Harold E. Van Wart[a]

[a]Inflammatory Diseases Unit, Roche Bioscience, Palo Alto, Calif., and [b]Department of Medicine, Washington University, St. Louis, Mo., USA

Summary

There are currently no therapies that inhibit the progressive destruction of alveoli in emphysema. This process is characterized by the degradation of lung elastin by elastases. While early attention was focused on the role of neutrophil elastase in the disease, more recent evidence supports a strong rationale for macrophage elastase, a member of the matrix metalloproteinase family.

Role of Proteases in the Pathophysiology of Emphysema

Emphysema is a degenerative lung disease characterized by the destruction of the alveoli. The disease is caused primarily by cigarette smoking, which results in an accumulation of both neutrophils and macrophages in the respiratory bronchioles and alveolar spaces. The prevailing hypothesis for the pathogenesis of emphysema is a protease-antiprotease imbalance in the lung parenchyma [1]. The focus has been on the role of elastases capable of destroying the elastic fibers that comprise the alveoli. Traditionally, elastin has been recognized as a matrix component that is extremely resistant to proteolysis, signifying a key role for specific elastases in elastin destruction. The physiological consequence of alveolar destruction is a decrease in the elastic recoil of the lungs resulting in hyperinflation and impaired pulmonary function. Perhaps more importantly, loss of elastic fiber attachments of the small airways predisposes to airway collapse with consequent airflow obstruction.

The protease-antiprotease hypothesis was initially formulated in response to the observation that a subset of prematurely emphysematous patients possessed homozygous deficiency for α_1-protease inhibitor, a protein that inhibits serine proteases including neutrophil elastase. The hypothesis was supported further by animal models in which emphysema-like changes were induced upon administration of elastolytic enzymes [1]. Historically, emphasis had been placed on the role of neutrophil elastase as the primary mediator of matrix destruction because α_1-protease inhibitor is the natural inhibitor of this elastase. However, an elastase from murine macrophages was purified and characterized in 1981 [2]. Several years later, the human macrophage enzyme was identified [3]. In contrast to neutrophil elastase, macrophage elastase (ME) is a metalloprotease, more specifically a member of the matrix metalloproteinase (MMP) family.

Macrophage Elastase and the MMP Family

The MMPs, also referred to as the matrixins, are a family of metalloproteases that has become recognized for its ability to degrade matrix macromolecules. The MMPs contain an active-site zinc atom that is chelated by the three histidine residues that are part of the HEXXH + H motif. They also contain a conserved methionine residue that forms part of a 1,4-turn and whose side chain creates a hydrophobic environment for the zinc-binding site. Thus, the MMPs are part of the larger 'metzincin' family. All of the MMPs also have a conserved cysteine-switch

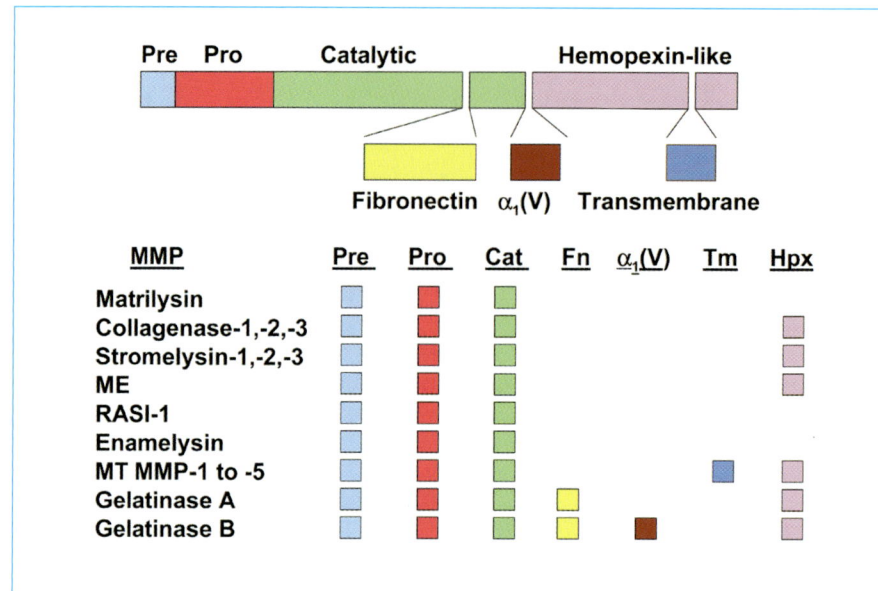

Fig. 1. Domain structure of the MMP family.

motif involved in the latency of the pro-MMP zymogens [4]. The MMPs also share the property that they are inhibited by one of the four naturally occurring tissue inhibitors of metalloproteinases (TIMPs) [5]. The members of the family differ with regard to their domain structure (fig. 1). The MMPs are classified either by their protein substrate specificity, as for ME which is named after its ability to degrade elastin, or by shared structural features, such as the transmembrane domain that distinguishes the five known membrane-type MMPs. While MMPs have attracted most interest, based on their ability to degrade components of the extracellular matrix, other nonmatrix substrates exist for these enzymes. For example, several MMPs, including ME, can cleave and inactivate α_1-protease inhibitor [6–9]. Thus, the MMPs can modulate the activities of serine proteases such as neutrophil elastase.

Macrophage Elastase and Emphysema

Macrophages comprise over 90% of the inflammatory cells in the lungs of smokers. With the discovery that macrophages produce ME, its potential role in emphysema has been investigated. Increased expression of ME has been found in lung samples from emphysema patients, supporting the possible involvement of the enzyme in the pathophysiology of the disease [10]. Stronger support for the role of ME in emphysema was obtained by generating a knockout mouse in which the ME gene was deleted. In contrast to wild-type mice, ME(−/−) mice did not develop emphysema in a murine smoke-induced emphysema model [11]. This model mimics the human disease in that it is triggered by cigarette smoke and is slowly progressing. An additional, unexpected finding was a reduction in the number of macrophages that normally accumulate in the lung after smoke exposure. Subsequent research suggests that ME-generated elastin fragments chemotactically attract macrophages into the lung and also induce ME expression [unpubl. obs.]. Thus, ME is the central mediator in a cycle of elastin degradation and macrophage recruitment. In addition, ME may also play a pathological role by augmentation of neutrophil elastase activity through inactivation of α_1-protease inhibitor [6, 7]. More recently, the role of macrophages in the development of emphysema has been demonstrated in rats that have been chronically exposed to cigarette smoke [12].

Synthetic MMP Inhibitors

The catalytic zinc atom in the MMPs binds the carbonyl group of the scissile peptide bond (P_1-P_1') of the substrate and activates it for hydrolysis. The specificity of the individual MMP for its substrate is determined by the degree of complementarity between the specificity pockets on the enzyme ($S_n...S_n'$) and the residues in the substrate ($P_n....P_n'$). Typically, synthetic inhibitors contain a zinc-chelating group (e.g., a carboxylate or a hydroxamate moiety) attached to a pharmacophore that binds favorably in the S_n pockets on either the primed or nonprimed side of the enzyme [13]. The S_1' subsite is the best defined substrate recognition feature of the MMPs and has played a prominent role in the design of potent, selective inhibitors. MMP inhibitors have been proposed as therapies for a variety of disease indications including arthritis, cancer, multiple sclerosis, congestive heart failure. Since emphysema is a disease of lung elastin degradation that may be caused by ME, inhibitors of ME have therapeutic potential in the treatment of the disease.

Inhibition of Smoke-Induced Emphysema by MMP Inhibitors

To investigate the role of MMPs in an animal model of emphysema, two orally bioavailable synthetic inhibitors (RS-113456 and RS-132908) have been tested in the murine smoke-induced emphysema model. In this model, mice are exposed to chronic cigarette smoke, resulting in alveolar destruction as measured by changes in the mean linear intercept of lung tissue that has been fixed at constant pressure. The changes are consistent with the pathology observed in the lungs of human smokers, although human lungs also exhibit destruction of bronchioles, a structure not present in mouse lungs. In mice, an increase of approximately 50% in the number of lung macrophages can be observed as early as 1 month after smoke exposure. After 6 months of smoke exposure, there is an approximate 3-fold increase in the number of macrophages. After 1 month of smoke exposure, the expression of ME in the lungs of these mice is increased as well. The mice start to develop alveolar destruction after 6 weeks and this continues throughout the 6 months of smoke exposure.

The inhibition constants for the two inhibitors are listed in table 1. Both compounds are potent (<1.2 nM) inhibitors of both human and murine ME. RS-132908 was administered in a preventive protocol in which the compound was dosed at 50 mg/kg b.i.d. throughout the entire six month smoking period. In contrast, RS-113456 was administered in a treatment protocol in which the mice were allowed to establish their emphysema in three months of smoking, after which the compound was dosed at 50 mg/kg b.i.d. for the remaining 3 months of smoking. At 6-week intervals, study groups were sacrificed and the mean linear intercepts and lung macrophage contents were determined, as shown in figures 2 and 3, respectively.

RS-132908 markedly inhibited the smoke-induced increase in mean linear intercept at every 6-week observation and produced a 74% inhibition at the end of 6 months of smoke exposure (fig. 2). Likewise, there was a reduction in macrophage accumulation within the lung tissue, which also reached about 75% inhibition after 6 months (fig. 3). These results are consistent with the postulated roles for ME in the development of emphysema. In the treatment protocol, RS-113456 was also extremely

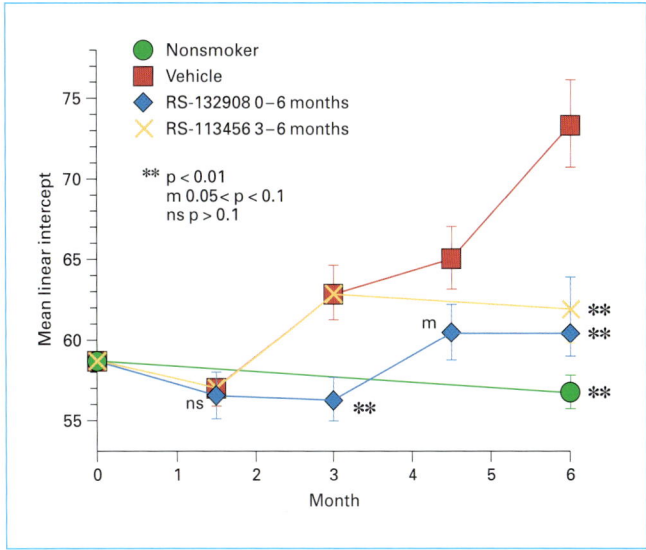

Fig. 2. Effect of MMP inhibitors on smoke-induced emphysema. Groups of fifteen C57BL/6 mice, 12 weeks of age, were exposed to the smoke from two nonfiltered cigarettes for 6 days a week, up to 6 months. Study drugs were administered orally by gavage at a dose of 50 mg/kg b.i.d. The mice were sacrificed, the lungs inflated to 25 cm H$_2$O pressure in formalin and fixed. Histologic sections were prepared from the lungs. Airspace enlargement was quantified by determining the mean linear intercept (Lm) by point counting of midsagittal sections.

Table 1. In vitro inhibition profile of test compounds

Enzyme	K_i, nM	
	RS-132908	RS-113456
ME	0.12	0.033
Murine ME	0.58	1.2
Collagenase-1	360	70
Collagenase-3	0.23	0.17
Gelatinase B	0.41	0.065
Stromelysin-1	12	5.2
MT-MMP-1	0.30	0.089

K_i values were determined in a continuous fluorogenic assay. All enzymes tested were recombinant human enzymes except where noted. MT-MMP-1 = Membrane-type MMP-1.

efficacious. The compound completely blocked further disease progression as measured by mean linear intercept changes. Interestingly, it also reduced the interstitial macrophage concentration by the same amount as RS-132908, even though this compound was only dosed for the last 3 months. These studies indicate that MMP inhibitors have the potential to block progression in established

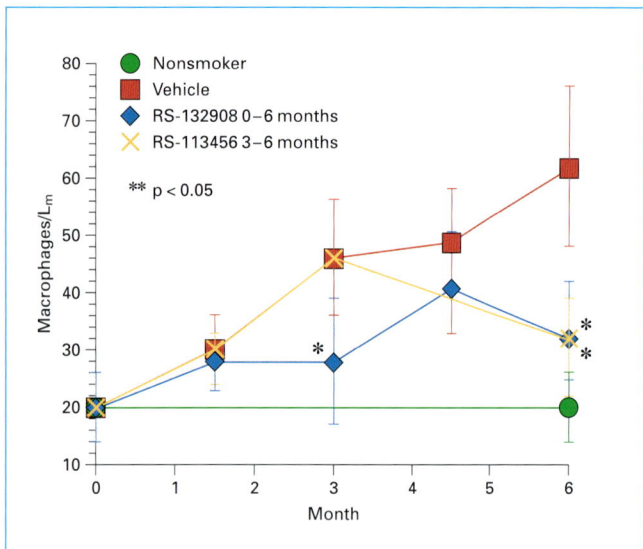

Fig. 3. Effect of MMP inhibitors on macrophage accumulation in the lung. Interstitial macrophage accumulation in the lung was determined by identifying macrophages by murine Mac-3 (rat antibody against mouse Mac-3 protein; PharMingen, San Diego, Calif., USA) immunostaining. Cell counts were determined by counting five random high-power fields at ×400. The positive-staining macrophage counts were normalized to airspace area.

disease. These data provide strong preclinical support for a role of MMPs in the development of emphysema. Experiments with more selective ME inhibitors will be required to pinpoint ME as the dominant MMP in this process.

Conclusions

It has long been recognized that elastases may play a prominent role in promoting the destruction of alveoli in human emphysema. Initially, attention was focused on neutrophil elastase because of the genetic susceptibility of patients deficient in α_1-protease inhibitor. However, these patients represent a small fraction of those with emphysema and it is possible that the role of neutrophil elastase is over-represented in this population. The more recent discovery of ME and the observation that ME (–/–) knockout mice are resistant to smoke-induced emphysema have raised the possibility that ME may be an important mediator of the disease. The efficacy observed with the MMP inhibitors in the murine emphysema model provides strong support for this concept and indicates that MMP inhibitors may have therapeutic potential in treatment of the disease.

References

1 McElvaney NG, Crystal RG: Proteases and lung injury; in Crystal RG, West JB (eds): The Lung, ed 2., Philadelphia, Lippincott, 1997, pp 2205–2278.
2 Banda MJ, Werb Z: Mouse macrophage elastase: Purification and characterization as a metalloproteinase. Biochem J 1981;193:589–605.
3 Shapiro SD, Kobayashi DK, Ley TJ: Cloning and characterization of a unique elastolytic metalloproteinase produced by human alveolar macrophages. J Biol Chem 1993;268:23824–23829.
4 Van Wart HE, Birkedal-Hansen H: The cysteine switch: A principle of regulation of metalloproteinase activity with potential applicability to the entire matrix metalloproteinase family. Proc Natl Acad Sci USA 1990;87:5578–5582.
5 Birkedal-Hansen H, Moore WGI, Bodeen MK, Windsor LJ, Birkedal-Hansen B, DeCarlo A, Engler JA: Matrix metalloproteinases: A review. Crit Rev Oral Biol Med 1993;4:197–250.
6 Banda MJ, Clark EJ, Werb Z: Limited proteolysis by macrophage elastase inactivates human α-proteinase inhibitor. J Exp Med 1980;152:1563–1570.
7 Gronski TJ, Martin RL, Kobayashi DK, Walsh BC, Holman MC, Huber M, Van Wart HE, Shapiro SD: Hydrolysis of a broad spectrum of extracellular matrix proteins by human macrophage elastase. J Biol Chem 1997;272:12189–12194.
8 Sires UI, Murphy G, Baragi VM, Fliszar CJ, Welgus HG, Senior RM: Matrilysin is much more efficient than other matrix metalloproteinases in the proteolytic inactivation of α-antitrypsin. Biochem Biophys Res Commun 1994;204:613–620.
9 Desrochers PE, Jeffrey JJ, Weiss SJ: Interstitial collagenase (matrix metalloproteinase-1) expresses serpinase activity. J Clin Invest 1991;87:2258–2265.
10 Shapiro SD: The pathogenesis of emphysema: The elastase:antielastase hypothesis 30 years later. Proc Assoc Am Physicians 1995;107:346–352.
11 Hautamaki RD, Kobayashi DK, Senior RM, Shapiro SD: Requirement for macrophage elastase for cigarette smoke-induced emphysema in mice. Science 1997;277:2002–2004.
12 Ofulue AF, Ko M: Effects of depletion of neutrophils or macrophages on development of cigarette smoke-induced emphysema. Am J Physiol 1999;277:L97–L105.
13 Brown PD: Synthetic inhibitors of Matrix metalloproteinases; in Parks WC Mecham RP (eds): Matrix Metalloproteinases. San Diego, Academic Press, 1998, pp 243–261.

Robert L. Martin
Roche Pharmaceuticals
3401 Hillview Ave., Mail Stop A1-4
Palo Alto, CA 94304 (USA)
Tel. +1 650 855 5670, Fax +1 650 496 3500
E-Mail robert-v.martin@roche.com

Allergen- and IgE-Directed Therapies

Allergen, IgE and Mast-Cell-Directed Therapies: An Overview

Mark Larché   A. Barry Kay

Department of Allergy and Clinical Immunology, Imperial College School of Medicine, National Heart and Lung Institute, London, UK

Summary

In addition to traditional drug development strategies, a number of current approaches focus on modulation of the immune response to allergens or, the allergens themselves. Disease-modulating specific immunotherapy has been used for many years and has been shown to be efficacious, although this form of treatment is slow and carries the risk of systemic adverse reactions. The identification of naturally occurring allergen isoforms of the native protein which do not bind IgE has led to modification of a number of allergens by site-directed mutagenesis. Such proteins have a reduced or absent interaction with IgE whilst retaining much of their ability to stimulate T cells. The improved safety profile of such molecules may result in larger, more efficacious doses of protein being given with improved safety. Fragments of allergen molecules, such as peptides, are also under development, employing a similar rationale of destroying IgE binding epitopes whilst retaining T cell determinants. Neutralization of specific molecules in the inflammatory cascade is currently being addressed with 'humanized' monoclonal antibodies and soluble receptors/receptor antagonists, directed towards IgE, cytokines such as IL-4 and IL-5, and cell surface molecules such as CD23.

Atopic allergic diseases, including allergic rhinoconjunctivitis, allergic asthma and atopic dermatitis, represent a particular therapeutic problem since their prevalence has increased dramatically in recent decades. The market for new and more effective medicaments for allergic disease is both substantial and increasing. For this reason, the pharmaceutical and academic communities have invested heavily in research and development in this area which represents one of the largest group of chronically symptomatic patients, particularly in the developed world.

Therapy of allergic diseases can be classified into palliative and disease modulating. The former, which describes drugs such as anti-histamines and glucocorticosteroids, forms the largest sector of the market. Disease-modulating therapy such as specific immunotherapy (SIT), otherwise known as desensitization, is more restricted despite its clinical efficacy, largely as a result of the requirement of the patient that he or she make a substantial and ongoing time commitment to his other treatment.

There is a need to develop both improved drugs for palliation and also, and arguably more importantly, to develop novel disease-modulating therapies which may act, not only to relieve symptoms but also, to impact upon the burden of this group of diseases on the population as a whole.

Currently, the development of novel therapies appears to be following a number of parallel routes (fig. 1). The first consists of approaches which seek to modify and improve SIT by the use of modified allergen molecules or fragments thereof. The second approach has been to target specific molecules which have been identified as pivotal in the allergic cascade (e.g. cytokines, chemokines, IgE, costimulatory molecules). The third, which is covered elsewhere in this text, is the use of medicinal chemis-

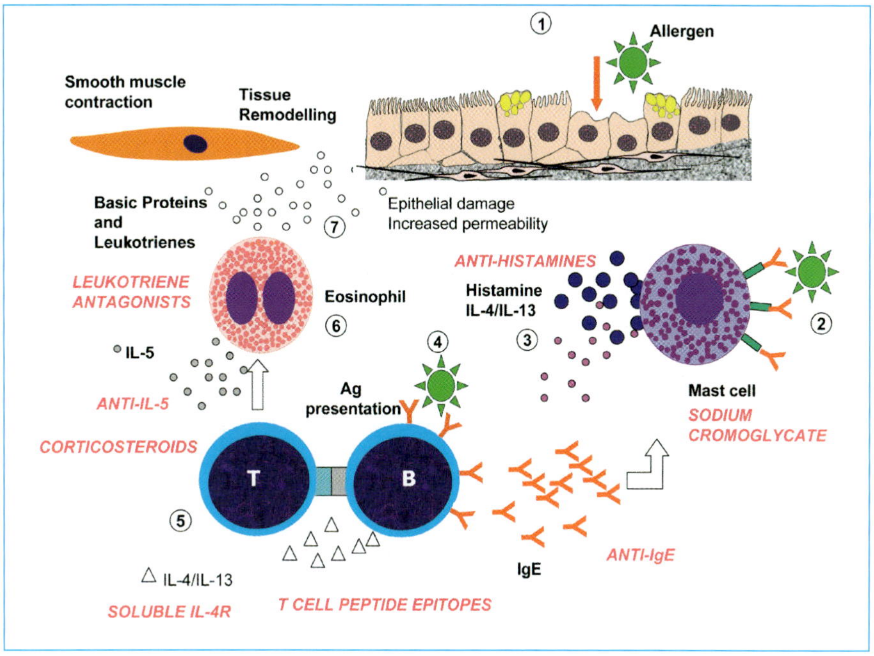

Fig. 1. Allergic inflammation results from allergen impact on mucosal surfaces [1]. Cross-linking of allergen-specific IgE [2] leads to the release of histamine, IL-4, IL-13 from mast cells [3]. Whole allergen is taken up by antigen-presenting cells [4] and peptides are presented to T cells, resulting in T cell activation [5] and elaboration of cytokines. Eosinophil recruitment [6] leads to the release of toxic proteins and mediators such as leukotrienes [7], causing bronchoconstriction and epithelial cell damage. Current therapeutic approaches, some of which are discussed in this section, are shown in *italics*.

try to develop compounds which block important steps in the generation of allergic inflammatory responses (e.g. leukotriene inhibitors, phosphodiesterase inhibitors). Finally, immunization with bacterial products or modified bacterial DNA sequences is been developed as a potential method for switching Th2-type responses to Th1. The reviews in this section relate specifically to the targeting of allergen molecules, IgE and the low-affinity IgE receptor for the treatment of allergic diseases.

Second-Generation Specific Immunotherapy

Traditional whole-allergen SIT has been employed to treat allergic diseases for almost a century [1]. It has been demonstrated to be highly effective in carefully selected patients [2], but demands a considerable commitment from both patient and clinician in terms of time. This form of therapy, by virtue of the fact that the patient is injected with the very substance to which he or she is allergic, also carries the risk of systemic side effects such as anaphylaxis, which when severe can be life-threatening. Anaphylaxis and related adverse events associated with this form of therapy arise as a result of cross-linking of specific IgE antibodies on the surface of mast cells leading to degranulation and the release of histamine, cytokines such as IL-4 and IL-5 and leukotrienes. All of these mediators have been identified as important contributors to both acute and chronic allergic inflammation.

Allergens and Allergoids

One approach has been to exploit the fact that relatively minor changes to the amino acid sequence of an allergen molecule (such as may be found in some allergen isoforms for example) can result in a substantially reduced ability to bind IgE [3–7]. Similarly, other approaches which disrupt the integrity of the three-dimensional structure of the allergen have been developed as second-generation immunotherapeutics. Whole allergen molecules have been treated with formaldehyde in order to modify lysine residues and cross-link amino acid side chains [8–10]. In common with point mutation of the whole protein, the allergoid approach spares the majority of T cell epitopes within the allergen molecule, a property which is believed to be essential for the success of SIT.

Peptides and Fragments

Disruption of allergen structure through the generation of peptide fragments is also being pursued as a potential avenue for developing efficacious therapies with improved safety profiles. A number of groups have evaluated the safety and clinical efficacy of two peptides derived from the major cat allergen Fel d 1 [11–14]. Clinical results were modest but established proof of concept, which has been further supported by the work of Muller et al. [15] in bee-venom-allergic individuals. Studies from our own group described later in this section suggest that the use of carefully selected peptides derived from the amino acid sequence of allergens may be both safe and highly efficacious in the treatment of allergic disorders, particularly asthma. The clear advantage of allergen-specific approaches to therapy, over targeting inflammation in general (for example with glucocorticosteroids) or individual components of the allergic cascade (anti-cytokine antibodies or small molecule receptor antagonists) is that the effect of the therapy is restricted to the specific immune response underlying the disease, rather than by inhibiting the synthesis or actions of one or more non-specific components of the response.

Therapeutic Targets in Allergic Disease

Allergic diseases are complex and multifactorial in their aetiology. In general, allergic inflammation involves multiple cell types and the synthesis, release and action of a number of soluble mediators. Choosing which of these to target for therapy has presented a significant challenge. Many previous approaches focussing on a single mediator have failed to impress clinically. Identifying the events that initiate allergic inflammation is difficult but recently a number of strategies have been developed which are currently undergoing evaluation in clinical trials.

Antibodies to IgE

The concept of an inhibitor of IgE that blocks binding to high-affinity IgE receptors but lacks the ability to trigger degranulation of IgE-synthesized cells has been achieved by the generation of non-anaphylactogenic anti-IgE antibodies [16]. Humanized monoclonal antibodies which bind IgE, either in soluble or receptor-bound form, but are non-anaphylactogenic, have been shown to reduce serum IgE levels dramatically and have also been demonstrated to be efficacious in both the control of allergic sypmtoms and reduction in the use of anti-allergic medication [17, 18]. The results of clinical studies with anti-IgE antibodies are discussed later in this section.

Antibodies to CD23

CD23 is a pleiotropic molecule which is crucial in the regulation of IgE synthesis [19]. In addition to FcεRI, IgE also binds to CD23 which is referred to as the low-affinity IgE receptor or FcεRII. A number of ligands other than IgE have been identified which interact with CD23 such as CD21. Following triggering through the CD23-CD21 axis, basophils were shown to release histamine [20]. Interaction of CD23 with CD11b and CD11c on monocytes resulted in release of pro-inflammatory cytokines (IL-1β, IL-6 and TNF-α, together with increased production of nitrite-oxidative metabolites [21]. Elevated soluble CD23 levels have been shown in the serum of allergic subjects [22] including allergic asthmatics [23]. CD23 has also been shown to regulate antigen-induced bronchoconstriction in a murine model [24]. Anti-CD23 (Fab) antibodies were shown to significantly reduce allergen-induced bronchoconstriction [24]. CD23-mediated allergen focussing has also been implicated as a mechanism by which allergen processing and presenting is enhanced in allergic individuals, leading to more vigorous T cell responses [25]. Thus, results indicate that blockade of CD23 function may prove efficacious in the treatment of allergic asthma.

Conclusions

The rising prevalence of allergic diseases such as asthma highlights the requirement for more effective therapy. Current strategies include the modification of well-established approaches such as SIT, together with the specific targeting of mediators of the allergic inflammatory response such as IgE. Clinical data from a number of programmes have demonstrated efficacy, and direct comparisons between the most effective of these approaches will ultimately determine whether traditional pharmacotherapy, such as anti-histamines and glucocorticosteroids, can be improved upon in the near future.

References

1 Noon L: Prophylactic inoculation against hay fever. Lancet 1911;i:1572.
2 Durham SR, Walker SM, Varga E-M, Jacobson MR, O'Brien F, Noble W, Till SJ, Hamid QA: Nouri-Aria KT: Long-term clinical efficacy of grass-pollen immunotherapy. N Engl J Med 1999;341:468–475.
3 Valenta R, Vrtala S, Focke-Tejkl M, Bugajska-Schretter, Ball T, Twardosz A, Spitzauer S, Gronlund H, Kraft D: Genetically engineered and synthetic allergen derivatives: Candidates for vaccination against type I allergy. Biol Chem 1999;380:815–824.
4 Pauli G, Purohit A, Oster JP, de Blay F, Vrtala S, Niederberger V, Kraft D, Valenta R: Clinical evaluation of genetically engineered hypoallergenic rBet v 1 derivatives. Int Arch Allergy Immunol 1999;118:216–217.
5 Smith AM, Chapman MD: Reduction in IgE binding to allergen variants generated by site-directed mutagenesis: Contribution of disulfide bonds to the antigenic structure of the major house dust mite allergen Der p 2. Mol Immunol 1996;33:399–405.
6 Takai T, Yokota T, Yasue M, Nishiyama C, Yuuki T, Mori A, Okudaira H, Okumura Y: Engineering of the major house dust mite allergen Der f 2 for allergen-specific immunotherapy. Nat Biotechnol 1997;15:754–758.
7 Schramm G, Kahlert H, Suck R, Weber B, Stuwe HT, Muller WD, Bufe A, Becker WM, Schlaak MW, Jager L, Cromwell O, Fiebig H: 'Allergen engineering': Variants of the timothy grass pollen allergen Phl p 5b with reduced IgE-binding capacity but conserved T cell reactivity. Immunology 1999;162:2406–2414.

8 Norman PS, Lichtenstein LM, Kagey-Sobotka A, Marsh DG: Controlled evaluation of allergoid in the immunotherapy of ragweed hay fever. J Allergy Clin Immunol 1982;70:248–260.
9 Marsh DG, Lichtenstein LM, Campbell DH: Studies on 'allergoids' prepared from naturally occurring allergens. I. Assay of allergenicity and antigenicity of formalinized rye group component. Immunology 1970;18:705–722.
10 Bousquet J, Hejjaoui A, Soussana M, Michel FB; Double-blind, placebo-controlled immunotherapy with mixed grass-pollen allergoids. IV. Comparison of the safety and efficacy of two dosages of a high-molecular-weight allergoid. J Allergy Clin Immunol 1990;85:490–497.
11 Norman PS, Ohman JL, Long AA, Creticos PS, Gefter MA, Shaked Z, Wood RA, Eggleston PA, Hafner KB, Rao P, Lichtenstein LM, Jones NH, Nicodemus CF: Treatment of cat allergy with T-cell reactive peptides. Am J Respir Crit Care Med 1996;154:1623–1628.
12 Simons F, Imada M, Li Y, Watson W, Hayglass K: Fel d 1 peptides: Effect on skin tests and cytokine synthesis in cat-allergic human subjects. Int Immunol 1996;8:1937–1945.
13 Maguire P, Nicodemus C, Robinson D, Aaronson D, Umetsu DT: The safety and efficacy of ALLERVAX CAT in cat-allergic patients. Clin Immunol 1999;93:222–231.
14 Pene J, Desroches A, Paradis L, Lebel B, Farce M, Nicodemus CF, Yssel H, Bousquet J: Immunotherapy with Fel d 1 peptides decreases IL-4 release by peripheral blood T cells of patients allergic to cats. J Allergy Clin Immunol. 1998;102:571–578.
15 Muller U, Akdis CA, Fricker M, Akdis M, Blesken T, Bettens F, Blaser K: Successful immunotherapy with T-cell epitope peptides of bee venom phospholipase A2 induces specific T-cell anergy in patients allergic to bee venom. J Allergy Clin Immunol 1998;101:747–754.
16 Heusser C, Jardieu P: Therapeutic potential of anti-IgE antibodies. Curr Opinion Immunol 1997;9:805–814.
17 Fahy JV, Fleming HE, Wong HH, Liu JT, Su JQ, Reimann J, Fick RB Jr, Boushey HA: The effect of an anti-IgE monoclonal antibody on the early- and late-phase responses to allergen inhalation in asthmatic subjects. Am J Respir Crit Care Med 1997;155:1828–1834.
18 Milgrom H, Fick RB Jr, Su JQ, Reimann JD, Bush RK, Watrous ML, Metzger WJ, for the rhuMAb-E25 Study Group: Treatment of allergic asthma with monoclonal anti-IgE antibody. N Engl J Med 1999;341:1966–1973.
19 Sutton BJ, Gould HJ: The human IgE network. Nature 1993;366:421–428.
20 Bacon K, Gauchat JF, Aubry JP, Pochon S, Graber P, Henchoz S, Bonnefoy JY: CD21 expressed on basophilic cells is involved in histamine release triggered by CD23 and anti-CD21 antibodies. Eur J Immunol 1993;23:2721–2724.
21 Lecoanet-Henchoz S, Gauchat JF, Aubry JP, Graber P, Life P, Paul-Eugene N, Ferrua B, Corbi AL, Dugas B, Plater-Zyberk C, et al: CD23 regulates monocyte activation through a novel interaction with the adhesion molecules CD11b-CD18 and CD11c-CD18. Immunity. 1995;3:119–125.
22 Yanagihara Y, Sarfati M, Marsh D, Nutman T, Delespesse G: Serum levels of IgE-binding factor (soluble CD23) in diseases associated with elevated IgE. Clin Exp Allergy 1990;20:395–401.
23 Matsumoto K, Taki F, Miura M, Matsuzaki M, Takagi K: Serum levels of soluble IL-2R, IL-4, and soluble Fc epsilon RII in adult bronchial asthma. Chest 1994;105:681–686.
24 Dasic G, Juillard P, Graber P, Herren S, Angell T, Knowles R, Bonnefoy JY, Kosco-Vilbois MH, Chvatchko Y: Critical role of CD23 in allergen-induced bronchoconstriction in a murine model of allergic asthma. Eur J Immunol 1999;29:2957–2967.
25 van Neerven RJ, Wikborg T, Lund G, Jacobsen B, Brinch-Nielsen A, Arnved J, Ipsen H: Blocking antibodies induced by specific allergy vaccination prevent the activation of CD4+ T cells by inhibiting serum-IgE-facilitated allergen presentation. J Immunol 1999;163:2944–2952.

Mark Larché, PhD
Department of Allergy & Clinical Immunology
Imperial College School of Medicine
National Heart & Lung Institute
Dovehouse Street, London SW3 6LY (UK)
Tel. +44 20 7351 8181, Fax +44 20 7376 3138
E-Mail m.larche@ic.ac.uk

Allergen Immunotherapy

Duncan R. Wilson   Stephen R. Durham

Upper Respiratory Medicine, Imperial College School of Medicine, National Heart and Lung Institute, London, UK

Summary

Allergen injection immunotherapy is highly effective in selected patients with IgE-mediated allergic disease. Immunotherapy is the only treatment in current use that can improve the long-term outcome of allergic disease following its discontinuation. The probable mechanism of action is through alteration of the Th1/Th2 T lymphocyte balance either by inducing unresponsiveness (anergy) or immune deviation in favour of Th1, responses. Alternative routes of administration may improve further on safety and broaden the availability of immunotherapy.

Allergen immunotherapy involves the administration of gradually increasing doses of standardized allergenic extracts to selected patients suffering from IgE-mediated allergic conditions with the aim of modifying the immune response to future contact with the allergen, resulting in reduction of symptoms.

Subcutaneous Allergen Immunotherapy

Efficacy of Immunotherapy. Bee/Wasp Venom. Hymenoptera venom immunotherapy is highly effective in patients with a history of bee or wasp sting-induced anaphylaxis [1], up to 65% of whom would have a similar, potentially fatal reaction if stung again. Large local reactions and mild systemic reactions following a sting are less likely to recur and are not an indication for immunotherapy. Following 3 years of venom immunotherapy, follow-up studies confirm 90% protection against a future anaphylactic reaction for at least 5 years after discontinuation [2].

Seasonal Allergens. Injection immunotherapy is highly effective in patients with seasonal allergic rhinitis caused by pollens such as grass [3], birch [4] ragweed [5] and *Parietaria* [6]. A number of hay fever sufferers also experience seasonal asthma. Several studies have demonstrated improvement in seasonal asthma symptoms [7] and bronchial hyperresponsiveness [8] following pollen immunotherapy. Studies comparing allergen immunotherapy with pharmacotherapy are needed. Three to four years of grass pollen immunotherapy treatment results in a sustained improvement in hay fever symptoms and a marked reduction in requirements for anti-allergic medication that persists for 3 years after withdrawal of treatment [9] (fig. 1).

Perennial Allergens. Perennial rhinitis and asthma are frequently associated with sensitivity to house-dust mite and domestic pets. For such patients, allergen avoidance measures combined with pharmacotherapy represent first-line management. In general immunotherapy may be less effective for perennial disease in which specific allergens may be only one of the determinants. The efficacy of immunotherapy in patients with mite-sensitive asthma was confirmed in a meta-analysis of 20 randomized controlled trials [10] in which the odds for symptomatic improvement, combining all allergens, was 3.2 (95% CI 2.2–4.9). Clinical improvement has been shown to be accompanied by inhibition of late asthmatic responses and decreased bronchial hyperresponsiveness [11]. Within the United Kingdom immunotherapy is not recommended for perennial asthma because of the increased risks in this group.

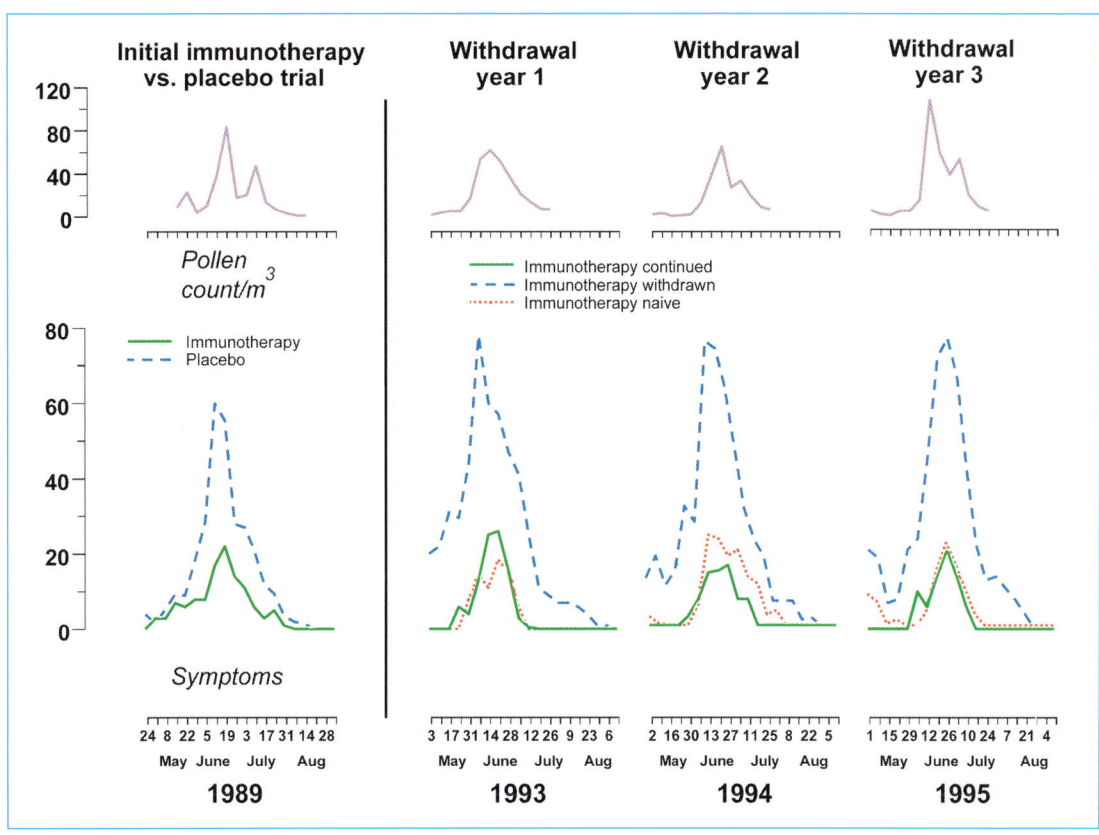

Fig. 1. Median weekly pollen counts and symptom scores for placebo-controlled trial of immunotherapy (1989) and 3 years of double-blind placebo-controlled treatment withdrawal. From Durham et al. [9].

Immunotherapy with a standardized cat extract resulted in a marked reduction in symptoms during controlled cat exposure with an accompanying reduction in peak flow response and conjunctiva and skin sensitivity [12]. Immunotherapy was also highly effective in patients with cat-induced asthma [13] and had long-term effects on bronchial hyperreactivity [14].

Safety of Immunotherapy. Large (>5 cm) local swellings occasionally occur early (<1 h) or late (1–24 h) after injections. These are usually not troublesome and require no treatment. Systemic reactions include rashes, pruritis and hypotension; these usually occur within 30 min. Anaphylaxis is an extremely rare complication of injection immunotherapy. In 1986, the British Committee on Safety of Medicines reported 26 deaths associated with immunotherapy over 30 years [15], these occurred almost exclusively in individuals for whom the indication for immunotherapy was bronchial asthma. Major factors in these fatalities were the performance of immunotherapy by untrained operators without immediate access to epinephrine. Injection immunotherapy must therefore be performed by trained personnel with access to adequate resuscitation facilities. Patients should remain under observation for at least 30 min after injections. Signs of systemic reaction should be identified early and treated with 0.5 mg (0.5 ml of 1:1,000) intramuscular epinephrine (adjusted in children).

Mechanism of Immunotherapy. Serum Immunoglobulins. A consistent pattern of changes in serum immunoglobulin concentrations is seen during immunotherapy. IgE levels rise after up-dosing then steadily fall over several years [16]. In contrast, allergen-specific IgG4 antibodies increase rapidly and remain raised throughout the course of treatment. It has been proposed that IgG4 may act as a 'blocking antibody' – competing with cell membrane-bound IgE for allergen. The lack of any correlation with clinical response to immunotherapy questions this proposed role for increases in IgG4, which may simply reflect high allergen exposure during immunotherapy [17].

Mediators and Effector Cells. Following successful immunotherapy, there is a reduction in both mast-cell-associated mediators [18] and eosinophil recruitment and

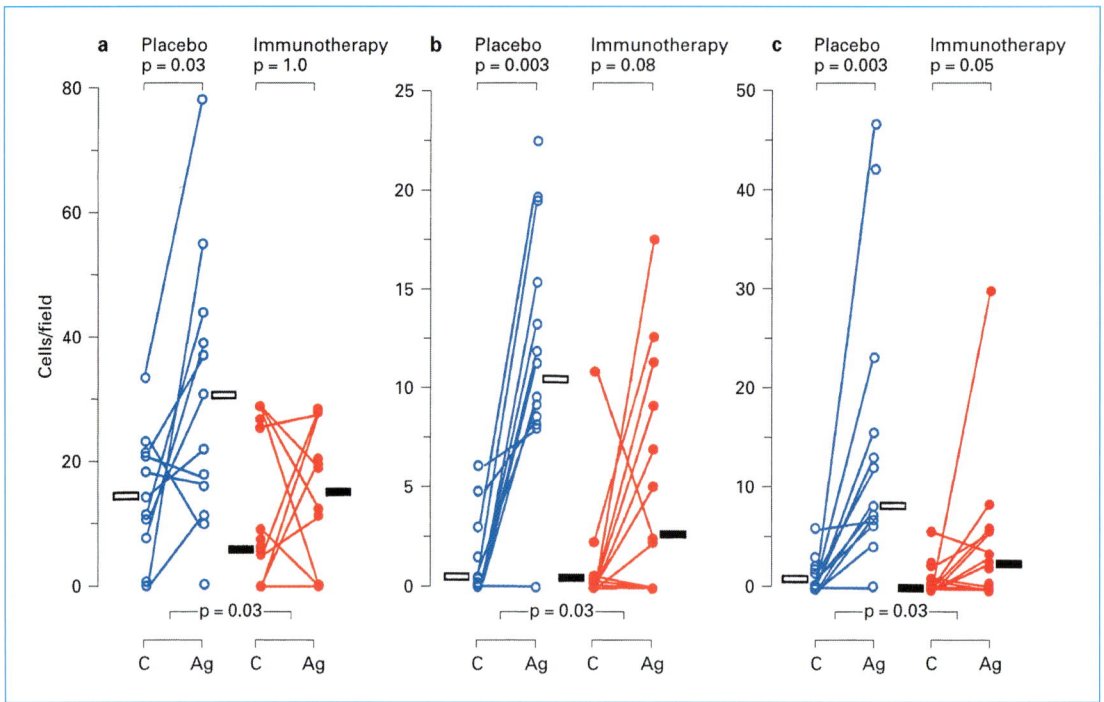

Fig. 2. Cellular infiltration with CD4+ T lymphocytes (**a**), MBP+ (**b**) and EG2+ (**c**) eosinophils 24 h after nasal provocation with allergen and control (allergen diluent) solution in immunotherapy-treated (●) and placebo-treated (○) subjects. From Durham et al. [21].

activation within target organs [19, 20]. Nasal biopsy studies have shown that both the late-phase response [21] and seasonal exposure [22] to pollen are associated with tissue eosinophilia which is inhibited by successful immunotherapy (fig. 2).

T Lymphocytes. The division of Th T lymphocytes into Th1 and Th2 subtypes is well established [23]. Th1-polarized T lymphocytes are important in the response to infection, they produce IFN-γ and promote IgG production by B lymphocytes. Th2 T lymphocytes produce the cytokines IL-4, which is an important signal to B cells to switch to IgE production, and IL-5, which plays a vital role in eosinophil recruitment, activation and survival.

Alterations of serum antibodies and effector cells after specific immunotherapy may occur as a consequence of modulation of the T cell response to allergen. Studies in peripheral blood have shown a decrease in allergen-induced T cell proliferation and a decrease in IL-4 production following immunotherapy [24]. The inhibition of allergen-induced late nasal responses by grass pollen immunotherapy is associated with an increase in IFN-γ mRNA expression in the nasal mucosa [21]. Prolonged immunotherapy (4–7 years) results in decreased IL-4 expression in biopsies from allergen-induced late cutaneous responses [9]. The increased IL-5 mRNA expression observed in the nasal mucosa of hay fever sufferers during natural seasonal pollen exposure is inhibited by immunotherapy. This down regulation correlates closely with the clinical response to immunotherapy and the reduction in tissue eosinophilia [22]. Taken together, these findings suggest that alteration of the Th2/Th1 T cell balance may occur either as a consequence of immune deviation (Th2 to Th1) or down-regulation of Th0/Th2 responses (anergy) (fig. 3)

Alternative Routes for Allergen Immunotherapy

The injection route for administering immunotherapy can be inconvenient and may rarely be associated with serious systemic reactions. For these reasons, alternative routes have been explored. Oral allergen administration was ineffective in 4 of 7 published studies [25] and has largely been abandoned. There have been few studies of the bronchial route, and unacceptable side effects limit further progress. A majority of studies of nasally administered immunotherapy have demonstrated efficacy in both seasonal and perennial allergic rhinitis with a dose re-

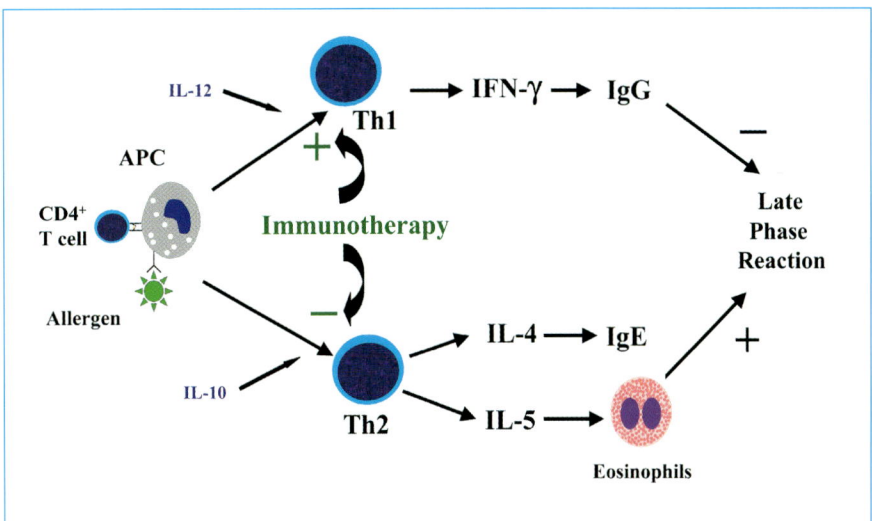

Fig. 3. Possible mechanism of allergen immunotherapy: alteration of Th1 / Th2 balance in favour of Th1 either by downregulation of Th2 response (anergy) or immune deviation (Th2 to Th1).

sponse [25]. The occurrence of local side effects of itching and sneezing when allergen is placed directly in the nose may possibly limit the acceptability of this route.

Sublingual-swallow immunotherapy, using high doses of grass or *Parietaria* pollen allergens that can be self-administered at home after initial up-dosing, has been studied in many recent trials. In a majority, improvements were seen in symptoms or medication requirements during the relevant pollen season with few adverse effects [25]. Further studies comparing the sublingual route with conventional injection immunotherapy and pharmacotherapy are required.

Adjuvants

Adjuvants have been administered with allergen vaccines in an attempt to either delay absorption from the injection site, e.g. alum in depot preparations, or to augment the immune response. Freund's adjuvant can induce production of IL-12 by macrophages in animal models, which drives a Th1 immune response. It is possible that IL-12 itself administered in low doses, with the allergen, may prove effective as an adjuvant although this potential role may be limited by toxicity.

Allergoids

Allergoids are chemically modified allergens in which agents such as formaldehyde or glutaraldehyde are used to cross-link within and between proteins to minimize IgE-binding potential and therefore the risk of anaphylaxis, whilst retaining T cell epitopes. Although a number of studies have demonstrated efficacy with these vaccines, there remain problems of standardization following chemical modification, and further controlled studies are required.

References

1 Hunt KJ, Valentine MD, Sobotka AK, Benton AW, Amodio FJ, Lichtenstein LM: A controlled trial of immunotherapy in insect hypersensitivity. N Engl J Med 1978;299:157–161.

2 Lerch E, Muller UR: Long-term protection after stopping venom immunotherapy: Results of re-stings in 200 patients. J Allergy Clin Immunol 1998;101:606–612.

3 Varney VA, Gaga M, Frew AJ, Aber VR, Kay AB, Durham SR: Usefulness of immunotherapy in patients with severe summer hay fever uncontrolled by antiallergic drugs. BMJ 1991; 302:265–269.

4 Petersen BN, Janniche H, Munch EP, Wihl JA, Bowadt H, Ipsen H, Lowenstein H: Immunotherapy with partially purified and standardized tree pollen extracts. I. Clinical results from a three-year double-blind study of patients treated with pollen extracts either of birch or combinations of alder, birch and hazel. Allergy 1988 Jul;43:353–362.

5 Lowell F, Franklin W: A double-blind study of the effectiveness and specificity of injection therapy in ragweed hay fever. N Engl J Med 1965;273:675–679.

6 D'Amato G, Kordash TR, Liccardi G, Lobefalo G, Cazzola M, Freshwater LL: Immunotherapy with Alpare in patients with respiratory allergy to *Parietaria* pollen: A two-year double-blind placebo-controlled study. Clin Exp Allergy 1995;25:149–158.

7 Creticos PS, Reed CE, Norman PS, Khoury J, Adkinson NF Jr, Buncher CR, Busse WW, Bush RK, Gadde J, Li JT, Richerson HB, Rosenthal RP, Solomon WR, Steinberg P, Yunginger JW: Ragweed immunotherapy in adult asthma. N Engl J Med 1996;334:501–506.

8 Walker SM, Pajno G, Torres-Lima M, Wilson DR, Durham SR: Grass pollen immunotherapy improves quality of life in seasonal rhinitis and reduces peak seasonal asthma and bronchial hyperresponsiveness. J Allergy Clin Immunol 2000;105(1pt2);S68.
9 Durham SR, Walker SM, Varga E-M, Jacobson MR, O'Brien F, Noble W, Till SJ, Hamid QA, Nouri-Aria KT: Long-term clinical efficacy of grass pollen immunotherapy. N Engl J Med 1999;341:468–475.
10 Abramson MJ, Puy RM, Weiner JM: Is allergen immunotherapy effective in asthma? A meta-analysis of randomized controlled trials. Am J Respir Crit Care Med 1995;151:969–974.
11 Van Bever HP, Stevens WJ: Effect of hyposensitization upon the immediate and late asthmatic reaction and upon histamine reactivity in patients allergic to house dust mite *(Dermatophagoides pteronyssinus)*. Eur Respir J 1992; 5:318–322.
12 Varney VA, Edwards J, Tabbah K, Brewster H, Mavroleon G, Frew AJ: Clinical efficacy of specific immunotherapy to cat dander: A double-blind placebo-controlled trial. Clin Exp Allergy 1997;27:860–867.
13 Alvarez-Cuesta E, Cuesta-Herranz J, Puyana-Ruiz J, Cuesta-Herranz C, Blanco-Quiros A: Monoclonal antibody-standardized cat extract immunotherapy: Risk-benefit effects from a double-blind placebo study. J Allergy Clin Immunol 1994;93:556–566.
14 Hedlin G, Heilborn H, Lilja G, Norrlind K, Pegelow KO, Schou C, Lowenstein H: Long-term follow-up of patients treated with a three-year course of cat or dog immunotherapy. J Allergy Clin Immunol 1995; 96(6 pt 1):879–885.

15 Committee on Safety of Medicines. Desensitising vaccines. BMJ 1986;293:948.
16 Lichtenstein LM, Ishizaka K, Norman PS, Hill BM: IgE antibody measurements in ragweed hay fever. Relationship to clinical severity and the results of immunotherapy. J Clin Invest 1973;52:472–482.
17 Djurup R, Osterballe O: IgG subclass antibody response in grass pollen allergic patients undergoing specific immunotherapy. Prognostic value of serum IgG subclass antibody levels early in immunotherapy. Allergy 1984;39:433–441.
18 Creticos PS, Adkinson NF Jr, Kagey-Sobotka A, Proud D, Meier HL, Naclerio RM: Nasal challenge with ragweed pollen in hay fever patients. J Clin Invest 1985;76:2247–2253.
19 Furin MJ, Norman PS, Creticos PS, Proud D, Kagey-Sobotka A, Lichtenstein LM, Naclerio RM: Immunotherapy decreases antigen-induced eosinophil cell migration into the nasal cavity. J Allergy Clin Immunol 1991;88:27–32.
20 Rak S, Bjornson A, Hakanson L, Sorenson S, Venge P: The effect of immunotherapy on eosinophil accumulation and production of eosinophil chemotactic activity in the lung of subjects with asthma during natural pollen exposure. J Allergy Clin Immunol 1991;88:878–888.

21 Durham SR, Ying S, Varney VA, Jacobson MR, Sudderick RM, Mackay IS, Kay AB, Hamid QA: Grass pollen immunotherapy inhibits allergen-induced infiltration of CD4+ T lymphocytes and eosinophils in the nasal mucosa and increases the number of cells expressing messenger RNA for interferon-gamma. J Allergy Clin Immunol 1996;97:1356–1365.
22 Durham SR, Wilson DR, Walker SM, O'Brien F, Nouri-Aria KT: Grass pollen immunotherapy inhibits seasonal increases in eosinophils and interleukin-5 mRNA positive cells in the nasal mucosa. J Allergy Clin Immunol 2000; 105(1 pt 2);S366.
23 Mosmann TR, Cherwinski H, Bond MW, Giedlin MA, Coffman RL: Two types of murine helper T cell clone. I. Definition according to profiles of lymphokine activities and secreted proteins. J Immunol 1986;136:2348–2357.
24 Secrist H, Chelen CJ, Wen Y, Marshall JD, Umetsu DT: Allergen immunotherapy decreases interleukin-4 production in CD4+ T cells from allergic individuals. J Exp Med 1993; 178:2123–2130.
25 Bousquet J, Lockey RF, Malling H-J: WHO position paper. Allergen Immunotherapy: Therapeutic vaccines for allergic diseases Allergy 1998;53(supp 44):1–42.

Dr. Duncan Wilson
Upper Respiratory Medicine
Imperial College School of Medicine at the
National Heart and Lung Institute
Dovehouse Street
London SW3 6LY (UK)
Tel. +44 171 351 8912, Fax +44 171 351 8949
E-Mail duncw_99@syahoo.co.uk

Peptide Immunotherapy

William L.G. Oldfield   A. Barry Kay   Mark Larché

Department of Allergy and Clinical Immunology, Imperial College School of Medicine, National Heart and Lung Institute, London, UK

Summary

Allergic disease is a major cause of morbidity in the developed world. Current treatments are only partially effective and traditional whole allergen immunotherapy carries the risk of anaphylaxis. Allergen-derived T cell peptide epitopes offer the possibility of modulating the immune response to allergen with only minimal side effects. This chapter will review the rationale behind the use of peptides for immunotherapy and the current evidence from both in vitro and in vivo systems concerning their mechanism of action and efficacy.

Allergic diseases are increasing in prevalence, especially in westernized countries, with 10–20% of the population suffering from some form of atopic disorder. They are characterized by the inappropriate synthesis of IgE specific to common aeroallergens (in the United Kingdom these include house dust mite, grass and tree pollen, and dander from furry animals, notably cats and dogs) and food substances, e.g. cow's milk. Important examples of atopic disorders include allergic asthma, allergic conjunctivo-rhinitis and atopic dermatitis.

The management of allergic disease comprises allergen avoidance, usually in combination with pharmacotherapy, e.g. corticosteroids (topical and systemic) and anti-histamines. Standard allergen avoidance techniques are often ineffective as the common aeroallergens are widespread, especially in temperate climates. For example, the domestic cat is a common pet in the UK and even after removal of the cat from the relevant environment, cat antigen has been shown to persist for months to years [1]. Also, clinically significant amounts of cat allergen have been demonstrated in environments, e.g. schools, hospitals that have never contained a cat [2, 3].

Current conventional treatments for aeroallergen-induced disease include topical corticosteroids, inhaled bronchodilators, and anti-histamines. These treatments work reasonably well in cases of mild to moderate disease but often fail to completely suppress symptoms, especially in the case of severe disease, and to be most effective must be taken on a regular basis. Understandably, many patients are reluctant to do this and only take their medication on exposure to a cat when the inflammatory cascade has already been triggered, further reducing efficacy.

Once allergen avoidance and conventional pharmacological treatments have been tried, the only current option for resistant disease is whole-allergen immunotherapy. This has been shown to be efficacious and have a prolonged duration of action [4] but misgivings remain owing to the potential for inducing IgE-mediated anaphylaxis and problems with the standardization of allergen extracts. Consequently, current efforts are being directed towards developing an alternative to whole-allergen immunotherapy for pharmacologically resistant disease.

The Allergic Response

The response to allergen challenge in a previously sensitized individual can be divided into two phases: the early response occurring within minutes and generally complete within 1 h and the late response which starts about 3 h after allergen exposure, peaks at 6–9 h and has generally resolved by 24 h. The early response is caused by intact allergen molecules cross-linking preformed IgE on the surface of mast cells leading to cellular degranulation and release of preformed mediators including histamine, together with lipid mediators such as leukotrienes and prostaglandins. This reaction is manifested in the skin as the 'wheal and flare' reaction and in the lung as bronchoconstriction. In severe cases these mediators can lead to the syndrome of anaphylaxis (fig. 1).

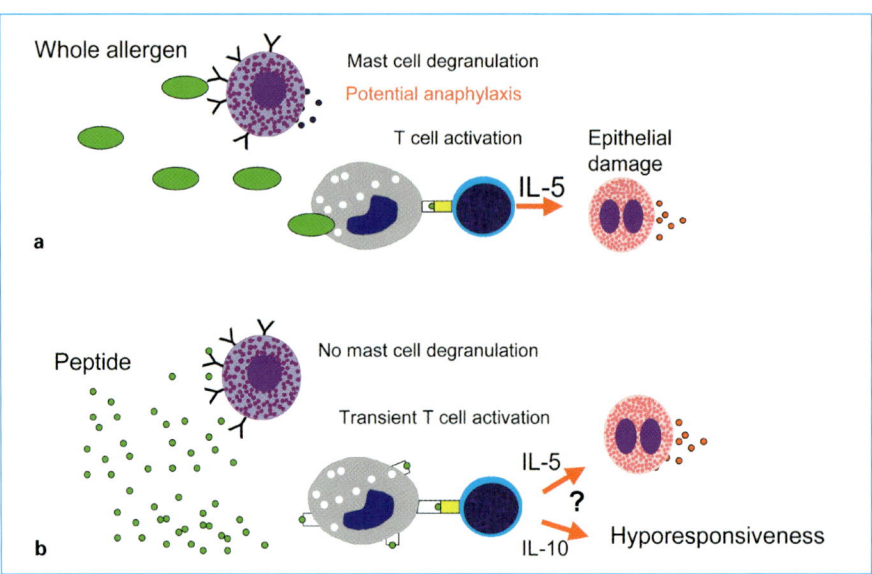

Fig. 1. Encounter with whole allergen results in IgE-dependent activation of mast cells with the potential for anaphylaxis. Additionally, allergen is taken up by antigen-presenting cells and presented to T cells which subsequently play a role in the recruitment of other inflammatory cells such as eosinophils. Allergen-derived peptides are generally too small to cross-link adjacent IgE molecules on the surface of the mast cell, even if they are capable of being recognized as a B cell epitope. Peptides remain able to interact with T cells through MHC-restricted presentation. At high doses, peptides induce hyporesponsiveness to allergen.

The mechanisms underlying the initiation and maintenance of late-phase reactions are less well defined but are likely to involve a number of cell types and soluble mediators. In contrast to the early phase, the late allergic reaction is associated with allergen-derived peptides being presented to T cells. The activated T cells secrete cytokines in a Th2 pattern (IL-4, 5, 13) which subsequently influence other cells in the inflammatory cascade and promote the Th2 phenotype. The ability to dissociate antibody and TCR-mediated allergen recognition suggests that small allergen-derived T cell peptides, whilst unable to cross-link IgE due to the loss of their three-dimensional conformational determinants, may still interact with allergen-specific T cells inducing cell activation or tolerance depending on the mode of presentation. However, the allergic late-phase response is not solely dependent on the T cell pathway since cutaneous late-phase reactions can be transferred by IgE or injection of anti-IgE [5, 6].

In vitro Studies

The first demonstration that antigen-derived peptides could alter the phenotype of T cells utilized influenza virus haemagglutinin-specific human Th0 T cell clones [7]. T cell anergy to whole-antigen challenge was induced following exposure of the clones to supraoptimal doses of peptide in the absence of antigen-presenting cells. These findings were subsequently confirmed in a murine model and it was demonstrated that the state of unresponsiveness could be reversed by the addition of IL-2 [8].

Subsequently, similar results have been obtained in a murine model of cat allergy [9]. Peptides derived from the major cat allergen, Fel d 1, were administered via a subcutaneous route. Following in vivo peptide-induced tolerization, T cells were isolated from lymph nodes and shown to have a reduced proliferative response to whole allergen and decreased IL-2 production.

Other studies in mice have demonstrated the induction of T cell tolerance following peptide challenge via the mucosal route [10]. It has also been demonstrated that administration of peptides derived from house dust mite allergen to mice via the intranasal route initially induces transient T cell activation [11]. This was followed by T cell hyporesponsiveness to whole antigen as demonstrated by decreased proliferative responses and IL-2/3 production. Interestingly, the tolerance induced via the mucosal route was more short-lived than that induced via the subcutaneous route.

The ability to modulate T cell function has also been demonstrated for altered peptide ligands (analogues of wild-type peptides in which one or more residues have undergone conservative substitution). The first demonstration of this phenomenon utilized a murine Th clone. An altered peptide ligand was identified that induced IL-4 production and was capable of B cell help but did not induce proliferation [12]. The proliferative response could be restored by addition of IL-1. Subsequently, also utilizing a murine Th1 clone, APLs, that are themselves incapable of inducing clonal proliferation, have been shown to induce unresponsiveness to the immunogenic peptide on subsequent stimulation [13].

The mechanism underlying the ability to dissociate different components of T cell effector functions remains unclear. Altering individual residues of a peptide alters the affinity of the MHC-peptide complex for the T cell receptor and consequent TCR triggering. An altered peptide ligand capable of inducing partial T cell activation of a murine clone has been shown to cause changes in the pattern of phosphorylation of the TCR ζ chain and failure of ZAP-70 kinase activation [14]. Thus, the effect of APLs may be mediated by alterations in intracellular signalling following peptide-TCR ligation.

In vivo Studies

As discussed, mucosal administration of peptide is an effective method of inducing T cell tolerance. Administration of a peptide containing the immunodominant T cell epitope of the house dust mite allergen Der p 1 to naïve or primed mice caused suppression of the T cell response to not only the dominant peptide but also to the minor flanking epitopes [15]. This suggests effective peptide therapy will not require peptides spanning the entire allergen but that rather a few select peptides can be used.

An early study in man utilized three peptides derived from PLA_2, the major bee venom allergen [16]. All five patients studied demonstrated an increase in the peptide-specific IgG4:IgE ratio and tolerated a subcutaneous challenge with PLA_2 without systemic side effects following peptide therapy. Three out of the five patients also tolerated a subsequent rechallenge with live bee sting.

Further studies have involved the treatment of patients with cat-allergic asthma with Fel d 1 derived peptides. The first study utilized two peptides (each 27 residues long) spanning the centre of chain 1 of Fel d 1 [17]. Subcutaneous administration of the peptides on a weekly basis for 4 weeks caused a reduction in allergic symptoms at the highest dose used. A number of adverse reactions (both early and late) were noted during the study following the first injection of peptide. The early reactions were probably caused by an IgE-mediated mechanism as the peptides used were long enough to cross-link adjacent IgE molecules on the surface of mast cells. The late reactions may have been a result of the transient T cell activation seen following initial peptide challenge [11].

However, a subsequent study utilizing the same peptides did not show any improvement in cutaneous sensitivity to allergen and there was no change in the allergen-specific T cell phenotype following treatment [18]. A third study showed that peptide treatment resulted in a slight improvement in lung function but only in those subjects with impaired function at baseline. This study was characterized by a high incidence of both early and late side effects [19]. In vivo studies assessing the effect of these peptides showed a dose-dependent decrease in IL-4 production by peptide-specific T cell lines although there was no change in cytokine production by whole-allergen-specific lines [20]. Importantly, no change in the proliferative responses to either peptide or whole allergen were seen. A subsequent study confirmed this reduction in IL-4 production and also showed that there was no change in IFN-γ, IgE or IgG levels [21]. Importantly, the reduction in IL-4 production did not correlate with the improvement in bronchial hyperresponsiveness to whole cat allergen.

Haselden et al. [22] also utilized a human cat-allergic asthma model. In this study, however, the peptides used were much shorter (16/17 residues) and were demonstrated to have no histamine-releasing activity suggesting that they were incapable of cross-linking IgE. Isolated late asthmatic reactions were induced in a proportion of subjects on initial peptide challenge suggesting transient T cell activation. These reactions were attenuated on subsequent rechallenge implying the development of hyporesponsiveness or functional tolerance. Development of isolated late allergic reactions was shown to be mediated by an MHC class II-restricted mechanism. This implies that for peptide-based immunotherapy to be effective in an outbred population, the peptides used must take into account the differing HLA haplotypes seen in that population.

The overall mechanism of action behind the induction of a clinical effect by allergen-derived peptides is unclear. Animal studies suggest the induction of an anergic state is responsible, but this is not borne out by human studies. The mechanisms underlying the induction of clinical hyporesponsiveness to whole allergen by allergen-derived T cell peptide epitopes in man remain unclear, but may include one or more of the following possibilities:
- induction of T cell anergy
- change in the T cell phenotype from Th2 to Th1/Th0
- induction of a regulatory T cell population
- activation-induced cell death

Safety Issues

There is mounting evidence that allergen-derived peptide therapy will provide a safer alternative to traditional whole-allergen immunotherapy. As discussed, whole-allergen immunotherapy is extremely effective in a number of allergic diseases but, due to the presence of intact, three-dimensional B cell epitopes, the risk of adverse reactions including anaphylaxis, albeit rare, remains. Short, allergen-derived peptides, however, have a much lower risk of inducing IgE-mediated anaphylaxis since there is a smaller chance of them cross-linking adjacent IgE molecules on the mast cell surface and many conformational determinants are removed. However, linear B cell epitopes do exist, as may peptide-specific IgE, so the risk of anaphylaxis remains, although is much reduced.

Additionally, a second issue associated with peptide-based immunotherapy follows the observation that induction of T cell tolerance by peptides is initially preceded by transient T cell activation. This is distinct from an IgE-mediated event and manifests as a response delayed in time similar to an allergic late-phase reaction. This isolated late phase reaction is markedly attenuated on subsequent peptide readministration due to the onset of T cell hyporesponsiveness. Future protocols may possibly circumvent this response by commencing treatment at a very low dose that does not elicit a clinical reaction and updosing over a period of weeks to allow tolerance to develop.

Conclusion

In conclusion, there is now strong supportive evidence from both animal and human models that allergen-derived peptides will provide a viable alternative to whole-allergen immunotherapy in the treatment of severe allergic disease. To be maximally effective, the peptides will need to be capable of being presented by the differing MHC class II restriction elements present in an outbred population. To reduce IgE-dependent side effects, the peptides need to be as short as possible to minimize any IgE cross-linking ability. Also, treatment protocols will need to consider the initial phase of T cell activation that occurs on peptide challenge by starting at a very lose dose, thus allowing T cell tolerance to develop in the absence of overt clinical symptoms of late-phase reactions.

References

1 Wood RA, Chapman MD, Adkinson NF, Eggleston PA: The effect of cat removal on allergen content in household-dust samples. J Allergy Clin Immunol 1989;83:730–734.

2 Munir AKM, Einarsson R, Schou C, Dreborg SKG: Allergens in school dust. I. The amount of the major cat (Fel d I) and dog (Can f I) allergens in dust from Swedish schools is high enough to probably cause perenial symptoms in most children with asthma who are sensitised to cat and dog. J Allergy Clin Immunol 1993;91:1067–1074.

3 Custovic A, Fletcher A, Pickering CAC, Francis HC, Green R, Smith A, Chapman M, Woodcock A: Domestic allergens in public places. III. House dust mite, cat, dog, and cockroach allergens in British hospitals. Clin Exp Allergy 1998;28:53–59.

4 Durham SR, Walker SM, Varga E-M, Jacobson MR, O'Brien F, Noble W, Till SJ, Hamid QA, Nouri-Aria KT: Long-term clinical efficacy of grass-pollen immunotherapy. N Eng J Med 1999; 341:468–475.

5 Dolovich J, Hargreave FE, Chalmers R, Shier KJ, Gauldie J, Bienenstock J: Late cutaneous allergic responses in isolated IgE-dependent reactions. J Allergy Clin Immunol 1973;52:38–46.

6 Solley GO, Gleich GJ, Jordon RE, Schroeter AL: The late phase of the immediate wheal and flare skin reaction. Its dependence upon IgE antibodies. J Clin Invest 1976;58:408–420.

7 Lamb J, Skidmore B, Green N, Chiller J, Feldman M: Induction of tolerance in influenza virus-immune T lymphocyte clones with synthetic peptides of influenza haemagglutinin J Exp Med 1983;157:1434–1447.

8 Schwartz RH: Costimulation of T lymphocytes: The role of CD28, CTLA-4, and B7/BB1 in interleukin-2 production and immunotherapy. Cell 1992;71:1065–1068.

9 Briner T, Kuo M, Keating K, Rogers B, Greenstein J: Peripheral T-cell tolerance induced in naïve and primed mice by subcutaneous injection of peptides from the major cat allergen Fel d 1. Proc Natl Acad Sci USA 1993;90:7608–7612.

10 Hoyne G, O'Hehir R, Wraith D, Thomas W, Lamb J: Inhibition of T cell and antibody responses to house dust mite allergen by inhalation of the dominant T cell epitope in naïve and sensitized mice. J Exp Med 1993;178:1783–1788.

11 Hoyne GF, Askonas BA, Hetzel C, Thomas WR, Lamb JR: Regulation of house dust mite responses by intranasally administered peptide: Transient activation of CD4+ T cells precedes the development of tolerance in vivo. Int Immunol 1996;8:335–342.

12 Evavold B, Allen P: Separation of IL-4 production from Th proliferation by an altered T cell receptor ligand. Science 1991;252:1308–1310.

13 Sloan-Lancaster J, Evavold B, Allen P: Induction of T cell anergy by altered T cell receptor ligand on live antigen presenting cells. Nature 1993;363:156–159.

14 Sloan-Lancaster J, Shaw AS, Rothbard JB, Allen PM: Partial T cell signalling: Altered phospho-ζ and lack of zap70 recruitment in APL-induced T cell anergy. Cell 1994; 79:913–922.

15 Hoyne G, Callow M, Kuo M-C, Thomas W: Inhibition of T cell responses by feeding peptides containing major and cryptic epitopes. Studies with the Der p 1 allergen. Immunology 1994;83:190–195.

16 Muller U, Akdis CA, Fricker M, Akdis M, Blesken T, Bettens F, Blaser K: Successful immunotherapy with T cell epitope peptides of bee venom phospholipase A_2 induces specific T cell anergy in patients allergic to bee venom. J Allergy Clin Immunol 1998;101:747–754.

17 Norman PS, Ohman JL, Long AA, Creticos PS, Gefter MA, Shaked Z, Wood RA, Eggleston PA, Hafner KB, Rao P, Lichtenstein LM, Jones NH, Nicodemus CF: Treatment of cat allergy with T-cell reactive peptides. Am J Respir Crit Care Med 1996;154:1623–1628.

18 Simons F, Imada M, Li Y, Watson W, Hayglass K: Fel d 1 peptides: Effect on skin tests and cytokine synthesis in cat-allergic human subjects. Int Immunol 1996;8:1937–1945.

19 Maguire P, Nicodemus C, Robinson D, Aaronson D, Umetsu DT: The safety and efficacy of ALLERVAX CAT in cat-allergic patients. Clin Immunol 1999;93:222–231.

20 Marcotte GV, Braun CM, Norman PS, Nicodemus CF, Kagey-Sobotka A, Lichtenstein LM, Essayan DM: Effects of peptide therapy on ex vivo T-cell responses J Allergy Clin Immunol 1998;101:506–513.

21 Pene J, Desroches A, Paradis L, Lebel B, Farce M, Nicodemus CF, Yssel H, Bousquet J: Immunotherapy with Fel d 1 peptides decreases IL-4 release by peripheral blood T cells of patients allergic to cats. J Allergy Clin Immunol 1998;102:571–578.

22 Haselden BM, Kay AB, Larché M: Immunoglobulin E-independent, major histocompatibility complex-restricted T cell peptide epitope-induced late asthmatic reactions. J Exp Med 1999;189:1885–1894.

Mark Larché, PhD
Department of Allergy and
Clinical Immunology
Imperial College School of Medicine
National Heart and Lung Institute
Dovehouse Street, London SW3 6LY (UK)
Tel. +44 20 7351 8181, Fax +44 20 7376 3138
E-Mail m.larche@ic.ac.uk

Recombinant Allergens

Rudolf Valenta   Dietrich Kraft

Department of Pathophysiology, University of Vienna, Austria

Summary

An increasing number of hypoallergenic allergen derivatives is currently being produced by genetic engineering as well as by synthetic peptide chemistry and evaluated as candidate molecules for specific immunotherapy of type I allergy. One advantage of recombinant and synthetic hypoallergenic allergen derivatives is that they can be designed to simultaneously retain the immunogenic/tolerogenic properties of the wild-type allergens and to exhibit a strongly reduced allergenic activity. When used for immunotherapy, it may be expected that hypoallergenic allergen derivatives will exhibit a lower rate of anaphylactic side effects. Furthermore, hypoallergenic allergen derivatives can be used for component-resolved immunotherapy tailored according to the individual patient's sensitization profile. This chapter summarizes strategies for the production and evaluation of recombinant as well as of synthetic hypoallergenic allergen derivatives as candidate vaccines for type I allergy.

Diagnosis of allergy and specific immunotherapy are currently performed with allergen extracts consisting of difficult to standardize allergenic and non-allergenic components. It is thus not yet possible to treat patients according to their sensitization profile. During the last decade a constantly increasing number of recombinant allergen components has been produced by recombinant DNA technology [1]. Recombinant allergen components can now be used for component-resolved diagnosis (CRD) of type I allergy and thus allow to precisely establish the individual patient's sensitization profile [2]. Based on the diagnostic information obtained by CRD it is now possible to precisely select those allergen components for treatment against which the patient is sensitized. Furthermore, sequence, structural and epitope information gained via the molecular biological characterization of allergens open new possibilities to convert allergenic molecules into immunogenic/tolerogenic vaccines with low allergenic activity [3, 4]. This chapter describes strategies for the production and evaluation of hypoallergenic allergen derivatives by genetic engineering and synthetic peptide chemistry. We describe in detail rationales for selecting the correct allergen sources and technologies for the production of recombinant allergens. Next we deal with the characterization/evaluation of recombinant allergens and discuss strategies for the production of recombinant and synthetic hypoallergenic allergen molecules as well as their in vitro and in vivo evaluation. Finally, we summarize possible advantages of therapeutic strategies that are based on the use of synthetic and recombinant hypoallergenic allergen derivatives.

Selection of the Most Relevant Allergen Sources

It is well established that many allergen sources contain allergens which cross-react with structurally and thus immunologically related allergens present in other sources [5, 6]. Birch-pollen-allergic patients, e.g., can also exhibit IgE antibody reactivity and clinical symptoms to pollens of related trees belonging to the order *Fagales* (alder, hazel, hornbeam, oak) and plant-derived food (fruits, vegetables, spices). The reason for this phenomenon is that certain taxonomically related (e. g., birch and alder pollen) as well as unrelated (birch pollen, apple) allergen sources can contain allergens which are similar in terms of structure and epitopes [7–9]. The selection of relevant allergen sources and allergens therefore represents a key step before the production of recombinant allergens can be started. In this context the term 'relevant' means that a given allergen source and/or allergen is the one which contains most of the important B cell and T cell epitopes. Whether a certain allergen/allergen source contains the relevant IgE epitopes and thus represented the originally sensitizing agent can be easily determined by IgE competition experiments. It was demonstrated, for instance, that birch pollen allergens contained most of the IgE epitopes present in pollens of the order *Fagales* and thus may be sufficient for the diagnosis and treatment of birch pollen and associated allergies [10]. It was also shown that many patients with plant food allergy were originally sensitized to cross-reactive pollen allergens [11]. In this context, it is noteworthy that immunotherapy with birch pollen extract is sufficient to treat related pollen (e. g., alder, hazel) and plant food (e. g., apple) allergies [12, 13]. Figure 1 summarizes the process of selecting the relevant allergen sources and allergens. Using IgE competition studies performed with large numbers of patient sera, it is possible to determine those allergens/allergen sources which inhibit IgE binding to other related as well as unrelated allergens/allergen sources and which thus represent the originally sensitizing agents.

Production of Recombinant Allergens

After the relevant allergen sources have been identified, mRNA is isolated and cDNA synthesized (fig. 2). Allergen-encoding cDNAs can be either isolated directly with IgE antibodies from allergic patients using immunoscreening technology or by using DNA-based technologies (DNA-based screening, PCR-based approaches) [14]. The advantage of the immunoscreening procedure is that primarily those cDNAs are isolated that are produced as immunoreactive components in a foreign host organism. DNA-based technologies (e.g., PCR amplification of allergen-encoding cDNAs) are sometimes faster but can deliver cDNAs which code for molecules with low immunoreactivity [15]. On the other hand they may be the method of choice if it is difficult to express the recombinant allergen in hosts commonly used in the immunoscreening procedure (e.g., *Escherichia coli*). Next, the allergen-encoding cDNA is inserted in suitable vectors (viral, plasmid DNA) and can be produced as recombinant protein in various host organisms (e.g., prokaryotic, eukaryotic organisms) [16]. Basically, recombinant allergens can be produced in bacteria without post-translational modifications which, for most allergens, was sufficient to yield recombinant proteins equaling the immunological and biological properties of the natural proteins (fig. 3). For some allergens, it has turned out to be of advantage to express the proteins in eukaryotic organisms to obtain a post-translationally modified (e. g., glycosylated) protein which is correctly folded. Basically, both the prokaryotic and eukaryotic forms of expression represent well-established technologies whereas the purification of the recombinant allergens needs to be established for each component. This is however fairly easy for recombinant molecules because the biochemical properties of the molecules can be predicted according to the sequence of the allergen and it is also possible to produce recombinant allergens containing tags which allow single-step affinity-based purification procedures (e.g., his-tags). Whether a panel of recombinant allergens reflects the epitope complexity and thus equals a natural allergen extract can be easily evaluated by IgE binding and competition studies [10, 17–19].

Molecular, Immunological and Structural Analysis of Recombinant Allergens

If the cDNA sequence of an allergen has been determined it is possible to deduce the corresponding amino acid sequence. Knowledge about the allergen's primary sequence greatly facilitates the determination of B cell as well as of T cell epitopes. As indicated in figure 4, allergens may contain discontinuous B cell epitopes which comprise peptides or amino acids which are located on different portions of the molecule (fig. 4 AE, BC) or continuous B cell epitopes which represent peptides consisting of several amino acids in a row (fig. 4D). The availability of the allergen's cDNA sequence allows to determine continuous B cell epitopes using synthetic peptides or gene fragmentation technologies [20, 21]. The characterization of discontinuous epitopes is more difficult than that of continuous epitopes. It may be achieved by competition studies using monoclonal antibodies with defined epitope specificity [22] or by using structural biology methods (NMR or x-ray crystal determination of the three-dimensional allergen structure) [23]. The analysis of the allergen's three-dimensional structure is also greatly facilitated by recombinant DNA technology which allows to produce and purify large amounts of defined and folded proteins which can be labeled during protein expression for NMR analysis. Based on the amino acid sequence which can be deduced from the cDNA sequence of a cloned allergen, mapping of T cell epitopes can be easily achieved by using synthetic overlapping peptides spanning the complete allergen se-

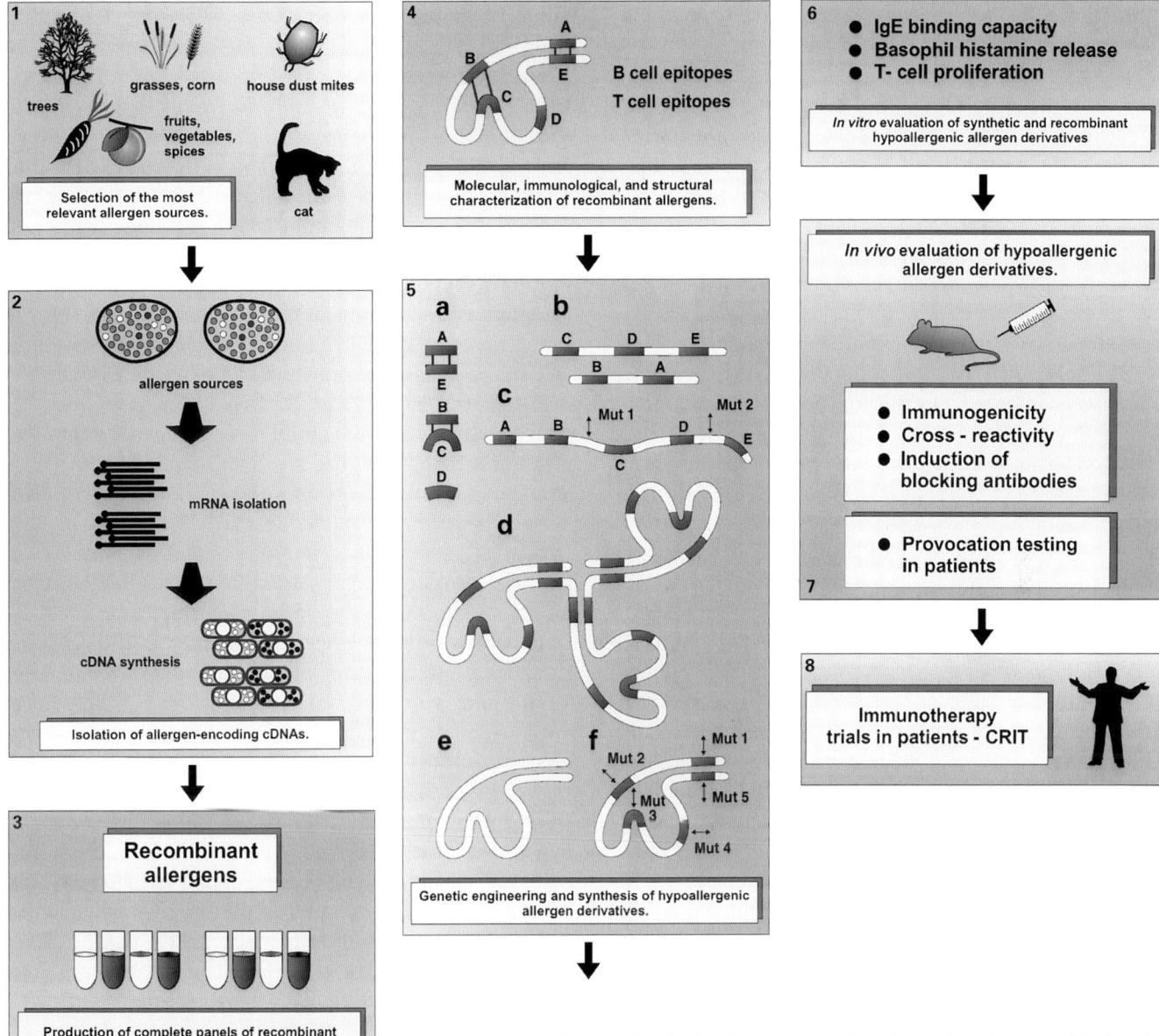

Fig. 1–8. Immunotherapeutics obtained by genetic engineering and synthetic peptide chemistry.

quence [24]. Using the purified recombinant allergen, it is easy to determine other important immunological characteristics (e.g., IgE binding capacity, frequency of IgE recognition, cross-reactivity, capacity to activate basophils and to induce biological responses in vivo) [25]. Taken together, it is obvious that recombinant DNA technology has greatly facilitated the molecular, immunological and structural characterization of allergens and provided us with defined molecules to investigate the mechanisms underlying allergen-specific immune responses.

Genetic Engineering and Synthesis of Hypoallergenic Allergen Derivatives

There are several possibilities how the molecular characterization of allergens by recombinant DNA technology can help improve allergen-specific immunotherapy. First, it is possible to produce recombinant allergens which can be used for refining the diagnosis of type I allergy. CRD will allow to precisely determine the allergic patient's sensitization profile and thus allow the selection of the correct allergens for treatment (component-resolved immunotherapy; CRIT) [2]. Second, it is possible to use recombinant DNA technology or synthetic peptide technology for the production of defined allergy vaccines. Third, and perhaps most importantly, molecular characterization of allergens will open new avenues towards the rational design and production of allergen derivatives with reduced allergenic activity [3, 4]. The use of such derivatives may allow to reduce anaphylactic side effects in the course of immunotherapy and it will allow to administer higher doses of the derivatives which may help to reduce the number of injections and result in a more effective modulation of the patient's immune response.

Recombinant DNA technology and synthetic peptide chemistry can be used for the reproducible production of well-defined hypoallergenic allergen derivatives (fig. 5) based on the knowledge gained through molecular, immunological and structural allergen characterization (fig. 4). Figure 5 shows some of the possible ways to produce recombinant or synthetic hypoallergenic allergen derivatives for immunotherapy. One possibility is to produce hypoallergenic allergen-derived peptides representing continuous, discontinuous or portions of IgE epitopes or T cell epitopes (fig. 5a). Another strategy is the production of recombinant allergen fragments which contain the entire sequence information of the allergens but fail to elicit allergenic activity because of the disruption of the proteins fold and thus of conformational IgE epitopes (fig. 5b). Mutations inserted into the allergen by site-directed mutagenesis outside the IgE epitopes may reduce the allergenic activity by changing the molecule's fold (fig. 5c). The construction of stable recombinant allergen oligomers may result in recombinant oligomers which, possibly due to reorientation and/or hiding of IgE epitopes, can be used as hypoallergenic allergy vaccines (fig. 5d). It is also possible to delete IgE epitopes from the allergen by deletion of the IgE-binding sites or by mutational change of the IgE epitopes (fig. 5e, f). The possibilities for reduction of the allergenic activity of a given allergen as depicted in figure 5 represent some examples which have been successfully applied [3, 4]. However, it should be stated that recombinant DNA technology and synthetic peptide chemistry will offer many more possibilities for reducing the allergenic activity of a given allergen molecule.

In vitro and in vivo Evaluation of Hypoallergenic Allergen Derivatives

In order to identify the hypoallergenic derivatives which represent the best-suited candidate molecules for immunotherapy, several assays are useful for evaluation. Some of these evaluation assays which are thought to determine the allergenic and immunogenic properties of allergen derivatives were applied almost 30 years ago by Marsh et al. [26] for chemically modified allergen extracts (allergoids). In vitro assays for the evaluation of hypoallergenic allergens are summarized in figure 6. They comprise the comparison of the wild-type recombinant allergen with the genetically modified or synthetic derivative regarding IgE binding capacity, induction of basophil histamine release and T cell proliferation. Promising features of a synthetic or recombinant allergen derivative are reduction of basophil histamine activity and preservation of T cell epitopes. The reduction of IgE binding capacity is desirable but hypoallergenic derivatives have been described which exhibited an IgE binding capacity that was almost comparable to that of the wild-type allergen. Those allergen derivatives with low allergenic activity in vitro need to be further evaluated in vivo. The in vivo evaluation must be performed in animals and by provocation testing in patients (fig. 7). Immunization/tolerization of animals (e.g., mice) should be performed under conditions which mimick as closely as possible the schedule intended for treatment of allergic patients (choice of adjuvant, route, frequency, dose of application). Treatment of animals should indicate whether the hypoallergenic derivative can induce an immune response or tolerize against the wild-type allergen. The latter can be evaluated, e.g. by testing whether the antibodies induced with the hypoallergenic derivative recognize the wild-type allergen and cross-react with as many as possible other allergens that are immunologically related to the wildtype allergen. In order to estimate whether the hypoallergenic derivative can induce protective (i.e., blocking antibodies) antibodies, it has to be evaluated whether the animal-derived antibodies can block the binding of patient's IgE to the wild-type allergen and prevent the allergen-induced histamine release from basophils of sensitized patients [27]. In this context it should be noted that, as has been previously shown for allergoids, too vigorous a reduction of the IgE binding capacity and allergenic activity may deliver a hypoallergenic derivative with too low an immunogenic activity which will fail to induce a protective immune response to the wild-type allergen [26]. Although the basophil histamine release represents a suitable assay to determine the allergenic potential of a hypoallergenic allergen derivative, we suggest extensive provocation testing in a representative number of patients in order to select the best hypoallergenic allergen derivative. Skin prick testing and intradermal testing of hypoallergenic derivatives have proven to be suitable provocation methods to compare the immediate reactions induced by hypoallergenic derivatives with those induced by the wild-type allergen [28, 29]. It may be also considered to study whether intradermal application of hypoallergenic derivatives may influence lung function because it has been reported that administration of non-allergenic peptides derived from the major cat allergen, Fel d 1, caused symptoms of bronchial asthma via T cell activation and induction of late-phase reactions [30]. The injection of hypoallergenic derivatives into skin blisters provides another convenient method for direct study of the capacity of modified allergens to activate T cells and eosinophils, and thus, to induce late phase reactions in vivo [31].

Immunotherapy Trials with Engineered and Synthetic Allergen Derivatives

There are at least two reasons why we suggest to perform a detailed evaluation of recombinant or synthetic hypoallergenic derivatives by all of the above-described in vitro and in vivo assays before immunotherapy trials (fig. 8) are started in patients. First, and most importantly, we believe that it is mandatory for ethical reasons to perform a thorough evaluation of the newly synthesized hypoallergenic molecules. The evaluation procedures described above aim to select the best vaccine candidates which will induce as little few unwanted side effects as possible, but retain most of the favourable features required for immunomodulation. Second, it has to be borne in mind that the performance of a clinical immunotherapy trial is laborious and cost intensive. Clinical trial preparations need to be produced under GMP conditions and extensive biochemical and biological evaluation will be required for the registration of new immunotherapy products.

Clinical immunotherapy trials should aim to evaluate the safety and efficacy of hypoallergenic allergen derivatives. In addition to evaluating end points, such as quality of life, it will be necessary to monitor as many objective parameters as possible to document the efficacy of the tested vaccine in a scientific manner. In this context, standardized methods are required to study whether vaccination will reduce symptoms induced by controlled provocation testing (e.g., skin testing, nasal provocation testing) with defined substances. At present, several recombinant and synthetic hypoallergenic allergen derivatives have been characterized extensively and will soon enter clinical immunotherapy trials. Their evaluation in immunotherapy trials will allow to study the immunological mechanisms underlying immunotherapy and tell us whether they represent an alternative to extract-based forms of immunotherapy.

Acknowledgments

This study was supported by grant Y078 GEN of the Austrian Science Fund and by the ICP programme of the Austrian Ministry of Science. We thank Anton Jäger, Vienna for preparing the illustrations.

References

1 Valenta R, Kraft D: Recombinant allergens for diagnosis and therapy of allergic diseases. Curr Opin Immunol 1995;7:751–756.
2 Valenta R, Lidholm J, Niederberger V, Hayek B, Kraft D, Grönlund H: The recombinant allergen-based concept of component-resolved diagnostics and immunotherapy (CRD and CRIT). Clin Exp Allergy 1999;29:896–904.
3 Singh MB, de Weerd N, Bhalla PL: Genetically engineered plant allergens with reduced anaphylactic activity. Int Arch Allergy Immunol 1999;119:75–85.
4 Valenta R, Vrtala S, Focke-Tejkl M, Bugajska-Schretter A, Ball T, Twardosz A, Spitzauer S, Grönlund H, Kraft D: Genetically engineered and synthetic allergen-derivatives: Candidates for vaccination against type I allergy. Biol Chem 1999;380:815–824.
5 Yman L: Botanical relations and immunological cross-reactions in pollen allergy, ed 2. Uppsala, Pharmacia, 1982.
6 Valenta R, Steinberger P, Duchêne M, Kraft D: Immunological and structural similarities among allergens: Prerequisite for a specific and component-based therapy of allergy. Immunol Cell Biol 1996;74:187–194.
7 Ipsen H, Bowadt H, Janniche H, Nüchel-Petersen B, Munch EP, Wihl JA, Loewenstein H: Immunochemical characterization of reference alder (Alnus glutinosa) and hazel (Corylus avellana) pollen extracts and the partial immunochemical identity between the major allergens of alder, birch and hazel pollens. Allergy 1985;40:510–518.
8 Halmepuro L, Loewenstein H: Immunological investigation of possible structural similarities between pollen antigens and antigens in apple, carrot and celery tuber. Allergy 1985;40:264–272.
9 Valenta R, Kraft D: Type I allergic reactions to plant-derived food: A consequence of primary sensitization to pollen allergens. J Allergy Clin Immunol 1995;97: 893–895.
10 Niederberger V, Pauli G, Grönlund H, Fröschl R, Rumpold H, Kraft D, Valenta R, Spitzauer S: Recombinant birch pollen allergens (rBet v 1 and rBet v 2) contain most of the IgE epitopes present in birch, alder, hornbeam, hazel, and oak pollen: A quantitative IgE inhibition study with sera from different populations. J Allergy Clin Immunol 1998;102:579–591.
11 Kazemi-Shirazi L, Pauli G, Purohit A, Spitzauer S, Fröschl R, Hoffmann-Sommergruber R, Breiteneder H, Scheiner O, Kraft D, Valenta R: Quantitative IgE inhibition experiments with purified recombinant allergens indicate pollen-derived allergens as the sensitizing agents responsible for many forms of plant food allergy. J Allergy Clin Immunol 1999;105: 116–125.

12 Petersen BN, Janniche H, Munch EP, Wihl JA, Bowadt H, Ipsen H, Lowenstein H: Immunotherapy with partially purified and standardized tree pollen extracts. I. Clinical results from a three-year double-blind study of patients treated with pollen extracts either of birch or combinations of alder, birch and hazel. Allergy 1988;43:353–362.
13 Asero R: Effects of birch pollen-specific immunotherapy on apple allergy in birch pollen hypersensitive patients. Clin Exp Allergy 1998; 28:1368–1373.
14 Breitenbach M, Valenta R, Breiteneder H, Pettenburger K, Scheiner O, Rumpold H, Kraft D: Introduction to cDNA-cloning of plant allergens; in Sehon AH, Kraft D, Kunkel G (eds): Epitopes of Atopic Allergens. Brussels, UCB Institute of Allergy, 1990;57–61.
15 Breiteneder H, Ferreira F, Hoffmann-Sommergruber K, Ebner C, Breitenbach M, Rumpold H, Kraft D, Scheiner O: Four recombinant isoforms of Cor a I, the major allergen of hazel pollen, show different IgE binding properties. Eur J Biochem 1993;212:355–362.
16 Valenta R, Twardosz A, Vrtala S, Kraft D: Large scale production and quality criteria of recombinant allergens. Arb Paul Ehrlich Inst Bundesamt Sera Impfstoffe, Frankfurt, in press.
17 Valenta R, Duchêne M, Vrtala S, Birkner T, Ebner C, Hirschwehr R, Breitenbach M, Rumpold H, Scheiner O, Kraft D: Recombinant allergens for immunoblot diagnosis of tree-pollen allergy. J Allergy Clin Immunol 1991;88: 889–894.
18 Valenta R, Vrtala S, Ebner C, Kraft D, Scheiner O: Diagnosis of grass pollen allergy with recombinant timothy grass *(Phleum pratense)* pollen allergens. Int Arch Allergy Immunol 1992;97:287–294.
19 Niederberger V, Laffer S, Fröschl R, Kraft D, Rumpold H, Kapiotis S, Valenta R, Spitzauer S: IgE antibodies to recombinant pollen allergens (Phl p 1, Phl p 2, Phl p 5, and Bet v 2) account for a high percentage of grass pollen-specific IgE. J Allergy Clin Immunol 1998;101: 258–264.
20 Vant Hof W, Driedijk PC, Van den Berg M, Beck-Sickinger AG, Jung G, Aalberse RC: Epitope mapping of the *Dermatophagoides pteronyssinus* house dust mite major allergen Der p II using overlapping synthetic peptides. Mol Immunol 1991;28:1225–1232.
21 Greene WK, Cyster JG, Chua KY, O'Brien RM, Thomas WR: IgE and IgG binding of peptides expressed from fragments of cDNA encoding the major house dust mite allergen Der p I. J Immunol 1991;147:3768–3773.
22 Lebecque S, Dolecek C, Laffer S, Visco V, Denepoux S, Pin JJ, Guret C, Boltz-Nitulescu G, Weyer A, Valenta R: Immunologic characterization of monoclonal antibodies that modulate human IgE binding to the major birch pollen allergen Bet v 1. J Allergy Clin Immunol 1997;99:374–384.
23 Paterson Y, Englander SW, Roder H: An antibody binding site on cytochrome c defined by hydrogen exchange and two-dimensional NMR. Science 1990;249:755–759.
24 Ebner C, Szepfalusi Z, Ferreira F, Jilek A, Valenta R, Parronchi P, Maggi E, Romagnani S, Scheiner O, Kraft D: Identification of multiple T cell epitopes on Bet v 1, the major birch pollen allergen, using specific T cell clones and overlapping peptides. J Immunol 1993;150: 1047–1054.
25 Valenta R, Laffer S, Vrtala S, Grönlund H, Elfman L, Sperr WR, Valent P, Ferreira F, Mayer P, Liehl E, Heiss S, Steiner R, Eichler HG, Susani M, Kraft D: Recombinant allergens. Steps on the way to diagnosis and therapy of type I allergy; in Sehon et al (eds): New Horizons in Allergy Immunotherapy. New York, Plenum Press, 1996, pp 185–196.
26 Marsh DG, Lichtenstein LM, Campbell DH: Studies on 'allergoids' prepared from naturally occurring allergens. Immunology 1970;18: 705–722.
27 Vrtala S, Ball T, Spitzauer S, Pandjaitan B, Suphioglu C, Knox B, Sperr W R, Valent P, Kraft D, Valenta R: Immunization with purified natural and recombinant allergens induces mouse IgG1 antibodies that recognize similar epitopes as human IgE and inhibit the human IgE-allergen interaction and allergen-induced basophil degranulation. J Immunol 1998;160: 6137–6144.
28 Pauli G, Purohit A, Oster JP, de Blay F, Vrtala S, Niederberger V, Kraft D, Valenta R: Comparison of genetically engineered hypoallergenic rBet v 1 derivatives with rBet v 1 wildtype by skin prick and intradermal testing: Results obtained in a French population. Clin Exp Allergy 2000;30:1076.
29 van Hage-Hamsten M, Kronqvist M, Zetterström O, Johansson E, Niederberger V, Vrtala S, Grönlund H, Grönneberg R, Valenta R: Skin test evaluation of genetically engineered hypoallergenic derivatives of the major birch pollen allergen, Bet v 1. Results obtained with a mix of two recombinant Bet v 1 fragments and rBet v 1 trimer in a Swedish population before the birch pollen season. J Allergy Clin Immunol 1999;104:969–977.
30 Haselden BM, Kay BA, Larche M: Immunoglobulin E-independent major histocompatibility complex-restricted T cell peptide epitope-induced late asthmatic reactions. J Exp Med 1999;189:1885–1894.
31 Nopp A, Halldén G, Lundahl J, Johansson E, Vrtala S, Valenta R, Grönneberg R, van Hage-Hamsten M: Genetically engineered hypoallergenic derivatives of the major birch pollen allergen, Bet v 1, induce less eosinophilic activity in skin chamber fluids collected from birch pollen allergic patients than rBet v 1 wild type. J Allergy Clin Immunol, in press.

Rudolf Valenta
Department of Pathophysiology, AKH
University of Vienna, Währinger Gürtel 18–20
A–1090 Vienna (Austria)
Tel. +43 1 40400 5108, Fax +43 1 40400 5130
E-Mail Rudolf.Valenta@akh-wien.ac.at

Anti-IgE Antibody

Homer A. Boushey[a]   Robert Fick[b]   John V. Fahy[a]

[a] Department of Medicine, University of California, San Francisco, Calif., and [b] Genentech, Inc., S. San Francisco, Calif., USA

Summary

This brief review summarizes the rationale for selecting IgE as a target appropriate for specific therapy, the development and preclinical testing of a selective monoclonal anti-IgE antibody, the demonstration of its safety and efficacy in a clinical model, and, finally, the demonstration of the antibody's safety and efficacy in a large clinical trial.

A century has passed since it was first recognized that a soluble factor in serum is capable of transferring wheal and flare reactions to intradermal injection of allergen, but it was not until 1968 that IgE was recognized as the antibody responsible [1]. With the demonstration of a strong association between increased serum levels of IgE and bronchial hyperreactivity and skin test reactivity to allergens [2, 3], IgE came to be regarded as playing a central role in the pathogenesis of diseases associated with immediate hypersensitivity reactions, like anaphylaxis, allergic rhinitis and asthma. The mechanisms by which IgE plays this central role are thought to depend on its binding to high-affinity receptors (FcεRI receptors) on mast cells and basophils, and perhaps also to low affinity receptors (FcεRII receptors) on macrophages, dendritic cells, B lymphocytes, and other cells. On exposure to a specific allergen, allergen molecules crosslink adjacent Fab components of IgE on the cell surface, activating intracellular signal transduction. In mast cells, this cascade leads to the release of histamine, tryptase, and other preformed mediators. Antigen-antibody bridging also leads to the synthesis and release of other chemicals, including prostaglandin D_2, leukotrienes, and cytokines like TNF-α and IL-4 and IL-5. These compounds in turn cause vascular leakage, smooth muscle contraction, mucus secretion, and the attraction and activation of lymphocytes, eosinophils, neutrophils and other inflammatory cells.

Anti-IgE Antibody Development

The development of a therapeutic anti-IgE antibody was complicated, for anti-IgE antibodies directed against Fab components of the molecule – where allergen binding occurs – are themselves potent stimuli of mast cell degranulation and, therefore, of anaphylaxis. This complication was overcome by developing a monoclonal antibody that recognizes IgE at the same site as the high-affinity receptor for IgE (fig. 1) [4, 5]. These anti-IgE antibodies form complexes with free, unbound IgE but not with IgG or IgA. They were shown to lower serum free IgE in rodents and to block passive sensitization of lung fragments by serum from sensitized individuals. They thus appear to block the binding of IgE to its receptors on effector cells, like mast cells and basophils, but not to trigger the activation of these cells. Humanized versions of these murine monoclonal anti-IgE antibodies – rhuMab-E25 and CGP 51901 – were developed by grafting the variable immunoglobulin region of murine origin onto a 'backbone' of the constant region of human IgG1 [6]. This reduced the immunogenicity of the monoclonal antibody and enabled examination of the role of IgE in human disease.

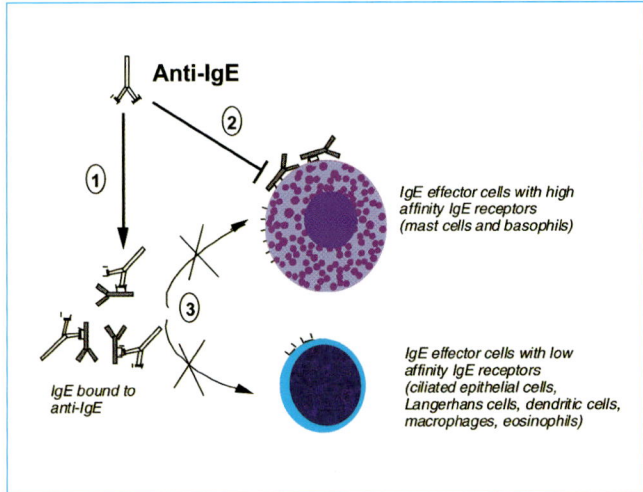

Fig. 1. Schematic of the mechanism of action of anti-IgE antibody. 1: Anti-IgE binds free IgE, and faciliates its removal via the reticuloendothelial system; 2: anti-IgE *does not* bind IgE already bound to high- or low-affinity IgE receptors on effector cells and is not anaphylactogenic; 3: IgE complexed to anti-IgE is unavailable to bind to receptors on IgE effector cells; leading ultimately to their 'disarmament'. From Fahy [5], with permission.

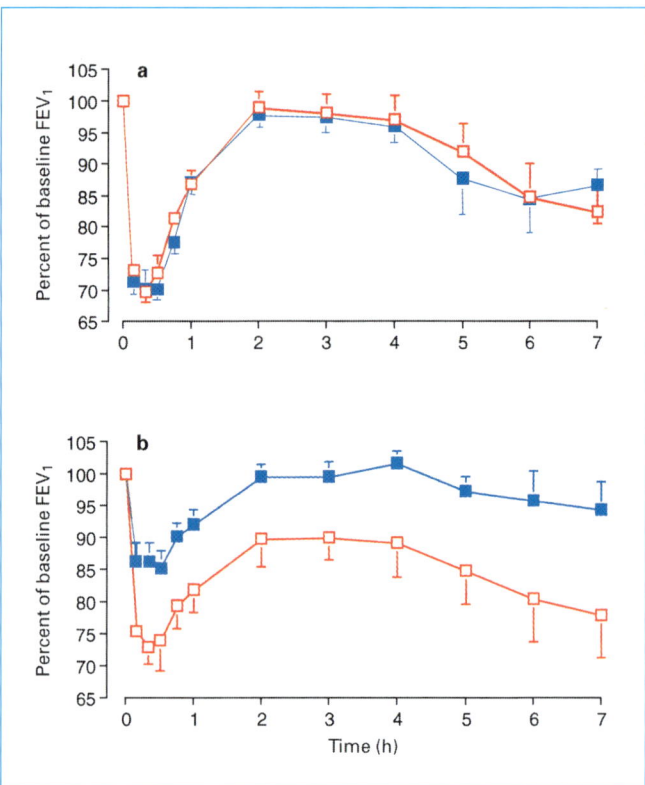

Fig. 2. Effects of anti-IgE on early- and late-phase responses to inhaled allergen in 18 allergic asthmatic subjects. FEV_1 is plotted as a percent of baseline. The early- and late-phase responses at baseline (□) and after treatment (■) were similar in the placebo group (**a**) but were significantly reduced in the rhuMAb-E25 group (**b**). From Fahy et al. [9], with permission.

Safety and 'Proof-of-Concept' Testing

Repeated injection of allergic human subjects with E25, a humanized anti-IgE antibody, did not provoke anaphylaxis and lowered serum free IgE levels by >99% [7]. Furthermore, this treatment also reduced basophil FcεRI density by 96% and antigen-stimulated histamine release from basophils by 90% [7]. These actions seem ideal for inhibiting IgE-mediated responses to allergen. The effects of E25 treatment were then examined in allergic human subjects, by analyzing its effects on the airway responses to allergen challenge. Two concurrent studies were undertaken. One examined the effects of E25 treatment on the dose of allergen needed to provoke an early (within 15 min) fall in the forced expired volume in 1 s (FEV_1), and the other examined the effects of treatment on both the early and the late (4–8 h) bronchoconstriction provoked by inhalation of allergen. In neither study did E25 provoke anaphylaxis in any subject; in both studies, the treatment lowered serum free IgE to unmeasurably low levels. The first study showed the dose of allergen required to cause immediate bronchoconstriction more than doubled after 4 weeks of treatment [8]. The second study, which examined the effects of 9 weeks of treatment [9], showed significant reductions in the early and late responses to allergen challenge (fig. 2). This study also showed E25 treatment to reduce the number of circulating eosinophils and the increases in bronchial reactivity and in sputum eosinophilia provoked by allergen challenge.

Animal Studies of E25

The availability of the murine form of anti-IgE antibody also allowed the study of the role of IgE in the eosinophilic inflammation of the airways provoked by antigen challenge in sensitized mice. Coyle et al. [10] showed that giving an anti-IgE antibody to dust-mite-sensitized mice 6 h before airway challenge significantly reduced the influx of eosinophils into the airways. Anti-IgE treatment also inhibited the production of IL-4 and IL-5, but not IFN-γ, by lung lymphocytes. Interestingly, allergen challenge of mice pretreated with anti-CD23 or of mice deficient in CD23 also caused little influx of eosinophils in BAL samples 24 h later. These findings suggest that IgE-dependent mechanisms are important in the induction of

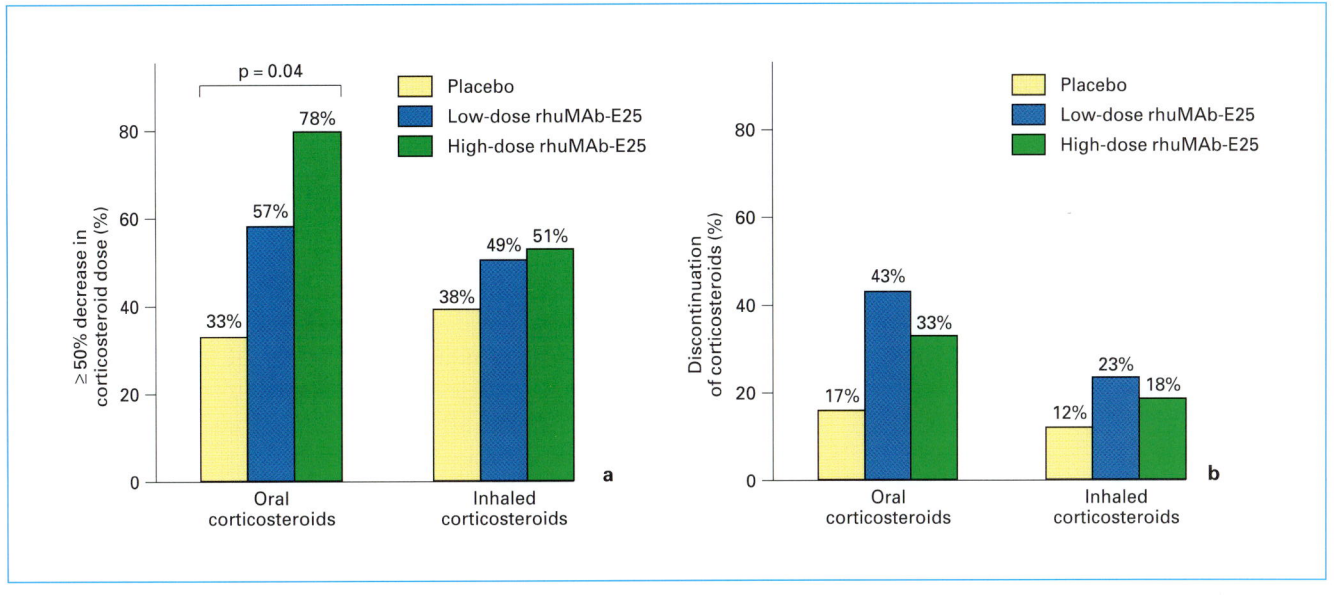

Fig. 3. Results of efforts to taper the dose of corticosteroids. **a** Percentage of subjects in each group who were able to reduce their daily corticosteroid dose by at least 50% at 20 weeks. **b** Percentage of subjects in each group who were able to discontinue corticosteroid therapy. In the placebo, low-dose, and high-dose groups, 12, 14, and 9 subjects, respectively, were taking oral corticosteroids and 93, 92, and 97 subjects were taking inhaled corticosteroids. Subjects who left the study had their last recorded dose carried forward. rhuMAb-E25 = Recombinant humanized monoclonal antibody E25. From Milgrom et al. [15], with permission.

the characteristic Th2 cytokine response to allergen and the subsequent infiltration of eosinophils into the airways. They further suggest that the low-affinity IgE receptor, CD23 (FcεRII), may be important in mediating the airway eosinophilia initiated by antigen-IgE binding. Support for this idea comes from the finding that CD23 mediates IgE-dependent antigen focusing by human B lymphocytes [11].

Clinical Trials

The first large clinical trial of the efficacy of the humanized, monoclonal anti-IgE antibody, E25, examined the effects of repeated dosing on the severity of symptoms of allergic rhinitis [12]. This study confirmed that the symptoms of rhinitis correlated with antigen-specific IgE levels and also that E25 caused no important toxicity while reducing serum free IgE levels. But because the doses were not individualized for each subject's baseline IgE level, serum free IgE was reduced to undetectable levels in only 11 of the 181 given active treatment. The quartile of subjects with the highest E25:IgE dosing (lowest baseline IgE) had little or no increase in symptoms during the ragweed season. Indeed, because the number of IgE antibodies that must be activated to provoke the release of 50% of basophil histamine is only 1,000 per cell [13], and because the number of FcεRI receptors per basophil is estimated at between 0.5×10^4 and 1.0×10^6 [14], it is calculated that serum free IgE must be lowered by >99%. Using this reasoning, the dose of E25 was adjusted according to the subjects' baseline IgE levels in subsequent studies.

When given as regular treatment to patients with moderate to severe asthma requiring regular treatment with inhaled or oral corticosteroids, E25 again showed safety and efficacy [15]. A double-blind, prospective study of >300 patients compared the effects of placebo and of two doses of E25 given as adjunctive therapy. Treatment with 'low dose' or 'high dose' E25 (2.5 or 5.8 μg/kg per ng IgE/ml) was given every 2 weeks for 20 weeks. In both active treatment groups, serum free IgE dropped rapidly and remained low over the course of the study (low-dose group = 18.0 ng/ml; high-dose group = 10.2 ng/ml). Both active treatments significantly improved morning peak flow, quality of life scores, the need for rescue treatments with albuterol, and the severity of asthma symptoms. Active treatment also enabled significant reduction in the dose requirements for corticosteroid treatment (fig. 3). Apart from a slight increase in urticaria, adverse events were no more frequent in the active treatment groups than in the placebo group. Another large study has shown

E25 to be effective in adults and children with ragweed allergic rhinitis [16]. Patients randomized to receive E25 demonstrated a 24 and 39% improvement in the nasal and ocular symptoms, respectively, and a 54% reduction in use of rescue medications [15]. Other studies of E25 in adults and children with moderately severe asthma have just been completed [17, 18]. Both confirm the safety and efficacy of the antibody, and add the important demonstration of a significant reduction in the frequency of asthma exacerbations, both when E25 was given as therapy adjunctive to corticosteroids and later when corticosteroid treatment was tapered.

Discussion

Studies of a highly selective monoclonal anti-IgE antibody in human subjects confirm that IgE plays an important role in asthma and allergic rhinitis. Treatment with anti-IgE antibody reduces both the early and late airway responses to allergen challenge, and brings about significant improvement in asthma control in patients with chronic corticosteroid-dependent asthma. But careful examination of these studies can raise questions as to whether the role of IgE wholly mediates the response to allergen. In the study by Boulet et al. [8], the effects of E25 on the provocative dose of allergen were no greater after 8 weeks than after 4 weeks of treatment. And in the large study by Milgrom et al. [15], the clinical effects were as great with low-dose as with high-dose treatment. Neither study was designed to examine the dose and time dependency of the effects of E25, however, and it is possible that cells armed with IgE persist in the airways for long periods after serum free IgE has been reduced to undetectable levels. Still, the apparent absence of dose and time dependency of the inhibitory effects of anti-IgE monoclonal antibody treatment raises the possibility that other, non-IgE-dependent mechanisms may also contribute to the responses to allergen challenge and to the pathophysiologic disturbances responsible for chronic asthma. The extraordinary specificity of action of this monoclonal antibody may make possible the study of the hypothesis that IgE *amplifies* sensitivity to allergens, but is not necessarily its sole mechanism.

Studies of B-cell-deficient mice have demonstrated that pulmonary eosinophilia and airway hyperresponsiveness can be induced in the absence of immunoglobulins [19, 20]. It has also been shown that nasal eosinophilia can be induced in IgE-deficient mice [21]. Other studies have shown that cloned Th2 cells [22] and even IL-13 alone [23, 24] are sufficient to induce an asthma-like phenotype. In contrast, a study of mice selected for the production of large amounts of IgE showed that antibody neutralization of IgE reduced tissue eosinophilia, mucous metaplasia, and airway hyperreactivity [25]. It has even been shown that the role of IgE may depend on the conditions of sensitization and on the contribution of other mediators of eosinophilic infiltration, like IL-5 [26].

Definition of the role of IgE in human asthmatic responses will likely require study of the changes in responses at different time points of prolonged therapy with a range of doses. Animal studies will likely need to focus on the possible contribution of IgE to the changes that occur with repeated allergen inhalation over prolonged periods after initial sensitization, exploiting the power of genetic alterations to knock out or heighten expression of molecular mechanisms thought to play a critical role.

Conclusion

The importance of IgE in human asthma, inferred from studies of people with allergic disease, of sensitized animals, and of isolated tissues and cells, has been confirmed by studies of an exquisitely selective mechanism for reducing IgE treatment with a monoclonal antibody directed against the portion of IgE that binds to its receptors. The agent developed from humanization of a murine anti-IgE antibody, E25, has been proven safe and effective in reducing serum free IgE levels, in reducing the number of IgE receptors expressed on the surface of basophils, and in reducing the clinical severity of asthma, the frequency of exacerbations, and the corticosteroid requirements of patients with moderate or severe asthma. Clinical studies show E25 treatment to significantly improve asthma, but – at least in the patients studied so far – not to 'cure' it. This raises the possibility that IgE serves to amplify allergic reactions partially mediated by antibody-independent pathways. But even if IgE acts only as an amplifying mechanism, it is clear that this amplification is important in human disease. The development of a selective, apparently safe anti-IgE monoclonal antibody holds great promise not only as a research tool for defining the role of IgE in health and disease, but also as a novel treatment of asthma and allergic disease.

References

1 Bennich HH, Ishizaka K, Johansson SGO, et al: Immunoglobulin E, a new class of human immunoglobulin. Bull World Hlth Org 1968; 38:151–152.
2 Burrows B, Martinez FD, Halonen M, et al: Association of asthma with serum IgE levels and skin-test reactivity to allergens. N Engl J Med 1989;320:271–277.
3 Sears MR, Burrows B, Flannery EM, et al: Relation between airway responsiveness and serum IgE in children with asthma and in apparently normal children. N Engl J Med 1991;325:1067–1071.
4 Presta L, Shields R, O'Connell L, et al: The binding site on human immunoglobulin E for its high affinity receptor. J Biol Chem 1994; 269:26368–26373.
5 Fahy JV: Anti-IgE treatment strategy for asthma; in Yeadon M, Diamant Z (eds): Lung Biology in Health and Disease. New and Exploratory Therapeutic Agents for Asthma, edited by Lenfant C. New York, Dekker, in press.
6 Presta LG, Lahr SJ, Shields RL, et al: Humanization of an antibody directed against IgE. J Immunol 1993; 151:2623–2632.
7 MacGlashan DW, Bochner BS, Adelman DC, et al: Down-regulation of FcεRI expression on human basophils during in vivo treatment of atopic patients with anti-IgE antibody. J Immunol 1997;158:1438–1445.
8 Boulet L-P, Chapman KR, Cote J, et al: Inhibitory effects of an anti-IgE antibody E25 on allergen-induced early asthmatic response. Am J Respir Crit Care Med 1997;155:1835–1840.
9 Fahy JV, Fleming HE, Wong HH, et al: The effect of an anti-IgE monoclonal antibody on the early- and late-phase responses to allergen inhalation in asthmatic subjects. Am J Respir Crit Care Med 1997;155:1828–1834.
10 Coyle AJ, Wagner K, Bertrand C, et al: Central role of immunoglobulin (Ig) E in the induction of lung eosinophil infiltration and T helper 2 cell cytokine production: Inhibition by a non-anaphylactogenic anti-IgE antibody. J Exp Med 1996;183:1303–1310.
11 Pirron U, Schlunck T, Prinz JC, et al: IgE dependent antigen focusing by human B lymphocytes is mediated by the low affinity receptor for IgE. Eur J Immunol 1990;20:1547–1551.
12 Casale TB, Bernstein IL, Busse WW, et al: Use of an anti-IgE humanized monoclonal antibody in ragweed-induced allergic rhinitis. J Allergy Clin Immunol 1997;100:110–121.
13 MacGlashan DW, Peters SP, Warner J, et al: Characteristics of human basophil sulfidopeptide leukotriene release: Releasability defined as the ability of the basophil to respond to dimeric cross-links. J Immunol 1986;136:2231–2239.
14 Conroy MC, Adkinson NF, Lichtenstein LM: Measurement of IgE on human basophils: Relation to serum IgE and anti-IgE-induced histamine release. J Immunol 1977;118:1317–1324.
15 Milgrom H, Fick RB, Su JQ, et al: Treatment of allergic asthma with monoclonal anti-IgE antibody. N Engl J Med 1999;341:1966–1973.
16 Casale T, Condemi J, Miller SD, et al: rhuMAb-E25 in the treatment of seasonal allergic rhinitis (SAR). Ann Allergy Asthma Immunol 1999;82:75.
17 Busse W, Corren J, Lanier BQ, et al: rhuMAb-E25 (E25), a novel therapy for the treatment of allergic asthma (AA) (abstract). J Allergy Clin Immunol, in press.
18 Milgrom H, Nayak A, Berger W, et al: The efficacy and safety of rhuMAb-E25 (E25) in children with allergic asthma (AA) (abstract). J Allergy Clin Immunol, in press.
19 Corry DB, Grunig G, Hadeiba H, et al: Requirements for allergen-induced airway hyperreactivity in T and B cell-deficient mice. Mol Med 1998;4:344–355.
20 MacLean JA, Sauty A, Luster AD, et al: Antigen-induced airway hyperresponsiveness, pulmonary eosinophilia, and chemokine expression in B-cell-deficient mice. Am J Respir Cell Mol Biol 1999;20:379–387.
21 Van De Rijn M, Mehlhop PD, Judkins A, et al: A murine model of allergic rhinitis: Studies on the role of IgE in pathogenesis and analysis of the eosinophil influx elicited by allergen and eotaxin. J Allergy Clin Immunol 1998;102:65–74.
22 Kaminuma O, Mori A, Ogawa K, et al: Cloned Th cells confer eosinophilic inflammation and bronchial hyperresponsiveness. Int Arch Allergy Immunol 1999;118:136–139.
23 Wills-Karp M, Luyimbazi J, Xu X, et al: Interleukin-13: Central mediator of allergic asthma. Science 1998;282:2258–2261.
24 Grunig G, Warnock M, Wakil AE, et al: Requirement for IL-13 independently of IL-4 in experimental asthma. Science 1998;282:2261–2263.
25 Haile S, Lefort J, Eum SY, et al: Suppression of immediate and late responses to antigen by a non-anaphylactogenic anti-IgE antibody in a murine model of asthma. Eur Respir J 1999;13:961–969.
26 Hamelmann E, Tadeda K, Oshiba A, et al: Role of IgE in the development of allergic airway inflammation and airway hyperresponsiveness – a murine model. Allergy 1999;54:297–305.

Homer A. Boushey
Department of Medicine
University of California San Francisco
Box 0130, 1292-M, 505 Parnassus Avenue
San Francisco, CA 94143 (USA)
Tel. +1 415 476 8019, Fax +1 415 502 6235
E-Mail hab2@itsa.ucsf.edu

CD23

Daniel H. Conrad

Virginia Commonwealth University, Richmond, Va., USA

Summary

Model studies of transgenic animals overproducing CD23 as well as the demonstrated utility of LZ-EC-CD23 suggest that CD23 is indeed a potential target protein for use in type I allergic disease. CD23 may have increased potential in type I diseases such as asthma, where the level of improvement anti-IgE using anti-IgE is moderate. Agents that cause an increase in CD23 or injection of chimeric CD23 with the capacity to block IgE/FcεRI interactions both represent potential treatment modalities that warrant further investigation.

Human type I allergy, with the possible exception of certain idiopathic asthma situations, is a disease mediated by IgE. Thus, targeting IgE, either at the production level or by blocking binding to the high-affinity IgE receptor (FcεRI), is an attractive concept. As seen in the previous chapter, anti-IgE targeted to the site on the IgE molecule that interacts with the FcεRI has shown considerable promise in this regard, especially with respect to inhibiting binding to the FcεRI and is now being used clinically [1]. The low-affinity IgE receptor (FcεRII), also known as CD23, represents another IgE-binding molecule that has potential to block IgE-mediated disease. Since its discovery in 1978, CD23 has been proposed to play a role in controlling IgE production. Indeed the finding that IL-4 upregulated both IgE and CD23 synthesis leads to the attractive hypothesis that IL-4 induces both a positive effect, namely IgE production, and a negative regulator for the same, namely CD23. However, until recently, data supporting this concept have been limited.

Anti-CD23 Inhibits IgE Production

The initial evidence pointing for a role in IgE regulation came from the use of anti-CD23. Sherr et al. [2] demonstrated that both anti-CD23, as well as anti-IgE/IgE complexes inhibited IgE synthesis in human in vitro model systems involving either an IgE producing plasmacytoma line or B cells from atopic patients. In both cases, the IgE production observed was spontaneous rather than induced. Flores-Romo et al. [3] used a rabbit polyclonal anti-CD23 directed against the lectin domain and demonstrated that this antibody would inhibit an in vivo antigen-specific response in a rat model system. In both of these studies, the effect was limited to IgE in that synthesis of other Ig isotypes was not affected. Thus, these studies support a role for CD23 in IgE production, but do not provide a mechanism for this activity.

Mice Lacking or Overexpressing CD23

Several groups have produced $CD23^{-/-}$ animals. One of the initial studies reported an enhancement in antigen specific IgE production, subsequent to immunization with antigen-adjuvant [4]; however, other groups that analyzed different $CD23^{-/-}$ mice did not support this finding [5]. In more recent studies, $CD23^{-/-}$ mice have been shown to exhibit airway hyperresponsiveness, as well as elevated IgE responses, although an exact cause-effect hypothesis has yet to be proven [6]. Transgenic mice overproducing CD23 (CD23-tg) have also been produced. The initial animals utilized the Thy1 promoter, resulting in overexpression of CD23 primarily on T lym-

Fig. 1. Kinetics of Ag/alum response. CD23-tg (●) or littermate controls (▼) were immunized and boosted (arrow) with DNP-KLH in alum as described elsewhere [8] and bled on various days throughout the response. IgE (**a**) was essentially totally blocked over time with respect to that in littermate controls, and Ag-specific IgG1 (**b**) was also suppressed over time. The p values were determined by Student's t test. p < 0.05, statistically significant. Error bars are ± 1 SE. Reprinted from Payet et al. [8] with permission. Copyright 1999 The American Association of Immunologists.

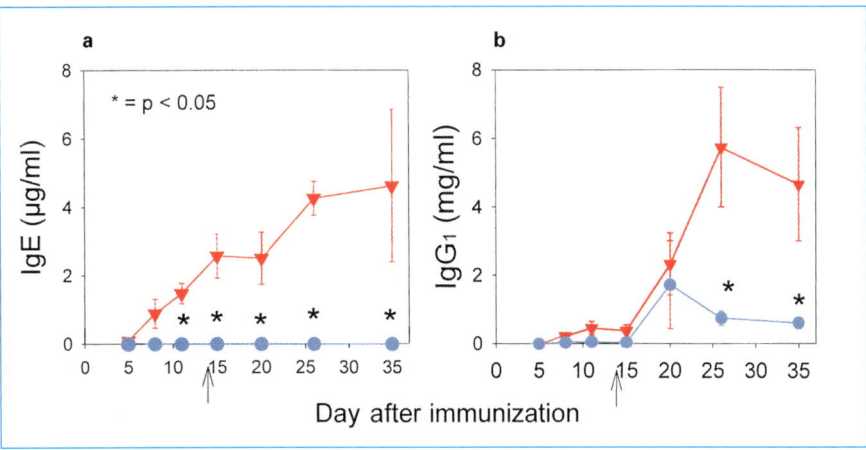

phocytes [7]. These animals exhibited an approximately 50% suppression of IgE production in response to antigen-adjuvant injections while responses to a stronger IgE stimulus, such as helminth infections, were not significantly affected. A second group of CD23-tg has been reported recently. In this case, CD23 expression was controlled by the MHC class I promoter combined with the Ig enhancer; a combination that resulted in overexpression primarily in the lymphoid compartment [8]. These animals exhibited a profound suppression of IgE production in response to antigen-adjuvant injection (fig. 1), and IgE responses to helminth infection were also significantly decreased. As can be seen in figure 1, antigen specific IgG1 responses were also decreased. Responses of other Ig isotypes were not significantly affected. In further studies, the mechanism of this suppression has been investigated. Adoptive transfer studies have indicated that a background cell, follicular dendritic cells, are potentially important for the observed suppression [M. Payet and D.H. Conrad, unpubl. data]. In other studies from this laboratory, IgE suppression had been observed in an in vitro model system where B cells were triggered to produce IgE in the presence of CHO cells overexpressing CD23 [9]. When combined with the CD23-tg adoptive transfer studies mentioned above, the results indicate that stimulation of Ig class switching, especially to IgE, is inhibited if the B lymphocytes are exposed to high levels of membrane CD23. This would suggest that an alternative allergy therapy strategy would be to induce elevated CD23 levels, especially on follicular dendritic cells. Since CD23 catabolism involves a metalloprotease digestion while at the cell surface, blocking this protease is one way of elevating CD23 levels. Christie et al. [10] demonstrated that the metalloprotease inhibitor batimistat had this ability namely CD23 degradation was inhibited and, interestingly, IgE levels in immunized mice treated with batimastat were suppressed.

Chimeric CD23 That Blocks FcεRI IgE Interaction

As mentioned above, CD23 is initially a membrane-bound molecule, but is cleaved while at the cell surface by (based on inhibitor studies) a membrane metalloprotease. The released fragment, termed soluble CD23 (sCD23) contains the entire lectin domain, and mutation analysis demonstrated that it is this lectin domain that interacts with IgE. However, in spite of an intact lectin domain, sCD23 interacts with IgE with at least an order of magnitude lower effective affinity than the membrane form. An explanation for this discrepancy comes from saturation binding analysis of IgE with membrane CD23 [11] in which a dual affinity was demonstrated. Beavil et al. [12] demonstrated that the stalk region of CD23 (defined as the domain in between the lectin and transmembrane domains) exhibited a heptad repeat pattern characteristic of molecules that form an α-helical coiled coil. The dual affinity of CD23 is explained by the multipoint interaction of two lectin domains with apparently different regions of the Cε3 domain of the IgE molecule (high affinity), while the lower affinity represents interaction with a single lectin domain. The finding that sCD23 exhibits only the low-affinity interaction suggests that the proteolytic cleavages, which are exclusively in the stalk domain, result in an equilibrium that greatly favors the monomeric molecule, which would be expected to interact with IgE with only a single low affinity. By this analysis, the high-affinity interaction is actually a result of avidity considerations in which at least two lectin domains interact with an IgE molecule. Proof of this

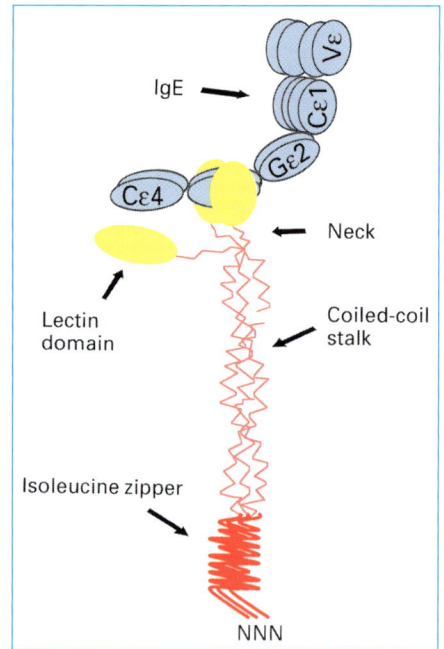

Fig. 2. Schematic representation of LZ-EC-C1M. The LZ-EC-C1M contains a modified isoleucine zipper motif attached to the amino terminus of the entire extracellular domain of CD23. The lectin head of CD23 consists of aa 189 to the end; the putative neck domain consists of aa 157–188, and the stalk domain contains aa 55–157. Reprinted from Kelly et al. [16] with permission. Copyright 1998 The American Association of Immunologists.

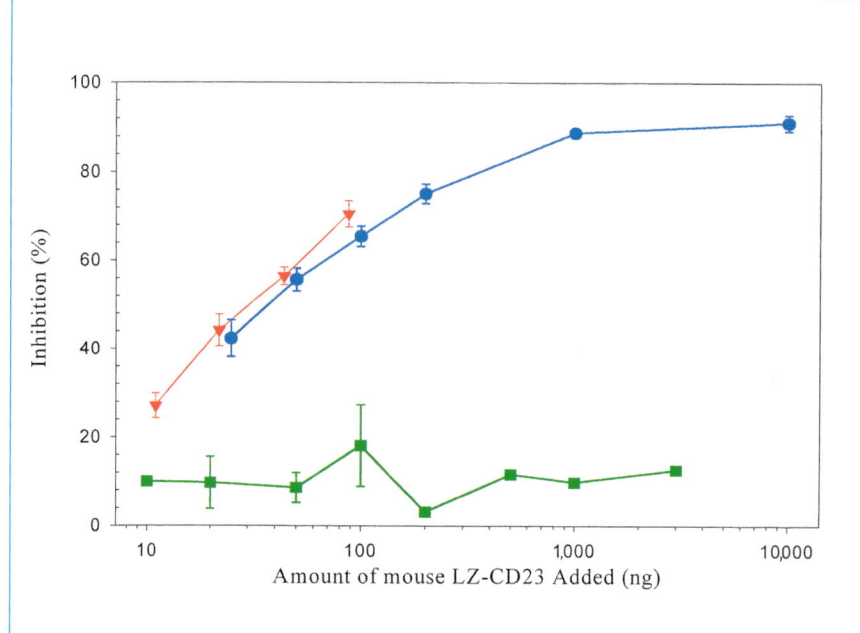

Fig. 3. Capacity of EC-CD23 vs LZ-EC-CD23 to inhibit ^{125}I-labeled mIgE binding to C57 mast cells. Increasing volumes of supernatant from LZ-EC-CD23-transfected COS cells (▼) or purified LZ-EC-CD23 (●) or EC-CD23 (■) (both prepared in *E. coli*) were added to C57 mast cells in a binding assay as described elsewhere [16]. Percentage inhibition of ^{125}I-IgE binding was calculated as follows: (cpm experimental – cpm 100-fold excess of unlabeled IgE)/(cpm control with no inhibitor – cpm 100-fold excess of unlabeled IgE) × 100. Reprinted from Kelly et al. [16] with permission. Copyright 1998 The American Association of Immunologists.

model awaits analysis of crystal structure, but the model fits current data.

Initial attempts to produce a soluble CD23 with full IgE binding activity were directed at using the entire extracellular region of CD23 (termed EC-CD23), produced by removing the DNA that codes for the cytoplasmic and transmembrane domains, placing the truncated cDNA in an appropriate expression vector in frame with a leader sequence and analyzing the secreted molecule. Alternatively, the molecular engineering product was produced in *Escherichia coli* and renatured from inclusion bodies. EC-CD23 was found to exhibit an intermediate affinity for IgE when compared to native sCD23 and membrane CD23 [13]. This indicates that the transmembrane and cytoplasmic domains help in some manner to stabilize the oligomeric structure, potentially by simply restricting the mobility of the molecule by the constraint of being membrane-bound. Utilizing the finding by McGrew et al. [14] that adding the sequence coding for a modified leucine zipper to the amino terminus of soluble CD40 ligand was a very effective way to produce trimeric soluble CD40 ligand, a similar trimeric construct was produced with CD23. The modified leucine zipper is the GCN4 sequence (which in its native form is a dimer) in which isoleucines are substituted for leucines; this modification has been shown by X-ray crystallography to result in α-helical coiled coil trimer formation when the modified protein is produced [15]. Addition of the modified leucine zipper motif to the amino terminal end of EC-CD23 (fig. 2) resulted in a molecule that interacted with IgE at least as effectively as membrane bound CD23. Indeed this chimera, termed LZ-EC-CD23, was shown to be an effective inhibitor of the IgE/FcεRI interaction [16] (fig. 3), suggesting that this chimera could have potential clinical utility in much the same manner as the anti-IgE described earlier. Experiments to determine if the LZ-EC-CD23 chimera will both inhibit IgE synthesis as well as inhibit IgE/FcεRI interaction are under way as an influence on both activities would represent an advantageous situation.

References

1 Chang TW: The pharmacological basis of anti-IgE therapy. Nat Biotechnol 2000;18:157–162.
2 Sherr E, Macy E, Kimata H, Gilly M, Saxon A: Binding the low affinity FcεR on B cells suppresses ongoing human IgE synthesis. J Immunol 1989;142:481–489.
3 Flores-Romo L, Shields J, Humbert Y, Graber P, Aubry J-P, Gauchat J-F, Ayala G, Allet B, Chavez M, Bazin H, Capron M, Bonnefoy J-Y: Inhibition of an in vivo antigen-specific IgE response by antibodies to CD23. Science 1993; 261:1038–1041.
4 Yu P, Kosco-Vilbois M, Richards M, Köhler G, Lamers MC, Kohler G: Negative feedback regulation of IgE synthesis by murine CD23. Nature 1994;369:753–756.
5 Fujiwara H, Kikutani H, Suematsu S, Naka T, Yoshida K, Tanaka T, Suemura M, Matsumoto N, Kojima S, Kishimoto T, Yoshida N: The absence of IgE antibody-mediated augmentation of immune responses in CD23-deficient mice. Proc Natl Acad Sci USA 1994;91:6835–6839.
6 Cernadas M, De Sanctis GT, Krinzman SJ, Mark DA, Donovan CE, Listman JA, Kobzik L, Kikutani H, Christiani DC, Perkins DL, Finn PW: CD23 and allergic pulmonary inflammation: Potential role as an inhibitor. Am J Respir Cell Mol Biol 1999;20:1–8.
7 Texido G, Eibel H, Le Gros G, Van der Putten H: Transgene CD23 expression on lymphoid cells modulates IgE and IgG1 responses. J Immunol 1994;153:3028–3042.
8 Payet ME, Woodward EC, Conrad DH: Humoral response suppression observed with CD23 transgenics. J Immunol 1999;163:217–223.
9 Cho SW, Kilmon MA, Studer EJ, Van der Putten H, Conrad DH: B cell activation and Ig, especially IgE, production is inhibited by high CD23 levels in vivo and in vitro. Cell Immunol 1997;180:36–46.
10 Christie G, Barton A, Bolognese B, Buckle DR, Cook RM, Hansbury MJ, Harper GP, Marshall LA, McCord ME, Moulder K, Murdock PR, Seal SM, Spackman VM, Weston BJ, Mayer RJ: IgE secretion is attenuated by an inhibitor of proteolytic processing of CD23 (FcεRII). Eur J Immunol 1997;27:3228–3235.
11 Dierks SE, Bartlett WC, Edmeades RL, Gould HJ, Rao M, Conrad DH: The oligomeric nature of the murine FcεRII/CD23: Implications for function. J Immunol 1993;150:2372–2382.
12 Beavil AJ, Edmeades RL, Gould HJ, Sutton BJ: α-Helical coiled-coil stalks in the low-affinity receptor for IgE (FcεRII/CD23) and related C-type lectins. Proc Natl Acad Sci USA 1992; 89:753–757.
13 Bartlett WC, Kelly AE, Johnson CM, Conrad DH: Analysis of murine soluble FcεRII: Sites of cleavage and requirements for dual affinity interaction with IgE. J Immunol 1995;154: 4240–4249.
14 McGrew JT, Leiske D, Dell B, Klinke R, Krasts D, Wee SF, Abbott N, Armitage R, Harrington K: Expression of trimeric CD40 ligand in *Pichia pastoris*: Use of a rapid method to detect high-level expressing transformants. Gene 1997;187:193–200.
15 Harbury PB, Kim PS, Alper T: Crystal structure of an isoleucine-zipper trimer. Nature 1994;371:80–83.
16 Kelly AE, Woodward EC, Chen B-H, Conrad DH: Production of a chimeric form of CD23 that is oligomeric and blocks IgE binding to the FcεRI. J Immunol 1998;161:6696–6704.

Daniel H. Conrad
PO Box 980678, MCV Station
Richmond, VA 23298 (USA)
Tel. +1 804 828 2311, Fax +1 804 828 9946
E-Mail dconrad@hsc.vcu.edu

T Cell Immunomodulation

T Cell Immunomodulation: An Overview

Athanasios Koulis   Douglas S. Robinson

Allergy and Clinical Immunology, Imperial College School of Medicine, National Heart and Lung Institute, London, UK

Summary

There is now good evidence that atopic allergic asthma is driven by allergen-specific Th2-type T cells. Corticosteroids and other immunosuppressive drugs reduce T cell activation and cytokine production, but at the risk of side effects. Recent advances in understanding the immunology of Th2 cells gives the opportunity of specific immunomodulation to control asthma and allergy. Approaches include cytokine modulation of the Th1/Th2 balance, specific allergen or peptide immunotherapy, with or without adjuvants, and targeting Th2 T cells through co-stimulatory molecules, chemokine receptors or IL-1R family receptors.

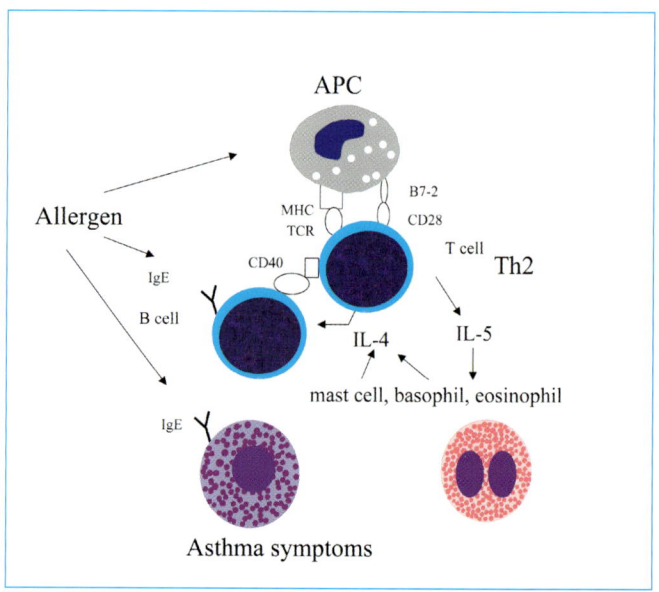

Fig. 1. The Th2 hypothesis of asthma. Allergen is taken up by APCs (possibly via high-affinity IgE receptors) and processed into peptide fragments. These are then complexed with MHC class II molecules and interact with CD4 T cells with a T cell receptor recognizing that particular complex. A second signal is required to activate the T cell: this co-stimulation can be via CD28/CD80 or CD86, CD40 and CD40 ligand or other pathways. Th2 cell production of IL-4 is required for B cell switching to IgE production, and IL-5 activates and prolongs survival of eosinophils. Many potential targets for therapy stem from this model.

Atopic allergic asthma is thought to be a chronic inflammatory airway disease driven by Th2-type CD4+ T lymphocytes (fig. 1). The signature Th2 cytokines are IL-4, essential for IgE switching of B lymphocytes, and IL-5, which acts selectively in eosinophil maturation, survival and activation [1, 2]. In addition to the CD4+ Th2 model of asthma, CD8+ Tc2 T cells may also play a role [3], and T cells may also contribute to airway hyperresponsiveness through mechanisms not dependent on IL-4 or IL-5 [4, 5]. If allergic asthma is driven by T cells responding to allergen, then this is an attractive target for specific therapeutic intervention.

The current mainstay of asthma therapy is corticosteroid treatment, which is associated with a reduction of T cell activation in the airway, and in T cell expression of Th2 cytokines including IL-4 and IL-5 [6, 7]. Although inhaled corticosteroids are generally effective and well tolerated, there are theoretical long-term safety concerns, and these agents control inflammation, but do not alter the underlying immune reactivity predisposing to atopic airway inflammation. Thus strategies for the immunodulation of T cell responses are attractive since they may offer the prospect of long-term disease modification and prevention.

There is less information on non-atopic asthma although both occupational and intrinsic asthma are characterized by airway T cell activation and eosinophilia, by

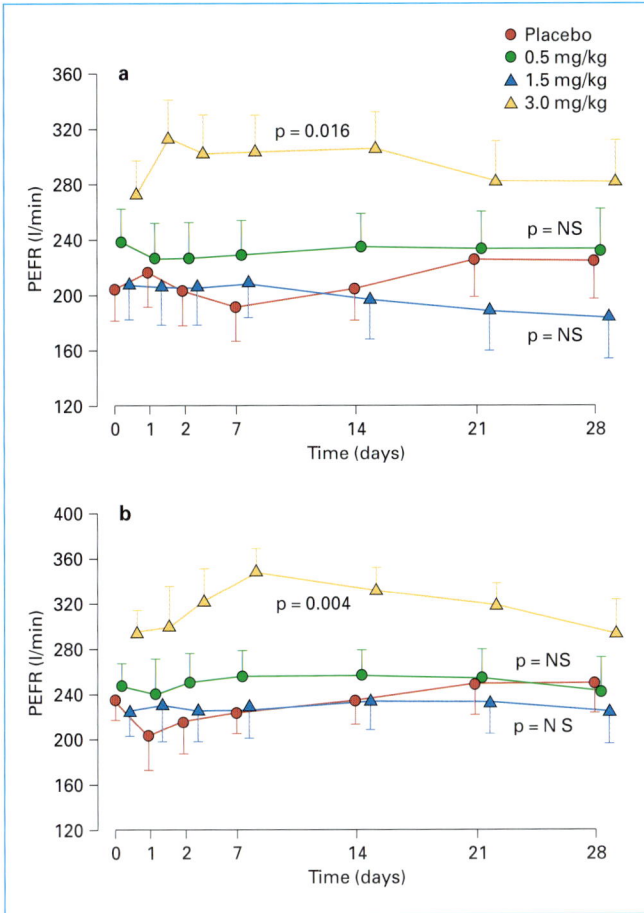

Fig. 2. Effect of anti-CD4 monoclonal antibody in chronic, steroid-dependent asthma. In a double-blind, dose ranging study, four groups of patients with severe asthma were randomized to a single infusion of placebo or three doses of humanized anti-CD4 (keliximab). At the highest dose there was a sustained and statistically significant improvement in have morning (**a**) and evening (**b**) peak expiratory flow rate (PEFR) [19].

a similar increase in bronchial mucosal expression of IL-4 and IL-5 and evidence of local IgE synthesis [8]. In COPD, biopsy studies also show a T cell infiltrate, with variable contribution from neutrophils and eosinophils in different patients [9].

Approaches to T Cell Modulation

Cytokines That Modulate Th1/Th2 Development or Phenotype Expression. IL-12 drives Th1 expansion from naïve T cells in vitro, and in vivo, and reduces Th2 cell cytokine production [10]. In murine models IL-12 blocks airway hyperresponsiveness and eosinophilia to inhaled antigen challenge [11]. However, preliminary data on IL-12 in humans did not show efficacy on allergen challenge [Kips J., abstract, presented at European Respiratory Society Annual Congress, Madrid 1999].

IL-4 is critical for the development of Th2 cells [10], and blockade of IL-4 via a soluble IL-4 receptor has recently been shown to be effective in clinical asthma in a phase 1 study [12].

Immunoregulatory Cytokines. IL-10 acts to reduce antigen-presenting cell (APC) MHC class II expression and thus inhibits T cell activation [13]. In the mouse, it was described to specifically inhibit Th2 responses, to reduce proliferation and cytokine production by both human Th1 and Th2 cells, to influence APC and exert a direct activity on T cells. IL-10-gene-deleted mice develop spontaneous colitis, suggesting an important role for this cytokine in homoeostatic immune regulation. Pilot studies reported in other chapters in this book did not show any inhibitory activity on the allergen-induced late asthmatic response.

Transforming growth factor-β (TGF-β) has a number of properties that make it a strong anti-inflammatory and immunoregulatory agent [14]. Depending on the cell type, TGF-β downregulates the activity of a number of G1 cyclins and associated cyclin-dependent kinases. It has anti-proliferative effects on both Th1 and Th2 cells, B cells, CD8+ cells, NK cells and macrophages.

Th2-Specific Transcription Factors. Th1- or Th2-specific transcription factors (e.g. GATA-3 for IL-5 and Th2 responses [15]) have been described in murine and some human systems. These too are potential targets for intervention, although lack of specificity and involvement in other gene activation mechanisms may limit their clinical use.

Co-Stimulation. Activation of T cells relies on two signals: one delivered via the T-cell-receptor-engaging peptide/MHC complex, and a second signal termed 'co-stimulation'. Engagement of the TCR without co-stimulation can lead to antigen-specific non-responsiveness upon re-challenge, termed 'anergy'. Blockade of T cell co-stimulation via anti-CD80 [16], CD86 [17] or with CTLA-4-Ig, also inhibited airway hyperresponiveness and eosinophilia in mouse models of airway challenge, and blocked antibodies to CD4. Antibodies to CD86 could inhibit allergen-induced responses of both blood and airway T cells from atopic asthmatics [18]. More directly targeting the T cell, a dose finding study of humanized anti-CD4 in severe asthma showed significant improvement in peak flow and symptoms (fig. 2) [19]. The problem with this approach is that it will block all T cell responses and thus may cause immunosuppression.

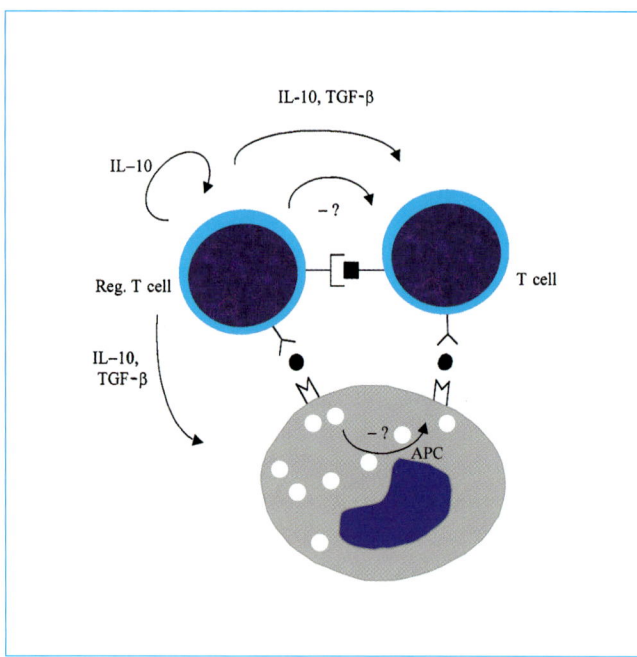

Fig. 3. T cell immunomodulation. Regulatory T cells suppress T cell proliferation and cytokine production via the secretion of IL-10, TGF-β and via a contact-dependent pathway. T cell-T cell and T cell-antigen-presenting cell interactions may be mediated by CTLA4-CD80/86 or via a yet unknown set of molecules (Reg. T cell: Tr1 or Th3 or CD4+ CD25+).

Specific Blockade of Th2 Co-Stimulation. Recent evidence suggests that there may be Th2-specific co-stimulation, via inducible co-stimulator, at least in certain circumstances, and this could be a target in Th2-mediated disease [20]. Allergen immunotherapy and peptide-induced non-responsiveness are reviewed elsewhere in this volume [37].

Targeting Specific Th1 or Th2 Surface Markers. Recent data suggest that there is interaction with the innate immune response (via macrophage, dendritic cell or NK cell activation in an antigen non-specific fashion) that may specifically amplify the Th1 or Th2 limbs of an effector response via particular members of the IL-1 receptor family and Toll-like receptors. Thus IL-18 is an IL-1-like molecule that amplifies Th1 responses [21], whereas T1/ST2 is an IL-1R family member, selectively expressed by Th2 cells, that can amplify a Th2 response [22]. Similarly, different sets of chemokines acting on different chemokine receptors may recruit Th1 or Th2 cells. Th2 cells have been reported to express CCR3 [23], CCR4 [24] and CCR8 [25].

Immunosuppressive Drugs. Cyclosporin A interferes with IL-2 transcription, and thus T cell activation, by inhibiting the transcription factor NFAT, and also inhibits transcription of other T cell cytokines, including IL-5. Cyclosporin A was shown to improve lung function, to have a steroid-sparing role in severe steroid-dependent asthma, and to be able to reduce allergen-induced late asthmatic reactions. Other immunosuppressive drugs, including methotrexate, azathioprine and gold, have been shown to have some clinical efficacy in severe steroid-dependent asthma [26]. Intravenous immunogobulin was ineffective in placebo-controlled trials. Although these approaches carry the risk of side effects and are not applicable to most asthmatics, they provide support for the concept that the CD4 T cell is a drug target in asthma.

Immune Deviation and Regulatory T Cells

Allergen Immunotherapy. Allergen injection immunotherapy (AII) is a very effective treatment for some allergic diseases, particularly bee or wasp venom anaphylaxis or hay fever. As reviewed elsewhere in this book, it has been suggested that AII may modulate allergen-specific T cell responses from a predominantly Th2 phenotype towards a Th1 or Th0 pattern [27]. A number of adjuvants have been suggested to increase this effect, including CpG oligonucleotides and mycobacterial products.

Another pattern seen in studies of AII is induction of CD4+CD25+ T cells that show low proliferative responses to allergen, but produce IL-10 and suppress proliferative and cytokine responses of other T cells [28]. These may be regulatory T cells (fig. 3).

Regulatory T Cells. In recent years years, the role of immunosuppression by specific subsets of T cells has gained significant ground. Several regulatory T cell subsets have been described:
- Human and mouse Tr1 clones derived from cells stimulated in the presence of IL-10 [29]. These cells had low proliferative capacity, and produced high levels of IL-10 and moderate amounts of TGF-β and IFN-γ. Additionally, human Tr1 clones secreted high levels of IL-5. These Tr1 clones were shown to be antigen specific, suppress the proliferation of CD4+ T cells in response to antigen via IL-10 production and the mouse clones could prevent colitis induced in SCID mice by the pathogenic CD4+CD45RB[high] splenic T cell subset.
- Murine Th3 clones were derived after feeding antigen to induce oral tolerance and could suppress autoimmune encephalomyelitis in mice [30]. These T cells produce TGF-β with various amounts of IL-4 and IL-10. Th3 cells were also induced in multiple sclerosis patients following oral myelin treatment [31].

- A CD4+CD25+ regulatory T cell population has been defined in mice [32, 33]. Traditionally, CD25 has been used as a marker of activated cells. However, CD4+CD25+ T cells isolated from the periphery or thymus of unstimulated animals are naturally anergic and suppress T cell proliferation. They produce little or no cytokines, and anergy can be removed by the addition, in vitro, of exogenous IL-2. They are antigen specific during activation but their effector function is antigen non-specific. Removal of this subset results in the induction of various autoimmune diseases in mice. More recent work has shown the suppression to be partially IL-10 dependent and CTLA-4 mediated. A T cell population, CD38+CD45RB^{low}, with immune regulatory properties was further characterized to be CD4+CD45RB^{low}CD38+CD25+ as the subset with the regulatory potential [34].
- Suppressor T cells were initially described to be CD8+ T cells. This T cell population suppresses the proliferative response of autologous CD4+ T cells in vitro and is distinguished from the cytolytic CD8+CD28+ cells by their lack of CD28 expression [35]. The T suppressor cells prevent the APCs from upregulating B7 molecule expression in response to T helper signals. APCs exposed to the suppressor T cells render other T helper cells anergic. This is due to the inhibition of the CD40 signalling pathway in APCs [36]. In effect, the T suppressor lymphocytes inhibit the NF-κB-mediated transcription of the CD86 gene in APCs.

The role of these various regulatory T cell populations in humans remains to be established. However, if such a population can be induced by AII, this raises the possibility that specific induction of allergen-specific regulatory T cells may allow allergen specific control of allergen disease, including asthma.

T Cell Modulation in COPD. The role of T cells in COPD is much less well established. CD1-restricted T cells have been described for some bacterial antigens and it is possible that such responses to chronic respiratory infection may play a role. However, the failure of inhaled corticosteroids to impact on lung function or COPD symptoms raises doubt about the relevance of T-cell-directed therapy in this condition. A minority of smokers progress to COPD and a minority of aspergillus-sensitive subjects progress to bronchiectasis or allergic bronchopulmonary aspergillosis. The role of immunogenetics in these responses remains to be determined.

Conclusion

Better understanding of the immunology of T cell activation in atopic asthma has led to a number of exciting novel approaches to therapy, some of which are nearing clinical trials. The next 10 years should see dramatic developments in the control of allergic disease, including asthma, and in our understanding of the role of the immune response in other airway diseases including COPD.

References

1 Mosmann TR, Cherwinski H, Bond MW, Gieldin MA, Coffman RL. Two types of murine helper T cell clones. Definition according to profiles of lymphokine activities and secreted proteins. J Immunol 1986;136:2348–2357.

2 Robinson DS, Hamid Q, Sun Ying, Tsicopoulos A, Brakans J, Bentley AM, Corrigan CJ, Durham SR, Kay AB: Predominant TH2-like bronchoalveolar T-lymphocyte population in atopic asthma. N Engl J Med 1992;326:298–304.

3 Mosmann TR, Sad S: The expanding universe of T-cell subsets: Th1, Th2 and more. Immunol Today 1996;17:139–146.

4 Hogan SP, Matthaei KI, Young JM, Koskinen A, Young IG, Foster PS: A novel T cell-regulated mechanism modulating allergen-induced airways hyperreactivity in BALB/c mice independently of IL-4 and IL-5. J Immunol 1998; 161:1501–1509.

5 Haselden BM, Barry Kay A, Larche M: Immunoglobulin E-independent MHC-restricted T cell peptide epitope-induced late asthmatic reactions. J Exp Med 1999;189:1885–1894.

6 Robinson D, Hamid Q, Ying S, Bentley A, Assoufi B, Durham S, Kay AB: Prednisolone treatment in asthma is associated with modulation of bronchoalveolar lavage cell interleukin-4, interleukin-5 and interferon-gamma cytokine gene expression. Am Rev Respir Dis 1993; 148:401–406.

7 Leung DY, Martin RJ, Szefler SJ, Sher ER, Ying S, Kay AB, Hamid Q: Dysregulation of interleukin 4, interleukin 5, and interferon gamma gene expression in steroid-resistant asthma. J Exp Med 1995;181:33–40.

8 Humbert M, Menz G, Ying S, Corrigan CJ, Robinson DS, Durham SR, Kay AB: The immunopathology of extrinsic (atopic) and intrinsic (non-atopic) asthma: More similarities than differences. Immunol Today 1999;20:528–533.

9 Jeffery PK: Differences and similarities between chronic obstructive pulmonary disease and asthma. Clin Exp Allergy 1999;29(suppl 2): 14–26.

10 O'Garra A: Cytokines induce the development of functionally heterogeneous T helper cell subsets. Immunity 1998;8:275–283.

11 Gavett SH, O'Hearn DJ, Li X, Huang SK, Finkelman FD, Wills-Karp M: Interleukin 12 inhibits antigen-induced airway hyperresponsiveness, inflammation, and Th2 cytokine expression in mice J Exp Med 1995;182:1527–1536.

12 Borish LC, Nelson HS, Lanz MJ, Claussen L, Whitmore JB, Agosti JM, Garrison L: Interleukin-4 receptor in moderate atopic asthma. A phase i/ii randomized, placebo-controlled trial. Am J Respir Crit Care Med 1999;160:1816–1823.

13 Moore KW, O'Garra A, de Waal Malefyt R, Vieira P, Mosmann TR: Interleukin-10. Annu Rev Immunol 1993;11:165–190.
14 Prud'homme GJ, Piccirillo CA: The inhibitory effects of transforming growth factor-beta-1 in autoimmune diseases. J Autoimm 2000;14:23–42.
15 Zhang DH, Yang L, Cohn L, Parkyn L, Homer R, Ray P, Ray A: Inhibition of allergic inflammation in a murine model of asthma by expression of a dominant-negative mutant of GATA-3. Immunity 1999;11:473–482.
16 Harris N, Peach R, Naemura J, Linsley PS, Le Gros G, Ronchese F: CD80 costimulation is essential for the induction of airway eosinophilia. J Exp Med 1997;185:177–182.
17 Tsuyuki S, Tsuyuki J, Einsle K, Kopf M, Coyle AJ: Costimulation through B7-2 (CD86) is required for the induction of a lung mucosal T helper cell 2 (TH2) immune response and altered airway responsiveness. J Exp Med 1997; 185:1671–1679.
18 Larche M, Till S, Haselden BM, North J, Barkans J, Kay AB, Robinson DS: Co-stimulation through CD86 is involved in airway antigen presenting cell and T cell responses to allergen in atopic asthmatics. J Immunol 1998;161: 6375–6382.
19 Kon OM, Sihra BS, Compton CH, Leaonard TB, Kay AB, Barnes NC: Randomised, dose-ranging, placebo-controlled study of chimeric antibody to CD4 (keliximab) in chronic severe asthma. Lancet 1998;352:1109–1113.
20 Hutloff A, Dittrich AM, Beler KC, Eljaschewitsch B, Kraft R, Anagnoastopoulos I, Kroczek RA: ICOS is an inducible T-cell co-stimulator structurally related to CD28. Nature 1999; 397:263–266.
21 Robinson D, Shibuya K, Mui A, Zonin F, Murphy E, Sana T, Hartley SB, Menon S, Kastelein R, Bazan F, O'Garra A: IGIF does not drive Th1 development but synergizes with IL-12 for interferon γ production and activates IRAK and NFκB. Immunity 1997;7:571–581.
22 Lohning M, Stroehmann A, Coyle AJ, Grogan JL, Lin S, Gutierrez-Ramos JC, Levinson D, Radbruch A, Kamradt T: T1/ST2 is preferentially expressed on murine Th2 cells, independent of interleukin 4, interleukin 5, and interleukin 10, and important for Th2 effector function. Proc Natl Acad Sci USA 1998;95:6930–6935.
23 Sallusto F, Mackay CR, Lanzavecchia A: Selective expression of the eotaxin receptor CCR3 by human T helper 2 cells. Science 1997; 277:2005–2007.
24 Bonecchi R, Bianchi G, Bordignon PP, D'Ambrosio D, Lang R, Borsatti A, Sozzani S, Allavena P, Gray PA, Mantovani A, Sinigaglia F: Differential expression of chemokine receptors and chemotactic responsiveness of type 1 T helper cells (Th1s) and Th2s. J Exp Med 1998; 187:129–134.
25 Zingoni A, Soto H, Hedrick JA, Stoppacciaro A, Storlazzi CT, Sinigaglia F, D'Ambrosio D, O'Garra A, Robinson D, Rocchi M, Santoni A, Zlotnik A, Napolitano M: The chemokine receptor CCR8 is preferentially expressed in Th2 but not Th1 cells. J Immunol 1998;161:547–551.
26 Kon OM, Kay AB: Anti-T cell strategies in asthma. Inflamm Res 1999;48:516–523.
27 Durham SR, Till SJ: Immunologic changes associated with allergen immunotherapy. J Allergy Clin Immunol 1998;102:157–164.
28 Akdis CA, Blaser K: IL-10-induced anergy in peripheral T cell and reactivation by microenvironmental cytokines: Two key steps in specific immunotherapy. FASEB J 1999;13:603–609.
29 Groux H, O'Garra A, Bigler M, Rouleau M, Antonenko S, de Vries JE, Roncarolo MG: A CD4+ T-cell subset inhibits antigen-specific T-cell responses and prevents colitis. Nature 1997;389:737–742.
30 Chen Y, Kuchroo VK, Inobe J-L, Hafler DA Weiner HL: Regulatory T cell clones induced by oral tolerance: Suppression of autoimmune encephalomyelitis. Science 1994;265:1237–1240.
31 Fukaura H, Kent SC, Pietrusewicz MJ, Khoury SJ, Weiner HL, Hafler DA: Induction of circulating myelin basic protein and proteolipid protein-specific transforming growth factor β-1 secreting T cells by oral administration of myelin in multiple sclerosis patients J Clin Invest 1996;98:70–77.
32 Thornton AM, Shevach EM: CD4+CD25+ immunoregulatory T cells suppress polyclonal T cell activation in vitro by inhibiting interleukin 2 production. J Exp Med 1998;88:287–296.
33 Itoh M, Takahashi T, Sakaguchi N, Kuniyasu Y, Shimizu J, Otsuka F, Sakaguchi S: Thymus and autoimmunity: Production of CD25+ CD4+ naturally anergic and suppressive T cells as a key function of the thymus in maintaining immunologic self-tolerance. J Immunol 1999; 162:5317–5326.
34 Read S, Mauze S, Asseman C, Bean A, Coffman R, Powrie F: CD38+ CD45RB[low] CD4+ T cells: A population of T cells with immune regulatory activities in vitro. Eur J Immunol 1998; 28:3435–3447.
35 Damle NK, Engleman EG. Antigen-specific suppressor T lymphocytes in man. Clin Immunol Immunopathol 1998;53:S17–S24.
36 Liu Z, Tugulea S, Cortesini R, Lederman S, Suciu-Foca N: Inhibition of CD40 signalling pathway in antigen presenting cells by T suppressor cells. Hum Immunol 1999;60:568–574.
37 Larché M, Kay AB: Allergen, IgE and mast-cell-directed therapies: An overview; in Barnes P, Hansel T (eds): New Drugs for Asthma, Allergy and COPD. Prog Respir Res. Basel, Karger, 2001, vol 31, pp 182–185.

Douglas S. Robinson
Allergy and Clinical Immunology
Imperial College School of Medicine at the
National Heart and Lung Institute
London SW3 6LY (UK)
Tel. +44 207 351 8116, Fax +44 207 376 3138
E-Mail d.s.robinson@ic.ac.uk

Costimulatory Molecules in T Cell Activation

Anthony J. Coyle   Jose-Carlos Gutierrez-Ramos

Millennium Pharmaceuticals Inc., Cambridge, Mass., USA

Summary

It is now well established that activation and differentiation of T cells play a critical role in the pathogenesis of allergic airway disease. Upon encounter with the specific antigen, naïve T helper precursor cells become activated, an event that is regulated not only by engagement of the TCR with the peptide presented in the context of MHC class II molecules but by a number of costimulatory signals. The most important costimulatory signal delivered to resting T cells occurs upon CD28 engagement by B7 molecules. However, largely as a consequence of the unraveling of the human genome, it is now becoming clear that other related members not only of the CD28/B7 family, but also the IL-1 and TNF receptor family also play important roles in providing both unique and complementary signals required for optimal T cell activation.

CD28 and CTLA-4 and Their Counterligands B7-1 and B7-2

CD28 and its related family member, CTLA-4, are homodimeric glycoproteins of the immunoglobulin superfamily. Signaling through CD28 either with specific antibodies or via its natural ligand B7-1 (CD80) or B7-2 (CD86) is required for IL-2 production, IL-2 receptor expression and cell cycle progression. B7-1 and B7-2 are also members of the immunoglobulin superfamily that exhibit approximately 25% identity in the Ig-V- and C-like extracellular domain, but exhibit pronounced differences in their cytoplasmic domains. Nevertheless, despite these differences, both proteins exhibit similar tertiary structure and functionally appear to have overlapping functions. B7-1 and B7-2 bind to CD28 with lower affinity and to CTLA-4 with much higher affinity. B7-2 is constitutively expressed on dendritic cells and is rapidly upregulated compared to B7-1. These observations have led to the hypothesis that B7-2 interactions are required for the initial T cell costimulation whereas B7-1:CD28 interactions are more involved in the sustained T cell activation. The importance of CD28:B7 interactions is illustrated in mice deficient for CD28 which show strong impairment of proliferation in vitro after stimulation with anti-TCR antibodies, allostimulation and specific antigen [1, 2].

A large number of studies have attempted to address the importance of CD28-mediated costimulation using a variety of in vivo model systems. These data have suggested that CD28 engagement is critical in determining susceptibility to disease progression following infection with *Leishmania major* [3], in the maintenance of long-term allograft survival [4], for mediating experimental autoimmune encephalomyelitis [5], for T-cell-dependent antibody production [6] and in the development of allergic lung disease [7, 8].

In contrast to CD28, the second member of this family of molecules, CTLA-4, delivers a negative signal to the activated T cell, opposing CD28-mediated costimulation [9]. The importance of this pathway is further illustrated in mice deficient in CTLA-4 which exhibit profound lymphoproliferative defects characterized by polyclonal T cell activation and a high frequency of cells expressing activation/memory T cell antigens [10]. More recently, CTLA-4 engagement has been demonstrated to augment antitumor immunity, to regulate autoimmune diabetes [11] and to provide an important signal leading to T cell tolerance [12]. Many of the in vivo studies cited above have concluded that CD28 plays a critical role in the T-cell-mediated process by making use of the chimeric receptor CTLA-4-Fc which binds with high affinity to B7-1 and B7-2 and hence inhibits CD28: B7 interactions. However, it is important to note that this protein would also inhibit the negative/anergy signal provided by CTLA-4: B7 and hence some of these data should be interpreted with caution.

Recent in vitro experiments have suggested that the dependency on CD28/B7-mediated costimulation is greatly influenced by the antigenic experience of the T cell. Although antigen inexperienced CD4+ T cells require CD28-mediated signaling for IL-2 production and clonal expansion, optimal activation of recently activated T helper subsets occurs independent of CD28 ligation [13]. Likewise, while CTLA-4-Ig is effective in inhibiting a number of immune responses in vivo when administered at the time of initial T cell activation, delaying CTLA-4-Ig treatment has, in some situations, been reported to be ineffective. Likewise, although CTLA-4-Ig is effective in inhibiting primary immune responses, some studies have shown that secondary immune responses cannot be fully suppressed by administration of CTLA-4-Ig, consistent with B7-1 and 2 independent activation of effector cells. In addition, there is evidence that the induction of a Th2 response does not require CD28 engagement [14]. Thus while CD28 plays an important role in T-cell-mediated activation, CD28 engagement by B7 molecules cannot fully account for all requirements of costimulatory molecules in T cell activation.

Inducible Costimulator and B7-Related Protein-1

Recently, the third member of the CD28 family has been identified and termed 'inducible costimulator' (ICOS) [15]. ICOS, unlike CD28, is induced upon activation of T cells. In situ analysis of lymph node cells supports these findings revealing increased expression in the T cell paracortex region during contact hypersensitivity responses [16]. In vitro, ICOS delivers a CD28-independent signal for IFN-γ, IL-4 and IL-10, but not for IL-2 production [15, 16]. ICOS binds its own unique counter-receptor, B7-related protein-1 (B7RP-1) [16] which has 20% homology to B71 and B7-2 and is expressed on macrophages and B cells, but not dendritic cells. Cross-linking ICOS upregulates CD40 ligand expression and facilitates T-B interactions [16]. These data are consistent with observations in mice transgenic for B7RP-1 which devel-

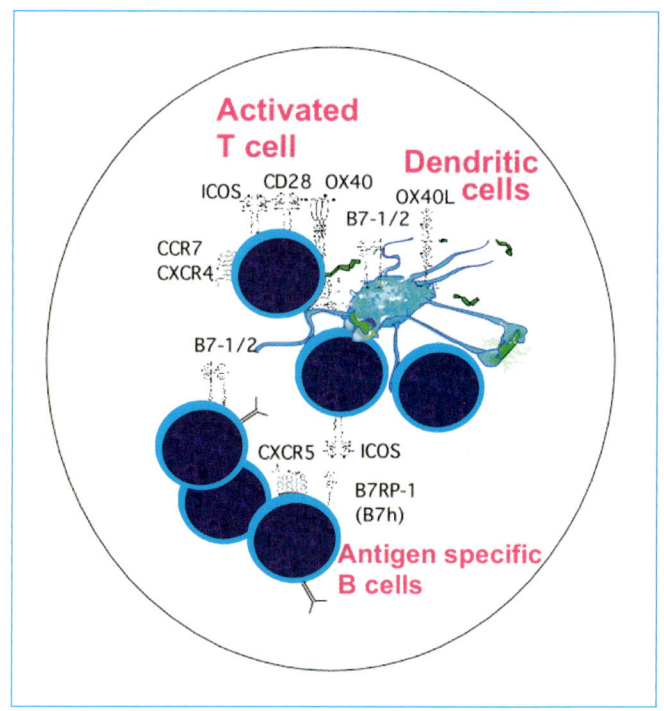

Fig. 1. Costimulatory pathways for T cell activation. Recently activated cells express CD40L and other members of the TNF family, such as OX40, and migrate to either B cell areas in the germinal center to provide help of B cell maturation or migrate to inflamed tissues. In a secondary immune response, the frequency of antigen-specific T cells is dramatically increased and molecules such as ICOS expressed on either recently activated T cells or memory cells may play a more important role than CD28 by interacting through its ligand, B7RP-1, expressed on B cells.

op B cell hyperplasia, plasmacytosis and hypergammaglobulinemia [16]. Furthermore, administration of B7RP-1-Fc augments the effector response during a cutaneous hypersensitivity reaction. Based on the requirement of stimulation for ICOS induction and the expression of its ligand on B cells, raising the possibility that ICOS plays a more important role than CD28 in secondary immune responses, where a clear CD28-independent response has been described (fig. 1). ICOS is an important costimulatory receptor for both recently activated cells and for Th2, but not Th1 effector cells [17]. The contribution of ICOS to effective T-cell-mediated immune responses and the function consequences of ICOS inhibition would be critically influenced by both the nature of the immune response and the timing of intervention with anti-ICOS blockade strategies. This hypothesis is supported by the recent demonstration that B7RP-1-Ig enhances responses in a model of cutaneous hypersensitivity when administered at the time of challenge, but not during the initial sensitization phase and regulates IgG1 production more profoundly during a secondary immunization [16, 17]. In addition, ICOS has also been reported to be expressed on CD4+CD44hiCD69low cells – cells best defined as memory T cells [16], which undergo rapid expansion on antigen re-exposure, independent of B7 and CD40 ligation [18]. Clearly the identification of ICOS has important implications for regulating the function of previously activated T cells and/or memory cells. Recent data from our laboratory suggested that engagement of ICOS regulates T-cell-dependent eosinophilic inflammation in a murine model of asthma and as such, may provide novel therapies for the treatment of allergic airway disease.

PD-1 and B7H-1

Recently, a fourth member of the B7 family has been identified and termed B7H-1 [19] B7H-1 gene encodes for a putative type 1 transmembrane protein containing four cysteine residues that are conserved in B7-1, B7-2 and B7RP-1. B7H-1 is more widely expressed than B7-1 and B7-2 suggesting that its function may extend above and beyond the immune system. The ligand for B7H-1 has recently been identified as PD-1, a 55-kD transmembrane protein containing an immunoreceptor tyrosine-based inhibitory motif induced in lymphocytes and monocytic cells following activation. PD-1 exhibits 24% homology to CTLA-4 in the extracellular domain. Ligation of PD-1 results in inhibition of T cell proliferation and attenuation of cytokine production. These results support previous observations that mice deficient in PD-1 develop a characteristic lupus-like proliferative arthritis and glomerulonephritis response [20]. The role of PD-1 and B7H-1 in allergic responses awaits further characterization. However, these observations suggest that in addition to CTLA-4, B7 interactions, PD-1:B7H-1 are also involved in the maintenance of peripheral self-tolerance by serving as a negative regulator of immune responses. whereas CD28 and ICOS provide positive costimulatory signals (fig. 2).

TNF and TNF-Receptors

Recently, members of the TNF:TNF receptor families that include OX40, OX40L, RANK:RANKL and 4-1BB:4-1BBL have been implicated as regulators of T cell function. OX40 is expressed on activated T cells whereas its ligand has a broader pattern of expression and is present on T cells, B cells and dendritic cells. In vivo, administration of an OX40 antibody results in a severely impaired IgG response [21]. However, mice deficient in OX40 generate normal antibody responses and CTL responses. In

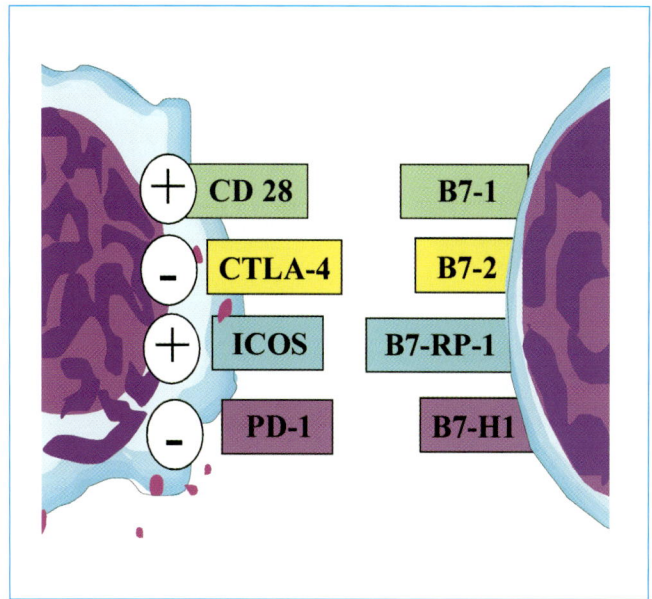

Fig. 2. The CD28 and B7 family members. CD28 and CTLA-4 bind to both B7-1 and B7-2 expressed on dendritic cells and B cells. ICOS binds to its own unique ligand, B7RP-1, which is expressed on both resting and activated B cells, whereas PD-1 binds the recently identified B7 homologue B7-H1. While CD28 and ICOS ligation results in a positive costimulatory signal, activation of CTLA-4 and PD-1 results in an attenuation of T cell activation and may provide an important signal for peripheral tolerance.

contrast, OX40 is important for the induction of CD4+, but not CD8+ effector cells [21, 22]. Thus OX40 is an important molecule for Th function, although it remains to be clarified whether OX40 plays an important role in the mechanisms leading to the induction of allergic inflammation. In contrast, the 41BB-41BBL is currently believed to be more important for an effective CTL rather than Th cell responses [23]. RANK (receptor activator for NK-κB) is expressed by dendritic cells and is upregulated by CD40L and suggested to play a role in T cell tolerance [24]. The function of this molecule awaits further analysis.

Members of the IL-1 Receptor Superfamily

The IL-1 receptor/Toll-like receptor (IL-1R/TLR) superfamily comprises a diverse family of cell surface receptors defined by a characteristic conserved sequence in its cytosolic regions termed the Toll/IL-1 receptor domain (TIR), which function in inflammation and host defense against microbial pathogens. Two members of the IL-1R superfamily now add to the chemokine receptors CCR3, CCR4 CCR5 and CCR8 as shown as being differentially

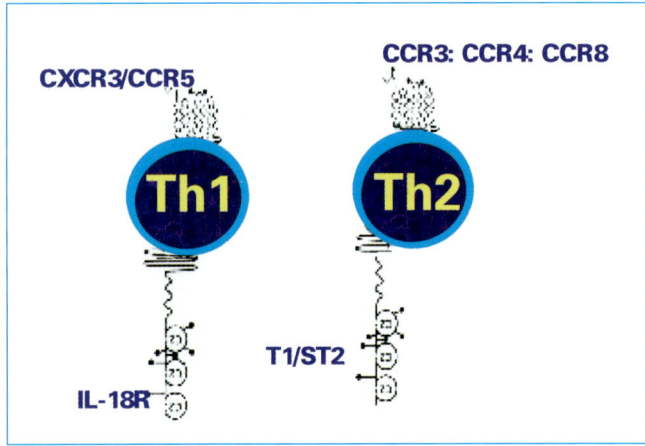

Fig. 3. T-cell-subset-specific surface receptors. In addition to the chemokine receptors CXCR3/CCR5 and CCR3/CCR4/CCR8 which are expressed on Th1 and Th2 cells, the IL-1 receptor superfamily members, IL-18 receptor and the orphan receptor T1/ST2 are also differentially expressed and regulate T cell effector function.

expressed on T cell populations (fig. 3). The IL-18 receptor (originally identified as IL-1-related protein) is expressed on Th1 cells [25] whereas T1/ST2 is expressed on Th2 cells [26, 27]. The IL-18 receptor is expressed on activated Th1 cells and regulates IFN-γ secretion, IL-12Rβ2 expression and Th1-mediated inflammation in vivo [24]. T1/ST2, originally identified as a gene induced by serum stimulation of fibroblasts, has more recently been demonstrated to be overexpressed on Th2 effector cells in vitro and in vivo [26, 27]. Inhibition of T1/ST2 attenuates Th2-driven responses in vivo and inhibits eosinophilic inflammation of the airways [27]. T1/ST2 is more than a useful stable marker for identifying Th2 cells and functions as an important receptor for optimal cytokine production from Th2 cells. Taken together, our data add to the growing appreciation that members of the IL-1R superfamily including the IL-18 receptor, TRL-2, TRL-4 and now T1/ST2, are critical.

Conclusions

The mechanisms by which T cells migrate from the blood to secondary lymph organs, interact with B cells and dendritic cells and acquire effector or memory function is now beginning to be understood. It is anticipated that, as a consequence of our increasing appreciation of events that regulate this response, we will be able to design better therapeutic agents to selective target T cells in diseases such as allergic asthma, while protective immune responses against pathogens remain intact. If the clinical experience of these agents is as promising as in other inflammatory diseases, such as rheumatoid arthritis and psoriasis, the way we approach management of the asthmatic condition may change over the coming years.

References

1 Green JM, Turka LA, June CH, Thompson CB: CD28 and staphylococcal enterotoxin synergize to induce MHC-independent T-cell proliferation. Cell Immunol 1992;145:11–20.
2 Shahinian A, Pfeffer K, Lee KP, Kundig TM, Kishihara K, Wakeham A, Kawai K, Ohashi PS, Thompson CB, Mak TW: Differential T cell costimulatory requirements in CD28-deficient mice. Science 1993;261:609–612.
3 Corry DB, Reiner SL, Linsley PS, Locksley RM: Differential effects of blockade of CD28-B7 on the development of Th1 or Th2 effector cells in experimental leishmaniasis. J Immunol 1994;9:4142–4148.
4 Sayegh MH, Akalin E, Hancock WW, Russell ME, Carpenter CB, Linsley PS, Turka LA: CD28-B7 blockade after alloantigenic challenge in vivo inhibits Th1 cytokines but spares Th2. J Exp Med 1995;5:1869–1874.
5 Cross AH, Girard TJ, Giacoletto KS, Evans RJ, Keeling RM, Lin RF, Trotter JL, Karr RW: Long-term inhibition of murine experimental autoimmune encephalomyelitis usin CTLA-4-Fc supports a key role for CD28 costimulation. J Clin Invest 1995;6:2783–2789.
6 Linsley PS, Wallace PM, Johnson J, Gibson MG, Greene JL, Ledbetter JA, Singh C, Tepper MA: Immunosuppression in vivo by a soluble form of the CTLA-4 T cell activation molecule. Science 1992;257:792–795.
7 Tsuyuki S, Tsuyuki J, Einsle K, Kopf M, Coyle AJ: Costimulation through B7-2 (CD86) is required for the induction of a lung mucosal T helper cell 2 (TH2) immune response and altered airway responsiveness. J Exp Med 1997;9:1671–1679.
8 Keane-Myers A, Gause WC, Linsley PS, Chen SJ, Wills-Karp M: B7-CD28/CTLA-4 costimulatory pathways are required for the development of T helper cell 2-mediated allergic airway responses to inhaled antigens. J Immunol 1997;158:2042–2049.
9 Walunas TL, Lenschow DJ, Bakker CY, Linsley PS, Freeman GJ, Green JM, Thompson CB, Bluestone JA: CTLA-4 can function as a negative regulator of T cell activation. Immunity 1994;1:405–413.
10 Tivol EA, Borriello F, Schweitzer AN, Lynch WP, Bluestone JA, Sharpe AH: Loss of CTLA-4 leads to massive lymphoproliferation and fatal multiorgan tissue destruction, revealing a critical negative regulatory role of CTLA-4. Immunity 1995;3:541–547.
11 Luhder F, Hoglund P, Allison JP, Benoist C, Mathis D: Cytotoxic T lymphocyte-associated antigen 4 (CTLA-4) regulates the unfolding of autoimmune diabetes. J Exp Med 1998;187:427–432.
12 Perez VL, Van Parijs L, Biuckians A, Zheng XX, Strom TB, Abbas AK: Induction of peripheral T cell tolerance in vivo requires CTLA-4 engagement. Immunity 1997;4:411–417.
13 Schweitzer AN, Sharpe AH: Studies using antigen-presenting cells lacking expression of both B7-1 (CD80) and B7-2 (CD86) show distinct requirements for B7 molecules during priming versus restimulation of Th2 but not Th1 cytokine production. J Immunol 1998;6:2762–2771.

14 Brown DR, Green JM, Moskowitz NH, Davis M, Thompson CB, Reiner SL: Limited role of CD28-mediated signals in T helper subset differentiation. J Exp Med 1996;3:803–810.
15 Hutloff A, Dittrich AM, Beier HC, Eljaschewitsch B, Kraft R, Anagnostopoulos I, Kroczek RA: ICOS is an inducible T-cell co-stimulator structurally and functionally related to CD28. Nature 1999;397:263–266.
16 Yoshinaga SK, Whoriskey JS, Khare SD, Sarmiento U, Guo J, Horan T, Shih G, Zhang M, Coccia MA, Kohno T, Tafuri-Bladt A, Brankow D, Campbell P, Chang D, Chiu L, Dai T, Duncan G, Elliott GS, Hui A, McCabe SM, Scully S, Shahinian A, Shaklee CL, Van G, Mak TW, Senaldi G: T-cell co-stimulation through B7RP-1 and ICOS. Nature 1999;402: 827–832.
17 Coyle AJ, Lehar S, Lloyd CM, Delaney T, Tian J, Manning S, Nguyen T, Burwell T, Scheider H, Gonzalo JA, Gosselin M, Rudolph-Owen L, Rudd CE, Gutierrez-Ramos JC: The CD28 related molecule ICOS is required for effective T cell dependent immune responses. Immunity 2000;13:95–105.
18 London CA, Lodge MP, Abbas AK: Functional responses and costimulator dependence of memory CD4+ T cells. J Immunol 2000;164: 265–272.
19 Dong H, Zhu G, Tamada K, Chen L: B7H-1, a third member of the B7 family, costimulates T cell proliferation and interleukin 10 secretion. Nat Med 1999;5:1365–1369.
20 Nishimura H, Nose M, Hiai H, Minato N, Honjo T: Development of lupus-like autoimmune diseases by disruption of the PD-1 gene encoding an ITIM motif-carrying immunoreceptor. Immunity 1999;11:141–151.
21 Chen AI, McAdam AJ, Buhlmann JE, Scott S, Lupher ML, Greenfield EA, Baum PR, Fanslow WC, Calderhead DM, Freeman GJ, Sharpe AH: OX40 ligand has a critical costimulatory role in dendritic cell: T cell interactions. Immunity 1999;11:689–698.
22 Kopf M, Ruedl C, Schmitz N, Gallimore A, Lefrang K, Ecabert B, Odermatt B, Bachmann MF: OX-40-deficient-mice are defective in Th cell proliferation but are competent in generating B cell and CTL responses after virus infection. Immunity 1999;11:699–708.
23 DeBenedette MA, Wen T, Bachmann MF, Ohashi PS, Barber BH, Stocking KL, Peschon JJ, Watts TH: Analysis of 4-1BB ligand (4-1BBL)-deficient mice and of mice lacking both 4-1BBL and CD28 reveals a role for 4-1BBL in skin allograft rejection and in the cytotoxic T cell response to influenza virus. J Immunol 1999;163:4833–4841.
24 Anderson DM, Maraskovsky E, Billingsley WL, Dougall WC, Tometsko ME, Roux ER, Teepe M, Dubose RF, Cosman D, Galibert L: A homologue of the TNF receptor and its ligand enhance T-cell growth and dendritic-cell function. Nature 1997;390:175–178.
25 Xu D, Chan WL, Leung BP, Hunter D, Schulz K, Carter RW, McInnes IB, Robinson JH, Liew FY: Selective expression and functions of interleukin 18 receptor on T helper (Th) type 1 but not Th2 cells. J Exp Med 1998;188:1485–1492.
26 Xu D, Chan WL, Leung BP, Huang FP, Wheeler R, Piedrafita D, Robinson JH, Liew FY: Selective expression of a stable cell surface molecule on type 2 but not type 1 helper T cells. J Exp Med 1998;187:787–794.
27 Coyle AJ, Lloyd C, Tian J, Nguyen T, Eriksson C, Wang L, Ottoson P, Persson P, Delaney T, Lehar S, Lin S, Poisson L, Meisel C, Kamradt T, Bjerke T, Levinson D, Gutierrez-Ramos JC: Crucial role of the interleukin 1 receptor family member T1/ST2 in T helper cell type 2-mediated lung mucosal immune responses. J Exp Med 1999;190:895–902.

Dr. A.J. Coyle
Millennium Pharmaceuticals Inc.
45-75 Sidney St., Cambridge, MA 02139 (USA)
Tel. +1 617 679 7347, Fax +1 617 551 8910
E-Mail Coyle@mpi.com

GATA-3: A Th2-Selective Target

Anuradha Ray   Prabir Ray

Department of Medicine, Pulmonary and Critical Care Section, Yale University School of Medicine, New Haven, Conn., USA

Summary

It is now generally accepted that the inflammatory responses that mediate airway tissue damage in asthma arise from aberrant T cell-mediated immune responses to a range of inhaled allergens. CD4+ T-cells producing IL-4, IL-5 and IL-13, classified as Th2-type cells, appear to dominate the allergen-specific response in asthmatics. Recent studies highlight a critical role for the transcription factor GATA-3 in Th2 cell differentiation and allergic airway inflammation. Since GATA-3 is largely expressed in a Th2-restricted fashion in adults, targeting GATA-3 expression in asthma will have one distinct advantage over existing treatment modalities which is selectivity. Thus, inhibition of GATA-3 expression/function will not cause general immunosuppression but will block both the generation and effector function of Th2 cells.

CD4+ T Cells in the Etiology of Asthma

The secreted products of T cells play a central role in orchestrating the unique inflammatory response seen in asthma. T cells are not a homogeneous class of cells. Based on which profile of cytokines they secrete in response to antigenic stimulation, T cells are classified as Th1 when they produce IFN-γ and lymphotoxin, Th2, when they secrete IL-4 and IL-5 and Th0 when they secrete a combination of Th1 and Th2 cytokines [1, 2]. Cytokine expression profiles of allergen-specific T cell clones isolated from atopics are skewed toward a Th2-like profile [3]. CD4+ T cells producing IL-4, IL-5 and IL-13 have been identified in bronchoalveolar lavage fluid and airway biopsies from asthmatics. Th2 lymphocytes are increased in the airways of allergic asthmatics after antigen challenge [4, 5]. The identification of Th2 cells in the airways of asthmatics, and the validation of their importance in the development of airway eosinophilia, airway hyperresponsiveness and serum IgE levels in animal models has established the crucial role of Th2 cells in the induction of the inflammatory response that results in asthma [6]. How the T cell system gets locked into the Th1 or the Th2 pathway is currently an area of intense scientific investigation in many laboratories.

Cytokine-Induced Initiation of Molecular Programming in Th2 Cells

Cytokines provide a potent stimulus for Th1/Th2 differentiation. It is also clear that cytokine production by Th1 and Th2 cells is regulated at the level of cytokine gene transcription. Recent studies have demonstrated that regulation of cytokine gene transcription involves an interplay between chromatin structure, tissue-specific transcription factors and probabilistic gene activation [6]. It has been shown that naive T cells have a closed chromatin configuration around the IL-4/IL-5/IL-13 and IFN-γ gene loci. After naïve CD4+ T cells are induced to differentiate by antigen and cytokine, rapid chromatin remodeling and CpG demethylation occurs with the acquisition of a characteristic cell-specific open chromatin structure [7]. This, in turn, results in occupancy of the accessible DNA by Th2-specific transcription factors that are induced/activated as a result of stimulation of naïve cells by antigen and cytokine. Synergism between these tissue-specific transcription factors and more generally expressed transiently induced/activated factors induces transcription of Th2 genes. It appears that the open chromatin configuration and the expression of tissue-specific transcription factors are maintained in the polarized cells. During subsequent antigenic stimulation of the memory/effector cells, transcription factors such as AP-1 are rapidly induced which synergize with preexisting tissue-specific factors causing active transcription of the IL-4/IL-5/IL-13 gene locus in Th2 cells.

Transcription Factor GATA-3

Almost 10 years ago, GATA-3 was first described as a transcription factor that interacted with the TCR-α gene enhancer [8]. Six members (GATA-1 to -6) of the GATA family of proteins have been identified to date. Based on their expression profile and structure, the GATA proteins may be classified as hematopoietic (GATA-1 to -3) or non-hematopoietic (GATA-4 to -6). In adults, GATA-3 expression is largely restricted to T cells which express low levels of the protein in the resting state. While GATA-3-binding sites have been identified in multiple T-cell-specific genes, such as the TCR-α, -β, and -δ genes and the CD8α gene, it is unclear whether GATA-3 is critical for the expression of these genes. However, as discussed below, GATA-3 plays an essential role at two levels in T cell biology – T cell development and Th2 differentiation.

GATA-3: A Critical Factor in Early T Cell Development

Targeted disruption of the GATA-3 gene in mice results in embryonic death on day 12 with massive internal bleeding, failure of fetal liver hematopoiesis and defects in the central nervous system [9]. The lethal effect of the GATA-3 null mutation was bypassed using the RAG2 complementation system in conjunction with GATA-3–/– ES cells. While the GATA-3–/–/RAG-2–/– chimeric mice had normal B cell populations, they had no double-positive or single-positive cells in the thymus and no mature T cells in the periphery [10]. Molecular analysis of the T cell defects in the GATA-3–/–/RAG 2–/– mice demonstrated that GATA-3 is required at the very early steps of T cell development in the generation/survival of the double-negative thymocyte population [10]. The targets of GATA-3 in the early T cell progenitors are presently unknown. Taken together, these initial studies demonstrated that despite the presence of multiple GATA family proteins, GATA-3 is not a functionally redundant family member.

GATA-3: A Th2-Specific Factor

Exposure of naïve CD4+ T cells to IL-4 in conjunction with antigen presented by antigen-presenting cells (APCs) initiates a cellular differentiation program involving the activation of multiple transcription factors that ultimately results in the generation of Th2 cells. Among all of these factors, GATA-3 is the only Th2-specific factor. The initial response in the cascade of events triggered upon IL-4 receptor engagement is the nuclear translocation of the transcription factor STAT6 that induces to a dramatic increase in the expression of the GATA-3 gene. Using the IL-5 gene as a model system for Th2-specific gene transcription, our laboratory demonstrated the critical importance of a double GATA-3-binding site in the IL-5 promoter for its activation in T cells [11]. Using established clones as well as Th1 or Th2 cells generated from naïve CD4+ T cells, our laboratory demonstrated Th2-specific expression of GATA-3 [12]. Th2-specific expression of GATA-3 was also demonstrated using representational differential analysis of Th1 and Th2 cells [13]. GATA-3 mRNA expression is substantially increased at 48 h during Th2 development and plateaus thereafter [12]. In contrast, no such increase is seen in developing Th1 cells and there is actually a progressive decline in GATA-3 message in developing Th1 cells [12].

GATA-3: A Negative Regulator of Th1 Development

An important consideration in discussions of Th1/Th2 differentiation is cross-regulation between the two subsets, which results in apparent exclusivity of one type of immune response during infection or in disease. For example, during the course of differentiation, IFN-γ produced by Th1 cells facilitates Th1 development but inhibits Th2 cell proliferation, whereas IL-4 and IL-10 produced by Th2 cells amplify the Th2 pathway but inhibit Th1 differentiation. To determine the functional significance of GATA-3 downregulation in Th1 cells, GATA-3 was forcibly overexpressed in Th1 cells using retroviral gene transfer methods [14, 15]. These studies showed that overexpression of GATA-3 in developing but not committed Th1 cells results in inhibition of IFN-γ production [14, 15] and extinction of IL-12Rβ2 expression [14]. The lack of any effect of GATA-3 in already differentiated Th1 cells argues against direct effects of GATA-3 on the IFN-γ promoter [14]. Thus, by inhibiting IFN-γ and IL-12Rβ2 expression, GATA-3 provides a mechanism for commitment to the Th2 phenotype. In striking contrast to αβ T cells, however, γδ T cells, polarized to the γδ2 phenotype, express high levels of IL-12Rβ2 despite high levels of GATA-3 expression and absence of IFN-γ production [16]. While the general profile of GATA-3 expression is similar under Th1 and Th2 conditions in αβ and γδ T cells, the net outcome of GATA-3 expression is different in αβ and γδ T cells in regard to IL-12Rβ2 expression. The persistence of IL-12Rβ2 expression in γδ2-type cells is in accordance with dominance of IL-12 over IL-4 in γδ T cells in contrast to IL-4 dominance in αδ T cells.

Different Levels of GATA-3 Control in Th2 Cells

It is becoming increasingly clear that GATA-3 controls Th2 cytokine expression at multiple levels (fig. 1). First, GATA-3 rather than Stat6 may be the principal chromatin-remodeling factor around the IL-4/IL-5/IL-13 locus in cells stimulated with antigen and IL-4 [17]. Second, GATA-3 directly activates the IL-5 promoter [11, 12, 18] and has been shown to bind a distal enhancer in the IL-4 gene by chromatin immunoprecipitation experiments [Anjana Rao, pers. commun.]. Possibly, this site and other potential GATA-3 binding elements dispersed throughout the IL-4 locus provide sites of action for GATA-3 in regulation of IL-4 and IL-13 gene expression. It should be noted that GATA-3 does not activate the IL-4 promoter [18, 19]. Third, GATA-3 appears to function in a feedback positive autoregulatory loop in an IL-4/STAT6-independent fashion to upregulate its own expression thus stabilizing the Th2 phenotype [17]. A second Th2-specific factor, c-Maf, has also been shown to be crucial for IL-4 gene expression with direct effects on the IL-4 promoter [20]. However, unlike GATA-3, c-Maf does not appear to be important for IL-5 and IL-13 production [21]. While the Th2-specific factors such as GATA-3 and c-Maf are essential and determine the tissue specificity of gene expression, the concomitant activation of more general factors such as NF-κB, AP-1, NF-AT and C/EBPβ is required for high-level expression of the Th2 cytokine genes.

GATA-3 in Asthma

The relevance of GATA-3 expression in Th2 gene expression is also evident in human studies. A significant increase in GATA-3 expression was demonstrated in asthmatic airways compared to that in control subjects [22]. The increase in GATA-3 expression in these asthmatics correlated significantly with IL-5 expression and airway hyperresponsiveness [22]. While the studies in humans clearly showed increased GATA-3 expression in asthma, the initial animal studies did not conclusively indicate that GATA-3 was sufficient for the expression of all Th2 cytokine genes. Thus, it was unclear whether GATA-3

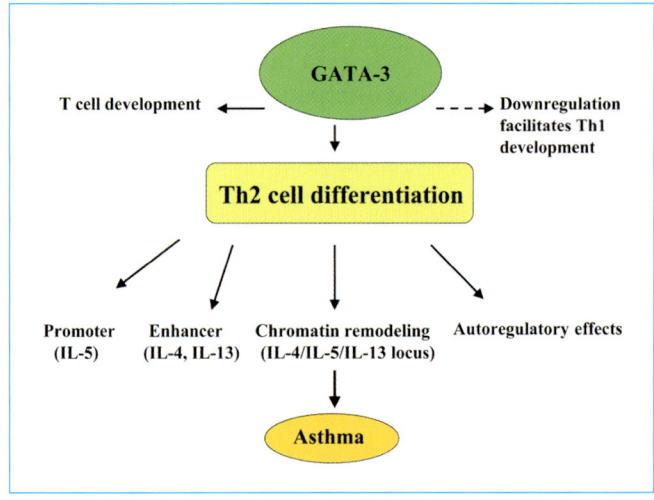

Fig. 1. The multiple roles of GATA-3 in T cell responses.

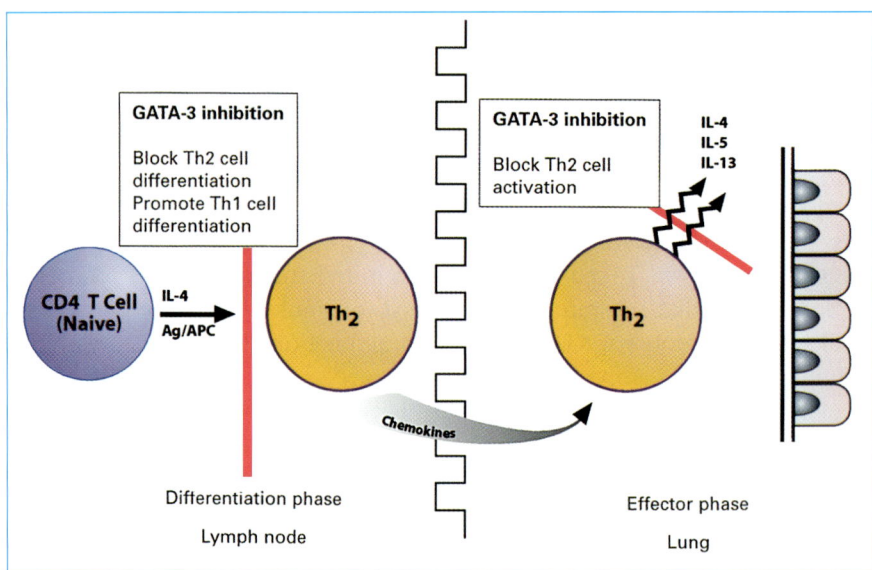

Fig. 2. GATA-3, a potential target in asthma therapy.

inhibition would block the production of all the key Th2 cytokines, IL-4, IL-5 and IL-13, that have been implicated in asthma. Since embryonic lethality in GATA-3-null mice precluded their analysis in animal models of allergic inflammation, a dominant-negative mutant of GATA-3 was used to address the importance of GATA-3 in Th2 cytokine gene expression in vivo [23]. Transgenic mice expressing a dominant-negative mutant of GATA-3 in an inducible and T cell-specific fashion were developed and analyzed in a murine model of allergic inflammation [23]. These studies demonstrated that inhibition of GATA-3 activity causes severe blunting of Th2 effects both locally in the lung (eosinophil influx, mucus production) as well as systemically (IgE production) [23].

GATA-3: A Candidate Target in Asthma Therapy

In summary, GATA-3 has two important roles in a dominant Th2 response: (1) it directly controls expression of Th2 cytokine genes and (2) by inhibiting IFN-γ production it facilitates rapid divergence of proliferating cells away from Th1. Since Th1 and Th2 responses are cross-regulatory, inhibition of GATA-3 activity will serve the dual purpose of inhibiting Th2 responses and facilitating Th1 responses by relieving inhibition of IFN-γ production. While blockade of STAT6 function will be effective only in the initial differentiation phase, inhibition of GATA-3 expression/function would thwart Th2 responses at multiple points. As shown in figure 2, targeting GATA-3 would inhibit new Th2 cell generation, promote Th1 cell generation and also block Th2 cytokine secretion from effector cells. Furthermore, uniquely, GATA-3 blockade will not affect other cell types and therefore will not cause general immunosuppression. Although targeting GATA-3 is not suitable in children due to the important role of this factor in thymocyte maturation, overall, studies of GATA-3 in mice and humans provide compelling reasons for targeting this master regulator of Th2 gene expression in therapies of asthma and allergic diseases in adults.

References

1 Mosmann TR, Coffman RL. TH1 and TH2 cells: Different patterns of lymphokine secretion lead to different functional properties. Annu Rev Immunol 1989;7:145–173.
2 Constant SL, Bottomly K: Induction of Th1 and Th2 CD4+ T cell responses: The alternative approaches. Annu Rev Immunol 1997;15:297–322.
3 Wierenga EA, Snoek M, de Groot C, et al: Evidence for compartmentalization of functional subsets of CD2+ T lymphocytes in atopic subjects. J Immunol 1990;144:4651–4656.
4 Walker C, Bode E, Boer L, Hansel TT, Blaser K, Virchow J Jr: Allergic and non-allergic asthmatics have distinct patterns of T-cell activation and cytokine production in peripheral blood and bronchoalveolar lavage. Am Rev Respir Dis 1992;146:109–115.
5 Robinson DS, Hamid Q, Ying S, et al: Predominant TH2-like bronchoalveolar T-lymphocyte population in atopic asthma. N Engl J Med 1992;326:298–304.
6 Ray A, Cohn L: Th2 cells and GATA-3 in asthma: New insights into the regulation of airway inflammation. J Clin Invest 1999;104:985–993.
7 Agarwal S, Rao A: Modulation of chromatin structure regulates cytokine gene expression during T cell differentiation. Immunity 1998;9:765–775.
8 Ho IC, Vorhees P, Marin N, et al: Human GATA-3: A lineage-restricted transcription factor that regulates the expression of the T cell receptor alpha gene. EMBO J 1991;10:1187–1192.
9 Pandolfi P, Roth ME, Karis A, et al: Target disruption of the GATA-3 gene causes severe abnormalities in the nervous system and in fetal liver hematopoiesis. Nature Genet 1995;11:40–44.
10 Ting C-N, Olson MC, Barton KP, Leiden JM: Transcription factor GATA-3 is required for development of the T-cell lineage. Nature 1996;384:474–478.
11 Siegel MD, Zhang D-H, Ray P, Ray A: Activation of the interleukin-5 promoter by cAMP in murine EL-4 cells requires the GATA-3 and CLE0 elements. J Biol Chem 1995;270:24548–24555.
12 Zhang D-H, Cohn L, Ray P, Bottomly K, Ray A: Transcription factor GATA-3 is differentially expressed in Th1 and Th2 cells and controls Th2-specific expression of the interleukin-5 gene. J Biol Chem 1997; 272:21597–21603.
13 Zheng W-P, Flavell RA: The transcription factor GATA-3 is necessary and sufficient for Th2 cytokine gene expression in CD4 T cells. Cell 1997;89:587–596.
14 Ouyang W, Ranganath SH, Weindel K, et al: Inhibition of Th1 development mediated by GATA-3 through an IL-4-independent mechanism. Immunity 1998;9:745–755.
15 Ferber IA, Lee HJ, Zonin F, et al: GATA-3 significantly downregulates IFN-gamma production from developing Th1 cells in addition to inducing IL-4 and IL-5 levels. Clin Immunol 1999;91:134–144.
16 Yin Z, Zhang DH, Welte T, et al: Dominance of IL-12 over IL-4 in gammadelta T cell differentiation leads to default production of IFN-gamma: Failure to down-regulate IL-12 receptor beta2-chain expression. J Immunol 2000; 164:3056–3064.
17 Ouyang W, Lohning M, Gao Z, et al: Stat6-independent GATA-3 autoactivation directs IL-4-independent Th2 development and commitment. Immunity 2000;12:27–37.
18 Zhang D-H, Yang L, Ray A: Differential responsiveness of the interleukin-5 (IL-5) and IL-4 genes to transcription factor GATA-3. J Immunol 1998;161:3817–3821.
19 Ranganath S, Ouyang W, Bhattacharya D, et al: GATA-3-dependent enhancer activity in IL-4 gene regulation. J Immunol 1998;161:3822–3826.
20 Ho I-C, Hodge MR, Rooney JW, Glimcher LH: The proto-oncogene c-*maf* is responsible for tissue-specific expression of interleukin-4. Cell 1996;85:973–983.
21 Kim JI, Ho I-C, Grusby MJ, Glimcher LH: The transcription factor c-Maf controls the production of IL-4 but not other Th2 cytokines. Immunity 1999;10:745–751.
22 Nakamura Y, Ghaffar O, Olivenstein R, et al: Gene expression of the GATA-3 transcription factor is increased in atopic asthma. J Allergy Clin Immunol 1999;103:215–222.
23 Zhang DH, Yang L, Cohn L, et al: Inhibition of allergic inflammation in a murine model of asthma by expression of a dominant-negative mutant of GATA-3. Immunity 1999;11:473–482.

Anuradha Ray, PhD
Pulmonary and Critical Care Medicine
Department of Medicine
Yale University School of Medicine
333 Cedar Street, 105 LCI
New Haven, CT 06520-8057 (USA)
Tel. +1 203 737 2705, Fax +1 203 785 3826
E-Mail anuradha.ray@yale.edu

Mycobacterial Immunization

Agents to Limit Asthma

Julian M. Hopkin

Experimental Medicine Unit, University of Wales, Swansea, UK

Summary

The recent surge in the prevalence of asthma in developed communities points to important environmental determinants of the condition, and to the possibility that their reversal will see a decline in the disease. This review considers the relationship between microbial exposures and atopic disorder, and in particular the epidemiologic and experimental data on the Th1-promoting and Th2-limiting properties of mycobacteria.

Microbial Exposure and Atopy: 'Th1/Th2 Balance'

Changing patterns of microbial exposure that have accompanied socio-economic development are one prime candidate mechanism for the rise in asthma. Asthma has risen in communities where standards of hygiene are high, where attack rates and mortality from different infectious diseases have greatly declined, and where mass public health immunization and frequent usage of antibiotics have become the norm [1].

One plausible mechanism for linking patterns of microbial exposure to asthma is through 'the balance' of Th1 and Th2 immune mechanisms [2]. The bronchial inflammation that characterizes asthma is driven by Th2 immune mechanisms, with prominent actions from IL-13, IL-5 and IL-4; moreover, the great majority of young asthmatics are also atopic, itself a disorder of exuberant Th2 immune mechanisms and excessive production of IgE to common environmental antigens including the house dust mite [1, 3]. Since Th1 and Th2 immune mechanisms are to a significant degree antagonistic [2], it can be envisaged that certain microbial exposures, that prominently promote Th1 immune mechanisms and increase IFN-γ levels within the immune system, may limit Th2 responses to allergens [4, 6]. Conversely, exposures that promote Th2 immune mechanisms and antibody production might have a deleterious effect; some of the public health immunizations currently administered may have this potential, but the case against them remains unproven and further work is required [7]. A number of epidemiological studies have noted an inverse association between exposure to potentially Th1-promoting infections and subsequent atopy – these include hepatitis A, *Toxocara canis*, *Helicobacter pylori* [8], measles (although its immunology is complex) [9], and the mycobacteria [10]. Further studies show that the use of antibiotic in early life predicts substantially more subsequent atopy – raising the possibility that removal of bowel microflora, with their potentially Th1-promoting effects, might also be able to 'release' Th2 atopic immune mechanisms [7, 11, 12].

Mycobacterial Exposure, Atopy and Asthma – The Epidemiology

The relationship between mycobacterial exposure and atopy in asthma is particularly interesting. In an epidemiologic study, we found a strong relationship between positive tuberculin responses in early life, indicative of exposure and response to mycobacteria, and less subsequent clinical asthma, rhinitis and eczema, lower IgE levels, and Th1 skewed cytokine profiles [10] (table 1). The prevalence of asthma in 12-year-old Japanese school children with a strong tuberculin response (Mantoux test response >10 mm to 2 tuberculin units, and likely due to natural *Mycobacterium tuberculosis* exposure) in early life, was only 28% of their tuberculin-negative counterparts; moreover, remission of atopic symptoms was observed with acquisition of positive tuberculin responses up to the age of 12 years [10].

Table 1. Odds ratio (OR) and 95% confidence intervals (95% CI) for atopy (elevated total or allergen-specific IgE in serum) and asthma to the age of 12 years, according to tuberculin conversion in 867 Japanese school children [10]

Tuberculin response	Atopy		Asthma	
	OR	95% CI	OR	95% CI
Conversion to strong positive before 6 years	0.50	0.29–0.83	0.31	0.22–0.45
Conversion to strong positive at 6–12 years	0.43	0.25–0.83	0.42	0.24–0.56

Table 2. Symptoms, salbutamol use, and IFN-γ secretions in 40 adult subjects with grass-pollen-induced summer asthma and rhinitis: a masked placebo-controlled trial of immunization with killed *M. vaccae* (3 doses at monthly intervals through the spring) [24]

	Active immunization (n = 21)	Placebo immunization (n = 19)
Total symptom score	167.3	203.2
Chest symptom score	24.4	36.9
Salbutamol use (weekly group score)	4.8*	31.2
Mean (log pg/ml) IFN-γ secretion by PBMCs after incubation with tuberculin (after 2 immunisations)	1,784.4	669.0

* p = 0.45 on stepwise regression analysis.

Von Mutius et al. [13], using ecological methods in a large-scale international survey, have shown a step-wise increase of 25/100,000 in notification rates for tuberculosis, as one surrogate for mycobacterial exposure, relate to a step-wise decrease of 4.7% in the prevalence of wheeze [13].

Mycobacterial Exposure and Allergy: Experimental Approaches

Formal experimental data on the inverse link between mycobacterial exposure and allergy come from a set of murine experiments [14, 17]. They have uniformly shown impressive Th2 limiting properties of different mycobacterial preparations – including whole BCG and whole killed *Mycobacterium vaccae*. Mycobacterial impact on induced ovalbumin allergy included inhibition of IgE synthesis and of IL-5 production, inhibition of pulmonary eosinophilic infiltration, and the inhibition of fatal anaphylactic pulmonary reactions on inhaled allergen challenge. The degree of inhibition was influenced by the route of administration – BCG was most effective when instilled into the respiratory tract – as well as by dosage of mycobacterial product [14, 17]. These data accord with the strong Th1-promoting effects of the mycobacteria – with binding of their lipoproteins to Toll-like receptors on antigen-presenting cells and leading to prominent IL-12 synthesis and hence Th1 immune responses with prominent IFN-γ secretion [18, 19]. The findings also accord with parallel observations of the inhibition of allergic lung inflammation in a mouse model of asthma by bacterial CpG oligodeoxynucleotides [20].

Mycobacterial Immunization to Limit Atopy and Asthma in Man?

The epidemiologic and experimental data point to the possibility that the mycobacteria or their products could be used as immunizing agents to prevent or restrain Th2 immune mechanisms and hence asthma in man.

Endeavours to retrospectively examine the relationship between the receipt of BCG immunization, as part of public health policies, and its relationship to subsequent atopy have produced inconclusive results. BCG immunization at 14 years of age seems to confer little benefit [21]. The same has been observed for BCG immunization given at variable timings up to 6 months of age [22], whereas administration of BCG on the first day of life has been associated with less subsequent atopy [23]. I suspect that retrospective analyses may not be good enough to critically test this idea, because of the presence of many unrecorded confounding variables, both environmental and genetic.

Prospective, 'Proof-of-Concept' Experimental Approaches Are Now Needed in Man

We have conducted preliminary clinical experiments with killed *M. vaccae* in a masked placebo control study of adults with grass-pollen-induced asthma and rhinitis (table 2) [24]. Receipt of killed *M. vaccae* (as three intradermal inoculations of 10^9 organisms) was associated with fewer asthmatic symptoms and significantly less use of bronchodilator relief medication during the pollen season; the mean weekly total dose of salbutamol was 4.8 in *M. vaccae* recipients, and 31.2 in the placebo recipients. Over the same spell, active immunization showed a trend to enhance IFN-γ secretion by mononuclear cells in response to tuberculin antigens, but no clear evidence of other re-ordering of Th1/Th2 immune cytokine balance was observed. Further clinical testing is required in order to address the repeatability of such symptomatic benefit following immunization. These trials are in progress.

Future Directions

In principle, the impact of mycobacterial exposure in limiting Th2 immune disorder should be greatest in early life, that is, before the development of substantial burdens of Th2-driven cells and the development of clinical disease [3]. One early experiment, which might provide valuable 'proof of concept' data and offer safety, would be the critical testing of neonatal BCG immunization. Such a prospective clinical trial should take account of other important environmental determinants, (maternal smoking and breast-fed infant, receipt by the infant of public health immunizations and antibiotics), and also genetic variables that impinge on Th2 and Th1 immune signalling and which are relevant to atopy and asthma [25].

If the concept of limitation of Th2 immune mechanisms by mycobacterial exposure can be experimentally established in man then there are real prospects for serious limitation of atopic disorder and asthma in the future. But the approach will need nicely judged decisions on route of exposure, and the nature of the mycobacterial product and its dosage. In the murine experiments, administration of BCG via the respiratory route provided the greatest inhibition of respiratory allergy [15]. It is possible that the use of whole mycobacteria may provide more potent effects than isolated mycobacterial molecular products – and more predictable safety. The object should be to limit Th2 responses to allergens, but without causing exaggerated Th1 priming of the whole immune system and which might predispose to autoimmunity. Finally the approach of mycobacterial immunization will have to squarely face the prospect that genetic factors may limit certain individuals' responses to this approach [25], and that environmental factors (including receipt of public health vaccines and of antibiotics) could confound the approach in others.

Conclusion

Current data, epidemiological and experimental, point to exciting possibilities for mycobacterial immunization in the limitation of atopy and asthma. But there is a testing time ahead, if these possibilities are to be realized.

References

1 Hopkin JM: Mechanisms of enhanced prevalence of asthma and atopy in developed countries. Curr Opin Immunol 1997;6:788–792.
2 Mosmann TR, Sad S: The expanding universe of T-cell subsets: Th1, Th2 and more. Immunol Today 1996;3:138–146.
3 Yabuhara A, Macaubas C, Prescott SL, Venaille TJ, Holt BJ, Habre W, Sly PD, Holt PG: Th2-polarised immunological memory to inhalant allergens in atopics is established during infancy and early childhood. Clin Exp Allergy 1997;11:1261–1269.
4 Randolph DA, Carruthers, CJ, Szabo SJ, Murphy KM, Chaplin DD: Modulation of airway inflammation by passive transfer of allergen-specific Th1 and Th2 cells in a mouse model of asthma. J Immunol 1999;4:2375–2383.
5 Li XM, Chopra RK, Chou TY, Schofield BH, Wills-Karp M, Huang SK: Mucosal IFN-gamma gene transfer inhibits pulmonary allergic responses in mice. J Immunol 1996;8:3216–3219.
6 Gavett SH, O'Hearn DJ, Li X, Finkelman FD, Wills-Karp M: Interleukin 12 inhibits antigen-induced airway hyperresponsiveness, inflammation, and Th2 cytokine expression in mice. J Exp Med 1995;5:1527.
7 Farooqi IS, Hopkin JM: Early childhood infection and atopic disorder. Thorax 1998;53:927–932.
8 Matricardi PM, Rosmini F, Ferigno L, et al: Exposure to foodborne and orofecal microbes versus airborne viruses in relation to atopy and allergic asthma: epidemiological study. BMJ 2000;320:412–416.
9 Shaheen SO, Aaby P, Hall AJ, et al: Measles and atopy in Guinea-Bissau. Lancet 1996;347:1792–1796.
10 Shirakawa T, Enomoto T, Shimazu, Hopkin JM: The inverse association between tuberculin responses and atopic disorder. Science 1997;275:77–79.
11 Wickens K, Pearce N, Crane J, Beasley P: Antibiotic use in early childhood and the development of asthma. Clin Exp Allergy 1999;29:766–771
12 Pulverer G, Koh L, Beuth J: Immunomodulatory effects of antibiotics influencing digestive flora. Pathol Biol Paris 1993;41:753–758.
13 Von Mutius, Pearce N, Beasley R, Cheng S, von Ehrenstein O, Bjorksten G, Weiland S: International patterns of tuberculosis and the prevalance of symptoms of asthma, rhinitis and eczema. Thorax, in press.
14 Wang EC, Rook GAW: Inhibition of established allergic response to ovalbumin in BALB/c mice by killed *Mycobacterium vaccae*. Immunology 1998;93:307–313.
15 Erb KJ, Holloway JW, Sobeck A, Moll H, Le Gros G: Infection of mice with *Mycobacterium bovis*-bacillus Calmette-Guérin (BCG) suppresses allergen-induced airway eosinophilia. J Exp Med 1998;4:561–569.
16 Herz U, Gerhold K, Gruber C, Braun A, Wahn U, Renz H, Paul K: BCG infection suppresses allergic sensitization and development of increased airway reactivity in an animal model. J Allergy Clin Immunol 1998;5:867–874.
17 Sano K, Haneda K, Tamura G, Shirato K: Ovalbumin (OVA) and *Mycobacterium tuberculosis* bacilli cooperatively polarize anti-OVA T-helper (Th) cells toward a Th1-dominant phenotype and ameliorate murine tracheal eosinophilia. Am J Respir Cell Mol Biol 1999;6:1260–1267.
18 Brightbill, HD, Libraty DH, Krutzik ST, Yang RB, Belisle JT, Bleharski JR, Maitland M, Norgard MV, Plevy SE, Smale ST, Brennan PJ, Bloom BR, Godowski PJ, Modlin RL: Host defence mechanisms triggered by microbial lipoproteins through toll-like receptors. Science 1999;285:732–736.
19 Ria F, Penna G, Adorini L: Th1 cells induce and Th2 inhibit antigen-dependent IL-12 secretion by dendritic cells. Eur J Immunol 1998;6:2003–2016.
20 Kline JN, Waldschmidt TJ, Businga TR, Lemish JE, Weinstock JV, Thorne PS, Krieg AM: Modulation of airway inflammation by CpG oligodeoxynucleotides in a murine model of asthma. J Immunol 1998;6:2555–2559.
21 Omenaas E, Jentoft HF, Vollmer WM, Buist AS, Bulsvik A: No relationship between tuberculin reactivity and atopy in BCG vaccinated young adults. Thorax, in press.
22 Alm JS, Lilja G, Pershagen G, Scheynius A: Early BCG vaccination and development of atopy. Lancet 1997;350:400–403.
23 Aaby P, Shaheen S, Hall A, Shiell A, Jensen H, Marchant A: Early BCG vaccination and reduction in atopy in Guinea-Bissau. Eur Respir J 1998;12(suppl 29)4S.
24 Hopkin JM: Asthma: Towards a Th-1 phenotype by vaccination. World Asthma Congress, Barcelona, 1998.
25 Shirakawa I, Deichmann KA, Izuhara I, Mao I, Adra CN, Hopkin JM: Atopy and asthma: Genetic variants of Il-4 and Il-13 signalling. Immunol Today 2000;21:60–64.

Prof. Julian M. Hopkin
Department of Experimental Medicine
University of Wales, Singleton Park
Swansea, West Glamorgan SA2 8PP (UK)
Tel. +44 1792 513 062, Fax +44 1792 513 054
E-Mail j.m.hopkin@swansea.ac.uk

CpG Oligodeoxynucleotides

Joel N. Kline[a] Arthur M. Krieg[a-c]

[a]University of Iowa, [b]Veterans Affairs Medical Center, Iowa City, Iowa, and
[c]Coley Pharmaceutical Group, Wellesley, Mass., USA

Summary

CpG oligodeoxynucleotides (ODNs) are a novel pharmacotherapeutic class with profound immunomodulatory properties. The mechanisms through which these agents work are incompletely understood, but it is clear that the oligonucleotides bind with both cytoplasmic and nuclear factors. In murine models, CpG ODNs can both prevent and treat the Th2-mediated inflammatory responses associated with asthma and atopy. This class of compounds is poised for human trials in asthma and allergy.

CpG ODNs: Discovery and Definition

CpG ODNs are a recently described class of pharmacotherapeutic agents that are characterized by the presence of an unmethylated CG dinucleotide in specific base-sequence contexts (CpG motif). These CpG motifs are not seen in eukaryotic DNA, in which CG dinucleotides are suppressed and, when present, usually methylated, but are present in bacterial DNA to which they confer immunostimulatory properties [1]. These immunostimulatory properties include induction of a Th1-type response with prominent release of IFN-γ, IL-12, and IL-18. CpG ODNs (18–24 bp in length) possess immunomodulatory properties similar to bacterial DNA.

Mechanism of Action of CpG DNA

Although there are cell surface proteins that can bind DNA, the immune stimulatory effects of CpG DNA require cell uptake [1, 2]. This DNA uptake is inducible and varies with cell type, but is sequence independent [3, 4]. Uptake probably involves both pinocytosis and endocytosis [4]. Although the nature of the intracellular receptor for CpG DNA is not yet clear, its intracellular location of the CpG receptor seems logical if this detection pathway evolved as a defense against intracellular pathogens. Several intracellular signaling pathways appear to be activated by CpG DNA. Within 7–10 min, the mitogen-activated protein kinases p38 and the c-Jun NH_2-terminal kinase are activated in human and murine B cells and macrophages [5, 6]. In addition, there is rapid generation of reactive oxygen species, which appears to be important in the activation of NF-κB [7, 8].

These signaling pathways converge on the nucleus, resulting in the activation of multiple transcription factors and increased expression of multiple inflammatory messengers [9–15]. Overall, the most highly produced cytokines in the response to CpG are the Th1-like cytokines such as IL-12, IL-18 and IFN-γ. However, CpG DNA also induces B cells to produce IL-10, which appears to act in a counter-regulatory fashion to limit the inflammatory response to CpG [14].

Need for Immunomodulatory Therapy

In recent years, the paradigm of asthma therapy has shifted from symptomatic relief of bronchospasm to treatment of airway inflammation. Despite this increased attention to the role played by inflammation in the pathogenesis of asthma, the prevalence, severity and morbidity ascribed to asthma have grown over the past two decades [16]. Immunotherapy, or the use of allergen and/or immunomodulating agents to alter the immune response to an antigen, is a potentially curative therapy. Development of better immunotherapy protocols has been hindered by the relatively low potency of therapeutic allergens and the risk of serious and potentially fatal adverse reactions. If more effective and safer immunotherapy were available for the treatment of asthma, this would be a significant tool in the armamentarium of the clinician: patients could develop clinical tolerance to exposure to allergens, reducing their need for chronic anti-inflammatory therapy.

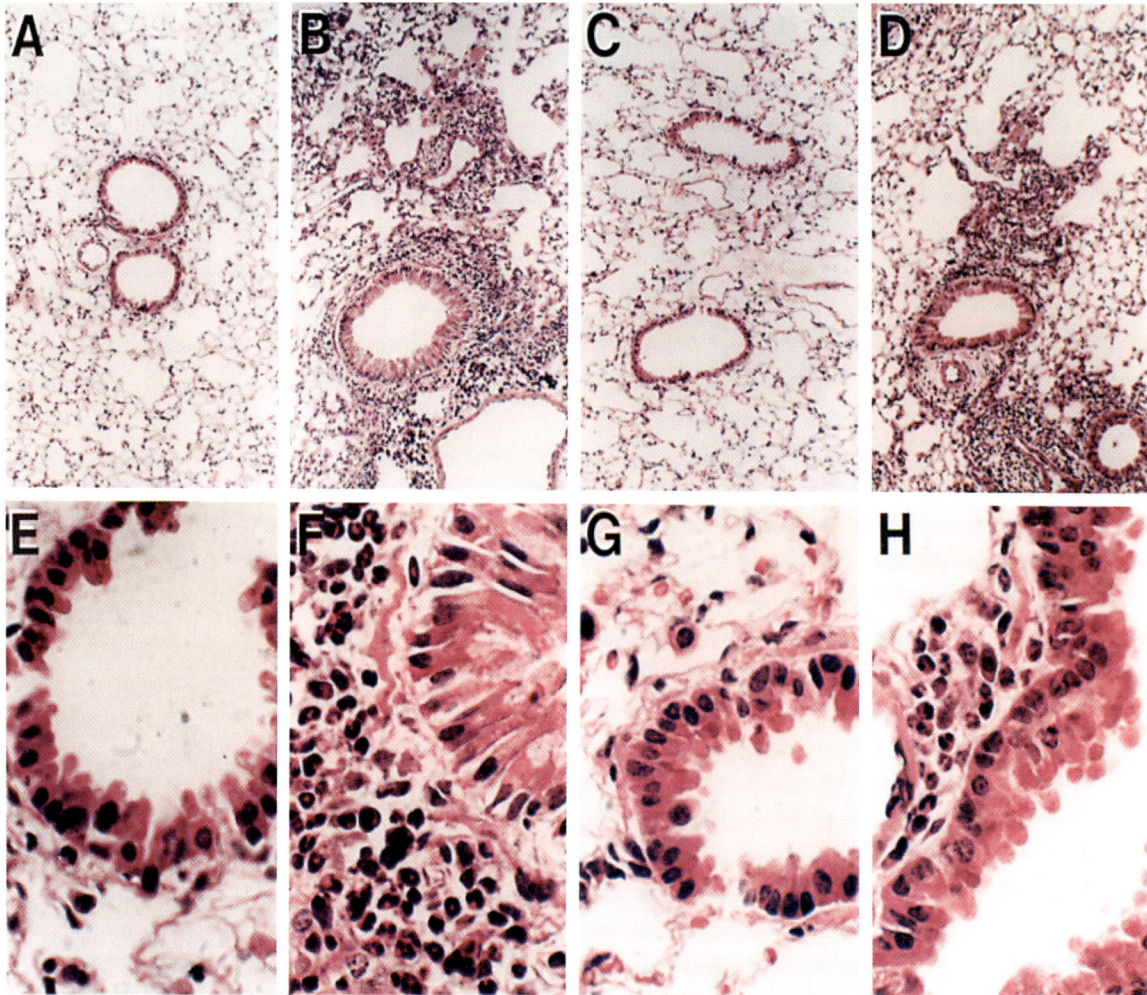

Fig. 1. HE-stained sections of murine lung. **A–D** ×160 (original magnification); **E–H** ×1,000 (original magnification). Saline control mice (**A**, **E**) demonstrate a bland parenchyma and bronchovascular bundle. In contrast, asthma control mice (**B**, **F**) display marked perivascular and peribronchial inflammatory infiltrate with eosinophils, lymphocytes, activated macrophages and other cells. This inflammation is nearly eliminated in the CpG-ODN-treated mice (**C**, **G**) but not in the control ODN-treated mice (**D**, **H**).

Preclinical Studies

Based on the epidemiologic data and our observations of the Th1 responses to CpG motifs, we hypothesized that administration of CpG ODNs may be an effective adjuvant in preventing manifestations of airway inflammation and altered physiologic responses in a murine model of asthma through suppression of Th2-mediated responses [17]. For these initial studies, we used a model in which C57BL/6 mice are sensitized to schistosome eggs and then challenged in the airways with soluble egg antigen (SEA) derived from the schistosome eggs. These mice developed marked airway eosinophilia, elevated BAL fluid IL-4 (table 1). Histopathologic examination (fig. 1) demonstrated peribronchial and perivascular infiltration of eosinophils, lymphocytes, activated macrophages and other inflammatory cells. Inflamed mice had exaggerated physiologic responses to inhaled methacholine (fig. 2). When mice received injections of CpG ODNs at the time of sensitization, all of these manifestations of asthmatic responses were abrogated (table 1, fig. 1, 2). This was associated with an induction of the Th1 cytokines, IL-12 and IFN-γ, in BAL fluid.

Because of the association between protection from eosinophilic airway inflammation and the induction of

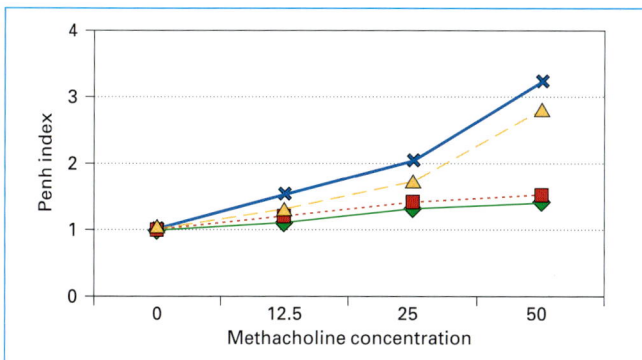

Fig. 2. Airway responses to methacholine inhalation challenge. Mice from various treatment groups are exposed to increasing concentrations of nebulized methacholine, after which they are assessed using a whole-body plethysmograph (Penh, Buxco). Asthma control mice (×——×) demonstrate marked bronchial hyperresponsiveness relative to saline control mice (♦——♦), this protection is nearly completely abrogated in the CpG-ODN-treated (■······■), but not the control ODN-treated mice (▲---▲).

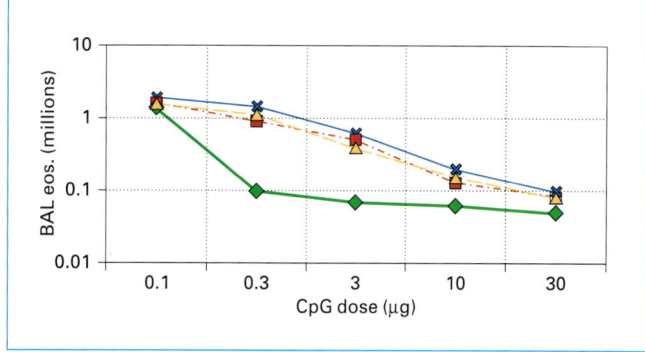

Fig. 3. CpG dose-response curve in inbred mice (♦——♦) and IFN-γ KO (□-·-□), IL-12 KO (△---△), and double (IFN-γ and IL-12) KO mice (×——×), all on C57 BL/6 background. Wild-type mice are substantially protected against the induction of airway eosinophilia when treated with amounts of CpG ODNs as low as 0.3 μg; for equivalent protection, the KO mice require at least one log greater amounts of CpG ODNs.

Table 1. Schistosome egg asthma model: effects of treatment with CpG ODNs

Treatment group	BAL eos. (× 10⁶)	BAL IL-4 pg/ml	BAL IFN-γ ng/ml	BAL IL-12 ng/ml	Serum IgE μg/ml
Saline control	ND	5 ± 1*	0.02 ± 0.01	0.6 ± 0.2	0.66 ± 0.38*
Asthma + control ODNs	2.2 ± 0.9	78 ± 18	0.12 ± .08	2.0 ± 0.8	3.04 ± 0.94
Asthma + CpG ODNs	0.4 ± 0.2*	23 ± 3*	0.42 ± 0.13*	5.5 ± 1.9*	1.04 ± 0.32*
Asthma control	3.5 ± 0.8	118 ± 29	0.02 ± 0.01	1.8 ± 0.7	4.10 ± 0.54

n = 6/group; ND = none detected; * $p < 0.01$ vs. asthma control mice.

Table 2. Effect of CpG ODNs on protection against airway eosinophilia and bronchial hyperreactivity in mice who were sensitized to schistosome eggs in the presence or absence of IFN-γ and/or IL-12, and in the presence or absence of CpG ODNs

Mouse type	Antibody T_x	CpG ODN T_x	BAL eos.	Penh$_{50}$
C57BL/6	–	–	1.6 ± 0.4 × 10⁶	3.6 ± 0.2
C57BL/6	–	+	0.2 ± 0.1 × 10⁶	1.2 ± 0.3
C57BL/6	anti-IFN-γ	+	0.1 ± 0.1 × 10⁶	1.1 ± 0.2
C57BL/6	Anti-IL-12	+	0.2 ± 0.3 × 10⁶	1.2 ± 0.2
IFN-γ KO	–	+	0.2 ± 0.3 × 10⁶	1.4 ± 0.2
IL-12 KO	–	+	0.3 ± 0.3 × 10⁶	1.3 ± 0.3
DKO	–	+	0.3 ± 0.2 × 10⁶	1.6 ± 0.3

Penh$_{50}$ = Penh index (fold increase over baseline) after inhalation of 50 mg/ml of methacholine.

Th1 cytokines in the airway, we next evaluated whether either IFN-γ or IL-12 was necessary for the protection offered by CpG ODNs [18]. For these studies, we used the same model of antigen-induced airway inflammation, but we carried out these studies in mice treated with anti-IFN-γ or anti-IL-12 antibodies as well as in mice whose gene for IFN-γ, IL-12, or both cytokines had been disrupted. To our surprise, we found that the administration of CpG ODNs was effective in preventing the development of both airway inflammation and of bronchial hyperresponsiveness in the absence of IFN-γ, IL-12, or both (table 2). When we carried out CpG dose-response studies, however, we found that there was approximately a log difference in sensitivity to the protective effects of CpG ODNs between wild-type inbred mice (C57BL/6) and mice deficient in either IFN-γ or IL-12 (also on a C57BL/6 background); the difference was even greater in double (IFN-γ and IL-12) knockout mice (fig. 3). These studies suggested to us that, although both of these Th1 cytokines played a role in the protection offered by CpG ODNs, neither alone nor in combination was essential for this protection. Undoubtedly there are redundant pathways through which these effects are mediated.

It was next important to determine whether CpG ODNs were effective in modulating attributes of asthma after the establishment of eosinophilic airway inflammation. For these studies, we adopted the schistosome-egg-induced murine model of asthma and administered ODNs, alone or in combination with antigen, at various time points. We first examined the effect of treatment fol-

Table 3. Effect of CpG treatment after sensitization on SEA-induced airway eosinophilia

Treatment	SEA (inhaled)	Harvest	BAL eos. ($\times 10^6$)
No treatment	weeks 2 and 3	week 3	2.6 ± 0.8
CpG week 1 (+ eggs)	weeks 2 and 3	week 3	0.6 ± 0.2
CpG week 2 (– eggs)	weeks 3 and 4	week 4	1.9 ± 0.6
CpG week 5	weeks 3, 4, 6, 7	week 7	2.4 ± 0.7
CpG + SEA week 5	weeks 3, 4, 6, 7	week 7	3.2 ± 0.6
Saline (s.c.) weeks 4, 5, 6, 7	weeks 2, 3, 8, 9	week 9	2.9 ± 1.2
SEA (s.c.) weeks 4, 5, 6, 7	weeks 2, 3, 8, 9	week 9	1.2 ± 0.9
CpG + SEA (s.c.) weeks 4, 5, 6, 7	weeks 2, 3, 8, 9	week 9	0.2 ± 0.3

n = 6/group. All mice sensitized to schistosome eggs (i.p.) on days 0 and 7 (weeks 0 and 1).

lowing sensitization but before airway challenge, and found that a single administration of CpG ODNs and SEA, but not CpG ODNs alone, was effective in blocking the subsequent airway inflammatory response to inhaled antigen in previously sensitized mice (table 3). We next evaluated the response to treatment in mice who had been previously sensitized and challenged with antigen in the airways. Since a single treatment was ineffective in modulating eosinophilic airway inflammation (table 3), we instituted a course of immunotherapy treatment: 4-weekly subcutaneous injections of SEA in the presence or absence of ODNs. Following this therapy, mice were re-exposed to SEA. Mice treated with SEA injections demonstrated modest reductions in airway eosinophilia (table 3) compared with control mice (who received saline injections rather than active immunotherapy). Mice treated with SEA and CpG ODNs, however, had significant reductions in both airway eosinophilia (table 3) and bronchial hyperreactivity (not shown), suggesting that the CpG ODNs acted as an immunoadjuvant in downregulating established airway inflammation.

Conclusions

CpG ODNs have exhibited profound Th1-like immunomodulatory effects in both the prevention of antigen-induced asthma as well as treatment of previously established responses. These preclinical data have been reproduced by other groups, and there is strong support for the pursuit of clinical trials.

References

1 Krieg AM, Yi AK, Matson S, Waldschmidt TJ, Bishop GA, Teasdale R, Koretzky GA, Klinman DM: CpG motifs in bacterial DNA trigger direct B-cell activation. Nature 1995;374:546–549.
2 Manzel L, Macfarlane DE: Lack of immune stimulation by immobilized CpG-oligodeoxynucleotide. Antisense Nucleic Acid Drug Dev 1999;9:459–464.
3 Krieg AM, Gmelig-Meyling F, Gourley MF, Kisch WJ, Chrisey LA, Steinberg AD: Uptake of oligodeoxyribonucleotides by lymphoid cells is heterogeneous and inducible. Antisense Res Dev 1991;1:161–171.
4 Krieg AM: Uptake and localization of phosphodiester and chimeric oligonucleotides in normal and leukemic primary cells; in Akhtar S (ed): Delivery Strategies for Antisense Oligonucleotide Therapeutics. Boca Raton, CRC Press, 1995, pp 177–190.
5 Yi AK, Krieg AM: Rapid induction of mitogen-activated protein kinases by immune stimulatory CpG DNA. J Immunol 1998;161:4493–4497.
6 Hartmann G, Krieg AM: Mechanism and function of a newly identified CpG DNA motif in human primary B cells. J Immunol 2000;164: 944–953.
7 Yi AK, Klinman DM, Martin TL, Matson S, Krieg AM: Rapid immune activation by CpG motifs in bacterial DNA. Systemic induction of IL-6 transcription through an antioxidant-sensitive pathway. J Immunol 1996;157:5394–5402.
8 Stacey KJ, Sweet MJ, Hume DA: Macrophages ingest and are activated by bacterial DNA. J Immunol 1996;157:2116–2122.
9 Yi AK, Tuetken R, Redford T, Waldschmidt M, Kirsch J, Krieg AM: CpG motifs in bacterial DNA activate leukocytes through the pH-dependent generation of reactive oxygen species. J Immunol 1998;160:4755–4761.
10 Yi AK, Krieg AM: CpG DNA rescue from anti-IgM-induced WEHI-231 B lymphoma apoptosis via modulation of I kappa B alpha and I kappa B beta and sustained activation of nuclear factor-kappa B/c-Rel. J Immunol 1998; 160:1240–1245.
11 Yi AK, Hornbeck P, Lafrenz DE, Krieg AM: CpG DNA rescue of murine B lymphoma cells from anti-IgM-induced growth arrest and programmed cell death is associated with increased expression of c-myc and bcl-xL. J Immunol 1996;157:4918–4925.
12 Sweet MJ, Stacey KJ, Ross IL, Ostrowski MC, Hume DA: Involvement of Ets, rel and Sp1-like proteins in lipopolysaccharide-mediated activation of the HIV-1 LTR in macrophages. J Inflamm 1998;48:67–83.
13 Yi AK, Chang M, Peckham DW, Krieg AM, Ashman RF: CpG oligodeoxyribonucleotides rescue mature spleen B cells from spontaneous apoptosis and promote cell cycle entry. J Immunol 1998;160:5898–5906.
14 Redford TW, Yi AK, Ward CT, Krieg AM: Cyclosporin A enhances IL-12 production by CpG motifs in bacterial DNA and synthetic oligodeoxynucleotides. J Immunol 1998;161: 3930–3935.
15 Chace JH, Hooker NA, Mildenstein KL, Krieg AM, Cowdery JS: Bacterial DNA-induced NK cell IFN-gamma production is dependent on macrophage secretion of IL-12. Clin Immunol Immunopathol 1997;84:185–193.
16 Weiss KB, Gergen PJ, Hodgson TA: An economic evaluation of asthma in the United States. N Engl J Med 1992;326:862–866.
17 Kline JN, Waldschmidt TJ, Businga TR, Lemish JE, Weinstock JV, Thorne PS, Krieg AM: Modulation of airway inflammation by CpG oligodeoxynucleotides in a murine model of asthma. J Immunol 1998;160:2555–2559.
18 Kline JN, Krieg AM, Waldschmidt TJ, Ballas ZK, Jain V, Businga TR: CpG oligodeoxynucleotides do not require Th1 cytokines to prevent eosinophilic airway inflammation in a murine model of asthma. J All Clin Immunol 1999;104:1258–1264.

Joel N. Kline, MD
C33GH UIHC, 200 Newton Road
Iowa City, IA 52242 (USA)
Tel. +1 319 353 8551, Fax +1 319 353 6406
E-Mail joel-kline@uiowa.edu

CD8 T Cells: Potential Therapeutic Targets?

Theo A. Out[a,c]   Francina L. de Pater-Huijsen[a,b]   Henk M. Jansen[b]
Chris J. Corrigan[d]

[a]Clinical Immunology Laboratory and [b]Department of Pulmonology, Academic Medical Center, Amsterdam and [c]CLB Sanquin Blood Supply Foundation, Amsterdam, The Netherlands, and [d]Department of Respiratory Medicine and Allergy, Guy's, King's and St. Thomas' School of Medicine, London, UK

Summary

CD8 T cells differentiate to distinct subpopulations with unique functions. There are clear abnormalities in CD8 T cells both in asthma and in COPD when compared with healthy subjects. It is not clear whether CD8 T cells are protective or contribute to pathology. The role of CD8-specific T cell products, such as perforin, if any, in asthma and COPD is not understood. It is clearly impossible at present to formulate valid conclusions as to the possible role of CD8 T cell modulation for the therapy of asthma and COPD. A tailored therapeutic approach in different circumstances might be required.

Functional Spectrum of CD8 T Cells

T lymphocytes, which may be of the CD4 or CD8 phenotype in the circulation, regulate antigen-specific immune responses. CD4 T cells recognize antigenic peptides in the context of MHC class II molecules. CD8 T cells do so in the context of MHC class I molecules. As a rule, soluble antigens like proteins associate with MHC II and are handled by CD4 cells; intracellularly synthesized antigens such as those derived from intracellular microorganisms associate with MHC I and are handled by CD8 cells (fig. 1).

CD8 T cells are well known for their cytotoxic functions: they kill malignant-transformed and virus-infected cells. To this end they are equipped with two types of killing machinery. One involves Fas-ligand expressed at the cell surface; the other involves release of perforin and granzymes from intracellular granules. In addition, these cells produce high amounts of IFN-γ. These CD8 cells are

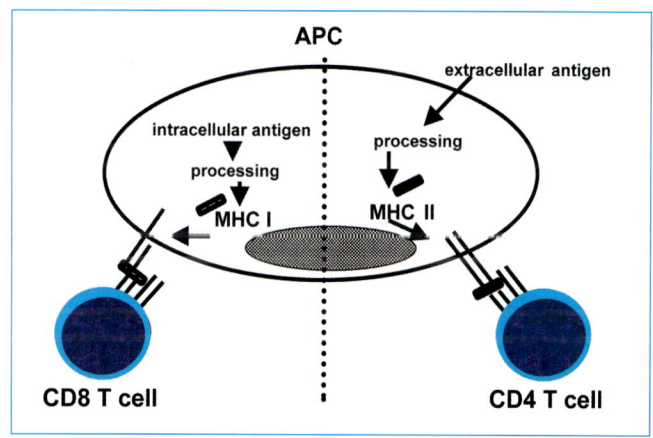

Fig. 1. CD8 T cells recognize antigen in the context of MHC I, CD4 T cells in the context of MHC II molecules.

now denoted as type 1, or Tc1. A distinct CD8 T-cell subset, termed Tc2, may have other regulatory functions, in particular the regulation of function of other immune cells by cytokine secretion. Tc2 CD8 T cells may produce IL-4 and IL-5. An IL-4 rich environment contributes to the shift of CD8 T cells from the Tc1 to the Tc2 phenotype [1].

Both Tc1 and Tc2 CD8 T cells can be functionally divided as naïve, memory and, at least in the case of Tc1, 'memory-effector' cells (fig. 2). These functional subsets can be discriminated on the basis of the surface marker

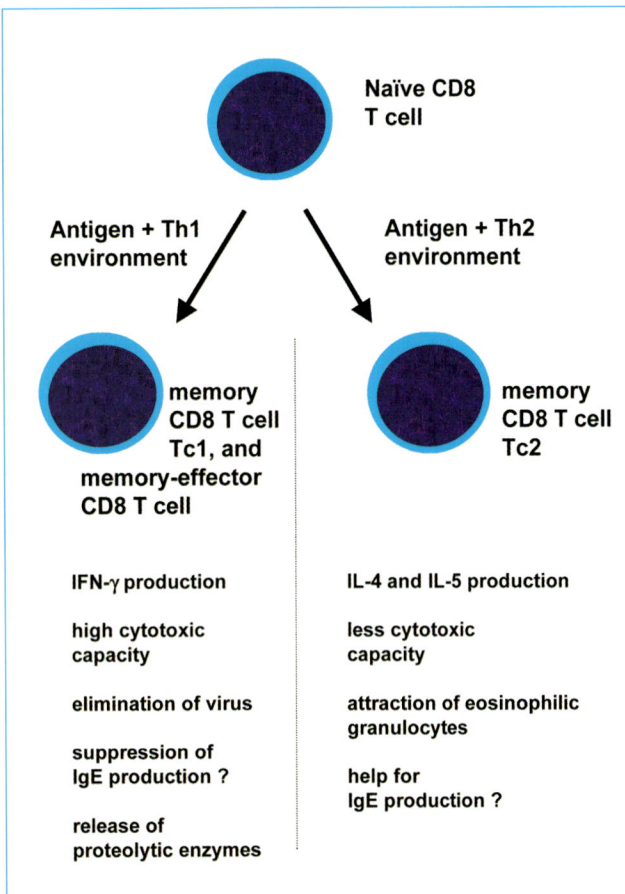

Fig. 2. Scheme of the development and the characteristics of CD8 T lymphocytes.

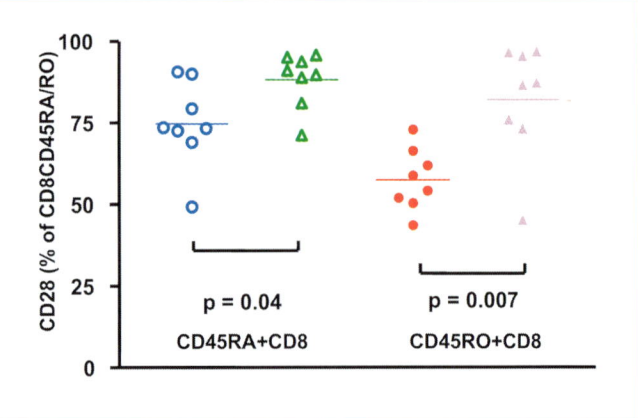

Fig. 3. CD8 T lymphocyte subpopulations in 8 patients with mild to moderate allergic asthma (median age, 25.5; range, 19–30 years) not using immunosuppressive therapy, and non-allergic healthy subjects (median age, 27.5; range, 20–39 years). Peripheral blood mononuclear cells were analysed by flow cytometry. Circles = asthma; triangles = healthy subjects; open symbols = CD8+CD45RA+; filled symbols = CD8+CD45RO+.

phenotypes CD45RA+CD27+CD28+, CD45RO+CD27+CD28+ and CD45RA+CD27–CD28–, respectively [2]. The latter population corresponds to the chemokine receptor CCR7– population that preferentially migrates into inflammatory tissues [3]. The CD45RA+CD27–CD28– cells have the same capacity for IFN-γ production as the CD45RO+ population, but fail to produce IL-4 [2, 3], at least in the peripheral blood. Mediators of cellular cytotoxicity are mainly expressed in the memory-effector subset [2, 3]. These cells have been demonstrated to contain antigen-specific cells recognizing among others viral antigens [2].

CD8 T Cells in Asthma

Activation of CD4 T cells appears to be a universal feature of asthma. In allergic asthma, these may be allergen-specific T cells. These cells are of a Th2 phenotype, producing relatively high amounts of IL-4 and IL-5, and low amounts of IFN-γ, and are typically seen in the inflamed airways of symptomatic asthma patients [4]. Interestingly, CD8, as well as CD4 T cells show expression of IL-4 and IL-5 mRNA and protein in the bronchial mucosa of both atopic and non-atopic asthmatics [4], suggesting that CD8 T cells may be a potential source of asthma-promoting cytokines. The activating stimulus for CD8 T cells is not clear.

In contrast to CD4 T cells, peripheral blood CD8 cells do not consistently show higher expression of activation markers such as CD25 in asthmatics than in controls. The CD8 T cells may show variable Th2 type cytokine expression [5, 6] and higher expression of perforin [7] as compared with controls. The latter matches with a higher percentage of CD8+CD28– [8], which was confirmed by our own findings, as shown in figure 3. Thus, there appears to be an increase in the CD8 memory-effector cell population in asthma.

Experimental allergen challenge results in significant increases in both the CD4 and the CD8 T cell populations in the airways [9, 10], and the numbers of CD8 T cells were negatively associated with the likelihood of a late-phase bronchoconstrictor response, suggesting a possible protective effect of CD8 T cells [9]. On the other hand, viral infection of the respiratory tract may exacerbate asthma, possibly by augmenting eosinophilic infiltration. This may reflect involvement of virus-specific Tc2 CD8 T cells.

CD8 T Cells in COPD

Recent studies have characterized the inflammatory cellular infiltrate in the central and peripheral airways of smokers with stable, chronic COPD, smokers with normal lung function and non-smoking controls [11–14]. COPD patients showed higher CD8 T cell numbers [11, 12]. However, it appeared that these findings may be related to smoking habits of the populations investigated [13, 14].

Studies in the peripheral blood of COPD patients have shown increased CD8 T cell numbers [15], which may be largely memory-effector CD8 cells, as defined by the membrane surface markers CD45RA+CD27–CD28– [16].

If CD8 T cells do contribute to airway inflammation in COPD, the mechanisms by which they do so, as well as the mechanisms of their initial activation, remain at present speculative.

Present Therapy

Drugs. Both CD4 and CD8 T cells are inhibited to a similar degree by phosphodiesterase inhibitors [17]. Dexamethasone and cyclosporin A inhibit re-expression of surface CD4, but not CD8, on activated T cells in vitro [18], which may reflect differential sensitivity of CD4 and CD8 T cells to these drugs. Further studies of the effects of glucocorticoids and other drugs on CD8 T cells in a disease setting in vivo are sorely needed.

Desensitization. Early studies have already suggested a possible role for CD8 T cells in favourable clinical responses to allergen immunotherapy [19].

Animal Models

Animal models have suggested prominent roles for CD8 T cells in the regulation of IgE synthesis. Repeated challenge of rats with ovalbumin resulted in the activation of CD8 T cells that could inhibit the development of IgE responses after adoptive transfer [20]. In virus infection models, the effects of CD8 T cells critically depended on the conditions chosen. CD8 T cells were essential in the induction of airway inflammation and airway hyperresponsiveness in a mouse model of intranasal administration of respiratory syncytial virus (RSV) [21]. In other models where the animals were vaccinated with polypeptides of RSV before the challenge, the CD8 T cells significantly contributed to suppression of airway inflammation [22]. It is difficult to translate these conditions of acute antigen challenges and acute infections with the chronic allergen exposure that underlies much of the pathophysiology in allergic asthma patients. There is no animal model that mimics the chronic airway inflammation and airway destruction with increased numbers of tissue CD8 T cells as found in COPD.

Anti-CD8 Antibody Therapy in Humans

Treatment with anti-CD8 antibodies has not as yet acquired a place in experimental or routine clinical practice. Experimental animal models have shown the potential of anti-human CD8 antibodies in depleting CD8 T cells. The humoral immune response and at least some aspects of cell mediated responses seem not to be affected by such treatment. In a patient with a chronic hepatitis C virus infection, CD8 T cell depletion resulted in improvement of the anti-viral immune response and clinical status [23]. On the other hand, in rhesus macaques, anti-CD8 treatment resulted in rapid emergence of a pathogenic strain of HIV-1 from an initially non-pathogenic virus [24].

With current knowledge, it would be difficult to formulate a cogent rationale for CD8 T cell depletion in asthma or COPD.

References

1 Byun DG, Demeure CE, Yang LP, Shu U, Ishihara H, Vezzio N, Gately MK, Delespesse G: In vitro maturation of neonatal human CD8 T lymphocytes into IL-4- and IL-5-producing cells. J Immunol 1994;153:4862–4871.

2 Hamann D, Roos MT, van Lier RA: Faces and phases of human CD8 T-cell development. Immunol Today 1999;20:177–180.

3 Sallusto F, Lenig D, Forster R, Lipp M, Lanzavecchia A: Two subsets of memory T lymphocytes with distinct homing potentials and effector functions. Nature 1999;401:708–712.

4 Humbert M, Menz G, Ying S, Corrigan CJ, Robinson DS, Durham SR, Kay AB: The immunopathology of extrinsic (atopic) and intrinsic (non-atopic) asthma: More similarities than differences. Immunol Today 1999;20:528–533.

5 Corrigan CJ, Hamid Q, North J, Barkans J, Moqbel R, Durham S, Kay AB: Peripheral blood CD4, but not CD8 T lymphocytes in patients with exacerbation of asthma transcribe and translate messenger RNA encoding cytokines which prolong eosinophil survival in the context of a Th2-type pattern: Effect of glucocorticoid therapy. Am J Respir Cell Mol Biol 1995;12:567–578.

6 Stanciu LA, Shute J, Promwong C, Holgate ST, Djukanovic R: Increased levels of IL-4 in CD8+ T cells in atopic asthma. J Allergy Clin Immunol 1997;100:373–378.

7 Arnold V, Balkow S, Staats R, Matthys H, Luttmann W, Virchow JC: Increase in perforin-positive peripheral blood lymphocytes in extrinsic and intrinsic asthma. Am J Respir Crit Care Med 2000;161:182–186.

8 Stanciu LA, Cho SH, Begishivilli B, Roberts K, Johnston SL: Circulating CD28+ CD4+ and CD8+ are decreased in and CD4+CD30+ increased in mild atopic asthmatics. Am J Respir Crit Care Med 1999;159:A101.

9 Gonzalez MC, Diaz P, Galleguillos FR, Ancic P, Cromwell O, Kay AB: Allergen-induced recruitment of bronchoalveolar helper (OKT4) and suppressor (OKT8) T-cells in asthma. Relative increases in OKT8 cells in single early responders compared with those in late-phase responders. Am Rev Respir Dis 1987;136:600–604.

10 Yurovsky VV, Weersink EJ, Meltzer SS, Moore WC, Postma DS, Bleecker ER, White B: T-Cell repertoire in the blood and lungs of atopic asthmatics before and after ragweed challenge. Am J Respir Cell Mol Biol 1998;18:370–383.

11 O'Shaughnessy T, Ansari CTW, Barnes NC, Jeffery PK: Inflammation in bronchial biopsies of subjects with chronic bronchitis: Inverse relationship of CD8+ T lymphocytes with FEV_1. Am J Respir Crit Care Med 1997;155:852–857.

12 Saetta M, Di Stefano A, Turato G, Facchini FM, Corbino L, Mapp CE, Maestrelli P, Ciaccia A, Fabbri LM: CD8+ T lymphocytes in positive peripheral airways of smokers with chronic obstructive pulmonary disease. Am J Respir Crit Care Med 1998;157:822–826.

13 Lams BE, Sousa AR, Rees PJ, Lee TH: Immunopathology of the small airway submucosa in smokers with and without chronic obstructive pulmonary disease. Am J Respir Crit Care Med 1998;158:1518–1523.

14 Lams BEA, Sousa AR, Rees PJ, et al: Immunopathology of the large airways submucosa in smokers with and without chronic obstructive pulmonary disease. Eur Respir J 2000;15:512–516.

15 De Jong JW, van der Belt-Gritter B, Koeter GH, Postma DS: Peripheral blood lymphocyte cell subsets in subjects with chronic obstructive pulmonary disease: Association with smoking, IgE and lung function. Respir Med 1997;91:67–76.

16 Out TA, Franssen R, Reijneke RMR, Jansen HM, Jonkers RE: Increased peripheral blood memory-effector CD8+ T lymphocytes in COPD (abstract). Am J Respir Crit Care Med 2000;161:A822.

17 Giembycz M, Corrigan CJ, Seybold J, Newton R, Barnes PJ: Identification of cyclic AMP phosphodiesterases 3, 4 and 7 in human CD4+ and CD8+ T-lymphocytes: Role in regulating proliferation and the biosynthesis of interleukin-2. Br J Pharmacol 1996;118:1945–1958.

18 Haczku A, Kay AB, Corrigan CJ: Inhibition of re-expression of surface CD4, but not CD8, on activated human T-lymphocytes by the immunosuppressive drugs dexamethasone and cyclosporine A: Correlation with inhibition of proliferation. Int J Immunopharmacol 1996;18:45–52.

19 Rocklin RE, Sheffer AL, Greineder DK, Melmon KL: Generation of antigen-specific suppressor cells during allergy desensitization. N Engl J Med 1980;302:1213–1219.

20 Sedgwick JD, Holt PG: Suppression of IgE responses in inbred rats by repeated respiratory tract exposure to antigen: Responder phenotype influences isotype specificity of induced tolerance. Eur J Immunol 1984;14:893–897.

21 Schwarze J, Makela M, Cieslewicz G, Dakhama A, Lahn M, Ikemura T, Joetham A, Gelfand EW: Transfer of the enhancing effect of respiratory syncytial virus infection on subsequent allergic airway sensitization by T lymphocytes. J Immunol 1999;163:5729–5734.

22 Hussell T, Baldwin CJ, O'Garra A, Openshaw PJ: CD8+ T cells control Th2-driven pathology during pulmonary respiratory syncytial virus infection. Eur J Immunol 1997;27:3341–3349.

23 Kiefersauer S, Reiter C, Eisenburg J, Diepolder HM, Rieber EP, Riethmuller G, Gruber R: Depletion of CD8+ T lymphocytes by murine monoclonal CD8 antibodies and restored specific T cell proliferation in vivo in a patient with chronic hepatitis C. J Immunol 1997;159:4064–4071.

24 Igarashi T, Endo Y, Englund G, Sadjadpour R, Matano T, Buckler C, Buckler-White A, Plishka R, Theodore T, Shibata R, Martin M: Emergence of a highly pathogenic simian/human immunodeficiency virus in a rhesus macaque treated with anti-CD8 mAb during a primary infection with a nonpathogenic virus. Proc Natl Acad Sci USA 1999;96:14049–14054.

T.A. Out, PhD
Clinical Immunology Laboratory
Academic Medical Center
B1 236, PO Box 22700
NL-1100 DE Amsterdam (The Netherlands)
Tel. +31 20 5662893, Fax +31 20 6091222
E-Mail t.a.out@amc.uva.nl

Macrocyclic Immunosuppressants

Thomas H. Keller[a] René Hersperger[b] Giovanni Della Cioppa[a]

[a]Novartis Horsham Research Center, Horsham, UK, and [b]Novartis Pharma, Basel, Switzerland

Summary

The clinical literature suggests that oral cyclosporin A can be effective in patients with severe steroid-dependent asthma, improving their clinical control and allowing a meaningful reduction of their daily dose of oral steroids. However, the safety profile is problematic, even in this severely asthmatic population. The development of locally active macrocyclic immunosuppressants for delivery by inhalation, such as IMM125 and MLD987, promises to provide a long-term therapy of asthma with a significantly improved side effect profile.

Rationale

One of the characteristic features of asthma is a persistent pulmonary inflammation, with increased numbers of eosinophils and activated T lymphocytes in the airways [1]. It is becoming increasingly clear that this process is driven by T cells with a type 2 cytokine phenotype (Th2), which migrate to the lung after antigen exposure or viral infection [2]. Th2-cell-derived cytokines play a number of important roles in the initiation and maintenance of the inflammatory process in asthma. For example, IL-4 is an essential cofactor for IgE production, while IL-5 mobilizes and activates eosinophils. Eosinophil degranulation products and mediators released from mast cells cause mucosal damage, mucus hypersecretion and bronchial hyperresponsiveness. Thus, modulating T cell activity in the lung with macrocyclic immunosuppressants, such as cyclosporin A (CsA), FK506, rapamycin or their analogues (fig. 1) might represent a valid approach for treating respiratory diseases such as chronic asthma.

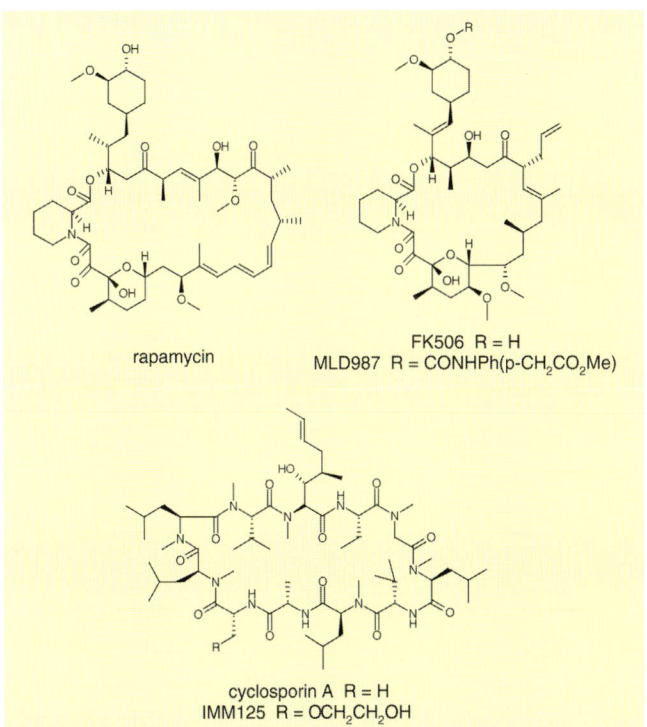

Fig. 1. Structures of macrocyclic immunosuppressants.

Molecular Mechanism of Action

CsA and FK506 elicit their biological action by binding to related intracellular receptors, cyclophilin and FKBP12 (collectively called immunophilins). The drug-receptor complexes then bind to the Ca^{2+} calmodulin-dependent protein phosphatase calcineurin (CNA), which results in allosteric inhibition of its phosphatase activity [3]. As a

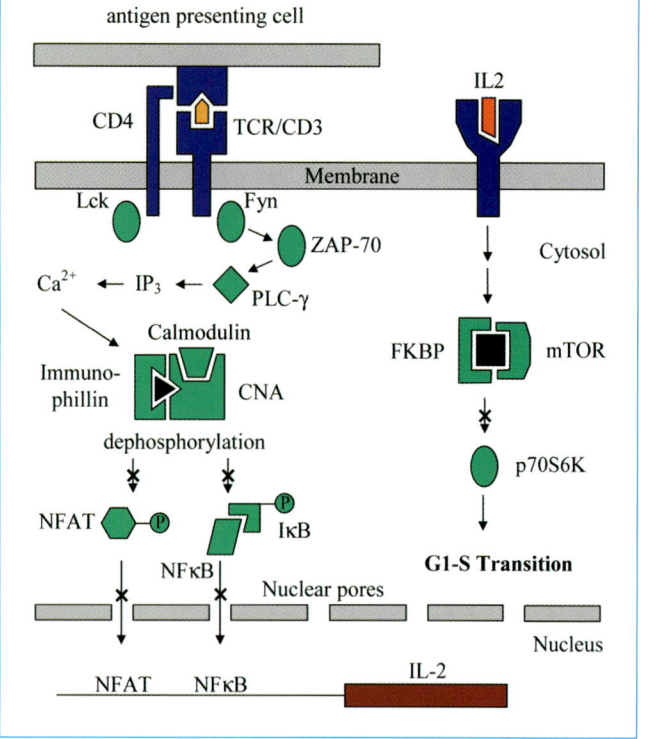

Fig. 2. Inhibition of signal transduction in T cells by CsA (▶), FK506 (▶) and rapamycin (■). For CsA and FK506 a generic mechanism is shown (see text and Bonham and Thomson [8]).

PHAS-I. It is still unclear how mTOR receives upstream signals and how exactly it transduces them to downstream signalling molecules [4].

Cellular Mechanism of Action

CsA and FK506 are powerful inhibitors of antigen-stimulated T cell activation and proliferation [5]. In addition, there is considerable evidence that the two agents can directly affect certain other cell types, the most important examples in the context of asthma being mast cells and eosinophils [5].

Besides its immunosuppressive properties, the effect of rapamycin on growth-factor-stimulated proliferation of a variety of cell types, such as smooth muscle cells and fibroblasts, has attracted considerable attention [6]. Airway remodelling, particularly hypertrophy and hyperplasia of airway smooth muscle and collagen deposition beneath the basement membrane, is a distinctive pathophysiological feature of asthma, which may lead to a gradual alteration of the airways and thus contribute to the decline in pulmonary function [7]. Rapamycin with its dual mode of action has the potential to affect both inflammation and the subepithelial fibrosis associated with chronic asthma.

Animal Models and Route of Administration

Immunosuppressants have been extensively studied in experimental models of asthma [8]. CsA and FK506 potently reduce antigen-induced pulmonary eosinophilia and bronchial hyperreactivity in models of allergic asthma in rodents [9]. Qualitatively similar effects were described for rapamycin, which effectively inhibited both leukocyte migration into BAL fluid and bronchial hyperreactivity in Sephadex-injected guinea pigs [10].

The use of these drugs for the treatment of respiratory diseases inevitably raises concerns related to systemic immunosuppression and the side effects associated with the chronic use of these compounds (see clinical studies). Local application and metabolic instability ('soft drugs') are strategies which have been used successfully to circumvent side effects in other drug categories, notably the inhaled glucocorticosteroids. A similar approach has been applied for the design of locally active immunosuppressants such as the cyclosporin analogue, IMM125, and the 'soft', metabolically labile ascomycin derivative, MLD987. Both compounds, when given locally by intratracheal application, dose-dependently inhibit eosinophil influx into BAL fluid of actively sensitized Brown-Norway rats following antigen challenge (fig. 3). Thus, there is convincing evidence from models of allergic asthma that

consequence, translocation of the transcription factor NF-AT from the cytoplasm to the nucleus is blocked (fig. 2), resulting in a failure to activate early genes necessary for T cell proliferation (e.g. IL-2). IMM125 and MLD987 (see below) produce their biological effects by the same molecular mechanisms as CsA and FK506, respectively.

Although both rapamycin and FK506 share the same intracellular target, FKBP12, they affect immunosuppression through different mechanisms. Whereas CsA and FK506 block the signal from the T cell receptor, rapamycin blocks/delays G_1 cell cycle progression by interrupting the signal from the IL-2 receptor [4]. In yeast, rapamycin depletes the pool of polysomes and abolishes protein translation via inhibition of the targets of rapamycin/FKBP12, TOR1 and TOR2, which are absolutely required for G_1 progression. The mammalian homologue mTOR seems to function in a similar way; however, compared to yeast, the mechanistic details seem to be considerably less straightforward. mTOR is a member of a novel family of phosphatidylinositol-3-kinase-related proteins, containing a C-terminal kinase domain which is required for signalling to the downstream targets p70 S6 kinase and inhaled immunosuppressants related to CsA, FK506 and rapamycin have potential as long-term therapy of asthma. Local application of these drugs should help to significantly reduce systemic immunosuppression and its associated side effects.

Clinical Studies

The first case report on the effect of oral CsA in clinical asthma was published in 1991 by Nizankowska et al. [11] of the University of Cracow, Poland. Low-dose oral CsA was added to the therapeutic regimen of a 42-year-old woman with very severe asthma poorly controlled in spite of a 15-year treatment with 20–30 mg oral prednisone per day on top of high-dose inhaled beclomethasone, aminophylline and fenoterol. Whereas previous attempts to reduce the dose of oral steroid had failed, 5 weeks after the addition of CsA, the tapering of oral prednisone was successfully started. At the end of the 11-month treatment period, the daily dose of oral prednisone had been reduced from 25 mg to 8.5 mg and at the same time the patient's asthma control and lung function had improved considerably. Other single case reports and small uncontrolled series followed throughout the 1990s [12–16], suggesting the efficacy of add-on low-dose oral CsA (3.5–5 mg/kg/day) in asthmatic patients in need of high-dose oral steroids who represent the extreme end of the spectrum of asthma severity. However, two other less welcome features also emerged. First, some patients showed a remarkable response while others did not respond at all. For example, in a series of 12 severely asthmatic patients [13], the dose of oral corticosteroids could be dramatically reduced in 6 patients, whereas in the remaining 6 all attempts to reduce oral steroids failed. In another series of 5 children with severe asthma [15], oral steroid reduction after addition of low-dose CsA was very successful in 3 young patients and a complete failure in 2. The second aspect which emerged was that even at the relatively low doses used to treat asthmatic patients, the safety and tolerability burden of oral CsA was troublesome: increased blood pressure, impaired renal function (elevated levels of serum creatinine) and hypertricosis were repeatedly reported.

Only three controlled clinical trials evaluating oral CsA in severe oral-steroid-dependent asthma have been published [17–19]. In the first [17], a double-blind cross-over study, CsA (5 mg/kg/day) and placebo were given, each for 3 months, in random sequence to 33 adults on a constant dose of oral prednisone and high-dose inhaled corticosteroids. The addition of CsA resulted in a 12% improvement in morning PEFR, an 18% improvement in

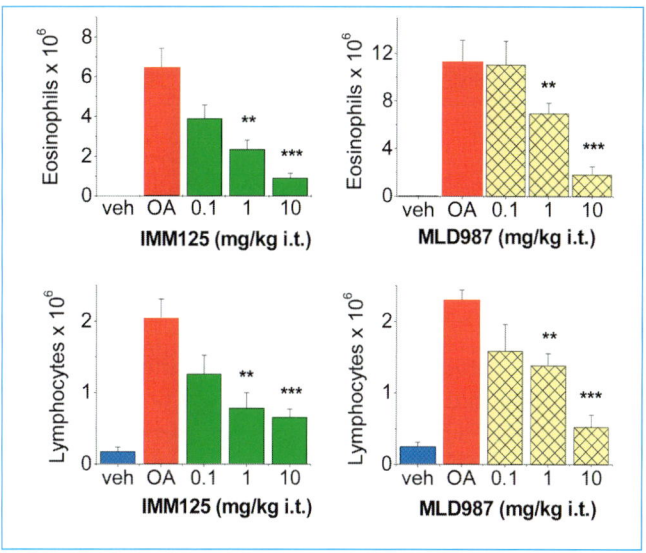

Fig. 3. Effect of IMM125 (mg/kg) and MLD987 (mg/kg) on ovalbumin (OA)-induced pulmonary leukocyte accumulation (mean ± SEM) in actively sensitized Brown Norway rats. Both compounds were administered intratracheally (i.t.), 1 h prior to and 24 h after antigen exposure. * $p < 0.05$, ** $p < 0.01$, and *** $p < 0.001$ indicate significant difference by comparison with vehicle (veh) and OA-treated animals.

FEV_1 and a 50% reduction in the frequency of asthma exacerbations. Interestingly, there was no improvement in symptom scores and rescue medication.

Steroid reduction was the primary objective of the second placebo-controlled trial which was a parallel-group study [18]. A total of 39 patients, all on both oral and high-dose inhaled corticosteroids received either oral CsA (5 mg/kg/day) or placebo for 9 months. The CsA group achieved a significantly greater oral steroid reduction compared to the placebo group, expressed as the lowest dose maintained for at least 2 weeks (mean: 3.5 vs. 7.5 mg/day) and the total dose taken during the 9-month treatment period (mean: ~2,500 vs. ~3,500 mg). At the same time, there was a trend toward reduced exacerbations and a significant increase in morning and evening PEFR. CsA gave no advantage over placebo with regard to FEV_1 and symptom scores. In the third controlled trial [19], results were less impressive. A total of 34 patients on oral steroids were randomized in a double-blind parallel group design to either CsA (starting dose: 2.5 mg/kg/day) or placebo for 8.5 months. After a 3-month fixed steroid dose period, steroid reduction was attempted over the last 5½ months. During the stable steroid phase, CsA patients showed a significant improvement compared to placebo in symptom scores and intake of rescue β_2-agonists, but

Table 1. Compounds in the process of development

	IMM125	MLD987	Rapamycin
Company	Novartis	Novartis	American Home Products
Status	phase II	preclinical	not registered for asthma or COPD
Administration	inhaled	inhaled	unknown
Comments	cyclosporin derivative	soft ascomycin derivative	WO-09214476 claims a novel rapamycin-containing formulation for asthma and COPD

no improvement in lung function. In the subsequent phase, the steroid reduction with CsA was not significantly greater than with placebo, and lung function worsened in patients receiving CsA.

The high variability in response between patients was confirmed in these controlled trials, as was the problematic safety and tolerability profile of low-dose oral CsA. Frequently documented adverse events in patients receiving CsA included increased systolic and diastolic blood pressure, increased serum potassium and decreased magnesium, increased serum creatinine and lowered glomerular filtration rate, high alkaline phosphatase and bilirubin levels, hypertricosis, paraesthesia and tremor. Most abnormalities disappeared or improved markedly shortly after discontinuation of CsA. However, reversibility after longer-term treatment with CsA remains unknown.

Development Status

Neither CsA nor FK506 are registered for asthma and there is no indication that they are in development for this indication either by the oral or the inhaled route. American Home Products patented a special formulation of rapamycin for use in respiratory diseases in 1992; however, its development status is unclear (table 1).

Of the two above-mentioned strategies undertaken to improve the risk-benefit ratio of this class of drugs, namely the development of metabolically labile compounds (such as the ascomycin derivative MLD987, Novartis), and the development of locally active drugs to be delivered in very low doses by inhalation (such as IMM 125, Novartis), the latter is about to complete a phase II proof-of-concept clinical trial at the time this chapter is being written.

References

1 Kon OM, Kay AB: T cells and chronic asthma. Int Arch Allergy Immunol 1999;118:133–135.
2 Robinson DS, Hamid Q, Ying S, Tsicopoulos A, Barkans J, Bentley AM, Corrigan C, Durham SR, Kay AB: Predominant TH2-like bronchoalveolar T-lymphocyte population in atopic asthma. N Engl J Med 1992;326:298–304.
3 Liu J, Farmer JD, Lane WS, Friedman J, Weissman I, Schreiber SL: Calcineurin is a common target of cyclophilin-cyclosporin A and FKBP-FK506 complexes. Cell 1991;66:807–815.
4 Abraham RT: Mammalian target of rapamycin: Immunosuppressive drugs uncover a novel pathway of cytokine receptor signaling. Curr Opin Immunol 1998;10:330–336.
5 Walker C: Immunomodulators; in Barnes PJ, Grunstein MM, Leff AR, Woolcock AJ (eds): Asthma. New York, Lippincott-Raven, 1997, vol 2, pp 1785–1803.
6 Dumont FJ, Su Q: Mechanism of action of the immunosuppressant rapamycin. Life Sci 1996;58:373–395.
7 Chetta A, Foresi A, Del Donno M, Bertorelli G, Pesci A, Olivieri D: Airways remodeling is a distinctive feature of asthma and is related to severity of disease. Chest 1997;111:852–857.
8 Bonham CA, Thomson AW: Immunosuppressants: Kay AB (ed): Allergy and Allergic Diseases. Oxford, Blackwell Science, 1997, vol 1, pp 642–663.
9 Nagai H, Yamaguchi S, Tanaka H, Inagaki N: Effect of some immunosuppressors on allergic bronchial inflammation and airway hyperresponsiveness in mice. Int Arch Allergy Immunol 1995;108:189–195.
10 Nogueira de Francischi J, Conroy DM, Maghni K, Sirois P: Inhibition by rapamycin of leukocyte migration and bronchial hyperreactivity induced by injection of Sephadex beads to guinea-pigs. Br J Pharmacol 1993;110:1381–1386.
11 Nizankowska E, Dworski R, Szczeklik A: Cyclosporin for a severe case of aspirin-induced asthma. Eur Respir J 1991;4:380.
12 Finnerty NA, Sullivan TJ: Effect of cyclosporine on costicosteroid dependent asthma. J Allergy Clin Immunol 1991;87:297A.
13 Szczeklik A, Nizankowska E, Dworski R, Domagala B, Pinis G: Cyclosporine for steroid dependent asthma. Allergy 1991;46:312–315.
14 Fukuda TF, Asakawa J, Motojima S, Makino S: Cyclosporine A reduces T lymphocyte activity and improves airway hyperresponsiveness in corticosteroid-dependent chronic severe asthma. Ann Allergy Asthma Immunol 1995;75:65–72.
15 Coren ME, Rosenthal M, Bush A: The use of cyclosporin in corticosteroid dependent asthma. Arch Dis Child 1997;77:522–523.
16 Reddington AE, Hardinge FM, Holgate ST, Howarth PH: Cyclosporine A treatment and airways inflammation in corticosteroid-dependent asthma. Allergy 1998;53:94–98.
17 Alexander AG, Barnes NC, Kay AB: Trial of cyclosporin in corticosteroid-dependent chronic severe asthma. Lancet 1992;339:324–328.
18 Lock SH, Kay AB, Barnes NC: Double-blind, placebo-controlled study of cyclosporin A as a corticosteroid-sparing agent in corticosteroid-dependent asthma. Am J Respir Crit Care Med 1996;153:509–514.
19 Nizankowska E, Soja J, Pinis G, Bochenek G, Sladek K, Domagala B, Pajak A, Szczeklik A: Treatment of steroid-dependent bronchial asthma with cyclosporin. Eur Respir J 1995;8:1091–1099.

Thomas H. Keller
Novartis Horsham Research Center
Wimblehurst Road
Horsham RH12 5AB (UK)
Tel. +44 1403 323122, Fax +44 1403 323837
thomas.keller@pharma.novartis.com

Cytokine-Directed Therapy

Cytokines: An Overview

K. Fan Chung

National Heart and Lung Institute, Imperial College School of Medicine, London, UK

Summary

Cytokines are likely to play important roles in the chronic inflammatory processes and airway wall remodelling of asthma and COPD. They have a wide variety of effects, including cell activation and proliferation, maturation of haematopoietic cells, chemoattraction and migration, adhesion, immune regulation and cell survival or apoptosis. In relation to asthma and COPD, cytokines may induce eosinophilic or neutrophilic airway inflammation, subepithelial fibrosis, goblet cell hyperplasia and increases in mucin expression, matrix metalloproteinases and bronchial hyperresponsiveness. Targetting specific cytokines may lead to much-needed novel therapies for asthma and COPD.

Cytokines are extracellular signalling proteins, usually less than 80 kD in size and many are glycosylated. They are produced by different cell types involved in cell-to-cell interactions, having an effect on closely adjacent cells, and therefore function in a predominantly paracrine fashion. They may also act at a distance (endocrine) and may have effects on the cell of origin (autocrine). A classification according to function is proposed in table 1.

The effects of an individual cytokine may be influenced by other cytokines released simultaneously from the same cell or from target cells following activation by the cytokine, and are mediated by binding to cell surface high-affinity receptors usually present in low numbers, which can be upregulated with cell activation. The receptors for many cytokines have been grouped into superfamilies based on the presence of common homology regions (table 1). Cytokines themselves may induce the expression of receptors which may change the responsiveness of both source and target cells. Some cytokines may stimulate their own production in an autocrine manner, whereas others stimulate the synthesis of different cytokines that have a feedback stimulatory effect on the first cytokine, resulting in an increase in its effects. The effects of cytokines are summarized in table 2, and have been recently reviewed [1]. This review will concentrate on the role of cytokines in asthma and COPD.

Table 1. Classification of cytokines and cytokine receptors

Cytokines	
Pro-inflammatory cytokines	IL-1α/β, TNFα/β, IL-6, IL-11, IFN-γ
Cytokines involved in atopy	IL-4, IL-13 (promoters); IFN-γ, IL-12 (inhibitors)
Cytokines of eosinophil chemoattraction and activation	IL-2, IL-3, IL-4, IL-5, GM-CSF, RANTES, eotaxin, MCP-3, MCP-4
Th2 cytokines	IL-4, IL-5, IL-10, IL-13
Cytokines involved in T cell chemoattraction	IL-16, RANTES, MIP-1α/β
Cytokines of neutrophil chemoattraction and activation	IL-8, IL-1α/β, TNFα/β
Anti-inflammatory cytokines	IL-10, IL-4, IL-13, IL-12, IL-1ra
Growth factors	PDGF, TGF-β, FGF, EGF, TNF-α, SCF
Cytokine receptors	
Cytokine receptor superfamily	IL-2Rβ- and γ-chains, IL-4R, IL-3R α- and β-chains, IL-5α- and β-chains, IL-6R, gp130, IL-12R, GM-CSFR; soluble forms by alternative splicing (e.g. IL-4R)
Immunoglobulin superfamily	IL-1R, IL-6R, PDGFR, M-CSFR
Protein kinase receptor superfamily	PDGFR, EGFR, FGFR
Interferon receptor superfamily	IFN-α/β receptor, IFN-γ receptor and IL-10 receptor
Nerve growth factor superfamily	NGFR, TNFR-I (p55), TNFR-II (p75)
Seven-transmembrane G-protein-coupled receptor superfamily	chemokine receptors

Table 2. Summary of effects of cytokines

Cytokine	Important cellular and mediator effects
Lymphokines	
IL-2	• eosinophilia in vivo
	• growth and differentiation of T cells
IL-3	• eosinophilia in vivo
	• pluripotent haematopoietic factor
IL-4	• ↑ eosinophil growth
	• ↑ Th2; ↓ Th1
	• ↑ IgE
	• ↑ mucin expression and goblet cells
IL-5	• eosinophil maturation
	• ↓ apoptosis
	• ↑ Th2 cells
	• BHR
IL-13	• activates eosinophils
	• ↓ apoptosis
	• ↑ IgE
	• ↑ mucin expression and goblet cells
IL-15	• as for IL-2
	• growth and differentiation of T cells
IL-16	• eosinophil migration
	• growth factor and chemotaxis of T cells (CD4+)
IL-17	• T cell proliferation
	• activates epithelia, endothelial cells, fibroblasts
Pro-inflammatory	
IL-1	• ↑ adhesion to vascular endothelium; eosinophil accumulation in vivo
	• growth factor for Th2 cells
	• B cell growth factor; neutrophil chemoattractant; T cell and epithelial activation
	• BHR
TNF-α	• activates epithelium, endothelium, antigen-presenting cells; monocytes/macrophages
	• BHR
	• ↑ IL-8 from epithelial cells
	• ↑ MMPs from macrophages
IL-6	• T-cell growth factor
	• B-cell growth factor
	• ↑ IgE
IL-9	• ↑ activated T cells and IgE from B cells
	• ↑ mast cell growth and differentiation
	• ↑ mucin expression and goblet cells
	• causes eosinophilic inflammation and BHR
Pro-inflammatory	
IL-11	• B cell growth factor
	• activates fibroblast
	• BHR
GM-CSF	• eosinophil apoptosis and activation; induces release of leukotrienes
	• proliferation and maturation of haematopoietic cells; endothelial cell migration
	• BHR
SCF	• ↑ VCAM-1 on eosinophils
	• growth factor for mast cells
Inhibitory cytokines	
IL-10	• ↓ eosinophil survival
	• ↓ Th1 and Th2
	• ↓ monocyte/macrophage activation; ↑ B cell; ↑ mast cell growth
	• ↓ BHR
IL-1ra	• ↓ Th2 proliferation
	• ↓ BHR
IFN-γ	• ↓ eosinophil influx after allergen
	• ↓ Th2 cells
	• activates endothelial cells, epithelial cells, alveolar macrophages/monocytes
	• ↓ IgE
	• ↓ BHR
IL-18	• ↓ via IFN-γ release
	• releases IFN-γ from Th1 cells
	• activates NK cells, monocytes
	• ↓ IgE
Growth factors	
PDGF	• fibroblast and airway smooth muscle proliferation
	• release of collagen
TGF-β	• ↓ T-cell proliferation
	• blocks IL-2 effects
	• fibroblast proliferation
	• chemoattractant for monocytes, fibroblasts, mast cells
	• ↓ Airway smooth muscle proliferation

Inflammation and Cytokines in Asthma

Asthmatic Inflammation. The chronic airway inflammation of asthma is characterized by an infiltration of T lymphocytes, eosinophils, macrophages/monocytes and mast cells, and sometimes neutrophils. An acute or chronic inflammation may be observed with acute exacerbations, with an increase in eosinophils and neutrophils in the airway submucosa and release of mediators, such as histamine and cysteinyl-leukotrienes, from eosinophils and mast cells to induce bronchoconstriction, airway oedema and mucus secretion. Changes in the resident cells are also observed, such as an increase in the thickness of the airway smooth muscle with hypertrophy and hyperplasia, more myofibroblasts with an increase in collagen deposition in the lamina reticularis, more vessels and an increase in goblet cell numbers in the airway epithelium.

Cytokines play an integral role in the coordination and persistence of the inflammatory process in the chronic inflammation of the airways (table 1).

Th2-Associated Cytokines. CD4+ T lymphocytes of the asthmatic airways express Th2 cytokines including IL-3, IL-4, IL-5, IL-10, IL-13 and GM-CSF. The primary signals that activate Th2 cells may be related to the presentation of a restricted panel of antigens in the presence of

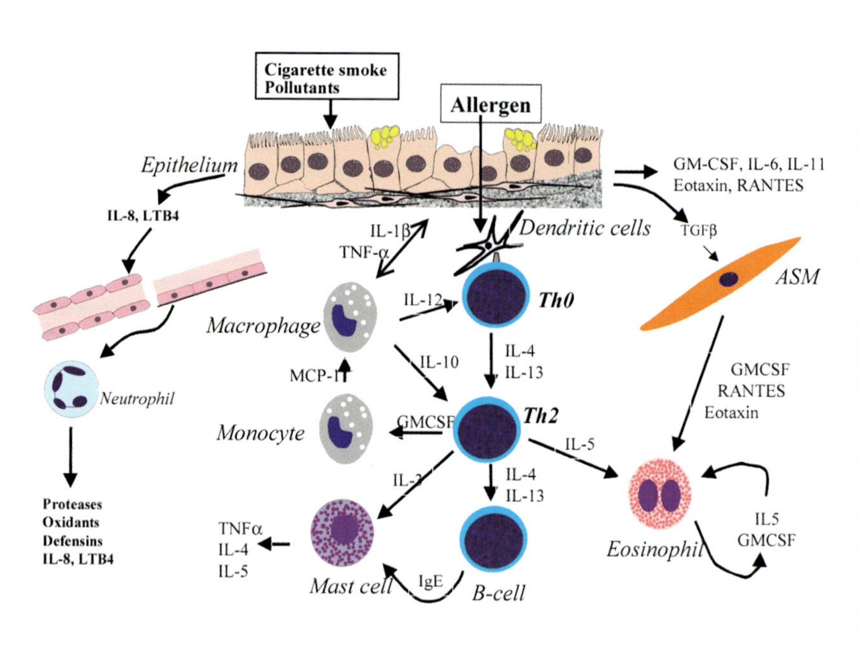

Fig. 1. Interactions of cells and cytokines in airway inflammation of asthma and COPD. In asthma, antigen presentation by dendritic cells to T cells with the subsequent polarization to Th2 cells appears to be an important initial process, but the roles of other cells such as airway epithelium, eosinophils, neutrophils, macrophages and airway smooth muscle (ASM) cells, are crucial as well. In COPD, the initiating factors include cigarette smoke and pollutants, with macrophages and airway epithelium inducing the release of chemotactic factors for neutrophils, which in turn are important effector cells for inflammation, tissue damage and repair.

appropriate cytokines. Dendritic cells are ideally suited to being the primary contact between the immune system and external allergens. Costimulatory molecules on the surface of antigen-presenting cells, in particular B7.2/CD28 interaction, may lead to proliferation of Th2 cells [2]. With the expression of IL-4, synthesis of IgE by B lymphocytes on immunoglobulin isotype switching occurs [3]. IgE produced in asthmatic airways binds to FcεRI receptors ('high-affinity' IgE receptors) on mast cells priming them for activation by antigen. The maturation and expansion of mast cells from bone marrow cells involve growth factors and cytokines such as SCF and IL-3 derived from structural cells. Bronchoalveolar mast cells from asthmatics show enhanced release of mediators such as histamine. Mast cells also elaborate IL-4 and IL-5 [4]. IL-4 also increases the expression of an inducible form of the low-affinity receptor for IgE (FcεRII or CD23) on B lymphocytes and macrophages [5]. IL-4 drives the differentiation of CD4+ Th precursors to Th2-like cells.

Antigen Presentation. Cytokines may play an important role in antigen presentation (fig. 1). Airway macrophages are usually poor at antigen presentation and suppress T-cell-proliferative responses (possibly via release of cytokines such as IL-1 receptor antagonist), but in asthma there is reduced suppression after exposure to allergen [6]. Both GM-CSF and IFN-γ increase the ability of macrophages to present allergen and express HLA-DR [7]. IL-1 is important in activating T lymphocytes and is an important costimulator of the expansion of Th2 cells after antigen presentation [8]. Airway macrophages may be an important source of 'first-wave' cytokines, such as IL-1, TNF-α and IL-6, which may be released on exposure to inhaled allergens via FcεRI receptors. These cytokines may then act on epithelial cells to release a 'second wave' of cytokines, including GM-CSF, IL-8 and RANTES which then leads to influx of secondary cells, such as eosinophils, which themselves may release multiple cytokines (fig. 1).

Eosinophil-Associated Cytokines. The differentiation, migration and pathobiological effects of eosinophils may occur through the effects of GM-CSF, IL-3, IL-5 and certain chemokines such as eotaxin [9, 10]. IL-5 and eotaxin also induce the mobilization of eosinophils and eosinophil precursors into the circulation [11]. Mature eosinophils may show increased survival in bronchial tissue [12]. Eosinophils themselves may also generate other cytokines such as IL-3, IL-5 and GM-CSF [13].

Cytokines such as IL-4 may also exert an important regulatory effect on the expression of adhesion molecules such as VCAM-1, both on endothelial cells of the bronchial circulation and on airway epithelial cells. IL-1 and TNF-α increase the expression of ICAM-1 in both vascular endothelium and airway epithelium [14]. Cytokines also play an important role in recruiting inflammatory cells to the airways.

Airway Wall Remodelling Cytokines. Proliferation of myofibroblasts and the hyperplasia of airway smooth muscle may occur through the action of several growth factors such as PDGF and TGF-β. They may be released from inflammatory cells in the airways, such as macrophages and eosinophils, but also by structural cells, such as airway epithelium, endothelial cells and fibroblasts. These growth factors may stimulate fibrogenesis by recruiting and activating fibroblasts or transforming myofibroblasts. Epithelial cells may release growth factors, since collagen deposition occurs underneath the basement membrane of the airway epithelium [15]. Growth factors may also stimulate the proliferation and growth of airway smooth muscle cells. PDGF and EGF are potent stimulants of human airway smooth muscle proliferation [16], and these effects are mediated via activation of tyrosine kinase and protein kinase C. Cytokines, such as TNF-α and FGF may also play an important role in angiogenesis of chronic asthma.

Inflammation and Cytokines in COPD

Inflammation in COPD. COPD is characterized by chronic obstruction of expiratory flow affecting peripheral airways, often associated with chronic bronchitis (mucus hypersecretion), and emphysema (destruction of airway parenchyma). Fibrosis, tissue damage with airway wall remodelling, and inflammation in the small airways appear to play an important role in patients with COPD, and accompanying emphysema leads to loss of lung elastic recoil, contributing to decreased expiratory flow. Increased numbers of neutrophils and macrophages are usually recovered in BAL fluid and in induced sputum, while in the small airways there is an increase in mucosal inflammatory cells comprised of mononuclear cells and CD8+ T cells, but without prominence of neutrophils [17]. During acute exacerbations of COPD, there is a prominence of eosinophils recovered in sputum or in bronchial biopsies, but without an increased expression of IL-5 in tissues [18]. Some patients with COPD have a preponderance of eosinophils in sputum, an observation that has been associated with significant improvement of FEV_1 with corticosteroid therapy [19].

Neutrophils are more prominent in COPD than in asthma. They have been implicated in causing tissue damage in COPD through the release of a number of mediators, including proteases such as neutrophil elastases and MMPs, oxidants and toxic peptides such as defensins. A primary role for macrophages is also proposed because of their capacity to produce several MMPs including MMP-1, MMP-9 and MMP-12 [20]. Expression of MMP-1 and MMP-9 mRNA was found to be enhanced in macrophages from patients with COPD [21]. Inhaled cigarette smoke may induce alveolar macrophages to produce macrophage metalloelastase which may induce chemotactic fragments that attract blood monocytes to the lung parenchyma. The role of the CD8+ T cell remains unclear, but they produce granzymes and perforin that may contribute to cell damage. One possibility is that these cells may be induced by certain viral infections, and virus-specific CD8+ T cells may produce IL-5.

Increased levels of TNF-α and IL-8 have been observed in induced sputum of patients with chronic bronchitis. TNF-α is produced by many cells including macrophages, T cells, mast cells and epithelial cells, but the principal source is the macrophage. The secretion of TNF-α by monocytes/macrophages is greatly enhanced by other cytokines, such as IL-1, GM-CSF and IFN-γ. TNF-α activates NF-κB that switches the transcription of the IL-8 gene from the airway epithelium. TNF-α increases the expression of the adhesion molecule, ICAM-1, which is increased in COPD [22]. TNF-α may activate macrophages to produce MMPs. This effect is inhibited by IL-10, which also enhances the release of tissue inhibitor of MMPs. TNF-α also stimulates bronchial epithelial cells to produce tenascin, an extracellular matrix glycoprotein.

IL-8, a CXC chemokine, is a mainly neutrophil chemoattractant and activator which induces a transient shape change, rise in intracellular calcium, exocytosis with release of enzymes and proteins from intracellular storage organelles, and respiratory burst. It also upregulates the expression of two integrins (CD11b/CD18 and CD11c/CD18) during exocytosis of specific granules. IL-8 activates neutrophil 5-LO with the formation of LTB_4 and 5-HETE. These properties of IL-8 support its potential role in COPD. Other CXC chemokines with a predominant neutrophilic action may also be released in COPD.

An increase in the expression of TGF-β and also of EGF in the epithelium and submucosal cells of patients with chronic bronchitis has been reported [23]; EGF is of interest since EGFR activation by TNF-α leads to the expression of mucin genes, in particular MUC5A [24]. These growth factors may be implicated in repair responses following injury, particularly to the epithelium. Growth factors such as TGF-β and EGF may be involved in fibroblast activation and proliferation leading to peribronchiolar fibrosis.

Conclusions

Cytokines play important roles in the chronic inflammatory processes and airway wall remodelling of asthma and COPD. They constitute important targets for novel therapies in these chronic conditions. There are several potential ways of inhibiting cytokine effects including blocking antibodies, small-molecule receptor antagonists, soluble receptors, altering the balance of certain cytokines, and antisense oligonucleotides. Inhibition of cytokines will be a promising way of obtaining efficacious drugs for asthma and COPD.

References

1 Chung KF, Barnes PJ: Cytokines in asthma. Thorax 1999;54:825–857.
2 Lenschow DJ, Walunas TL, Bluestone JA: CD28/B7 system of T cell costimulation. Annu Rev Immunol 1996;14:233–258.
3 Geha RS: Regulation of IgE synthesis in humans. J Allergy Clin Immunol 1992;90:143–150.
4 Bradding P, Roberts JA, Britten KM, et al: Interleukin-4, -5 and -6 and tumor necrosis factor-α in normal and asthmatic airways: Evidence for the human mast cell as a source of these cytokines. Am J Respir Cell Mol Biol 1994;10:471–480.
5 Vercelli D, Jabara HH, Lee BW, Woodland N, Geha RS, Leung DY: Human recombinant interleukin-4 induces FcεRII/CD23 on normal human monocytes. J Exp Med 1988;167:1406–1416.
6 Spiteri M, Knight RA, Jeremy JY, Barnes PJ, Chung KF: Alveolar macrophage-induced suppression of T-cell hyperresponsiveness in bronchial asthma is reversed by allergen exposure. Eur Respir J 1994;7:1431–1438.
7 Fischer HG, Frosch S, Reske K, Reske-Kunz AB: Granulocyte-macrophage colony-stimulating factor activates macrophages derived from bone marrow cultures to synthesis of MHC class II molecules and to augmented antigen presentation function. J Immunol 1988;141:3882–3888.
8 Chang TL, Shea CH, Urioste S, Thompson RC, Boom WH, Abbas AK: Heterogeneity of helper/inducer T lymphocytes: Lymphokine production and lymphokine responsiveness. J Immunol 1990;145:2803–2808.
9 Sanderson CJ, Warren DJ, Strath M: Identification of a lymphokine that stimulates eosinophil differentiation in vitro. Its relationship to interleukin 3, and functional properties of eosinophils produced in cultures. J Exp Med 1985;162:60–74.
10 Hallsworth MP, Litchfield TM, Lee TH: Glucocorticosteroids inhibit granulocyte-macrophage colony-stimulating factor and interleukin-5 enhanced in vitro survival of human eosinophils. Immunology 1992;75:382–385.
11 Collins PD, Griffiths-Johnson DA, Jose PJ, Williams TJ, Marleau S: Co-operation between interleukin-5 and the chemokine, eotaxin, to induce eosinophil accumulation in vivo. J Exp Med 1995;182:1169–1174.
12 Rothenberg ME, Owen WFJ, Siberstein DS: Human eosinophils have prolonged survival, enhanced functional properties and become hypodense when exposed to human interleukin. J Clin Invest 1988;81:1986–1992.
13 Moqbel R, Hamid Q, Ying S, et al: Expression of mRNA and immunoreactivity for the granulocyte/macrophage colony-stimulating factor (GM-CSF) in activated human eosinophils. J Exp Med 1991;174:749–752.
14 Tosi MF, Stark JM, Smith CW, Hamedani A, Gruenert DC, Infeld MD: Induction of ICAM-1 expression on human airway epithelial cells by inflammatory cytokines: Effects on neutrophil-epithelial cell adhesion. Am J Respir Cell Mol Biol 1992;7:214–221.
15 Brewster CEP, Howarth PH, Djukanovic R, Wilson J, Holgate ST, Roche WR: Myofibroblasts and subepithelial fibrosis in bronchial asthma. Am J Respir Cell Mol Biol 1990;3:507–511.
16 Hirst SJ, Barnes PJ, Twort CHL: Quantifying proliferation of cultured human and rabbit airway smooth muscle cells in response to serum and platelet-derived growth factor. Am J Respir Cell Mol Biol 1992;7:574–581.
17 Jeffery PK: Structural and inflammatory changes in COPD: A comparison with asthma. Thorax 1998;53:129–136.
18 Saetta M, Di SA, Maestrelli P, et al: Airway eosinophilia and expression of interleukin-5 protein in asthma and in exacerbations of chronic bronchitis. Clin Exp Allergy 1996;26:766–774.
19 Chanez P, Vignola AM, O'Shaugnessy T, et al: Corticosteroid reversibility in COPD is related to features of asthma. Am J Respir Crit Care Med 1997;155:1529–1534.
20 Shapiro SD: The macrophage in chronic obstructive pulmonary disease. Am J Respir Crit Care Med 1999;160:S29–S32.
21 Finlay GA, O'Driscoll LR, Russell KJ, et al: Matrix metalloproteinase expression and production by alveolar macrophages in emphysema (see comments). Am J Respir Crit Care Med 1997;156:240–247.
22 Riise GC, Larsson S, Lofdahl CG, Andersson BA: Circulating cell adhesion molecules in bronchial lavage and serum in COPD patients with chronic bronchitis. Eur Respir J 1994;7:1673–1677.
23 Vignola AM, Chanez P, Chiappara G, et al: Transforming growth factor-beta expression in mucosal biopsies in asthma and chronic bronchitis. Am J Respir Crit Care Med 1997;156:591–599.
24 Takeyama K, Dabbagh K, Lee HM, et al: Epidermal growth factor system regulates mucin production in airways. Proc Natl Acad Sci USA 1999;96:3081–3086.

Prof. K.F. Chung
National Heart and Lung Institute
Imperial College School of Medicine
Dovehouse St.
London SW3 6LY (UK)
Tel. +44 207 352 8121, Fax +44 207 351 8126
E-Mail f.chung@ic.ac.uk

TNF Antagonism

Neil D. McDonnell[a] Nicholas N. Abbott[a] Kendall M. Mohler[a]
Trevor T. Hansel[b] Johan C. Kips[c]

[a]Immunex Corporation, Seattle, Wash., USA, [b]NHLI Clinical Studies Unit, Imperial College, London, UK, and [c]Department of Respiratory Diseases, Ghent University Hospital, Ghent, Belgium

Summary

TNF antagonists such as soluble p75 receptor constructs and anti-TNF monoclonal antibodies are both currently licensed therapies for the treatment of rheumatoid arthritis (RA). Based on experimental studies in animals and the presence of elevated TNF levels in patients, there is also a strong rationale for TNF antagonism to be employed in asthma and COPD. In particular, TNF seems to play an important role in determining the severity of asthma. TNF antagonism might therefore be of particular interest for the treatment of severe persistent asthma as well as acute severe exacerbations. It might also constitute a novel anti-inflammatory therapy to control disease progression in COPD.

Rationale: TNF Involvement in Asthma and COPD

TNF is produced primarily by activated monocytes, macrophages, and lymphocytes as a homotrimer composed of three 17-kD TNF molecules (fig. 1). TNF is released from the cell membrane through the activity of the TNF-converting enzyme. TNF activity is mediated through binding to membrane-bound TNF receptors (p55 and p75 TNFR) found on a number of different cells, including leukocytes, dendritic cells, vascular endothelial cells and mesenchymal cells. One molecule of TNF must engage two or more TNFRs to initiate intracellular signal transduction. TNF activity is naturally regulated by the production of soluble TNFRs which render TNF biologically unavailable by preventing it from activating membrane-bound TNFRs.

TNF was originally described as a factor that induced necrosis of some tumors. It is now recognized to be an important proinflammatory cytokine with a large spectrum of activities. Ironically, despite its name, the role of TNF in anti-tumor immune surveillance is far from clear.

The pleiotropic activities of TNF include proinflammatory effects such as leukocyte recruitment through induction of adhesion molecules on vascular endothelial cells, and induction of cytokine and chemokine synthesis (fig. 2). Of special relevance to asthma and COPD is that TNF also has the potential to stimulate fibroblasts, myofibroblasts and smooth muscle cells, and to cause the induction and release of proteases [1, 2]. Through this range of activities, TNF could substantially contribute to the pathogenesis of the chronic inflammation and airway remodeling underlying asthma. As a result, TNF probably plays a substantial role in the pathogenesis of airway hyperreactivity (AHR). TNF also mediates acute phase responses with cachexia and pyrexia.

In vivo animal models confirm that exogenous administration of TNF can cause AHR and airway inflammation. Pretreatment with anti-TNF antibodies diminishes AHR and local neutrophilia following inhalation of endotoxin [3]. Anti-TNF has also proven efficacy in allergen challenge models of eosinophilia and AHR as well as hypersensitivity pneumonitis and pulmonary granuloma formation. As evidence for a role for TNF in mediating airway remodeling including fibrosis, it was found that expression of a TNF-α transgene in murine lung causes lymphocytic and fibrosing alveolitis [4].

Observations in man further support the hypothesis that TNF plays a substantial role in the pathophysiology of asthma and COPD. Elevated levels of TNF have been detected in sputum [5, 6], BAL fluid [7] and biopsies from asthmatics [8]. Inhalation of TNF causes AHR and increases sputum neutrophilia in healthy volunteers [9]. Genetic analysis further supports the role of TNF in child-

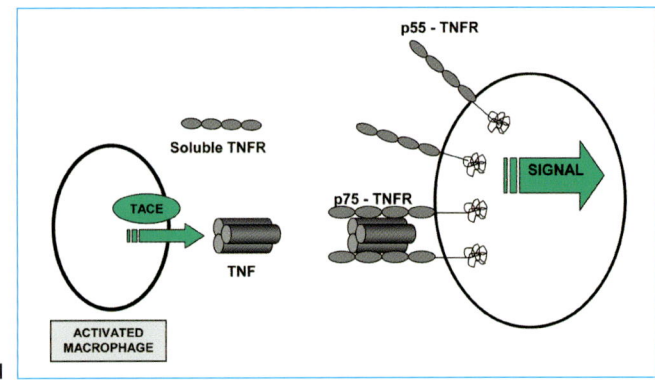

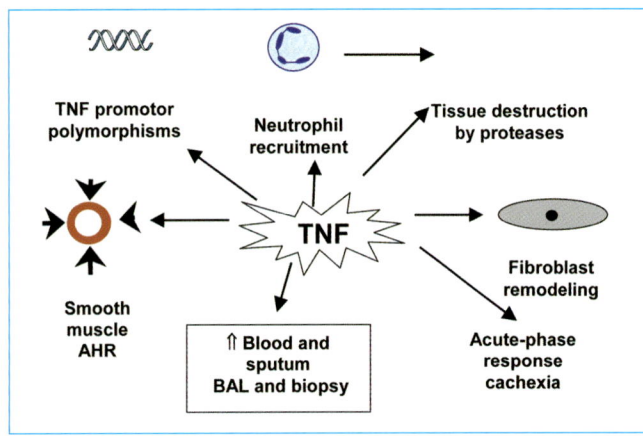

Fig. 1. TNF interactions with TNFR. TACE = TNF-converting enzyme.
Fig. 2. TNF action in asthma and COPD.

hood and adult asthma [10, 11]. The −308 TNF2 promotor polymorphism has been associated with the degree of AHR [12].

In addition, there is evidence to suggest that TNF might be an important element in determining the severity of asthma. Biopsy studies have shown increased numbers of neutrophils in the airways of patients with severe persistent asthma [13]. One of the major stimuli for neutrophil recruitment and endogenous TNF release is exposure to endotoxin [14]. The severity of asthma symptoms has been shown to correlate with endotoxin content of house dust [15]. Acute severe asthma exacerbations might also be largely TNF driven. Airways of patients who died of an asthma attack or who require ventilation due to status asthmaticus contain increased numbers of neutrophils [16–18]. BAL fluid collected from the latter group also contains increased levels of TNF [19].

Neutrophils have also been implicated in the pathogenesis of COPD. Sputum from COPD patients contains higher neutrophil numbers than that of smokers without airflow limitation [20]. In addition, elevated levels of TNF have been detected in serum in weight-losing COPD patients [21], while TNF is higher in sputum from patients with asthma than in that from smokers without airflow obstruction [5]. This elevation is resistant to the action of steroids [6]. Finally, TNF 5′ promotor gene polymorphisms also suggest a role for TNF in chronic bronchitis [22].

Table 1. TNF-blocking therapies

Product	Enbrel (etanercept)	Remicade (infliximab)	D2E7	PEG-TNFRI
Company	Immunex Wyeth	Centocor J & J	Knoll BASF	Amgen
Structure	Dimeric p75 TNFR:Fc IgG1	Chimeric (murine/human) anti-TNF MoAb	Humanized anti-TNF MoAb	PEGylated p55 TNFR monomer
Licensed Indications	RA Juvenile RA	RA Crohn's disease	(Investigational)	(Investigational)
Administration	s.c. twice weekly	2-hour i.v. infusion monthly to bimonthly	s.c. or i.v. weekly biweekly	s.c. weekly
Characteristics	Fully human, authentic glycosylation	Generally administered with MTX to prevent antibody formation	Not required to administer with MTX	Lower affinity for TNF than dimeric receptor

PEG = Polyethyleneglycol; MTX = methotrexate.

Therapeutic Approaches: Soluble TNFRs and Monoclonal Antibodies

To date, two general strategies have been employed to regulate TNF activity clinically: recombinant soluble TNFRs and monoclonal antibodies against TNF (table 1). Recombinant soluble TNFRs mimic the activity of naturally occurring soluble TNFRs, by binding to the receptor-binding domains of TNF and preventing interaction with membrane-bound TNFR. Etanercept (Enbrel®, Immunex) is a dimeric fusion molecule composed of two p75 TNFR moieties bound to the Fc portion of human IgG1. Etanercept has been shown to be effective in both adult [23, 24] and juvenile [25] rheumatoid arthritis (RA), has been shown to have disease-modifying activity in adult RA, and has shown preliminary activity in numerous other disease states including psoriatic arthritis and chronic heart failure. The dimeric structure of etanercept prolongs its pharmacokinetic half-life and improves its binding affinity and TNF-neutralizing capacity compared to monomeric p75 TNFR. Etanercept has the advantage of being fully human and thus relatively nonimmunogenic. A monomeric p55 TNFR fused to polyethylene glycol that also appears to be relatively nonimmunogenic has recently begun clinical development.

The second general strategy for TNF regulation has employed monoclonal antibodies against TNF. Decreased immunogenicity of murine monoclonal antibodies is achieved by creating a chimeric antibody, with a human Fc region and a murine Fab region, or by creating a humanized monoclonal antibody using a phage library. Infliximab (Remicade®, Centocor) is a chimeric anti-TNF antibody that retains some murine amino acid sequences. When given chronically, infliximab is typically administered with methotrexate to prevent development of human anti-chimeric antibodies. A fully human anti-TNF antibody, D2E7 (Knoll), is currently being studied in RA and appears to be effective in RA without requiring methotrexate.

Route of Administration

Current TNF inhibitors are given parenterally. Etanercept is administered subcutaneously twice weekly. Infliximab is administered via a 3-hour intravenous infusion every 4–8 weeks. The search continues for an orally bioavailable small molecule that specifically antagonizes TNF activity.

Clinical Experience in RA

The majority of the clinical experience obtained to date with TNF antagonists has been in patients with RA. Both etanercept and infliximab have shown encouraging efficacy in controlling signs and symptoms of RA and are important new treatments for this disease. In a randomized, double-blind, placebo-controlled trial, 59% of patients who had previously failed disease-modifying antirheumatic drugs responded to etanercept [23]. In patients with an inadequate response to methotrexate, 71% of those receiving etanercept + methotrexate responded [24]. Infliximab in combination with methotrexate has also shown activity in RA, with response rates ranging from 52 to 58% [27, 28]. Recent data have shown that both etanercept and the combination of infliximab and methotrexate have disease-modifying activity in RA, evident in the slowing of X-ray evidence of joint damage in patients receiving these agents [26, 29]. The substantial clinical efficacy and disease-modifying activity of etanercept and infliximab are powerful proofs of principle that these agents are viable means by which TNF-mediated diseases may be controlled.

Adverse Events

In controlled trials of etanercept, the only adverse events occurring more frequently in etanercept-treated patients than in placebo-treated patients were mild to moderate injection site reactions. In patients receiving infliximab, upper respiratory tract infections and headache are the most commonly reported adverse events. Occasionally, patients receiving infliximab experience infusion reactions consisting of headache, nausea, and rarely, hypotension and dyspnea. Because of the importance of TNF in host defense, both etanercept and infliximab are used with caution, if at all, in patients with active infection.

Clinical Studies in Asthma and COPD

To our knowledge, clinical studies have not been carried out in asthma or COPD with specific TNF-inhibiting therapies. As was explained above, TNF could contribute to the severity of persistent asthma and might play a key role in the mechanisms underlying acute severe exacerbations. It would therefore be of interest to focus initial proof-of-concept studies on a more severe spectrum of the disease.

COPD is also an attractive target for inhibitory therapy directed against TNF. In a proof-of-concept study, blood and sputum analysis could be used to monitor TNF levels and neutrophil numbers as a pharmacodynamic endpoint. In addition, as for any anti-inflammatory therapy against COPD, there is the need for longer-term studies to demonstrate effects on the exacerbation rate and decline in FEV_1, as part of the natural history of the disease.

Conclusions

TNF antagonism has proven to be remarkably effective in RA, and this provides a major impetus for this therapy to enter clinical studies in asthma and COPD. In addition, there are strong preclinical and clinical data to suggest that TNF could be an important mediator in both asthma and COPD. There is the urgent need to proceed to reliable exploratory proof of concept studies with TNF-directed therapy in both asthma and COPD.

References

1 Schwingshackl A, Duszyk M, Brown N, Moqbel R: Human eosinophils release matrix metalloproteinase-9 on stimulation with TNF-alpha. J Allergy Clin Immunol 1999;104:983–989.
2 Amrani Y, Panettieri RA Jr, Frossard N, Bronner C: Activation of the TNF alpha-p55 receptor induces myocyte proliferation and modulates agonist-evoked calcium transients in cultured human tracheal smooth muscle cells. Am J Respir Cell Mol Biol 1996;15:55–63.
3 Kips JC, Tavernier J, Pauwels RA: Tumor necrosis factor causes bronchial hyperresponsiveness in rats. Am Rev Resp Dis 1992;145:332–336.
4 Miyazaki Y, Araki K, Vesin C, Garcia I, Kapanci Y, Whitsett JA, et al: Expression of a tumor necrosis factor-alpha transgene in murine lung causes lymphocytic and fibrosing alveolitis. A mouse model of progressive pulmonary fibrosis. J Clin Invest 1995;96:250–259.
5 Keatings VM, Collins PD, Scott DM, Barnes PJ: Differences in interleukin-8 and tumor necrosis factor-alpha in induced sputum from patients with chronic obstructive pulmonary disease or asthma. Am J Respir Crit Care Med 1996;153:530–534.
6 Keatings VM, Jatakanon A, Worsdell YM, Barnes PJ: Effects of inhaled and oral glucocorticoids on inflammatory indices in asthma and COPD. Am J Respir Crit Care Med 1997;155:542–548.
7 Broide DH, Lotz M, Cuomo AJ, Coburn DA, Federman EC, Wasserman SI: Cytokines in symptomatic asthma airways. J Allergy Clin Immunol 1992;89:958–967.
8 Ackerman V, Marini M, Vittori E, Bellini A, Vassali G, Mattoli S: Detection of cytokines and their cell sources in bronchial biopsy specimens from asthmatic patients. Relationship to atopic status, symptoms, and level of airway hyperresponsiveness. Chest 1994;105:687–696.
9 Thomas PS, Yates DH, Barnes PJ: Tumor necrosis factor-alpha increases airway responsiveness and sputum neutrophilia in normal human subjects. Am J Respir Crit Care Med 1995;152:76–80.
10 Albuquerque RV, Hayden CM, Palmer LJ, Laing IA, Rye PJ, Gibson NA, et al: Association of polymorphisms within the tumour necrosis factor (TNF) genes and childhood asthma. Clin Exp Allergy 1998;28:578–584.
11 Chagani T, Pare PD, Zhu S, Weir TD, Bai TR, Behbehani NA, et al: Prevalence of tumor necrosis factor-alpha and angiotensin converting enzyme polymorphisms in mild/moderate and fatal/near-fatal asthma. Am J Respir Crit Care Med 1999;160:278–282.
12 Li KWTC, Mansur AH, Britton J, Williams G, Pavord I, Richards K, et al: Association between –308 tumour necrosis factor promoter polymorphism and bronchial hyperreactivity in asthma. Clin Exp Allergy 1999;29:1204–1208.
13 Wenzel SE, Szefler SJ, Leung DYM, Sloan SI, Rex MD, Martin RJ: Bronchoscopic evaluation of severe asthma: Persistent inflammation associated with high dose glucocorticoids. Am J Respir Crit Care Med 1997;156:737–743.
14 Michel O, Kips J, Duchateau J, Vertongen F, Robert L, Collet H, et al: Severity of asthma is related to endotoxin in house dust. Am J Respir Crit Care Med 1996;154:1641–1646.
15 Michel O, Nagy AM, Schroeven M, Duchateau J, Neve J, Fondu P, et al: Dose-response relationship to inhaled endotoxin in normal subjects. Am J Respir Crit Care Med 1997;156:1157–1164.
16 Carroll N, Carello S, Cooke C, James A: Airway structure and inflammatory cells in fatal attacks of asthma. Eur Respir J 1996;9:709–715.
17 Ordonez CL, Shaughnessy TE, Matthay MA, Fahy JV: Increased neutrophil numbers and IL-8 levels in airway secretions in acute severe asthma: Clinical and biologic significance. Am J Respir Crit Care Med 2000;161:1185–1190.
18 Lamblin C, Gosset P, Tillie-Leblond I, Saulnier F, Marquette CH, Wallaert B, et al: Bronchial neutrophilia in patients with noninfectious status asthmaticus. Am J Respir Crit Care Med 1998;157:394–402.
19 Tillie-Leblond I, Pugin J, Marquette CH, Lamblin C, Saulnier F, Brichet A, et al: Balance between proinflammatory cytokines and their inhibitors in bronchial lavage from patients with status asthmaticus. Am J Respir Crit Care Med 1999;159:487–494.
20 Peleman RA, Rytila PH, Kips JC, Joos GF, Pauwels RA: The cellular composition of induced sputum in chronic obstructive pulmonary disease. Eur Respir J 1999;13:839–843.
21 Takabatake N, Nakamura H, Abe S, Hino T, Saito H, Yuki H, et al: Circulating leptin in patients with chronic obstructive pulmonary disease. Am J Respir Crit Care Med 1999;159:1215–1219.
22 Huang SL, Su CH, Chang SC: Tumor necrosis factor-alpha gene polymorphism in chronic bronchitis. Am J Respir Crit Care Med 1997;156:1436–1439.
23 Moreland LW, Schiff MH, Baumgartner SW, Tindall EA, Fleischmann RM, Bulpitt KJ, et al: Etanercept therapy in rheumatoid arthritis. A randomized, controlled trial. Ann Intern Med 1999;130:478–486.
24 Weinblatt ME, Kremer JM, Bankhurst AD, Bulpitt KJ, Fleischmann RM, Fox RI, et al: A trial of etanercept, a recombinant tumor necrosis factor receptor: Fc fusion protein, in patients with rheumatoid arthritis receiving methotrexate. N Engl J Med 1999;340:253–259.
25 Lovell DJ, Giannini EH, Reiff A, Cawkwell GD, Silverman ED, Nocton JJ, Stein LD, Gedalia A, Ilowite NT, Wallace CA, Whitmore J, Finck BK: Etanercept in children with polyarticular juvenile rheumatoid arthritis. Pediatric Rheumatology Collaborative Study Group. N Engl J Med 2000;342:763–769.
26 Finck B, Martin R, Fleischmann R, Moreland L, Schiff M, Bathon J: A phase III trial of etanercept vs. methotrexate in early rheumatoid arthritis (ENBREL ERA-trial). Presentation to the 63rd Annual Scientific Meeting of the American College of Rheumatology, Boston 1999.
27 Maini RN, Breedveld FC, Kalden JR, Smolen JS, Davis D, Macfarlane JD, et al: Therapeutic efficacy of multiple intravenous infusions of anti-tumor necrosis factor alpha monoclonal antibody combined with low-dose weekly methotrexate in rheumatoid arthritis (see comments). Arthritis Rheum 1998;41:1552–1563.
28 Maini R, St CEW, Breedveld F, Furst D, Kalden J, Weisman M, et al: Infliximab (chimeric anti-tumour necrosis factor alpha monoclonal antibody) versus placebo in rheumatoid arthritis patients receiving concomitant methotrexate: A randomised phase III trial. ATTRACT Study Group. Lancet 1999;354:1932–1939.
29 Lipsky P, St Clair W, Furst D, et al: 54-week clinical and radiographic results from the ATTRACT trial: A phase III study of infliximab (Remicade™) in patients with active RA despite methotrexate. Presentation to the 63rd Annual Scientific Meeting of the American College of Rheumatology, Boston 1999.

Neil D. McDonnell, PharmD
Immunex Corporation
51 University Street
Seattle, WA 98101-2936 (USA)
Tel. +1 206 587 0430, Fax +1 206 223 5525
E-Mail mcdonnelln@immunex.com

GM-CSF Antagonists

William V. Williams

Clinical Pharmacology, SmithKline Beecham, Philadelphia, Pa., USA

Summary

GM-CSF is an important growth factor which shares many of the properties of cytokines and chemokines. GM-CSF is currently used therapeutically as a recombinant protein given parenterally to enhance the function and maturation of myeloid cells. GM-CSF has also been linked to a number of disease states characterized by hyperactivity of myeloid cells. In this review, the receptor interactions of GM-CSF will be described as well as the bioactivity of GM-CSF and its role in disease.

GM-CSF Receptor Interactions

GM-CSF is one of a group of prototypic 4-helix bundle cytokines which include IL-2, IL-3, IL-5, G-CSF, growth hormone, and many others. These 4-helix bundle cytokines exert their biological activity by binding to surface receptors and inducing receptor oligomerization with subsequent signal transduction. GM-CSF exists as a monomer in solution and appears to remain as a monomer upon receptor binding. The GM-CSF receptor (GMR) is comprised of an α-chain (GMRα), which is specific for GM-CSF [1], and a β-chain (βc), which can also associate with the IL-3 and IL-5 receptor α-chains [2]. GMRα, when expressed without βc, is able to bind GM-CSF with low affinity ($K_D \sim 2$–3 nM) while the heterodimeric receptor binds with much higher affinity ($K_D \sim 40$ nM) [1]. The high-affinity receptor (GMRα and βc) is the signal-transducing unit [3].

Signal transduction following GM-CSF binding to the heterodimeric GMR includes rapid phosphorylation of the Jak2 kinase via the cytosolic portion of the βc subunit [4]. Jak2 subsequently induces tyrosine phosphorylation of p95Vav [5]. Ras, Raf-1, MAP kinase, and S6 kinase are also activated via a distinct region of the cytosolic portion of βc [6]. Subsequent events lead to the activation of transcription factors including c-fos and c-jun, which associate to form the AP-1 enhancer complex, c-myc and Egr-1 [6]. AP-1 activation induces transcription of a number of cell growth genes, while Egr-1 is implicated in macrophage lineage commitment of hematopoietic precursor cells. One consequence of GM-CSF signal transduction is inhibition of apoptosis, and this is related to induction of AP-1 activity.

The GMRα exists in both membrane-bound and soluble forms [7]. The soluble form (sGMRα) is created via alternative splicing of GMα mRNA, which creates a receptor lacking the transmembrane region and possessing an altered carboxy terminus. Prior studies utilizing biosensors have shown that a soluble GMRα-Fc fusion protein binds GM-CSF with a rapid on rate and a relatively rapid off rate [8]. This would imply a need for high local concentrations of sGMRα for biological inhibitory function. The sGMRα is produced by a variety of cell types and tissues [7], most of which also produce the transmembrane form of sGMRα. Transcripts for tmGMRα predominate in the myelomonocytic cell lines, corneal fibroblasts, and unfractionated peripheral blood mononuclear cells. The tmGMRα/sGMRα transcript ratio appears roughly equal in human monocytes, T cells, bone marrow, and rheumatoid synovial tissue; while sGMRα transcripts predominate in synovial fibroblasts and osteoarthritis synovial tissue. While the biological function of sGMRα remains speculative in vivo, local production and inhibition of GM-CSF activity seem likely. The interaction of GM-CSF with its receptor is summarized in figure 1.

GM-CSF Bioactivity and Role in Disease

GM-CSF is produced by a variety of cell types, including macrophages, T cells, fibroblasts, and endothelial cells (table 1). The GMR is expressed predominately on cells of

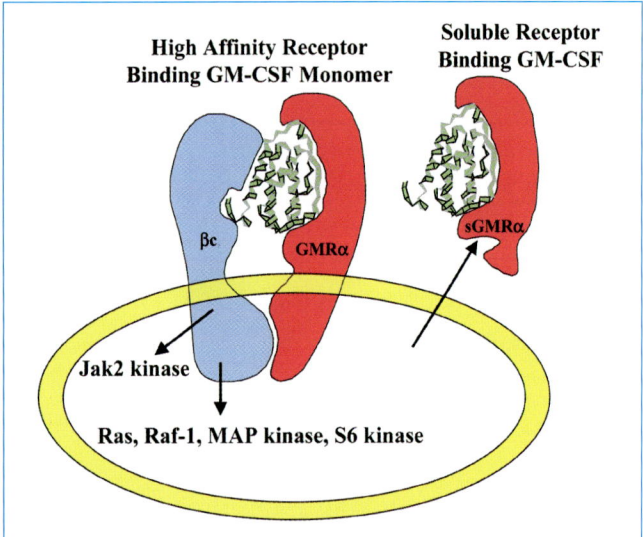

Fig. 1. Interaction of GM-CSF with its receptor. GM-CSF binds to a heterodimeric receptor comprised of an α-chain (GMRα) and a β-chain (βc). Signal transduction occurs via the βc chain and includes activation of a variety of intracellular kinases and other signaling molecules. The GMRα provides the major recognition site for GM-CSF and provides specificity for the interaction (βc is shared by the IL-3 and IL-5 receptors). A soluble form of the GMRα (sGMRα) is made by alternative splicing of the transcript, which lacks the transmembrane region and has an altered cytosolic domain. This may function as a local inhibitor of GM-CSF by binding it and competitively inhibiting cellular receptor binding.

Table 1. GM-CSF and GMR expression

Cell types which produce GM-CSF
- Macrophages, T cells, fibroblasts, endothelial cells

Cell types which express GMR and respond to GM-CSF
- Monocytes, tissue macrophages, dendritic cells, granulocytes

Cell types which express the soluble GMRα
- T cells, fibroblasts

Table 2. GM-CSF bioactivity

- Stimulation of granulocyte and macrophage differentiation
- Prevention of apoptosis of mature monocytes and tissue macrophages
- Induction of proliferation of mature monocytes and tissue macrophages
- Dendritic cell differentiation, survival and proliferation
- Activation of mature granulocytes and macrophages
- Increasing phagocytic and lytic activity
- Increasing class II MHC expression
- Enhancing antigen presentation
- Enhancing IL-1 production
- Stimulating macrophage tumoricidal activity
- Regulation of neutrophil adhesion and migration
- Induction of endothelial cell to migration and proliferation

From von Feldt et al. [9].

the myeloid lineage (table 1), including monocytes, tissue macrophages, dendritic cells, and granulocytes. Certain other cell types express the GMRα, such as T cells and fibroblasts, but in some cases this is predominately the sGMRα [7]. Thus, the predominant effects of GM-CSF occur in tissues with high expression of granulocytes and macrophages, such as the spleen, lymph nodes and liver. In disease states, this would include granulomas, inflammatory exudates, and immunologically active tissues such as rheumatoid synovium.

GM-CSF has a variety of biological functions (table 2). These have led to its use in patients with spontaneous or chemotherapy-induced leukopenia and aplastic anemia and as adjunct therapy in bone marrow transplantation. GM-CSF also has been used experimentally as a molecular adjuvant based on its ability to stimulate antigen presentation by macrophages and dendritic cells [10, 11]. Some of these effects are mediated by cell types other than granulocytes and macrophages, as eosinophil recruitment into areas of immune activation has been shown to be a key feature in some cases.

GM-CSF plays a significant role in pulmonary homeostasis. Mice which lack the GM-CSF gene (GM-CSF –/–) do not have any myelopoietic defects, presumably due to the redundancy of other growth factors which can take its place, but do develop a pulmonary pathology similar to human pulmonary alveolar proteinosis (PAP) [12, 13]. This defect is reversed by aerosolized GM-CSF [14], indicating the potential for therapeutic application if a similar defect is present in human PAP. GM-CSF-deficient mice are also susceptible to pulmonary group B streptococcal infection [15] with diminished production of superoxide radicals, hydrogen peroxide and lipid peroxidation, although phagocytosis is unaltered. PAP is also seen in mice with targeted deletion of βc, as well as a decrease in eosinophils (but not other myeloid cells) and increased susceptibility to parasitic infection [16]. These studies suggest an important role for GM-CSF in macrophage clearance of surfactant proteins in maintaining pulmonary homeostasis, as well as in parasitic and bacterial infections.

In human disease, a role for GM-CSF has been described in patients with PAP. This includes diminished

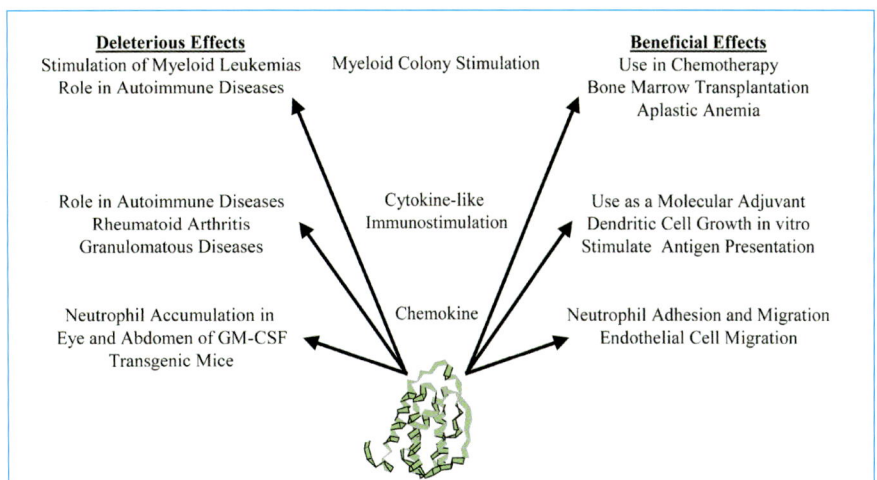

Fig. 2. Beneficial and deleterious effects of GM-CSF. The reported beneficial effects of GM-CSF are listed on the right side, with the deleterious effects shown on the left. In the middle, the properties of GM-CSF which induce these effects are listed (CSF, cytokine, chemokine).

production of GM-CSF [17], diminished responses to GM-CSF [18], and the presence of neutralizing antibodies to GM-CSF [19]. A defect in the expression of βc has been linked to certain cases of neonatal PAP [20].

These and other observations have led to the use of GM-CSF in the treatment of idiopathic PAP [21]. In this pilot study, 4 patients with PAP were treated with subcutaneous GM-CSF over 12 weeks, with escalating doses. Three of 4 patients showed improvement in symptoms, oxygenation, pulmonary function tests, and radiographically.

GM-CSF is also proposed to be important in the pathogenesis of several autoimmune and inflammatory conditions [reviewed in ref. 9]. Transgenic mice which overexpress the GM-CSF gene develop a wasting syndrome accompanied by neutrophil accumulation in the eye or within the abdomen. GM-CSF has been demonstrated to be the major cytokine responsible for induction of HLA-DR expression in the joints of rheumatoid arthritis (RA) patients. In addition, GM-CSF augments neutrophil-mediated cartilage degradation. The pathogenic role of GM-CSF in rheumatoid arthritis (RA) synovitis has been confirmed clinically. A subgroup of RA patients with Felty's syndrome (RA, neutropenia and splenomegaly) have been treated with GM-CSF [22]. This induces a flare-up of their arthritis, indicating that GM-CSF induces increased joint inflammation in RA, supporting its pathogenic role.

Studies with GM-CSF –/– mice indicate that they are nearly completely protected from the development of collagen-induced arthritis [23]. In this system, mice are immunized with xenogeneic type II collagen, inducing a cellular immune response against cartilage (where type II collagen is expressed). These mice subsequently develop a chronic arthritis pathologically and immunogenetically similar to human RA. The GM-CSF –/– mice immunized in this way only rarely develop arthritis, suggesting a key role of GM-CSF in the pathogenesis of inflammatory diseases.

GM-CSF Antagonist Development

These observations indicate potential clinical utility for GM-CSF agonists in developing immune responses, and GM-CSF antagonists in inhibiting autoimmune/inflammatory diseases. Development of agonists would be expected to be aided by antagonist development as a way to understand intermolecular interactions critical for receptor binding. To date, antagonist development has been more successful, and will be summarized here.

The role of GM-CSF in the pathogenesis of autoimmune and inflammatory diseases suggests that inhibition of GM-CSF bioactivity may ameliorate some of the aspects of these diseases. Several approaches exist for the development of GM-CSF antagonists, including the use of blocking antibodies or soluble receptors, using GM-CSF mutants with dominant negative activity, and the development of smaller pharmacophores with antagonist activity. Both soluble receptors and neutralizing monoclonal antibodies against TNF-α have been successfully used to treat RA and Crohn's disease, indicating that such an approach is feasible. Soluble GMRα is unlikely to be useful therapeutically due to its rapid dissociation rate [8], and construction of a stable high-affinity GMRα/βc construct has not yet been accomplished. Several neutralizing monoclonal antibodies against GM-CSF have been developed and could potentially be humanized for clinical use. This interesting approach has not yet been pursued.

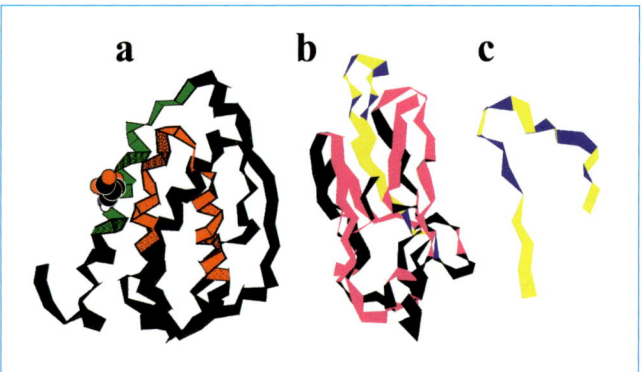

Fig. 3. GM-CSF antagonists. GM-CSF antagonists have been developed by several methods. **a** The structure of GM-CSF is shown using a ribbon for the GM-CSF backbone. The location of Glu21 on the A helix is shown with a CPK (ball) representation of the glutamic acid residue. Mutation of this residue produces biological antagonists. The locations of residues which have been used to develop antagonist peptides are shown, including those from the A helix (residues 17–31 in green) and the B and C helices (residues 54–78 in red). **b** A recombinant anti-GMR antibody light chain developed as described in the text is shown. The location of the inhibitory first hypervariable loop peptide is shown in yellow. **c** The predicted structure of the inhibitory peptide derived from the recombinant anti-GMR antibody light chain is shown.

The ability to develop GM-CSF analogs which act as antagonists or pharmacophores which interact with the GMR depends on understanding the geometry of the binding interaction of GM-CSF to the receptor. There have been two interaction sites on GM-CSF postulated, one for the GMRα and one for βc. The βc interaction site has been investigated by several groups, and appears to center on a glutamic acid residue on the 'A' helix, Glu21 (fig. 3a). Mutants of Glu21 inhibit binding of native GM-CSF to the low-affinity receptor but not to the high-affinity receptor and act either as partial agonists or full antagonists [24]. Such antagonists could have therapeutic potential, but have not yet been investigated clinically. It is possible that Glu21 interacts directly with His367 in the B'-C' loop of βc, which has been shown to be essential for high-affinity GM-CSF binding [25]. Tyr365 and Ile368 on the same loop are also implicated, as is Tyr421 on the F'-G' loop. Interestingly, synthetic peptides derived from the sequence of the GM-CSF A helix abolish the high affinity site on cells while leaving intact the low affinity site and act as biological antagonists (fig. 3a) [26]. While such small peptides have low affinity and are unlikely to be useful clinically, they do suggest the ability to develop small-molecular-weight analogs of this site, which could function as leads for structure-based drug design.

The GMRα interaction site is somewhat more controversial. By analogy with the growth hormone-receptor interaction, the D helix has been proposed as the interaction site with GMRα. However, studies using GM-CSF truncations, mutagenesis studies, mapping of neutralizing monoclonal antibodies, and synthetic peptide studies, as well as studies of cross-species hybrid molecules and studies with cells which express only GMRα to map binding epitopes with monoclonal antibodies, all suggest a central role for the C helix [reviewed in ref. 9]. Studies of a synthetic peptide derived from the B and C helices (fig. 3a) show biological inhibitory function, including blockade of receptor binding, and suggest that inhibition occurs via interaction with the GMRα [26].

An important role for residues on the C helix in GMRα recognition is supported by studies of GM-CSF mimics [27]. These include antibody and peptide mimics. An antibody mimic was developed by an anti-idiotype approach, utilizing polyclonal mouse anti-human GM-CSF as an immunogen in syngeneic mice to elicit anti-anti-GM-CSF which blocked the growth-promoting effects of GM-CSF. The lymphocytes from mice producing anti-anti-GM-CSF were used to develop a recombinant antibody library which expressed isolated kappa light chains. (Light chains were chosen as they are able to exist as stable homodimers, and eliminated the need for making separate libraries of heavy and light chains with linkers.) This library was probed with a neutralizing anti-GM-CSF monoclonal antibody, and a clone was selected which blocked GM-CSF binding and bioactivity (fig. 3b). Sequence and structural analysis of this clone showed that it mimicked the positioning of residues on the B and C helices of GM-CSF, predominately with residues from the first hypervariable loop of the recombinant light chain. A synthetic peptide from this first hypervariable loop was able to block GM-CSF binding and bioactivity (fig. 3b, c). While this peptide had low affinity, this approach suggests that it is possible to make small-molecular-weight antagonists of GM-CSF via binding to the receptor.

Together, these studies suggest several approaches for the development of GM-CSF antagonists. The application of this information to the development of small, high-affinity antagonists, or the use of biological agents which block GM-CSF activity will better define the role of GM-CSF in the pathogenesis of autoimmune and inflammatory diseases.

References

1 Gearing DP, King JA, Gough NM, Nicola NA: Expression cloning of a receptor for human granulocyte-macrophage colony-stimulating factor. EMBO J 1989;8:3667–3676.
2 Hayashida K, Kitamura T, Gorman DM, Arai K-I, Yokota T, Miyajima A: Molecular cloning of a second subunit of the human granulocyte-macrophage colony-stimulating factor (GM-CSF) receptor: Reconstitution of a high affinity GM-CSF receptor. Proc Natl Acad Sci USA 1990;87:9655–9659.
3 Sakamaki K, Miyajima I, Kitamura T, Miyajima A: Critical cytoplasmic domains of the common beta subunit of the human GM-CSF, IL-3 and IL-5 receptors for growth signal transduction and tyrosine phosphorylation. EMBO J 1992;11:3541–3549.
4 Sakamoto KM, Mignacca RC, Gasson JC: Signal transduction by granulocyte-macrophage colony-stimulating factor and interleukin-3 receptors. Receptors Channels 1994;2:175–181.
5 Matsuguchi T, Inhorn RC, Carlesso N, Xu G, Druker B, Griffin JD: Tyrosine phosphorylation of p95Vav in myeloid cells is regulated by GM-CSF, IL-3 and steel factor and is constitutively increased by p210BCR/ABL. EMBO J 1995;14:257–265.
6 Kwon EM, Sakamoto M: The molecular mechanism of action of granulocyte-macrophage colony-stimulating factor. J Investig Med 1996;44:442–446.
7 Williams WV, VonFeldt JM, Rosenbaum H, Ugen KE, Weiner DB: Molecular cloning of a soluble form of the granulocyte-macrophage colony stimulating factor receptor α-chain from a myelomonocytic cell line. Expression, biologic activity and preliminary analysis of transcript distribution. Arthritis Rheum 1994;37:1468–1478.
8 Monfardini C, Ramamoorthy M, Rosenbaum H, Fang Q, Godillot AP, Canziani G, Chaiken I, Williams WV: Construction and binding kinetics of a soluble granulocyte-macrophage colony stimulating factor receptor alpha chain-Fc fusion protein. J Biol Chem 1998;273:7657–7667.
9 Von Feldt JM, Monfardini C, Kieber-Emmons T, Voet D, Weiner DB, Williams WV: Granulocyte-macrophage colony stimulating factor (GM-CSF) mimicry and receptor interactions. Immunol Res 1994;13:96–109.
10 Dranoff G, Jaffee E, Lazenby A, Golumbek P, Levitsky H, Brose K, Jackson V, Hamada H, Pardoll D, Mulligan RC: Vaccination with irradiated tumor cells engineered to secrete murine granulocyte-macrophage colony-stimulating factor stimulates potent, specific, and long-lasting anti-tumor immunity. Proc Natl Acad Sci USA 1993;90:3539–3543.
11 Xiang Z, Ertl HC: Manipulation of the immune response to a plasmid-encoded viral antigen by coinoculation with plasmids expressing cytokines. Immunity 1995;2:129–135.
12 Dranoff G, Crawford AD, Sadelain M, Ream B, Rashid A, Bronson RT, Dickersin GR, Bachurski CJ, Mark EL, Whitsett JA, Mulligan RC: Involvement of granulocyte-macrophage colony-stimulating factor in pulmonary homeostasis. Science 1994;264:713–716.
13 Stanley E, Lieschke GJ, Grail D, Metcalf D, Hodgson G, Gall JAM, Maher DW, Cebon J, Sinickas V, Dunn AR: Granulocyte/macrophage colony-stimulating factor-deficient mice show no major perturbation of hematopoiesis but develop a characteristic pulmonary pathology. Proc Natl Acad Sci USA 1994;91:5592–5596.
14 Reed JA, Ikegami M, Cianciolo ER, Lu W, Cho PS, Hull W, Jobe AH, Whitsett JA: Aerosolized GM-CSF ameliorates pulmonary alveolar proteinosis in GM-CSF-deficient mice. Am J Physiol 1999;276:556–563.
15 LeVine AM, Reed JA, Kurak KE, Cianciolo E, Whitsett JA: GM-CSF-deficient mice are susceptible to pulmonary group B streptococcal infection. J Clin Invest 1999;103:563–599.
16 Nishinakamura R, Nakayama N, Hirabayashi Y, Inoue T, Aud D, McNeil T, Azuma S, Yoshida S, Toyoda Y, Arai K, et al: Mice deficient for the IL-3/GM-CSF/IL-5 beta c receptor exhibit lung pathology and impaired immune response, while beta IL3 receptor-deficient mice are normal. Immunity 1995;2:211–222.
17 Tchou-Wong K, Harkin T, Chi C, Bodkin M, Rom W: GM-CSF gene expression is normal but protein release is absent in a patient with pulmonary alveolar proteinosis. Am J Respir Crit Care Med 1997;156:1999–2002.
18 Carraway MS, Ghio AJ, Carter JD, Piantadosi CA: Detection of granulocyte-macrophage colony-stimulating factor in patients with pulmonary alveolar proteinosis. Am J Respir Crit Care Med 2000;161:1294–1299.
19 Kitamura T, Tanaka N, Watanabe J, Uchida K, Kanegasaki S, Yamada Y, Nakata K: Idiopathic pulmonary alveolar proteinosis as an autoimmune disease with neutralizing antibody against granulocyte/macrophage colony-stimulating factor. J Exp Med 1999;190:875–880.
20 Dirksen U, Nishinakamura R, Groneck P, Hattenhorst U, Nogee L, Murray R, Burdach S: Human pulmonary alveolar proteinosis associated with a defect in GM-CSF/IL-3/IL-5 receptor common β chain expression. J Clin Invest 1997;100:2211–2217.
21 Kavuru MS, Sullivan EJ, Piccin R, Thomassen MJ, Stoller JK: Exogenous granulocyte-macrophage colony-stimulating factor administration for pulmonary alveolar proteinosis. Am J Respir Crit Care Med 2000;161:1143–1148.
22 Hazenberg BP, Van Leeuwen MA, Van Rijswijk MH, Stern AC, Vellenga E: Correction of granulocytopenia in Felty's syndrome by granulocyte-macrophage colony-stimulating factor. Simultaneous induction of interleukin-6 release and flare-up of the arthritis. Blood 1989;74:2769–2770.
23 Campbell IK, Rich MJ, Bischof RJ, Dunn AR, Grail D, Hamilton JA: Protection from collagen-induced arthritis in granulocyte-macrophage colony-stimulating factor-deficient mice. J Immunol 1998;161:3639–3644.
24 Hercus TR, Bagley CJ, Cambareri B, Dottore M, Woodcock JM, Vadas MA, Shannon MF, Lopez AF: Specific human granulocyte-macrophage colony-stimulating factor antagonists. Proc Natl Acad Sci USA 1994;91:5838–5842.
25 Bagley CJ, Woodcock JM, Stomski FC, Lopez AF: The structural and functional basis of cytokine receptor activation: Lessons from the common β subunit of the granulocyte-macrophage colony-stimulating factor, interleukin-3 (IL-3) and IL-5 receptors. Blood 1997;89:1471–1482.
26 VonFeldt JM, Monfardini C, Fish S, Rosenbaum H, Kieber-Emmons T, Williams RM, Kahn SA, Weiner DB, Williams WV: Development of GM-CSF antagonist peptides. Peptide Res 1995;8:20–32.
27 Monfardini C, Kieber-Emmons T, VonFeldt JM, O'Malley B, Rosenbaum H, Godillot AP, Kaushansky K, Brown CB, Voet D, McCallus DE, Weiner DB, Williams WV: Recombinant antibodies in bioactive peptide design. J Biol Chem 1995;270:6628–6638.

William V. Williams, MD
Director of Clinical Pharmacology
SmithKline Beecham
51 North 39th Street
Philadelphia, PA 19104 (USA)
Tel. +1 215 823 3366, Fax +1 215 823 3219
E-Mail William_V_Williams@sbphrd.com

Interleukin-4 Antagonism

Larry Borish[a]   Jan M. Agosti[b]

[a]University of Virginia, Charlottesville, Va., and [b]Immunex Corporation, Seattle, Wash., USA

Summary

IL-4 receptor (IL-4R) is potentially a safe and effective treatment for asthma without the use of corticosteroids. Once-weekly inhaled dosing targeting the lungs will likely improve patient compliance, one of the greatest challenges facing the effective treatment of asthma. By inhibiting inflammation at a key central regulatory point and by treating the underlying cause of asthma, IL-4R may influence long-term disease progression. Additional studies of IL-4R are ongoing. Soluble IL-4R therapy revolutionizes our understanding of asthma and represents the next generation of asthma therapy.

IL-4 is critically important for the development of allergic inflammation. It is associated with induction of IgE secretion by B lymphocytes [1]. IgE-mediated immune responses are further enhanced by IL-4 through its ability to upregulate IgE receptors: the low-affinity IgE receptor (CD23) on B lymphocytes and monocytes and the high-affinity IgE receptor on mast cells and basophils [2]. IgE-dependent mast cell activation thereby induced by IL-4 plays a pivotal role in the development of immediate allergic reactions.

One of the most important activities of IL-4 in promoting cellular inflammation is its induction of VCAM-1 expression on vascular endothelium. Through the interaction of VCAM-1 with VLA-4, IL-4 is able to direct the migration of T lymphocytes, monocytes, basophils, and especially eosinophils to inflammatory loci [3]. IL-4 further promotes eosinophilic inflammation in asthma by increasing eotaxin expression and inhibiting eosinophil apoptosis. An additional mechanism of IL-4-induced airway obstruction is via mucus gene expression and hypersecretion [4].

A biological activity of IL-4 essential to allergic inflammation is its ability to drive the differentiation of Th0 lymphocytes into Th2 lymphocytes [5, 6]. These Th2 lymphocytes then secrete IL-4, IL-5, IL-9, and IL-13 and lose their capacity to produce IFN-γ. IL-4 knockout mice are unable to produce Th2 lymphocytes [7]. Mice which lack Stat6, a component of the IL-4 receptor (IL-4R) signaling pathway, also lack Th2 lymphocytes. In human studies, administration of IL-4 is associated with the generation of Th2 lymphocyte clones, whereas anti-IL-4 inhibits this effect. In contrast to IgE production and induction of VCAM-1, activities shared with the related cytokine IL-13, induction of Th2 lymphocytes is a unique biological activity of IL-4, since T lymphocytes only express IL-4 receptors and not IL-13 receptors.

IL-4 is also important in allergic immune responses because of its ability to prevent apoptosis of T lymphocytes. Activated T helper lymphocytes rapidly become apoptotic and are eliminated (activation-induced cell death). Several cytokines, including IL-2, IL-4, IL-7, and IL-15 are effective in preventing death of activated T cells [8]. Inhibition of apoptosis by IL-4 may be partially mediated by the ability of this cytokine to maintain levels of the survival-promoting protein Bcl-2 [8]. Apoptosis of T lymphocytes can be induced through signals mediated by FasL through the Fas receptor expressed on these cells. IL-4 downregulates cell surface Fas expression and this may explain persistence of inflammation in asthma. IL-4 blockade could promote apoptosis of Th2 lymphocytes and produce clinical benefits in asthma. Corticosteroids normally cause apoptosis in mature T helper cells and their induction of cell death is prevented by IL-4 [9]. IL-4 and IL-2 synergize to render lymphocytes refractory to the anti-inflammatory influences of corticosteroids. Through these mechanisms, the autocrine production of IL-4 by Th2 cells in the asthmatic lung may render these cells refractory to the beneficial influences of corticosteroids.

Table 1. Gene associated with IL-4 and IL-4 signaling linked to asthma and allergies

Gene	Polymorphism	Location	Reference
IL-4 promoter	A to G	−81	16
	C to T	−285	16
	C to T		17, 18
IL-4R	Ile to Val	+50	19
	Arg to Gln	+551	20
	Ser to Pro	+503	

Clinical Observations of IL-4 in Allergic Disease

IL-4 is increased in the serum and BAL fluid of allergic individuals [10, 11] and IL-4 production by peripheral blood mononuclear cells in response to dust mite antigen is significantly increased in atopic asthmatics [12]. Aerosol administration of IL-4 to patients with mild asthma produced a significant increase in AHR that was associated with an elevation in sputum eosinophils [13]. There are a variety of findings that suggest that atopic individuals have altered regulation in their IL-4 production. CD4+ T cell clones from atopics produce IL-4 and IL-5 in response to antigens that normally produce Th1 cytokines [14]. Atopic subjects have a higher frequency of IL-4-producing T cells [15].

Genetic Evidence for a Role for IL-4 in Asthma

Inherited abnormal production of IL-4 or hyperresponsiveness to this cytokine may further contribute to the pathophysiology of asthma. Genome searches and candidate gene approaches have linked atopy and asthma to both IL-4 and the IL-4R (table 1). Individuals genetically programmed to be hyperresponsive to IL-4 may be particularly responsive to treatment with an IL-4 antagonist.

Preclinical Studies Demonstrating the Role of IL-4 in Asthma

Neutralizing IL-4 with anti-IL-4 antibodies in mice prevents the development of allergen-specific IgE [21], and reduces eosinophilic inflammation [21] and airway reactivity [22]. Similarly, studies using IL-4 knockout mice have confirmed that IL-4 is necessary for allergen-specific IgE, pulmonary eosinophilia, and AHR. By inhibiting Th2 lymphocyte differentiation and promoting apoptosis of Th2 cells, IL-4 blockade inhibited the biological activities of IL-4 and reduced IL-5 production. Recombinant soluble IL-4R, which acts as a decoy for IL-4 binding and neutralizes IL-4 activity, has also been shown in murine models to block allergen-specific IgE production, AHR, and allergen-specific delayed-type hypersensitivity [23] and to inhibit VCAM-1 expression, eosinophil influx, and excessive mucus production [24]. These observations support important influences of IL-4, not only on allergen-specific IgE production, but also on the production of IL-5, eosinophilia, and AHR.

Approaches to Neutralizing IL-4 in Asthma

Several approaches are available to neutralize IL-4 in asthma. These include soluble IL-4R (fig. 1) and mutated IL-4 (IL-4 mutein). In addition, IL-4 protein can be inhibited using humanized rodent antibodies. A theoretical alternative approach would be to decrease IL-4 gene transcription with respirable anti-sense oligonucleotides (RASONs).

Soluble Cytokine Receptors as Therapeutic Agents

The IL-4R on the cell surface is a heterodimeric complex consisting of a specific high-affinity α-chain that binds to IL-4 and a second chain that can be either the common γ-chain shared with multiple cytokine receptors or the IL-13 receptor α-chain. Soluble forms of α-chain IL-4R occur naturally in patients with allergic inflammation and may represent an autoregulatory pathway for IL-4 inhibition [25]. Soluble IL-4R lacks the transmembrane and cytoplasmic domains so it cannot induce cellular activation (fig. 1). By acting as a decoy to bind to circulating IL-4 and neutralize its activity, its high specificity and affinity make it ideal as an IL-4 antagonist. Soluble recombinant human IL-4R (Nuvance™, Immunex Corporation) is the extracellular portion of the α-chain of the human receptor for IL-4, which is produced in a mammalian expression system. Since the amino acid sequences are identical to human sequences, soluble receptors are generally nonimmunogenic, unlike monoclonal antibodies, even chimerized or humanized monoclonal anti-

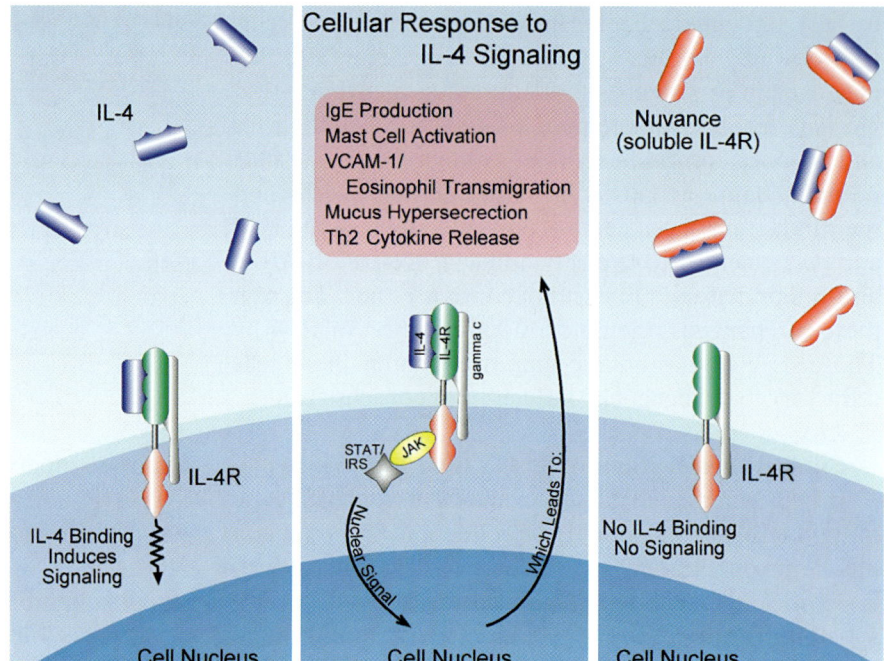

Fig. 1. Soluble IL-4R for the treatment of asthma.

bodies, which retain some murine sequences, or muteins which are mutated proteins. Another soluble receptor, Enbrel®, which is soluble TNF receptor, has been demonstrated to be safe and highly effective for long-term treatment of rheumatoid arthritis in adults and children.

Clinical Studies with Soluble IL-4R (Nuvance)

The promising data in preclinical studies led to preliminary investigations where IL-4R proved safe and effective in the treatment of patients with asthma [26, 27]. In the phase I study, 25 subjects with mild or moderate persistent asthma were withdrawn from their inhaled corticosteroids and randomized to placebo or IL-4R at 0.5 or 1.5 mg once by nebulizer [26]. There were no significant adverse events related to study drug. No patient developed antibodies to IL-4. Treatment with 1.5 mg IL-4R resulted in significantly better FEV_1 at 2 h after treatment and on days 2, 4 and 15 ($p < 0.05$). IL-4R was associated with statistically significant improvement in asthma symptom score ($p < 0.05$) and β_2-agonist use ($p < 0.05$). Scores on the third section of the AQLQ (patient's perception of general health and physical functioning) worsened in the placebo group and improved in the IL-4R 1.5-mg group ($p < 0.05$). Methacholine testing showed decreased sensitivity in 6 out of 8 patients tested in the 1.5-mg group. Exhaled NO scores were significantly improved among patients receiving IL-4R ($p < 0.05$), demonstrating an anti-inflammatory effect.

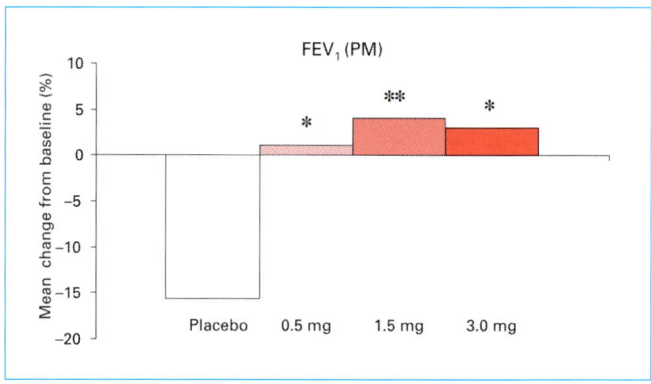

Fig. 2. FEV_1 (PM) percent change from baseline. FEV_1 (PM) was measured with Air Watch™ monitor at bedtime daily. Treatment with IL-4R 3.0 mg following discontinuation of inhaled corticosteroids prevented decline in FEV_1 (PM) (+3% IL-4R 3.0 mg versus –16% placebo; * $p = 0.01$) over the 3-month treatment period. * $p < 0.05$, ** $p < 0.01$ vs. placebo.

In the phase I/II randomized, double-blind, placebo-controlled study, 62 patients with moderate persistent asthma were randomized to twelve weekly nebulizations of 0.75, 1.5, or 3.0 mg of IL-4R (Nuvance) or placebo [27]. Before the study, patients documented dependence on inhaled corticosteroids by an exacerbation in asthma induced by one or two 50% reductions in inhaled corticosteroid dose at 2-week intervals. After the patients were restabilized on inhaled corticosteroids for 2 weeks, the inhaled corticosteroids were discontinued at the time that study medication was begun. IL-4R was safe and well tolerated. Antibodies to IL-4R occurred in <3%, which were nonneutralizing and resulted in no symptoms. Efficacy was demonstrated by a significant decline in FEV_1 observed in the placebo group (–0.4 liters; –13% predicted), which did not occur in the 3.0-mg treatment group (–0.1 liter; –2% predicted; p = 0.05 over the 3-month treatment period). Daily patient-measured FEV_1 (AM) also demonstrated a significant decline in the placebo group (–0.5 liter; –18% predicted), which did not occur in the 3.0-mg treatment group (–0.1 liter; p = 0.02 over the 3-month treatment period; –4% predicted). The FEV_1 (PM) also significantly improved and at high dose was 19% better than placebo (fig. 2). The efficacy of IL-4R was further confirmed by the absence of increase in asthma symptom score (Δ0.1) in the 3.0 mg treatment group compared to the placebo group (Δ1.4 over 1 month; p = 0.08).

References

1 Coffman RL, Ohara J, Bond MW, Carty J, Zlotnik A, Paul WE: B cell stimulatory factor-1 enhances the IgE response of lipopolysaccharide-activated B cells. J Immunol 1986;136: 4538–4541.
2 Pawankar R, Okuda M, Yssel H, Okumura K, Ra C: Nasal mast cells in perennial allergic rhinitis exhibit increased expression of the Fc epsilonRI, CD40L, IL-4, and IL-13, and can induce IgE synthesis in B cells. J Clin Invest 1997;99:1492–1499.
3 Moser R, Fehr J, Bruijnzeel PL: IL-4 controls the selective endothelium-driven transmigration of eosinophils from allergic individuals. J Immunol 1992;149:1432–1438.
4 Dabbagh K, Takeyama K, Lee HM, Ueki IF, Lausier JA, Nadel JA: IL-4 induces mucin gene expression and goblet cell metaplasia in vitro and in vivo. J Immunol 1999;162:6233–6237.
5 Hsieh CS, Heimberger AB, Gold JS, O'Garra A, Murphy KM: Differential regulation of T helper phenotype development by interleukins 4 and 10 in an alpha beta T-cell-receptor transgenic system. Proc Natl Acad Sci USA 1992;89: 6065–6069.
6 Seder RA, Paul WE, Davis MM, Fazekas de St Groth B: The presence of interleukin 4 during in vitro priming determines the lymphokine-producing potential of CD4+ T cells from T cell receptor transgenic mice. J Exp Med 1992;176: 1091–1098.
7 Kopf M, Le Gros G, Bachmann M, Lamers MC, Bluethmann H, Kohler G: Disruption of the murine IL-4 gene blocks Th2 cytokine responses. Nature 1993;362:245–248.
8 Vella A, Teague TK, Ihle J, Kappler J, Marrack P: Interleukin 4 (IL-4) or IL-7 prevents the death of resting T cells: stat6 is probably not required for the effect of IL-4. J Exp Med 1997; 186:325–330.
9 Xie H, Seward RJ, Huber BT: Cytokine rescue from glucocorticoid induced apoptosis in T cells is mediated through inhibition of Ikappa-Balpha. Mol Immunol 1997;34:987–994.
10 Daher S, Santos LM, Sole D, De Lima MG, Naspitz CK, Musatti CC: Interleukin-4 and soluble CD23 serum levels in asthmatic atopic children. J Invest Allergol Clin Immunol 1995; 5:251–254.

11 Walker C, Bauer W, Braun RK, Menz G, Braun P, Schwarz F, et al: Activated T cells and cytokines in bronchoalveolar lavages from patients with various lung diseases associated with eosinophilia. Am J Respir Crit Care Med 1994;150:1038–1048.
12 Leonard C, Tormey V, Burke C, Poulter LW: Allergen-induced cytokine production in atopic disease and its relationship to disease severity. Am J Respir Cell Mol Biol 1997;17:368–375.
13 Shi HZ, Deng JM, Xu H, Nong ZX, Xiao CQ, Liu ZM, et al: Effect of inhaled interleukin-4 on airway hyperreactivity in asthmatics. Am J Respir Crit Care Med 1998;157:1818–1821.
14 Parronchi P, De Carli M, Manetti R, Simonelli C, Piccinni MP, Macchia D, et al: Aberrant interleukin (IL)-4 and IL-5 production in vitro by CD4+ helper T cells from atopic subjects. Eur J Immunol 1992;22:1615–1620.
15 Chan SC, Brown MA, Willcox TM, Li SH, Stevens SR, Tara D, et al: Abnormal IL-4 gene expression by atopic dermatitis T lymphocytes is reflected in altered nuclear protein interactions with IL-4 transcriptional regulatory element. J Invest Dermatol 1996;106:1131–1136.
16 Song Z, Casolaro V, Chen R, Georas SN, Monos D, Ono SJ: Polymorphic nucleotides within the human IL-4 promoter that mediate overexpression of the gene. J Immunol 1996;156: 424–429.
17 Rosenwasser LJ, Borish L: Genetics of atopy and asthma: The rationale behind promoter-based candidate gene studies (IL-4 and IL-10). Am J Respir Crit Care Med 1997;156:S152–S155.
18 Burchard EG, Silverman EK, Rosenwasser LJ, Borish L, Yandava C, Pillari A, et al: Association between a sequence variant in the IL-4 gene promoter and FEV_1 in asthma. Am J Respir Crit Care Med 1999;160:919–922.
19 Mitsuyasu H, Izuhara K, Mao XQ, Gao PS, Arinobu Y, Enomoto T, et al: Ile50Val variant of IL4R alpha upregulates IgE synthesis and associates with atopic asthma (letter). Nat Genet 1998;19:119–120.

20 Hershey GKK, Friedrich MF, Esswein LA, Thomas ML, Chatila TA: The association of atopy with a gain-of-function mutation in the alpha subunit of the interleukin-4 receptor. N Engl J Med 1997;337:1720–1725.
21 Coyle AJ, Le Gros G, Bertrand C, Tsuyuki S, Heusser CH, Kopf M, et al: Interleukin-4 is required for the induction of lung Th2 mucosal immunity. Am J Respir Cell Mol Biol 1995;13: 54–59.
22 Corry DB, Folkesson HG, Warnock ML, Erle DJ, Matthay MA, Wiener-Kronish JP, et al: Interleukin 4, but not interleukin 5 or eosinophils, is required in a murine model of acute airway hyperreactivity. J Exp Med 1996;183: 109–117.
23 Renz H, Bradley K, Enssle K, Loader JE, Larsen GL, Gelfand EW: Prevention of the development of immediate hypersensitivity and airway hyperresponsiveness following in vivo treatment with soluble IL-4 receptor. Int Arch Allergy Immunol 1996;109:167–176.
24 Henderson W, Chi E, Maliszweski C: Soluble interleukin-4 receptor inhibits airway inflammation following allergen challenge in a mouse model of asthma. J Immunol 2000;164:1086–1095.
25 Benson M, Strannegard IL, Wennergren G, Strannegard O: Cytokines in nasal fluids from school children with seasonal allergic rhinitis. Pediatric Allergy Immunol 1997;8:143–149.
26 Borish L, Nelson H, Lanz M, Claussen L, Whitmore J, Agosti J, et al: Recombinant human interleukin-4 receptor in moderate atopic asthma: A randomized double-blind, placebo-controlled pilot study. Am J Respir Crit Care Med 1999;160:1816–1823.
27 Borish L, Nelson H, Corren J, Bensch G, Busse W, Whitmore J, Agosti J: Efficacy of soluble interleukin-4 receptor for the treatment of adults with asthma, in preparation.

L. Borish, MD
Allergy Division
University of Virginia Medical Center
Box 801355
Charlottesville, VA 22908 (USA)
Tel. +1 804 243 6570, Fax +1 804 924 5779
E-Mail lb4m@cms.mail.virginia.edu

Interleukin-13 Antagonism

Debra D. Donaldson[a]   Jack A. Elias[b]   Marsha Wills-Karp[c]

[a]Genetics Institute of Wyeth-Ayerst Research, Andover, Mass.; [b]Yale University, New Haven, Conn.; [c]Johns Hopkins University, Baltimore, Md., USA

Summary

The importance of IL-13 in the induction of AHR, mucus formation and airway remodeling in animal models of pulmonary disease is now well documented. Recent human genetic data associating genes of the IL-13 signaling pathway to allergic disease and data associating IL-13 with asthma confirm the animal model predictions. Together, these findings provide a compelling rationale for IL-13 antagonism as a therapeutic approach for the treatment of asthma and other inflammatory respiratory diseases.

Molecular Mechanism of Action

The interaction of cytokines with their receptors plays a pivotal role in induction and maintenance of inflammation [1]. Realizing the therapeutic potential of cytokine antagonism in asthma and COPD depends on understanding the contribution of particular cytokines in vivo to respiratory inflammation. For example, while the association of Th2 inflammation with the pathogenesis of asthma is well accepted, the exact role of particular Th2 cytokines and different subsets of inflammatory cells in this pathology is less clear [2, 3].

Human IL-13 is a 17-kD glycoprotein and is produced by Th2 T cells, macrophages, dendritic cells, NK2 cells, mast cells and basophils [4, 5]. Biologically active recombinant human IL-13 binds specifically to a low-affinity binding chain, IL-13Rα1, as well as to a high-affinity multimeric complex composed of IL-13Rα1 and IL-4R [4]. The high-affinity complex is expressed on a wide variety of hematopoietic and nonhematopoietic cell types. The participation of the IL-4R in both IL-4 and IL-13 receptor complexes explains some of the similarities in the functions of these cytokines [4] (fig. 1). Binding of IL-13 to IL-13Rα1 and IL-4R results in phosphorylation-dependent activation of JAK1 and JAK2 or TYK2, STAT6, and IRS1/2 proteins [6]. IL-13, and only IL-13, also binds an additional receptor chain, IL-13Rα2, which has not been shown to contribute to IL-13 signaling and may function specifically to attenuate the activity of IL-13 [5]. A soluble form of this receptor, which binds IL-13 with $100\times$ higher affinity than IL-13Rα1, has been identified in mouse serum [B. Jacobson, unpubl. obs.] and urine, suggesting that the natural form of this receptor may regulate IL-13 activity in vivo [5]. Potential roles for the IL-13Rα2 receptor in regulating IL-13 signaling are currently under study in IL-13Rα2-deficient mice (fig. 2).

Cellular Mechanism of Action

Many inflammatory cell types associated with the asthmatic phenotype, including Th2 T cells, synthesize and secrete IL-13. CD4+, CD8+, Th1, Th2, Th0 and naive CD45RA+ T cells have all been reported as sources of IL-13 following stimulation [4]. Many of these cells produce IL-4, however, CD45RA+ T cells and TH1 cells produce IL-13 but not IL-4. B cell tumors also secrete IL-13. For example, Hodgkin and Reed-Sternberg tumor cells, which may arise from germinal center B cells, secrete IL-13 which stimulates their growth in an autocrine fashion [7].

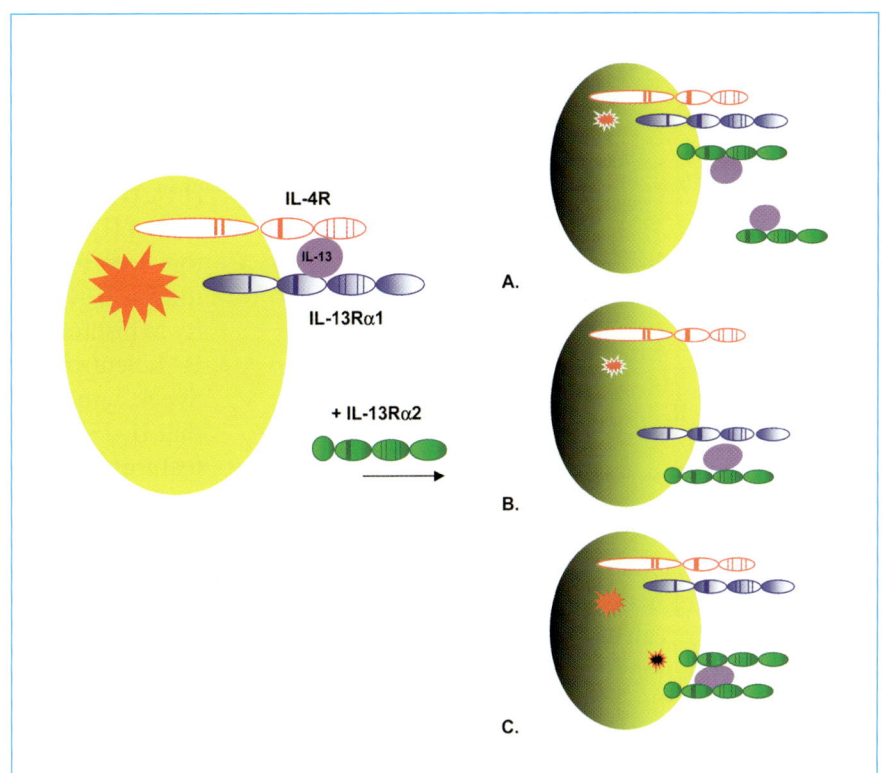

Fig. 1. Models for attenuation of IL-13 signaling via IL-13Rα2. **A** Competitive antagonist. **B** Sequester signaling chain. **C** Send a negative signal.

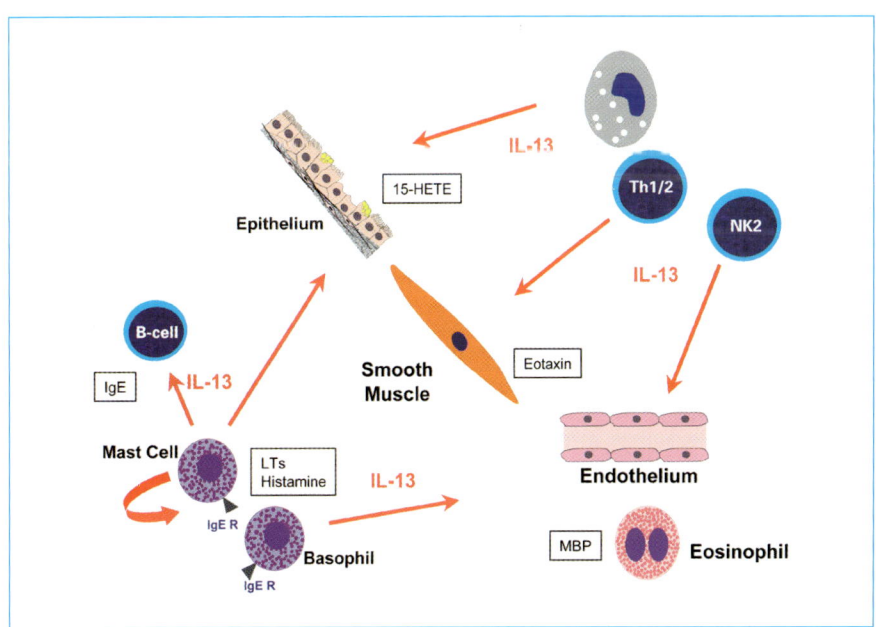

Fig. 2. IL-13: A central effector of allergic asthma.

IL-13 has been shown to regulate human B cell function and IgE synthesis in vitro in both normal individuals and patients with severe combined immunodeficiency [4]. The recent demonstration that IL-13 but not IL-4 contributes to isotype switching and IgM secretion from CD40-activated IgD+/CD38– naive B lymphocytes suggests that IL-13 may act earlier in B cell development than previously appreciated [8]. Interestingly, IL-4-independent induction of IgE has also recently been shown in transgenic mice expressing IL-13 [5]. A number of activi-

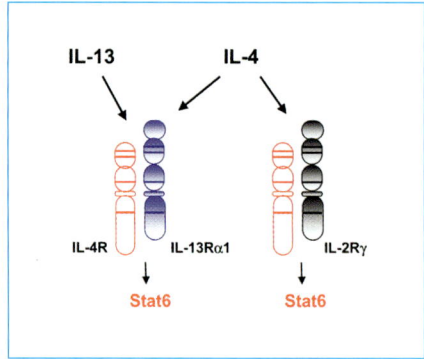

Fig. 3. IL-13 and IL-4 activate an IL-13 recepter complex.

ties of IL-13 on macrophages have been reported, including modulation of many cell surface proteins, inhibition of IL-12 secretion, calcium mobilization, and stimulation of giant cell formation [4, 9]. IL-13 has not been shown to act on T cells directly. However, IL-13 may impact T cell development indirectly through effects on monocyte/macrophages.

IL-13 has also been shown to regulate enzymes of the arachidonic acid pathway, NO production, VCAM expression, chemokine secretion and collagen production in fibroblasts, endothelial cells, smooth muscle cells and epithelial cells [4, 10] (fig. 3). These activities on nonhematopoietic cells likely contribute to the asthma-like phenotype seen when IL-13 is administered to the lung in vivo. More recent studies have demonstrated that IL-13 is also a potent stimulator of a variety of respiratory matrix metalloproteinases and cathepsins [T. Zheng, Z. Zhu, J.A. Elias, unpubl. obs.]. This provides mechanistic insights into pathways IL-13 could use in tissue remodeling in asthma and COPD.

Role for IL-13 in Animal Models of Allergy and Inflammation and Efficacy of sIL-13R

The potential role for IL-13 in vivo in airway disease has been studied by chronic or transient administration of IL-13 to the lung in murine and guinea pig models. Intranasal administration of recombinant IL-13, adenovirus expressing IL-13 and lung specific transgenic expression of IL-13 have been utilized in mice [6, 11; C. DeClercq and J. Sypek, unpubl. obs.]. Examination of these animals revealed pulmonary inflammation with mononuclear inflammatory cells and eosinophils, mucus formation, enhancement of IgE production and when measured, AHR. Of special interest, in a model of chronic lung-specific transgenic expression of IL-13, additional phenotypic changes relevant to asthma were also revealed. These changes included deposition of Charcot-Leyden-like crystals with airway obstruction, subepithelial fibrosis and induction of the eosinophil recruiting chemokine, eotaxin [11]. We have recently shown that intranasal administration of IL-13 to guinea pig induces a phenotype similar to that seen in mice. Tracheal nebulization of recombinant murine IL-13 resulted in a substantial increase in sensitivity to histamine stimulation of the airways with increased BAL neutrophil and eosinophil recovery [C. Lilly, and J. Sypek, unpubl. obs.]. Together, these studies demonstrate that IL-13 administration evoked most of the pathologic features of asthma and induced an inflammatory response similar to that associated with the asthmatic phenotype.

The impact of endogenous IL-13 production on animal models of inflammatory disease has been evaluated in IL-13-deficient mice, with antibodies to IL-13, and with high affinity soluble receptors [10, 12, 13]. IL-13-deficient mice have altered immune systems with impaired Th2 responses characterized by reduced production of Th2 cytokines in vitro and altered susceptibility to infections such as *Nippostrongylus* [5]. The effects of IL-13 deficiency in murine infectious disease models have been remarkably similar to studies in which IL-13 has been depleted with soluble receptor or antibodies to IL-13 [5].

The precise role of IL-13 in vivo has been well studied in normal animals where the impact of gene deficiency on immune development is not a variable. To this end, we have created a soluble form of the murine and human IL-13Rα2R, sIL-13R, by fusing the extracellular domain of the receptor to the Fc portion of human IgG1 [5]. In vitro, sIL-13R interferes with IL-13 binding to its signaling receptor and functions as a high-affinity antagonist. In vivo, administration of sIL-13R has been shown to completely block the expulsion of the intestinal nematode, *Nippostrongylus brasiliensis* [5]. Physiological responses within the gut which correlate with expulsion of parasites, such as goblet cell hyperplasia and mucus production have been shown to be IL-13 dependent and, are reminiscent of airway responses to airborne antigen in asthma, suggesting a common mediator [5].

Consistent with the hypothesis that IL-13 is a pivotal mediator of the asthmatic phenotype, sIL-13R has been shown to be highly efficacious in a number of murine asthma models. For example, sIL-13R administered therapeutically, prior to a second antigen challenge, completely blocked AHR to methylcholine, goblet cell hyperplasia, and mucus formation [5]. Systemic and intranasal routes of administration are equally effective. The effect of administration of sIL-13R has also been studied in schistosomiasis-induced liver fibrosis. Liver fibrosis associated with active hepatic egg deposition was significantly reduced by sIL-13R, suggesting a potential impact of IL-13 antagonism on remodeling in asthma and COPD [10, 14]. Taken together, these studies predict that disruption of IL-13 signaling may have significant therapeutic potential in asthma and other allergic diseases. In addition, the effects on mucus production and fibrosis suggest that IL-13 may be important in the pathogenesis of other inflammatory respiratory diseases as well.

Rationale for IL-13 Involvement in Human Asthma

The association of increased production of IL-13 has been well documented in atopic and nonatopic asthma, atopic dermatitis, allergic rhinitis and chronic sinusitis [1]. Decreased IL-13 expression following effective steroid therapy in rhinitis has also been reported. Variants in the IL-4R/STAT6 signaling pathway have been shown to genetically associate with asthma [15, 16]. Some variants may account for previously detected asthma susceptibility loci and showed functional effects in vitro.

Recently, a number of groups have described allelic variants in the *IL-13* gene, upstream of the coding region, within the coding region and in the 3' untranslated region of the message [17, 18]. These variants showed a strong association with asthma, elevated IL-13 levels or elevated IgE. Of particular interest is the Arg130/Gln substitution in the coding region of IL-13 noted by two groups and detected across multiple ethnic boundaries. Molecular modeling suggests potential biological impacts of this change including enhanced receptor binding and activation. Variants in the putative upstream promoter region of the gene or the 3' untranslated region of the message could lead to higher steady-state transcript levels which could result in elevated serum IL-13 levels. Effects on glycosylation of this glycoprotein should also be considered in terms of its impact on specific activity and serum half-life of IL-13 [19]. Further functional studies are anticipated but the current data strongly support *IL-13* as an atopy locus on 5q31.

Therapeutic Approach

A number of protein therapeutics might be employed to antagonize IL-13 or its receptor including administration of soluble receptors, anti-IL-13 monoclonal antibodies, antagonistic muteins, and anti-receptor antibodies [20, 21]. Potential advantages of dimeric sIL-13R include extended half-life in vivo and high-affinity binding to IL-13 with a fully human peptide sequence. Recent advances in particle formulation for large molecules and dry aerosol delivery systems may further enhance the value of sIL-13R and other large-molecule therapeutics [22, 23]. Reproducible, noninvasive, efficient pulmonary delivery of sIL-13R may allow treatment of a broad patient population with few side effects.

Suitable targets for small molecule antagonists of IL-13 include the IL-13 signaling receptor complex and signaling molecules such as STAT6. Identification of additional genes regulated by IL-13 and validation of their participation in pulmonary inflammation may provide further therapeutic opportunities for development of small molecules.

Conclusions

Results from recent in vivo studies and newly determined genetic associations have illuminated the role of IL-13 as a major mediator of the asthmatic response [24]. The ability of IL-13 administration to recapitulate all three aspects of the asthmatic triad, AHR, mucus production and remodeling, coupled with the efficacy of IL-13 antagonism in animal models is particularly exciting. The role of IL-13 in other types of respiratory disease and the potential of sIL-13R as a disease-modifying anti-asthmatic drug are currently under study in animal models.

References

1 Wills-Karp M: Immunologic basis of antigen-induced airway hyperresponsiveness. Annu Rev Immunol 1999;17:255–281.
2 Galli SJ: Complexity and redundancy in the pathogenesis of asthma: Reassessing the roles of mast cells and T cells. J Exp Med 1997;186: 343–347.
3 Drazen JM, Arm JP, Austen KF: Sorting out the cytokines of asthma (comment). J Exp Med 1996;183:1–5.
4 de Vries JE: The role of IL-13 and its receptor in allergy and inflammatory responses. J Allergy Clin Immunol 1998;102:165–169.
5 Finkelman FD, Wynn TA, Donaldson DD, Urban JF: The role of IL-13 in helminth-induced inflammation and protective immunity against nematode infections. Curr Opin Immunol 1999;11:420–426.
6 Gessner A, Rollinghoff M: Biological functions and signaling of the interleukin-4 receptor complexes. Immunobiology 2000;201:285–307.
7 Kapp U, Yeh WC, Patterson B, Elia AJ, Kagi D, Ho A, Hessel A, Tipsword M, Williams A, Mirtsos C, Itie A, Moyle M, Mak TW: Interleukin 13 is secreted by and stimulates the growth of Hodgkin and Reed-Sternberg cells. J Exp Med 1999;189:1939–1946.
8 Johansson B, Ingvarsson S, Bjorck P, Borrebaeck CA: Human interdigitating dendritic cells induce isotype switching and IL-13-dependent IgM production in CD40-activated naive B cells. J Immunol 2000;164:1847–1854.
9 DeFife KM, Jenney CR, McNally AK, Colton E, Anderson JM: Interleukin-13 induces human monocyte/macrophage fusion and macrophage mannose receptor expression. J Immunol 1997;158:3385–3390.
10 Chiaramonte MG, Donaldson DD, Cheever AW, Wynn TA: An IL-13 inhibitor blocks the development of hepatic fibrosis during a T-helper type 2-dominated inflammatory response. J Clin Invest 1999;104:777–785.
11 Zhu Z, Homer RJ, Wang Z, Chen Q, Geba GP, Wang J, Zhang Y, Elias JA: Pulmonary expression of interleukin-13 causes inflammation, mucus hypersecretion, subepithelial fibrosis, physiologic abnormalities, and eotaxin production. J Clin Invest 1999;103:779–788.
12 Bost K, Holton R, Cain T, Clements J: In vivo treatment with anti-interleukin-13 antibodies significantly reduces the humoral immune response against an oral immunogen in mice. Immunology 1996;87:633–641.
13 Matsukawa A, Hogaboam CM, Lukacs NW, Lincoln PM, Evanoff HL, Strieter RM, Kunkel SL: Expression and contribution of endogenous IL-13 in an experimental model of sepsis. J Immunol 2000;164:2738–2744.
14 Elias JA, Zhu Z, Chupp G, Homer RJ: Airway remodeling in asthma. J Clin Invest 1999;104: 1001–1006.
15 Shirakawa I, Deichmann KA, Izuhara I, Mao I, Adra CN, Hopkin JM: Atopy and asthma: Genetic variants of IL-4 and IL-13 signalling. Immunol Today 2000;21:60–64.
16 Ober C, Leavitt SA, Tsalenko A, Howard TD, Hoki DM, Daniel R, Newman DL, Wu X, Parry R, Lester LA, Solway J, Blumenthal M, King RA, Xu J, Meyers DA, Bleecker ER, Cox NJ: Variation in the interleukin 4-receptor alpha gene confers susceptibility to asthma and atopy in ethnically diverse populations. Am J Hum Genet 2000;66:517–526.
17 Graves PE, Kabesch M, Halonen M, Holberg CJ, Baldini M, Fritzsch C, Weiland SK, Erickson RP, von Mutius E, Martinez FD: A cluster of seven tightly linked polymorphisms in the IL-13 gene is associated with total serum IgE levels in three populations of white children. J Allergy Clin Immunol 2000;105:506–513.
18 Heinzmann A, Mao X, Akaiwa M, Kreomer RT, Gao P, Ohshima K, Umeshita R, Abe Y, Braun S, Yamashita T, Roberts MH, Sugimoto R, Arima K, Arinobu Y, Yu B, Kruse S, Enomoto T, Dake Y, Kawai M, Shimazu S, Sasaki S, Adra CN, Kitaichi M, Inoue H, Yamauchi K, Tomichi N: Genetic variants of IL-13 signalling and human asthma and atopy. Hum Mol Genet 2000;9:549–559.
19 Wicker LS: QTL influencing autoimmune diabetes and encephalomyelitis map to a 0.15-cM region containing *IL2*. Nat Genet 1999;21: 158–160.
20 Vaughan TJ, Osbourn JK, Tempest PR: Human antibodies by design. Nat Biotechnol 1998;16:535–539.
21 Grunewald SM, Werthmann A, Schnarr B, Klein CE, Brocker EB, Mohrs M, Brombacher F, Sebald W, Duschl A: An antagonistic IL-4 mutant prevents type I allergy in the mouse: inhibition of the IL-4/IL-13 receptor system completely abrogates humoral immune response to allergen and development of allergic symptoms in vivo. J Immunol 1998;160:4004–4009.
22 Patton J: Breathing life into protein drugs. Nat Biotechnol 1998;16:141–143.
23 Edwards DA, Ben-Jebria A, Langer R: Recent advances in pulmonary drug delivery using large, porous inhaled particles. J Appl Physiol 1998;85:379–385.
24 Corry DB: IL-13 in allergy: Home at last. Curr Opin Immunol 1999;11:610–614.

Debra Donaldson, MD
Immunology and Hemostasis
Genetics Institute, One Burtt Rd.
Andover, MA 01810 (USA)
Tel. +1 978 247 3604, Fax +1 978 247 1333
E-Mail ddonaldson@genetics.com

Interleukin-5 Antagonism

Maggie J. Leckie[a]   Christoph Walker[b]

[a]National Heart and Lung Institute, Clinical Studies Unit, Imperial College, London, and
[b]Novartis Research Centre, Horsham, UK

Summary

IL-5 inhibitors are being developed as specific anti-eosinophil directed therapies for the treatment of asthma and other allergic diseases. Strategies include blocking receptor binding, inhibiting release of cytokines from T cells, and using blocking monoclonal antibodies directed against IL-5. Several preclinical studies have been completed using monoclonal antibodies directed against IL-5, with promising results in terms of beneficial effects on airways hyperresponsiveness (AHR) and tissue eosinophilia. More recently, anti-IL-5 monoclonal antibodies have been administered to patients with mild allergic asthma using an allergen challenge model. Anti-IL-5 causes clear and long-term reduction in both blood and sputum eosinophils with no significant effect on either AHR or the late asthmatic reaction to inhaled allergen. Thus, IL-5 is an attractive target for anti-eosinophil-directed therapy, and further studies are ongoing to assess the efficacy of anti-IL-5 monoclonal antibodies in asthma.

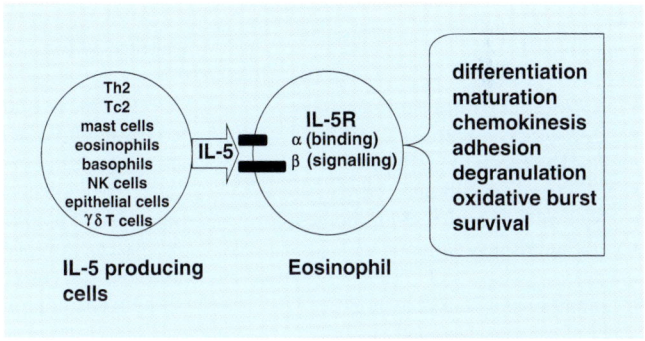

Fig. 1. IL-5-producing cells and IL-5 effector functions on eosinophils.

Eosinophils are implicated in the pathology of asthma and other allergic disorders [1, 2]. There is eosinophilic infiltration of the airways in patients with asthma, with a correlation between eosinophil number and activation state and severity of asthma, the late asthmatic reaction (LAR) and airways hyperresponsiveness (AHR). Airway wall remodelling is related to degranulation of eosinophils with the release of highly toxic granules, such as major basic protein. In addition, eosinophils are capable of inducing inflammation by both responding to and producing cytokines.

Thus, the prevention of eosinophil differentiation from progenitors in the bone marrow and the inhibition of tissue infiltration, activation and degranulation of these cells are currently regarded as promising therapeutic targets for the development of potential novel anti-asthma drugs. IL-5, amongst other cytokines, plays a key role in the development and activation of eosinophils. IL-5 is a haematopoietic growth factor composed of a dimeric core of two four-helix bundles formed by two identical polypeptide chains joined covalently by disulphide bonds [3]. A variety of cells produce IL-5 (fig. 1), the principal source of which is the Th2 cell [4]. IL-5 acts through a heterodimeric receptor composed of a cytokine-binding, ligand-specific α-chain (IL-5Rα) and a non-ligand-binding, high-affinity-receptor-forming and signal-transducing β-subunit (β-common) that is shared by the α-chains of the IL-3 and GM-CSF receptors [5].

Experiments in vivo clearly demonstrate the central role of IL-5 and indicate this cytokine as the major and possibly the only cytokine involved in the production of specific eosinophilia (table 1). Intravenous injection of recombinant IL-5 into mice or guinea pigs resulted in eosinophil production in the bone marrow and blood eosinophilia [6]. Similar results were found in mice overexpressing IL-5 which develop a long-lasting and selective

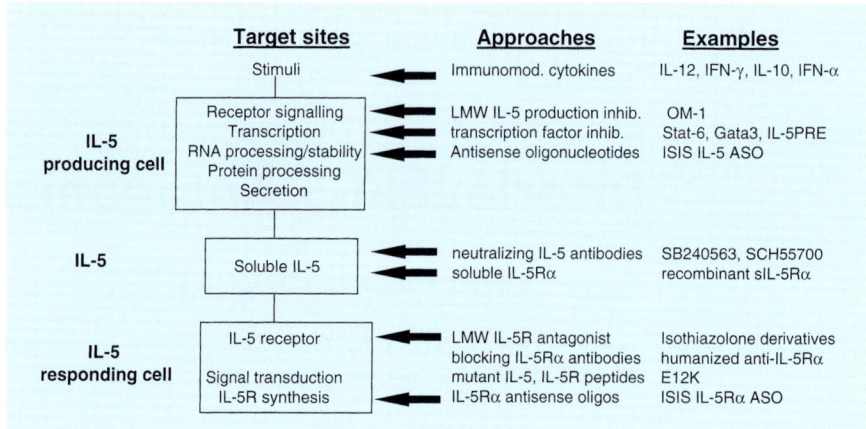

Fig. 2. Potential target sites to interfere with IL-5 production and effector function. LMW = Low-molecular-weight compound.

Table 1. Eosinophilia regulation by IL-5 in vivo

Experiment	Results
• IL-5 administration animals models	selective blood and tissue eosinophilia
• IL-5 knock-out mouse	no eosinophilia in response to antigens
• IL-5Rα knock-out mouse	no eosinophilia in response to antigens
• IL-5 transgenic mouse	selective blood eosinophilia
• Neutralizing anti-IL-5 antibodies	suppression of antigen-induced eosinophil infiltration and bronchial hyperreactivity
• IL-5 in asthma patients	increased expression of mRNA and proteins for IL-5 in bronchial mucosal biopsies, BAL and sputum, correlation with eosinophil number and clinical severity
• Inhalation of IL-5 in asthmatics	sputum eosinophilia, induction of bronchial hyperreactivity

blood eosinophilia [7]. In contrast, IL-5- and IL-5Rα-deficient mice are unable to produce increased numbers of eosinophils in response to specific antigens [8, 9]. Moreover, inhibition of the IL-5 response by using neutralizing antibodies prevents the terminal differentiation of eosinophils, suppresses the infiltration of mature eosinophils into inflamed tissues and reduces the induction of AHR in response to allergen exposure in actively allergen-sensitized animals [10, 11].

In humans, IL-5 is expressed during allergen-induced cutaneous late-phase reaction and is detectable in bronchial mucosal biopsies and BAL fluid of patients with asthma [4, 12]. Moreover, inhalation of IL-5 by asthmatics causes AHR and sputum eosinophilia [13]. All of these observations are consistent with a unique role of IL-5 in the production, activation and localization of eosinophils in allergic conditions. This cytokine is therefore considered as the prime target for therapeutic intervention in allergy and asthma.

Therapeutic Approaches (fig. 2)

IL-5 Production Inhibitors. Cytokines. The production of IL-5 may be inhibited by modulating the immune response to allergens by cytokines, such as IFN-α, IFN-γ, IL-12 or IL-10, creating a Th1 lymphocyte response [14]. However, none of these cytokines specifically target IL-5 and it is highly questionable whether cytokines themselves are useful drugs for the treatment of asthma due to their size, short half-life and potential side effect profile.

Low-Molecular-Weight IL-5 Production Inhibitors. The only IL-5-specific low-molecular-weight inhibitor described to date is OM-01 [15]. This synthetic compound efficiently suppresses IL-5 production without affecting the synthesis of IL-2 or IL-4. Moreover, OM-01 administered in vivo inhibits the late-phase eosinophil infiltration in a murine model of asthma.

Transcription Factors. Transcription factors exclusively expressed in IL-4- and IL-5-producing T-helper cells can be targeted. To date, several transcription factors (such as STAT6, GATA-3) have been implicated in Th2 cell differentiation or Th2 cell cytokine production, but none of these were found to selectively regulate IL-5 production [16]. A unique retarded complex binding to the so-called IL-5PRE site of the IL-5 promoter has been identified [17], and may be a useful target.

Antisense Oligonucleotides. Modified antisense oligonucleotides that are complementary to the mRNA encoding a specific protein have been developed and can be used therapeutically to inhibit its synthesis. This approach has been successfully applied using A1 adenosine receptors in an asthma model in rabbits, which resulted in beneficial therapeutic effects [18]. A similar strategy could therefore be used to block the synthesis of IL-5 or its receptor. Indeed, IL-5- and IL-5Rα-specific antisense oligonucleotides have been identified which selectively suppress the production of IL-5 and the expression of IL-5Rα, both in vitro and in vivo [J. Karras et al., and E. Trifilieff et al., unpubl. obs]. However, several issues such as delivery, cost, sequence specificity, cell uptake and cellular localization of antisense oligonucleotides may limit the use of these compounds as therapeutics.

IL-5 and IL-5 Receptor Antagonists. Low-Molecular-Weight IL-5R Antagonists. Inhibition of protein-protein interaction, such as binding of IL-5 to its receptor, present a difficult challenge to find or design low-molecular-weight inhibitors to interfere with the interaction, since there is usually a large area of contact involved. So far, only one study reported the identification of low-molecular-weight IL-5R antagonists [19]. However, the selective inhibition of IL-5 binding to its receptors by these isothiazolone derivatives was shown to involve the covalent modification of the sulphhydryl group of free cysteine residues in IL-5Rα, resulting in a decrease of the affinity for IL-5 and were therefore not progressed further.

Anti-IL-5 Antibodies. As already described above, animal models have shown that monoclonal antibodies directed against IL-5 can reduce eosinophilia, AHR and lung damage in response to a variety of antigens [10, 11].

Soluble IL-5Rα. Another approach to block the interaction of IL-5 with its receptor is the use of soluble IL-5R. This soluble protein binds IL-5 with only slightly reduced affinity compared to the membrane form of IL-5R. It acts as a selective IL-5 antagonist in vitro and suppresses the antigen induced infiltration of eosinophils into the bronchial lumen suggesting that sIL-5Rα may also exert IL-5 antagonizing activities in vivo [20].

Mutant IL-5. More recently, a single point mutant of IL-5 was identified, E12K, which binds IL-5R with almost wild-type affinity and is a potent antagonist in

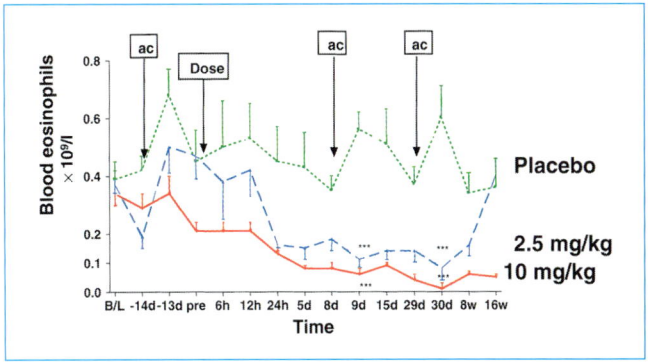

Fig. 3. Blood eosinophils following treatment anti-IL-5 monoclonal antibody. Ac = Allergen challenge; B/L = baseline. Time in hours (h), days (d) and weeks (w).

IL-5-induced proliferation and adhesion assays [21]. In contrast, E12K still mediates eosinophil survival, although with reduced potency compared to the wild-type protein.

Clinical Studies

There is limited experience with anti-IL-5 monoclonal antibody treatment in humans. Both SmithKline Beecham and Schering Plough have compounds which have completed early clinical trials. A single intravenous infusion of SB 240563, anti-IL-5 antibody (10 mg/kg) administered to 8 subjects with mild allergic asthma caused significant reduction in circulating eosinophil numbers which lasted for up to 16 weeks. This has clear implications for diseases associated with eosinophilia, such as atopic asthma, seasonal rhinitis and eczema. In addition, there was inhibition of the blood eosinophilia, which normally occurs following allergen challenge (fig. 3) and a marked reduction in sputum eosinophils for up to 30 days following treatment. Anti-IL-5 monoclonal antibody treatment does not completely ablate blood and tissue eosinophils; nevertheless, there is a theoretical risk that therapy may still impair host response to certain parasites and malignancies.

Despite significant reductions in blood and sputum eosinophils, there was no detectable effect on the allergen-induced LAR or AHR to histamine [22]. This provides the novel insight that eosinophils may not be a prerequisite for the LAR and AHR, and has relevance to the pathogenesis and treatment of asthma. The limited effects on the LAR and AHR following anti-IL-5 treatment may be due to the involvement of residual eosinophils as well as a number of other cell types such as allergen-specific T cells and mast cells. This has led to a questioning of the role of the eosinophil in human allergen challenge models of asthma, and in clinical asthma. A large-scale clinical study on the effect of multiple doses of anti-IL-5 on bone marrow, blood, skin and lung tissue eosinophils will provide further insight into the role of eosinophils in the clinical pathogenesis of allergy and asthma.

Conclusions

The unique role of IL-5 in eosinophil production, activation and localization makes this cytokine a prime target for therapeutic intervention in diseases characterized by eosinophilia and the development of drugs to neutralize the effect of IL-5 might represent a novel therapeutic approach in allergic diseases such as asthma.

Both preclinical and clinical studies using monoclonal antibodies have shown encouraging results in terms of effect on blood eosinophil numbers following allergen challenge. However, the lack of effect on either AHR or LAR to allergen in the clinical study questions the role of the eosinophil in the allergen challenge model of asthma, and the positive predictive value of preclinical studies.

References

1 Gleich GJ: The eosinophil and bronchial asthma: Current understanding. J Allergy Clin Immunol 1990;85:422–436.
2 Wardlaw AJ, Moqbel R, Kay AB: Eosinophils: Biology and role in disease. Adv Immunol 1995;60:151–266.
3 Milburn MV, Hassell AM, Lambert MH, Jordan SR, Proudfoot AE, Graber P, Wells TN: A novel dimer configuration revealed by the crystal structure at 2.4 Å resolution of human interleukin-5. Nature 1993;363:172–176.
4 Ying S, Durham SR, Corrigan CJ, Hamid Q, Kay AB: Phenotype of cells expressing mRNA for TH2-type (interleukin 4 and interleukin 5) and TH1-type (interleukin 2 and interferon gamma) cytokines in bronchoalveolar lavage and bronchial biopsies from atopic asthmatic and normal control subjects. Am J Respir Cell Mol Biol 1995;12:477–487.
5 Takatsu K, Takaki S, Hitoshi Y: Interleukin-5 and its receptor system: Implications in the immune system and inflammation. Adv Immunol 1994;57:145–190.
6 Palframan RT, Collins PD, Williams TJ, Rankin SM: Eotaxin induces a rapid release of eosinophils and their progenitors from the bone marrow. Blood 1998;91:2240–2248.
7 Dent LA, Strath M, Mellor AL, Sanderson CJ: Eosinophilia in transgenic mice expressing interleukin 5. J Exp Med 1990;172:1425–1431.
8 Foster PS, Hogan SP, Ramsay AJ, Matthaei KI, Young IG: Interleukin-5 deficiency abolishes eosinophilia, airways hyperreactivity, and lung damage in a mouse asthma model. J Exp Med 1996;183:195–201.
9 Yoshida T, Ikuta K, Sugaya H, Maki K, Takagi M, Kanazawa H, Sunaga S, Kinashi T, Yoshimura K, Miyazaki J, Takaki S, Takatsu K: Defective B-1 cell development and impaired immunity against *Angiostrongylus cantonensis* in IL-5R alpha-deficient mice. Immunity 1996; 4:483–494.

10 Mauser PJ, Pitman AM, Fernandez X, Foran SK, Adams GK, Kreutner W, Egan RW, Chapman RW: Effects of an antibody to interleukin-5 in a monkey model of asthma. Am J Respir Crit Care Med 1995;152:467–472.
11 Mauser PJ, Pitman A, Witt A, Fernandez X, Zurcher J, Kung T, Jones H, Watnick AS, Egan RW, Kreutner W, Adams GK: Inhibitory effect of the TRFK-5 anti-IL-5 antibody in a guinea pig model of asthma. Am Rev Respir Dis 1993; 148:1623–1627.
12 Kay AB, Ying S, Varney V, Gaga M, Durham SR, Moqbel R, Wardlaw AJ, Hamid Q: Messenger RNA expression of the cytokine gene cluster, interleukin 3 (IL-3), IL-4, IL-5, and granulocyte/macrophage colony-stimulating factor, in allergen-induced late-phase cutaneous reactions in atopic subjects. J Exp Med 1991;173:775–778.
13 Shi HZ, Xiao C-Q, Zhong D, Qin S-M, Liu Y, Liang GR, Xu H, Chen YG, Long XM, Xie ZF: Effect of inhaled interleukin-5 on airway hyperreactivity and eosinophilia in asthmatics. Am J Respir Crit Care Med 1998;157:204–209.
14 O'Garra A: Cytokines induce the development of functionally heterogeneous T helper cell subsets. Immunity 1998;8:275–283.
15 Okudaira H, Mori A, Mikami T, Kaminuma O, Ohmura T, Hoshino A, Suko M: Selective suppression of IL-5 synthesis by OM-01-pinpoint treatment of atopic diseases by IL-5 gene transcription inhibitor. Int Arch Allergy Immunol 1997;113:331–334.
16 Rincon M, Flavell RA: T-cell subsets: Transcriptional control in the Th1/Th2 decision. Curr Biol 1997;7:R729–R732.

17 Stranick KS, Payvandi F, Zambas DN, Umland SP, Egan RW, Billah MM: Transcription of the murine interleukin 5 gene is regulated by multiple promoter elements J Biol Chem 1995; 270:20575–20582.
18 Nyce JW, Metzger WJ: DNA antisense therapy for asthma in an animal model Nature 1997; 385:721–725.
19 Devos R, Plaetinck G, Cornells S, Guisez Y, Van der Heyden J, Tavernier J: Interleukin-5 and its receptor: A drug target for eosinophilia associated with chronic allergic disease. J Leukocyte Biol 1995;57:813–819.
20 Yamaguchi S, Nagai H, Tanaka H, Tsujimoto M, Tsuruoka N: Time course study for antigen-induced airway hyperreactivity and the effect of soluble IL-5 receptor. Life Sci 1994;54: L471–L475.
22 McKinnon M, Page K, Uings IJ, Banks M, Fattah D, Proudfoot AE, Graber P, Arod C, Fish R, Wells TN, Solari R: An interleukin 5 mutant distinguishes between two functional responses in human eosinophils. J Exp Med 1997;186: 121–129.
22 Leckie MJ, ten Brinke A, Lordan J, Khan J, Diamant Z, Walls CM, Cowley D, Hansel T, Djukanovic R, Sterk PJ, Holgate S, Barnes PJ: SB 240563, a humanised anti-IL-5 monoclonal antibody: initial single dose safety and activity in patients with asthma. Am J Respir Crit Care Med 1999;159:A624.

Maggie J. Leckie, MD
Clinical Studies Unit, 1st floor, Fulham Wing
Royal Brompton Hospital
Fulham Road, London SW3 6HP (UK)
Tel. +44 171 351 8977, Fax +44 171 351 8973
E-Mail m.leckie@ic.ac.uk

Interleukin-10

Satwant Narula   Francis Cuss

Department of Immunology and Allergy Drug Discovery, Schering-Plough Research Institute, Kenilworth, N.J., USA

Summary

Accumulating data suggest that several inflammatory respiratory diseases, such as asthma and cystic fibrosis, are associated with IL-10 deficiency. There is strong evidence from animal studies that endogenous IL-10 has an important immunoregulatory role in suppressing excessive inflammation in the lung. Regardless of the etiological role of IL-10 deficiency, there is little question that production of proinflammatory cytokines, such as IL-1, TNF, IL-6 and IL-8 is directly related to acute and chronic morbidity in many lung diseases. Thus, the effects of IL-10 may provide a physiological form of anti-inflammatory therapy which may ameliorate the morbidity of respiratory disease. Other activities of IL-10, particularly its potential antifibrotic effect, may offer other long term benefits. It is possible that local administration of IL-10 to the lung will be required for its full effectiveness.

IL-10 is a pleotrophic cytokine that inhibits a number of T cell, monocyte and macrophage functions leading to anti-inflammatory and immuno-suppressive effects in vivo. These biological activities have a number of potential therapeutic benefits, but this review will concentrate on the potential of IL-10 in respiratory diseases.

Discovery of and Physiochemical Characterization of IL-10

IL-10 was initially identified from mouse T helper subset 2 (Th2) clones as a factor inhibiting the production of IFN-γ by mouse T helper subset 1 clones (Th1) [1]. Initially named cytokine synthesis inhibitory factor to reflect this activity, murine IL-10 was cloned in 1990, followed by human IL-10 in 1991 [2, 3]. Murine and human IL-10 are similar in size (18.4 and 18.5 kD, respectively) and exist in solution as homodimers. They share an 81% homology at the nucleotide sequence and 73% homology in their amino acid sequence. Human IL-10 also has a strong homology to an open reading frame (BCRF1) in the genome of the Epstein-Barr virus (EBV) [3]. This may represent an early example of an infectious agent hijacking a cellular gene to evade host defenses.

IL-10 Synthesis. IL-10 is produced by a large array of cell types. Besides the CD4+ Th2 clones, IL-10 is produced by normal B cells and B cell lymphomas [4], Ly-1 B cells [5], activated mast cells [6], activated monocytes/macrophages [7], keratinocytes [8] and bronchial epithelium. Human IL-10 is produced by the CD45RA+ (naive) and CD45RO+ (memory) CD4+ T cell subsets as well as by CD8+ T cells [9].

IL-10 Receptor. IL-10 and its receptor fall within the IFN receptor family. Human IL-10 receptor was originally identified by cross-linking studies on human and murine cells [10]. Subsequently, both the mouse and human IL-10 receptor cDNA clones were identified [11, 12]. They share 70% sequence homology at the nucleotide level and 60% at the amino acid level. Both receptors can interact with EBV BCRF1 (viral IL-10) and while the mouse receptor can tolerate both the human and mouse ligand, this is not true of the human receptor which binds only human IL-10 and viral IL-10. CRFB4, a previously orphan member of the IFN receptor family has been identified as the second subunit of the IL-10 receptor complex [13]. The signaling pathway of IL-10 is typical of a cytokine, involving the JAK/STAT pathway [14–19]. IL-10 binding to its cognate receptor activates STAT1a, STAT3, JAK1 and Tyk2 [17, 19].

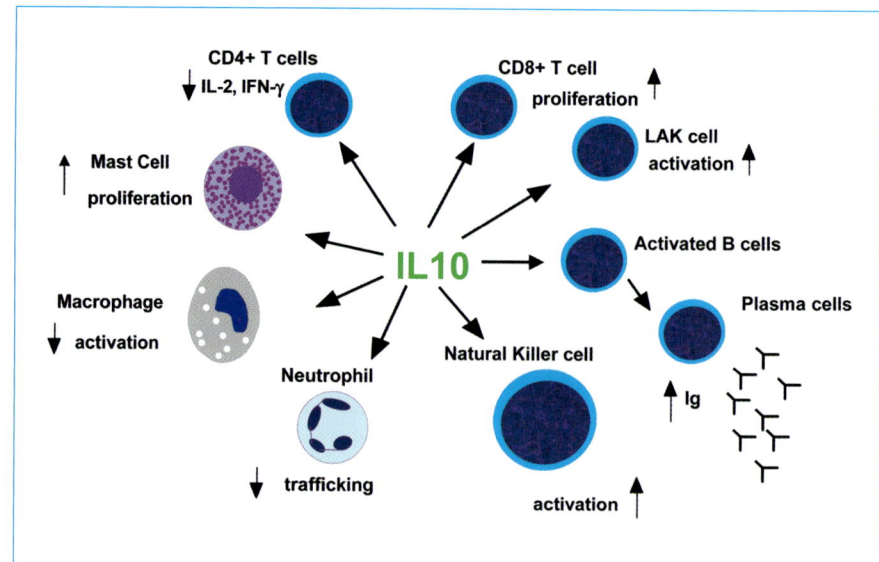

Fig. 1. Biological functions of IL-10.

Biological Characterization of IL-10

Effect of IL-10 on Various Cell Types. IL-10 is a very pleiotropic cytokine, having various effects on many cell types (fig. 1). Initially the primary activities of IL-10 were described as immunosuppressive and anti-inflammatory, but more recently in vitro studies indicate that IL-10 has the potential to be stimulatory in certain instances. The major effect of IL-10, clearly demonstrated both in vitro and in vivo, is its ability to downregulate macrophage activation. This includes inhibition of proinflammatory molecules, such as TNF, IL-1 and IL-6 and upregulation of anti-inflammatory regulators, such as IL-1 receptor antagonist and soluble TNF receptors [20–25]. Additionally, IL-10 downregulates MHC class II expression on antigen-presenting cells [26], thereby reducing antigen presentation and dampening T cell activation. Synthesis and release of IL-8 by polymorphonuclear cells is also inhibited by IL-10 [27–29]. B cells are also significantly responsive to IL-10, which enhances proliferation of activated B cells, resulting, in vitro, in increased secretion of IgM, IgG and IgA [30]. The stimulatory activity of IL-10 includes its ability to enhance pre-CTL proliferation and CTL activation [31]. It is also a chemotactic factor for CD8+ cells [32] and enhances the activation of natural killer cells and lymphokine-activated killer cells [33, 34].

IL-10 Knockout Mice. The fundamental role of IL-10 in modulating inflammatory responses was first suggested in studies of IL-10 (IL-10–/–) knockout mice [35]. Some of these mice are runted and anemic, and close investigation shows them to have chronic inflammatory bowel disease (IBD). The disease starts in the cecum of 3-week-old mice, progresses to involve the ascending and transverse colon, and finally even the small intestine of some aged IL-10–/– mice (animals kept in a pathogen-free environment do not get IBD, suggesting that IL-10 is functioning as an immunomodulator, suppressing pathogen-induced inflammation in the gastrointestinal tract) [36, 37]. Weanling mice treated with IL-10 fail to develop disease while adult IL-10–/– mice treated with IL-10 have a much reduced disease index [37]. Treatment of these mice with anti-IFN-γ antibody resulted in a marked reduction of the inflammation, confirming the role of Th1 responses in the pathogenesis of this disease. Additionally, transfer of IL-10–/– lamina propria lymphocytes and intraepithelial lymphocytes into Rag 2–/– mice transfers the disease, thus confirming the central role of T cells in disease pathogenesis [38, 39]. IL-10 has been shown to have a protective role in several other immunological models of IBD.

Subsequent studies have shown antigen-induced pulmonary inflammation to be more severe in IL-10–/– mice than in wild-type mice. IL-10–/– mice showed increased cell counts and eosinophilia in BAL fluid, again suggesting an endogenous immunosuppressive role for IL-10 [40]. Similarly, in a murine model of bronchopulmonary aspergillosis [41], with features of both IgE-mediated lung disease and hypersensitivity pneumonitis, Il-10–/– mice had exaggerated pulmonary inflammation and mortality compared to wild-type controls. In this study, both Th1 and Th2 responses appear to be suppressed by IL-10.

IL-10–/– mice infected chronically with Pseudomonas show many of the features of cystic fibrosis (CF) in humans. In three different studies, IL-10 deficiency resulted in severer inflammation and/or increased mortality [42–44] mimicking the differences between CF and wild-type mice with the same infection [45]. In each case, IL-10–/– mice had an equal or greater burden of bacteria than IL-10-sufficient animals, suggesting that higher IL-10 levels are not necessarily associated with poorer functioning of anti-bacterial defenses. Administration of IL-10 protein (rhIL-10) to mice with chronic Pseudomonas infection resulted in better weight retention, better survival and decreased lung inflammation, again with no increase in bacterial burden [44]. These data suggest that IL-10 may have a role in ameliorating the effects of chronic lung infection characteristic of CF.

Effects in Humans – Clinical Studies

IL-10 has been administered to over 1,000 human subjects and is generally well tolerated. Early studies were carried out in healthy human volunteers and reproduced the effects of IL-10 seen with human cells in vitro and mouse models in vivo. Administration of a single intravenous dose of IL-10 had a marked effect on circulating white blood cells over several hours, with values returning to baseline levels within 24–48 h [46]. The half-life of IL-10 in the circulation was approximately 2 h [47]. There was marked neutrophilia and lymphocytopenia, with both the CD4+ and CD8+ T cells decreasing in numbers [48]. Stimulation of cytokine production by LPS from ex vivo white blood cells was much reduced after IL-10 administration. TNF-α and IL-1β production were reduced and concentrations of IL-1RA were increased [46, 47, 49]. Neutrophil function was unaltered.

Rationale of IL-10 in Respiratory Disease

Asthma. Borish et al. [50] showed that constitutive IL-10 protein concentrations were reduced in BAL fluid from asthmatic compared to normal subjects and that IL-10 production from ex vivo monocytes, both constitutive and stimulated, was reduced in asthmatic subjects. Another study on monocyte differentiation in vitro suggests that IL-10 is required to obtain a 'suppressive' phenotype of macrophage and this macrophage population appears to be reduced in asthma [51]. John et al. [52] showed reduced basal IL-10 production in asthmatic subjects, but with a considerable increase in IL-10 after treatment with inhaled corticosteroids. These authors speculate that some of the therapeutic effects of corticosteroids in asthma may be due to stimulation of IL-10. Genotyping of asthmatic patients has suggested that there are polymorphisms in the promoter region of the IL-10 gene showing an association of low IL-10 haplotype and greater asthma severity [53] and increased IgE production [54].

In sensitized mice, exogenous administration of rIL-10 protein [55] or the IL-10 gene [56] can attenuate antigen-induced lung inflammation. A single intranasal administration of rmIL-10, concurrent to antigen challenge, significantly reduced eosinophil and neutrophil accumulation in the lung and TNF release from BAL fluid [55]. IL-10 gene therapy attenuated both cellular and physiological responses and reduced expression of inflammation cytokines such as TNF, IL-4 and IL-5, in the BAL fluid [56]. This effect was independent of Th1 cytokines such as IFN-γ.

Administration of antigen to allergic asthmatic subjects leads to bronchoconstriction, increased bronchial responsiveness and pulmonary inflammation. Inhibition of one or more of these effects by an investigational drug may indicate potential utility in clinical asthma, although absence of effect may not necessarily be predictive of lack of efficacy. In a recent double-blind study of a single parenteral dose of IL-10 there was no significant effect on the early or late bronchoconstrictor responses, on bronchial hyperresponsiveness or on inflammatory cells in BAL fluid [S. Lim and P. Barnes, pers. commun.]. It is possible that a higher single dose, multiple doses or local administration of IL-10 as used in the animal studies may be needed to show activity in humans. An accurate assessment of the effects of IL-10 awaits studies in clinical asthma.

Cystic Fibrosis. BAL fluid from subjects with CF contains less IL-10 than that of normal subjects, and bronchial epithelial cells from CF subjects secrete less IL-10 in vitro than those from normal donors [57–59]. Similarly, bronchial epithelial cells from uninfected CF mice also secrete less IL-10 in vitro than do cells from wild type mice, suggesting that decreased IL-10 production may be linked directly to defective CF transmembrane conductance regulator expression and/or function. IL-8 is an important, if not the major proinflammatory neutrophil chemoattractant in the CF lung [60, 61]. IL-8 and the other proinflammatory cytokines (IL-1, IL-6 and TNF) are greatly elevated in CF BAL fluid and are believed to be largely responsible for many manifestations of CF lung disease [58]. IL-10 inhibits production of all of these proinflammatory cytokines and, importantly, it inhibits all known sources of IL-8 production including epithelial cells, neutrophils and macrophages [62, 63]. It thus seems likely that decreased IL-10 production, especially by the bronchial epithelium, could contribute directly to the excessive pro-inflammatory cytokine and IL-8 production, accounting for the excessive inflammation in the CF lung.

COPD. In COPD, like other respiratory diseases, IL-10 levels in the airway are significantly reduced compared to normal controls [64]. Smokers also have lower concentrations than nonsmokers [64]. Pulmonary neutrophilic inflammation is a particularly prominent feature of COPD, and chemotactic cytokines secreted by neutrophils, such as IL-8, are important in maintaining the inflammation [61]. In vitro IL-10 is a potent inhibitor of neutrophil activation and release of proinflammatory cytokines and chemokines from neutrophils [62] and bronchial epithelium [63].

Following LPS administration to normal human volunteers there is a significant increase in proinflammatory cytokines and sequestration of neutrophils in the lungs as measured by granuloscintigraphy [49]. Granulocyte degranulation, as measured by plasma elastase/α_1-antitrypsin complexes, also occurs. Pretreatment with IL-10 shows a considerable reduction in all these parameters [49]. Administration of IL-10 1 h after LPS showed much more limited effects.

Recent data from a pilot study of IL-10 in patients with hepatitis C virus (HCV) infection suggest that IL-10 may also have anti-fibrotic effects. Patients with proven HCV infection, liver inflammation and fibrosis unresponsive to α-IFN, were treated with IL-10. Some showed significant improvements in liver fibrosis without effects on viremia [65]. If such an effect is confirmed, then IL-10 could have beneficial effects in conditions such as idiopathic pulmonary fibrosis where fibrosis is prominent or in other chronic lung diseases where airway remodeling may contribute to the long term outcome of the disease.

References

1 Fiorentino DF, Bond M, Mosmann TR: Two types of mouse helper T cell. IV. Th2 clones secrete a factor that inhibits cytokine production by Th1 clones. J Exp Med 1989;170:2081–2095.

2 Vieira P, de Waal-Malefyt R, Dang MN, et al: Isolation and expression of human cytokine synthesis inhibitory factor cDNA clones: Homology to Epstein-Barr virus open reading frame BCRF1. Proc Natl Acad Sci USA 1990; 88:1172–1176.

3 Moore KV, Vieira P, Fiorentino DF, et al: Homology of cytokine synthesis inhibitor factor (IL-10) to the Epstein-Barr virus gene BCRF1. Science 1990;248:1230–1234.

4 O'Garra A, Stapleton G, Dhar V, et al: Production of cytokines by mouse B cells: B lymphomas and normal B cells produce interleukin-10. Int Immunol 1990;2:821–832.

5 O'Garra A, Chang R, Go N, et al: Ly-1 B (B-1) cells are the main source of B cell-derived interleukin-10. Eur J Immunol 1992;22:711–717.

6 Thompson-Snipes L, Dhar V, Bond NW, et al: Interleukin-10: A novel stimulatory factor for mast cells and their progenitors. J Exp Med 1991;173:507–510.

7 Fiorentino DF, Zlotnik A, Mossmann TR, et al: IL-10 inhibits cytokine production by activated macrophages. J Immunol 1991;147:3815–3822.

8 Enk AH, Katz SI: Identification and induction of keratinocyte-derived IL-10. J Immunol 1992;149:92–95.

9 Yssel H, de Waal Malefyt R, Roncorolo M-G, et al: Interleukin 10 is produced by subsets of human CD4+ T cell clones and peripheral blood T cells. J Immunol 1992;149:2378–2384.

10 Tan JC, Indelicato S, Narula SK, et al: Characterization of interleukin-10 receptors on human and mouse cells. J Biol Chem 1993;268:21053–21059.

11 Ho AS-Y, Liu Y, Khan TA, et al: A receptor in interleukin-10 is related to interferon receptors. Proc Natl Acad Sci USA 1993;90:11267–11271.

12 Liu Y, Wei SH-Y, Ho AS-Y, et al: Expression cloning and characterization of a human interleukin-10 receptor. J Immunol 1994;152:1821–1829.

13 Kotenko, S, Krause, C, et al: Identification and function characterization of a second chain of the interleukin-10 receptor complex. EMBO J 1997;16:5894–5903.

14 Weber-Nordt RM, Meraz MA, Schreiber RD: LPS-dependent induction of IL-10 receptor expression on murine fibroblasts J Immunol 1994;153:3734–3744.

15 Weber-Nordt RM, Riley JK, Greenlund AC, et al: Stat3 recruitment by two distinct ligand-induced tyrosine phosphorylated docking sites in the IL-10 receptor intracellular domain. J Biol Chem 1996;271:27954–27961.

16 Finbloom DS, Winestock KD: IL-10 induces the tyrosine phosphorylation of tyk2 and Jak1 and the differential assembly of STAa and STAT3 complexes in human T cells and monocytes. J Immunol 1995;155:1079–1090.

17 Lai C, Ripperger J, et al: Receptors for interleukin (IL)-10 and IL-6 type cytokines use similar signaling mechanisms for inducing transcription through IL-6 response elements. J Biol Chem 1996;271:13968–13975.

18 Crawley J, Williams L, et al: Interleukin-10 stimulation of phosphatidylinositol 3-kinase and p70 S6 kinase is required for the proliferative but not the antiinflammatory effects of the cytokine. J Biol Chem 1996;271:16357–16362.

19 Ho AS-Y, Wei SH-Y Mui AL-F, et al: Functional regions of the mouse IL-10 receptor cytoplasmic domain. Mol Cell Biol 1995;15:5043–5053.

20 de Waal Malefyt R, Abrams J, Bennett B, et al: IL-10 inhibits cytokine synthesis by human monocytes: An autoregulatory role of IL-10 produced by monocytes. J Exp Med 1991;174:1209–1220.

21 Interleukin-10 inhibits cytokine production in vitro and in vivo and protects mice from lethal endotoxemia. Data on file at Schering-Plough Research Institute as P-5769 (December 1992).

22 Smith SR, Terminelli C, Kenworthy-Bott L, et al: The cooperative effects of TNF-α and IFN-γ are determining factors in the ability of IL-10 to protect mice from lethal endotoxemia. J Leukoc Biol 1994;55:711–718.

23 Howard M, Muchamuel T, Andrade S, Menon S, et al: Interleukin 10 protects mice from lethal endotoxemia. J Exp Med 1993;177:1205–1208.

24 Gerard C, Bruyns C, Marchant A, et al: IL-10 reduces the release of tumor necrosis factor and prevents lethality in experimental endotoxemia. J Exp Med 1993;177:547–550.

25 Fiorentino DF, Zlotnik A, Vieira P, et al: IL-10 acts on the antigen presenting cell to inhibit cytokine production by Th1 cells. J Immunol 1991;146:3444–3451.

26 de Waal Malefyt R, Haanen J, Spits H, et al: IL-10 and viral Il-10 strongly reduce antigen-specific human T cell proliferation by diminishing the antigen-presenting capacity of monocytes via downregulation of class II MHC expression. J Exp Med 1991;174:915–924.

27 Bazzoni F, Cassatella MA, Rossi F, et al: Phagocytosing neutrophils produce and release high amounts of the neutrophil activating peptide 1/interleukin 8. J Exp Med 1991;173:771–774.

28 Bazzoni F, Cassatella MA, Laudonna C, et al: Phagocytosis of opsonized yeast induces TNF-alpha mRNA and acccumulation and protein release by human polymorphonuclear leukocytes. J Leukoc Biol 1991;50:223–228.

29 Cassatella MA, Meda L, Bonora S, et al: Interleukin 10 (IL-10) inhibited the release of proinflammatory cytokines from human polymorphonuclear leukocytes. Evidence for an autocrine role of tumor necrosis factor and IL-in mediating the production of IL-8 triggered by lipopolysaccharide. J Exp Med 1993;178:2207–2211.

30 Rousset F, Garcia E, De France T, et al: Interleukin-10 is a potent growth and differentiation factor for abactivated human B cells. Proc Natl Acad Sci USA 1992;89:1890–1893.

31 Chen W-F, Zlotnik A: IL-10: A novel cytotoxic T cell differentiation factor. J Immunol 1991;47:528–534.

32 Hsu D-W, Moore KW, Spits H: Differential effects of IL-4 and IL-10 on IL-2 induced IFN-γ-synthesis and lymphokine-activated killer activity. Int Immunol 1992;4:563–569.

33 Schwarz M, Hamilton L, Tardelli L, Narula S, Sullivan L: Stimulation of cytolytic activity by interleukin-10. J Immunother 1994;16:95–104.

34 Cai G, Kastelein RA, Hunter CA: IL-10 enhances NK cell proliferation, cytotoxicity and production of IFN-gamma when combined with IL-18. Eur J Immunol 1999;29:2658–2665.

35 Berg DJ, Leach MW, Kuhn R, Rajewsky K, Muller W, Davidson NJ, Rennick D: Interleukin 10 but not interleukin 4 is a natural suppressant of cutaneous inflammation. J Exp Med 1995;182:99–108.

36 Kuhn R, Lohier J, Rennick D, et al: Interleukin-10 deficient mice develop chronic enterocolitis. Cell 1993;75:263–274.

37 Berg DJ, Davidson N, Kuhn R, et al: Enterocolitis and colon cancer in interleukin-10-deficient mice are associated with aberrant cytokine production and CD4+ TH1-like responses. J Clin Invest 1996;98:1010–1020.

38 Powrie F, Leach MW, Mauze S, et al: Inhibition of Th1 responses prevents inflammatory bowel disease in SCID mice reconstituted with CD45RB high CD4+ T cells. Immunity 1994;1:553–562.

39 Davidson NJ, Leach MW, Fort MM, Thompson-Snipes L, Kuhn W, Berg DJ, Rennick DM: T helper cell 1-type CD4+ T cells, but not B cells, mediate colitis in interleukin 10-deficient mice. J Exp Med 1996;184:241–251.

40 Tournoy KG, Kips JC, Pauwels RA: Absence of interleukin-10 aggravates allergic airway inflammation. Am J Respir Crit Care 1998;157:A701.

41 Grunig G, Corry DB, Leach MW, Seymour BWP, Kurup VP, Rennick DM: Interleukin-10 is a natural suppressor of cytokine production and inflammation in a murine model allergic bronchopulmonary aspergillosis. J Exp Med 1997;185:1089–1099.

42 Yu H, Hanes M, Chrisp CE, Boucher JC, Deretic V: Microbial pathogenesis in cystic fibrosis: Pulmonary clearance of mucoid Pseudomonas aeruginosa and inflammation in a mouse model of repeated respiratory challenge. Infect Immun 1998;66:280–288.

43 Stotland PK, Tam MF, Sapru K, Stevenson MM: Role of IL-10 in lung Pseudomonas aeruginosa infection in resistant and susceptible inbred mouse strains. Pediatr Pulmonol 1998;517:381.

44 Chmiel JF, Konstan MW, Knesebeck JE, Hilliard JB, Bonfield TL, Dawson DV, Berger M: IL-10 attenuates excessive inflammation in chronic pseudomonas infection in mice. Am J Respir Crit Care Med 1999;160:2040–2047.

45 van Heeckeren A, Walenga R, Konstan MW, Bonfield T, Davis PB, Ferkol T: Excessive inflammatory response of cystic fibrosis mice to bronchopulmonary infection with Pseudomonas aeruginosa. J Clin Invest 1997;100:2810-2815.

46 Huhn RD, Radwanski E, Gallo J, Affrime MB, Sabo R, Gonyo G, Monge A, Cutler DL: Pharmacodynamics of subcutaneous recombinant human interleukin-10 in healthy volunteers. Clin Pharmacol Ther 1997;62:171–180.

47 Radwanski E, Chakraborty A, Van Wart S, Huhn RD, Cutler DL, Affrime MB, Jusko WJ: Pharmacokinetics and leukocyte responses of recombinant human interleukin-10. Pharm Res 1998;15:1895–1901.

48 Huhn RD, Pennline K, Radwanski E, Clarke L, Sabo R, Cutler DL: Effects of single intravenous doses of recombinant human interleukin-10 on subsets of circulating leukocytes in humans. Immunopharmacology 1999;41:109–117.

49 Pajkrt D, Camoglio L, Tiel-van Buul MC, de Bruin D, Cutler DL, Affrime MB, Rikken G, van der Poll T, ten Cate JW, van Deventer SJ: Attenuation of proinflammatory response by recombinant human IL-10 in human endotoxemia: Effect of timing of recombinant human IL-10 administration. J Immunol 1997;158:3971–3977.

50 Borish L, Aarons A, Rumbyrt J, Cvietusa P, Negri J, Wenzel S: Interleukin-10 regulation in normal subjects and patients with asthma. J Allergy Clin Immunol 1996;97:1288–1296.

51 Tormey VJ, Leonard C, Faul J, Bernard S, Burke CM, Poulter LW: Dysregulation of monocyte differentiation in asthmatic subjects is reversed by IL-10. Clin Exp Allergy 1998;28:992–998.

52 John M, Lim S, Seybold J, Jose P, Robichaud A, O'Connor B, Barnes PJ, Chung KF: Inhaled corticosteroids increase interleukin-10 but reduce macrophage inflammatory protein-1alpha, granulocyte-macrophage colony-stimulating factor, and interferon-gamma release from alveolar macrophages in asthma. Am J Respir Crit Care Med 1998;157:256–262.

53 Lim S, Crawley E, Woo P, Barnes PJ: Haplotype associated with low interleukin-10 production in patients with severe asthma. Lancet 1998;352:113.

54 Hobbs K, Negri J, Klinnert M, Rosenwasser LJ, Borish L: Interleukin-10 and transforming growth factor-beta promoter polymorphisms in allergies and asthma. Am J Respir Crit Care Med 1998;158:1958–1962.

55 Zuany-Amorim C, Haile S, Leduc D, Dumarey C, Huerre M, Vargaftig BB, Pretolani M: Interleukin-10 inhibits antigen-induced cellular recruitment into the airways of sensitized mice. J Clin Invest 1995;95:2644–2651.

56 Stampfli MR, Cwiartka M, Gajewska BU, Alvarez D, Ritz SA, Inman MD, Xing Z, Jordana M: Interleukin-10 gene transfer to the airway regulates allergic mucosal sensitization in mice. Am J Respir Cell Mol Biol 1999;21:586–596.

57 Bonfield TL, Konstan MW, Berger M: Altered respiratory epithelial cell cytokine production in cystic fibrosis. J Allergy Clin Immunol 1999;104:72–78.

58 Bonfield TL, Panuska JR, Konstan MW, et al: Inflammatory cytokines in cystic fibrosis lungs. Am J Respir Crit Care Med 1995;152:2111–2118.

59 Bonfield TL, Konstan MW, Burfeind P, et al: Normal bronchial epithelial cells constitutively produce the anti-inflammatory cytokine IL-10 which is down-regulated in cystic fibrosis. Am J Respir Cell Mol Biol 1995;13:257–261.

60 Dean TP, Dai Y, Shute JK, et al: Interleukin-8 concentrations are elevated in bronchoalveolar lavage, sputum, and sera of children with cystic fibrosis. Pediatr Res 1993;34:159–161.

61 Richman-Eisenstat JB, Jorens PG, Heberg CA, et al: Interleukin-8: An important chemoattractant in sputum of subjects with chronic inflammatory airway diseases. Am J Physiol 1993;264:L413–L418.

62 Wang P, Wu P, Anthes JC, Siegel MI, Egan RW, Billah MM: Interleukin-10 inhibits interleukin-8 production in human neutrophils. Blood 1994;83:2678–2683.

63 Bonfield TL, Konstan MW, Berger M: Interleukin-10 suppresses IL-8 secretion by bronchial epithelial cells. Pediatr Pulmonol 1998;517:286.

64 Takanashi S, Hasegawa Y, Kanehira Y, Yamamoto K, Fujimoto K, Satoh K, Okamura K: Interleukin-10 level in sputum is reduced in bronchial asthma, COPD and in smokers. Eur Respir J 1999;14:309–314.

65 Nelson DR, Lauwers GY, Lau JY, Davis GL: Interleukin 10 treatment reduces fibrosis in patients with chronic hepatitis C: A pilot trial of interferon nonresponders. Gastroenterology 2000;118:655–660.

Satwant Narula
Department of Immunology and
Allergy Drug Discovery
Schering-Plough Research Institute
2015 Galloping Hill Road
Kenilworth, NJ 07033 (USA)
Tel. +1 908 740 7303, Fax +1 908 740 7305
E-Mail satwant.narula@spcorp.com

Interleukin-12, Interleukin-18 and Interferon-γ

Shannon Bryan[a]   Michiko Kobayashi[b]   Sanjiv Sur[c]

[a] National Heart and Lung Institute, Clinical Studies Unit, Imperial College, London, UK;
[b] Immunology and Hemostasis, Genetics Institute of Wyeth-Ayerst Research, Andover, Mass., USA, and
[c] Department of Internal Medicine, Division of Allergy and Immunology, NIAID Asthma Center, University of Texas Medical Branch, Galveston, Tex., USA

Summary

IL-12 has been shown to be instrumental in the development of T-helper type 1 (Th1) responses while inhibiting the generation of T-helper type 2 (Th2) responses that are thought to contribute to the inflammation present in asthma and allergy. This mechanism of action is largely due to its ability to induce Th1 cytokine production, namely interferon (IFN)-γ, from T cells and natural killer (NK) cells. IL-18 does not drive Th1 development independently, but rather potentiates IL-12-induced Th1 development and synergizes with IL-12 to induce maximal production of IFN-γ from T cells and NK cells. However, depending on the local milieu of IL-4 or IL-12, IL-18 can augment both Th1 and Th2 pathways. IFN-γ inhibits Th2 responses thereby decreasing inflammatory cytokine production. Therefore IL-12, IL-18 and IFN-γ have potential for therapeutic utilization in allergy and asthma, by promoting Th1 responses and suppressing Th2 responses which are believed to contribute to the pathogenesis of the disease.

Molecular Mechanisms of Action

IL-12 is a heterodimeric cytokine that binds with high affinity to its receptor expressed on T cells and natural killer (NK) cells, causing activation of tyrosine kinases JAK2 and TYK2, as well as nuclear translocation of signal transducers and activators of transcription (STAT) 3 and 4 that trigger the promoter regions for the interferon (IFN)-γ gene [1] (fig. 1). It has been shown that mice deficient in STAT4 produce reduced amounts of IFN-γ in response to IL-12 and have impaired Th1 activity, indicating that STAT4 is essential for IL-12 responses [2]. IFN-γ upregulates expression of the high-affinity IL-12 receptor, which is downregulated by the Th2 cytokine IL-4 [3].

IL-18 is a recently cloned cytokine synthesized by murine macrophages [4] and is a member of the IL-1 family. It is synthesized as a biologically inactive precursor molecule (pro-IL-18) and requires cleavage into an active molecule by the intracellular cysteine protease IL-1β-converting enzyme (ICE) or caspase-1. IL-18 signals through IL-1R-activating kinase (IRAK) and induces nuclear translocation of nuclear factor (NF)-κB [5] (fig. 1). It acts through an IL-18 receptor (IL-18R) complex which has been shown to be expressed selectively on murine Th1 cells but not on Th2 cells [6]. IL-12 upregulates the expression of the IL-18 receptor in both T and NK cells.

IFN-γ is produced by CD4+ and CD8+ T cells as well as NK cells and its receptor is expressed on T cells, B cells, monocytes/macrophages, dendritic cells, platelets and granulocytes as well as epithelial and endothelial cells. Binding of IFN-γ to the receptor activates STAT1 and induces a variety of genes in many cell types including T cells, NK cells and antigen-presenting cells (APCs). Inhibitory effects of IFN-γ are specific to Th2 cells and not Th1 cells, which do not express its receptor.

Cellular Mechanisms of Action (fig. 2)

Bacteria, bacterial products, intracellular pathogens and viruses rapidly induce IL-12 production by APCs, such as monocytes/macrophages, B lymphocytes and dendritic cells (fig. 2). IL-12 enhances the functions of acti-

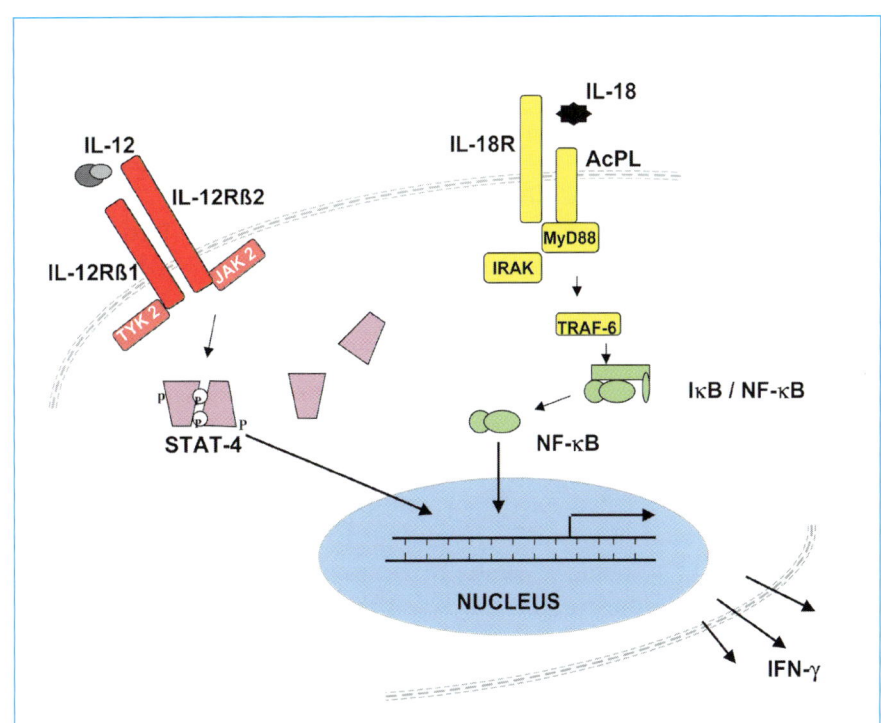

Fig. 1. IL-12 and IL-18 signalling pathways producing IFN-γ via activation of STAT4 and NF-κB.

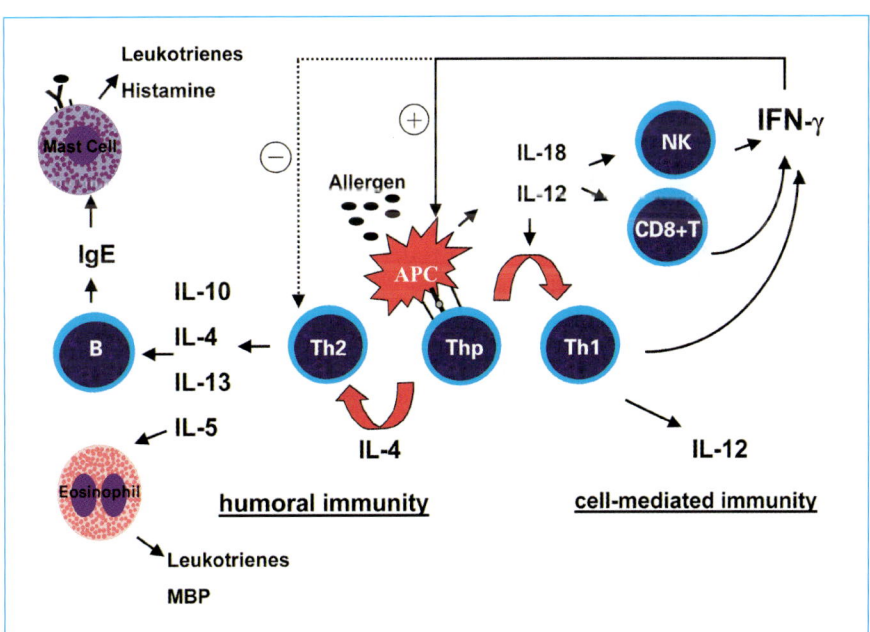

Fig. 2. Th1 and Th2 cell regulation, cytokine production and cellular effects.

vated T cells and NK cells, such as proliferation, cytotoxic activity and cytokine production. In particular, it stimulates both T cells and NK cells to secrete IFN-γ. IFN-γ then activates APCs, enhances IL-12 production, causes naïve T cells to differentiate into Th1 cells and inhibits Th2 responses [7, 8]. It primes T cells early to release IFN-γ, therefore regulating Th1 differentiation and suppressing Th2 responses.

IL-18 or IFN-γ-inducing factor (IGIF) can be synthesized by Kupffer cells and activated macrophages. This cytokine synergizes with IL-12 to induce IFN-γ production from Th1 cells, NK cells and B cells [9]. Together with IL-12, IL-18 induces anti-CD40-activated B cells to produce IFN-γ, which inhibits IL-4-dependent IgE production. IL-18 and IL-12 have synergistic effects on Th1 development, which is in part due to reciprocal upregulation of their receptors [9].

IFN-γ is able to activate APCs, T cells and NK cells and potentiate Th1 responses while suppressing Th2 responses. T cells from asthmatic subjects have been shown to produce reduced quantities of IFN-γ [10].

Animal Models

Intraperitoneal administration of IL-12 has been shown to suppress antigen-induced airway eosinophilia in sensitized mice [11]. Intranasal IL-12 administered to sensitized mice prevented airway hyperresponsiveness (AHR) and reduced airway eosinophilia after allergen challenge without systemic effects [12]. Doses of IL-12 administered early during allergen sensitization were found to be more effective in reducing IgE and inflammatory cytokine levels in animals than those given later in the sensitization process [13]. This finding has implications for IL-12 as a therapy for allergy or asthma as the timing relative to allergen exposure is crucial.

IL-18 –/– mice have been shown to have defective Th1 and NK cell responses suggesting a role for IL-18 in Th1 responses [14]. Mice deficient in IL-18 have decreased INF-γ production even though their levels of IL-12 are normal. However, in a study where IL-18 was given to sensitized mice before ovalbumin challenge, there was increased eosinophil recruitment into the lungs [15]. Similar findings in other studies have shown that IL-18 can induce a Th2 phenotype suggesting it plays a role in allergic sensitization [16]. Also, IL-18 levels in whole-lung homogenate from allergic mice have been found to be higher than those from non-allergic mice [17]. In the same study, administration of a neutralizing antibody against IL-18 prior to challenge increased bronchial eosinophilia. Paradoxically, administration of recombinant IL-18 at the time of allergen challenge also increased eosinophil numbers in both bronchoalveolar lavage (BAL) fluid and in the bronchus, and was associated with an increase in the level of eotaxin in the BAL fluid. Therefore there is a paradox in the relationship of IL-18 in allergy and asthma and this is yet to be clarified.

In IFN-γ knockout mice, IL-12 is pro-inflammatory, inducing an eosinophilia and increased serum IgE levels, indicating that IL-12 inhibits Th2 cells through the production of IFN-γ. It has been shown to inhibit eosinophil accumulation in the trachea of antigen-challenged mice. However, it also has been shown to exhibit some pro-inflammatory effects. Over-expression of IFN-γ was shown to be toxic when IL-12 was administered along with IL-18 [18] and IL-12 alone induced toxic effects in primates and mice which were largely due to induction of IFN-γ production.

Rationale

Cord blood from infants with a family history of atopy is deficient in IFN-γ production due to impaired IL-12 responses [19]. Reduced levels of IL-12 are found in blood from adults with allergic asthma [20], resulting in increased IgE and IL-5 production. Furthermore, IL-12 inhibits AHR and airway eosinophilia following antigen challenge in a number of animal models of allergen sensitization as above. Therefore, IL-12 appears to be a logical treatment for human allergic asthma.

IL-18 is downregulated in the lungs of asthmatics [21], but is expressed constitutively in normal lung epithelium. Since it acts in synergy with IL-12 in up-regulating IFN-γ production in animal studies, it too may be a possible therapy in altering the immune response in allergic disease. But given the above disparity between its anti-inflammatory and pro-inflammatory effects, it is difficult to justify its use in asthma until more information becomes available.

Clinical Studies in Humans

In a clinical study in patients with mild asthma, subcutaneous recombinant IL-12 was assessed for its effect on the late-phase response after inhaled allergen challenge as well as on AHR. A gradual dose escalation was carried out to minimize the side effects. There was no effect on AHR or the late-phase response. However, subcutaneous IL-12 significantly reduced blood eosinophils and prevented an increase in blood eosinophils after allergen challenge (fig. 3). A trend towards reduction in sputum eosinophils was noted. Side effects such as flu-like symptoms and raised liver transaminases occurred in some patients receiving IL-12, and these corresponded with the peak plasma levels of the drug about 3–4 h after administration. However, the frequency and severity of the side effects decreased with repeated administration of IL-12. Some major side effects were experienced in a few subjects receiving IL-12, for example cardiac arrhythmias, severe flu-like symptoms and abnormal liver function tests [unpubl. data]. In previous studies, administration of higher doses of intravenous IL-12 in the treatment of renal cancer was associated with severe schedule-dependent toxicity (hepatotoxicity, gastrointestinal bleeding, fever, chills and death in 2 patients) [22]. Subsequent

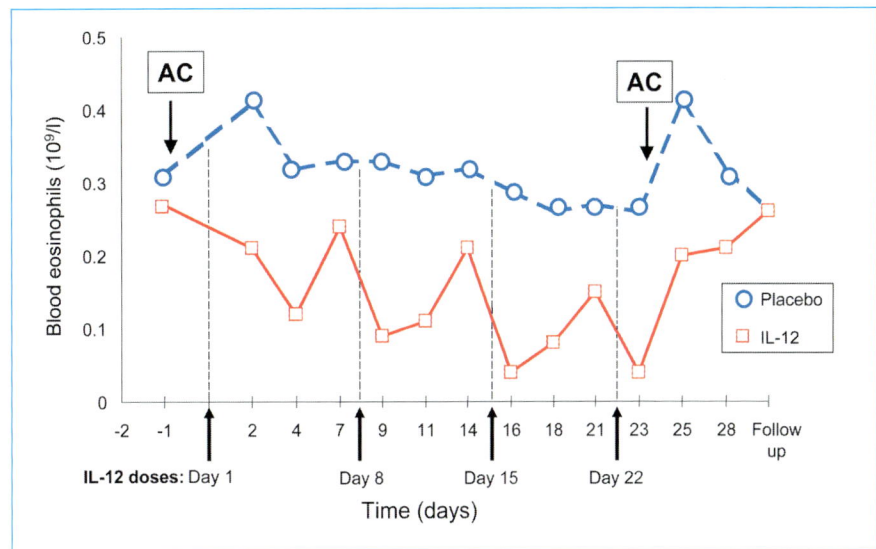

Fig. 3. Peripheral blood eosinophil levels in asthmatics after administration of systemic IL-12. AC = Allergen challenge.

studies have shown similar toxicity that is related to dose level. A further trial using nebulized IL-12 in a dose-rising study was performed in patients with mild asthma. The study was terminated after 8 subjects received a single 1-μg dose of inhaled IL-12. Adverse events such as coughing and wheezing and fluctuations in lung function were observed. Both placebo-treated and IL-12-treated patients suffered side effects and therefore the study was inconclusive, as the side effects could not be attributed to the nebulized IL-12. The threshold to terminate the study secondary to side effects was also very low to ensure safety, and therefore the efficacy of nebulized IL-12 has not yet been determined [unpubl. data].

To our knowledge, IL-18 has not been tested in human clinical trials yet.

Subcutaneous recombinant INF-γ was administered to subjects with ragweed allergy but had no significant effects on the symptom scores or serum IgE antibody to ragweed extract, indicating that treatment with IFN-γ is not useful in ragweed hayfever [23]. Systemic IFN-γ (intramuscular) caused side effects such as nausea, vomiting, fever and headache; however, nebulized IFN-γ was found to be well tolerated [24].

Route of Administration

Inhaled IL-12 may be an alternative to subcutaneous or other forms of systemic delivery of the drug in order to achieve high levels in the lungs and lower systemic levels, thus avoiding toxic effects. Nebulized IL-12 has been investigated in mice [12], which was shown to inhibit AHR. Further studies looking at mucosal administration of IL-12 have shown low systemic levels of IL-12 and good inhibition of airway eosinophilia as well as increasing IFN-γ expression in BAL fluid cells.

Conclusions

From studies that have been conducted in patients with asthma, it appears that IL-12 administered systemically at the doses used previously is too toxic for the treatment of mild asthma. However, these trials have been performed using systemic doses at the maximum tolerated dose, and the use of low-dose IL-12 has not yet been fully explored. Although there have been prior reports of adverse events associated with administration of IL-12, these have largely been with the use of high doses in the first studies, and in the more recent studies, lower doses have been explored. Following the introduction of gradual incremental dose increases, rh IL-12 has been used to safely treat several hundred patients. IL-12 may be useful if administered in nebulized or inhaled formulations at the same time as allergen sensitization to suppress allergic responses or to nebulize IL-12 during the allergic seasons to augment the immunomodulating potential of IL-12. Thus IL-12 remains a potential treatment for asthma and allergy if used as a vaccine adjuvant for inducing long-term immunomodulatory effects, rather than as an alternative for other anti-inflammatory drugs already known to be safe such as corticosteroids.

The role of IL-18 in asthma and allergy is complex, and more studies are required to assess the involvement of this cytokine in allergic inflammation. It appears to act as a bi-directional adjuvant in that it may synergize with IL-12 or IL-4, therefore amplifying either Th1 or Th2 responses. The use of IL-18 in conjunction with lower doses of IL-12 to reduce IL-12 toxicity may be a further option for using these cytokines to treat allergy.

Systematically administered, IFN-γ is unlikely to be a useful treatment for asthma or allergy because of its poor efficacy and significant side effects. However, further studies are ongoing investigating the use of nebulized IFN-γ.

References

1 Hasko G, Szabo C: IL-12 as a therapeutic target for pharmacological modulation in immune-mediated and inflammatory diseases: Regulation of T helper 1/T helper 2 responses. Br J Pharmacol 1999;127:1295–1304.
2 Kaplan MH, Sun Y, Hoey T, Grusby MJ: Impaired IL-12 responses and enhanced development of Th2 cells in Stat4-deficient mice. Nature 1996;382:174–177.
3 Szabo SJ, Dighe AS, Gubler U, Murphy KM: Regulation of the interleukin (IL)-12R β2 subunit expression in developing T helper 1 (TH1) and Th2 cells. J Exp Med 1997;185:817–824.
4 Okamura H, Tsutsi H, Komatsu T, Yutsudo M, Hakura A, Tanimoto T, Torigoe K, Okura T, Nukada Y, Hattori K: Cloning of a new cytokine that influences IFN-γ production by T cells. Nature 1995;378:88–91.
5 Matsumoto S, Tsuji-Takayama K, Aizawa Y, Koide K, Takeuchi M, Ohta T, Kurimoto M: Interleukin-18 activates NF-κB in murine T helper type 1 cells. Biochem Biophys Res Commun 1997;234:454–457.
6 Xu D, Chan WL, Leung BP, Hunter D, Schulz K, Carter RW, McInnes IB, Robinson JH, Liew FY: Selective expression and functions of interleukin 18 receptor on T helper (Th) type 1 but not Th2 cells. J Exp Med 1998;188:1485–1492.
7 Chung KF, Barnes PJ: Cytokines in asthma. Thorax 1999;54:825–857.
8 Trinchieri G: Interleukin-12: A cytokine at the interface of inflammation and immunity. Adv Immunol 1998;70:83–243.
9 Dinarello CA: IL-18: A new T_{H1}-inducing, proinflammatory cytokine and new member of the IL-1 family. J Allergy Clin Immunol 1999;103:11–24.
10 Koning H, Neijens HJ, Baert MR, Savelkoul HF, Savelkoul HF: T cell subsets and cytokines in allergic and non-allergic children. I. Analysis of IL-4, IFN-gamma and IL-13 mRNA expression and protein production. Cytokine 1997;9:416–426.
11 Iwamoto I, Kumano K, Kasai M, Kurasawa K: Interleukin-12 prevents antigen-induced eosinophil recruitment into mouse airways. Am J Respir Crit Care Med 1996;154:1257–1260.
12 Schwarze J, Hamelmann E, Cieslewicz G, Tomkinson A, Joetham A, Bradley K, Gelfand EW: Local treatment with IL-12 is an effective inhibitor of airway hyperresponsiveness and lung eosinophilia after airway challenge in sensitized mice. J Allergy Clin Immunol 1998;102:86–93.
13 Sur S, Lam J, Bouchard P, Sigounas A, Holbert D, Metzger WJ: Immunomodulatory effects of IL-12 on allergic lung inflammation depend on timing of doses. J Immunol 1996;157:4173–4180.
14 Takeda K, Tsutsui H, Yoshimoto T, Adachi O, Yoshida N, Kishimoto T, Okamura H, Nakanishi K, Akira S: Defective NK cell activity and Th1 response in IL-18 deficient mice. Immunity 1998;8:383–390.
15 Kumano K, Nakao A, Nakajima H, Hayashi F, Kurimoto M, Okamura H, Saito Y, Iwamoto I: Interleukin-18 enhances antigen-induced eosinophil recruitment into the mouse airways. Am J Resp Crit Care Med 1999;160:873–878.
16 Wild JS, Sigounas A, Sur N, Siddiqui MS, Alam R, Kurimoto M, Sur S: IFN-γ inducing factor (IL-18) increases allergic sensitization, serum IgE, Th2 cytokines, and airway eosinophilia in a mouse model of allergic asthma. J Immunol 2000;164:2701–2710.
17 Campbell E, Kunkel S, Strieter RM, Lukacs NW: Differential roles of IL-18 in allergic airway disease: Induction of eotaxin by resident cell populations exacerbates eosinophil accumulation. J Immunol 2000;164:1096–1102.
18 Okamura H, Kashiwamura S, Tsutsui H, Yoshimoto T: Regulation of interferon-gamma production by IL-12 and IL-18. Curr Opin Immunol 1998;10:259–264.
19 Prescott SL, Holt PG: Abnormalities in cord blood mononuclear cytokine production as a predictor of later atopic disease in childhood. Clin Exp Allergy 1998;28:1313–1316.
20 van der Pouw Kraan TCTM, Boeije LCM, de Groot ER, Stapel SO, Snijders A, Kapsenberg ML, Zee JS, Aarden LA: Reduced production of Il-12 and Il-12-dependent IFN-γ release in patients with allergic asthma. J Immunol 1997;158:5560–5565.
21 Cameron LA, Taha RA, Tsicopoulos A, Kurimoto M, Olivenstein R, Wallaert B, Minshall EM, Hamid Q: Airway epithelium expresses interleukin-18. Eur Respir J 1999;14:553–559.
22 Leonard JP, Sherman ML, Fisher GL, Buchanan LJ, Larsen G, Atkins MB, Sosman JA, Dutcher JP, Vogelzang NJ, Ryan JL: Effect of single-dose interleukin-12 exposure on interleukin-12-associated toxicity and interferon-γ production. Blood 1997;90:2541–2548.
23 Li JT, Yunginger JW, Reed CE, Jaffe HS, Nelson DR, Gleich GJ: Lack of suppression of IgE production by recombinant interferon gamma: A controlled trial in patients with allergic rhinitis. J Allergy Clin Immunol 1990;85:934–940.
24 Martin RJ, Boguniewicz M, Henson JE, Celniker AC, Williams M, Giorno RC, Leung D Y: The effects of inhaled interferon gamma in normal human airways. Am Rev Respir Dis 1993;148:1677–1682.

Dr. Shannon Bryan
Clinical Studies Unit
Royal Brompton Hospital
Fulham Road, London SW3 6HP (UK)
Tel. +44 207 351 8977, Fax +44 207 351 8973
E-Mail s.bryan@ic.ac.uk

Chemokine Receptor Inhibition

Chemokines: An Overview

Ian Sabroe   Timothy J. Williams

Imperial College, Division of Biomedical Sciences, South Kensington, UK

Summary

Chemokines, signalling via specific leukocyte chemokine receptors, are probably the major mediators of selective leukocyte recruitment, and hence must play a major role in inflammatory disease. Small molecule antagonists of leukocyte chemokine receptors are now in development and may prove to be effective inhibitors of recruitment of lymphocytes, monocytes and granulocytes in a wide variety of settings. Thus, these antagonists may prove to be useful treatments for diseases such as asthma and COPD.

Chemokines, Chemokine Receptors, and Their Roles in Leukocyte Recruitment

Inflammatory diseases such as asthma and COPD are characterized by the recruitment of leukocytes from the circulation into the lung. In asthma, eosinophils, neutrophils and lymphocytes all play a significant role in disease pathology. Similarly, neutrophil, monocyte and perhaps eosinophil recruitment are important in the pathology of COPD.

At sites of inflammation, leukocytes are recruited from the microcirculation in a three-stage process. The leukocytes initially interact with the vessel wall through selectin adhesion molecules. Upon encountering chemoattractants, leukocytes become tightly adherent to the vessel wall. Leukocyte diapedesis into tissues then follows along the chemoattractant concentration gradient (fig. 1). Pro-inflammatory mediators such as C5a, LTB_4 and PAF cause non-selective recruitment of these cells, but cannot account for the specific patterns of leukocyte infiltration

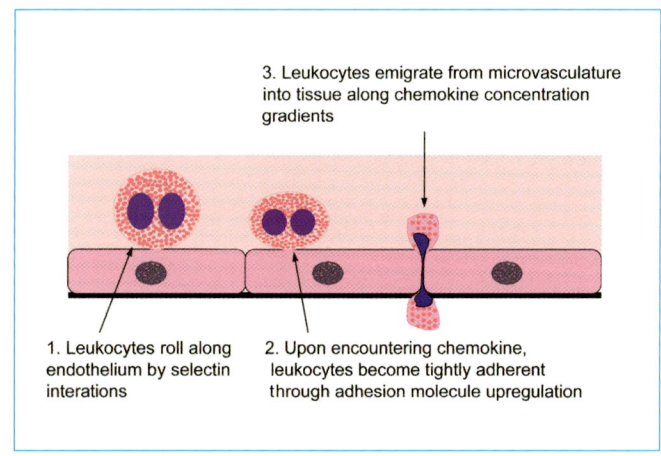

Fig. 1. Roles of chemokines in leukocyte recruitment.

observed in disease. The discovery in the last 12 years of a group of proteins capable of causing selective leukocyte recruitment, the chemoattractant cytokines (chemokines), brought about a major revolution in this field. To date, 39 chemokines have been identified; these molecules act selectively on specific members of the chemokine receptor family, expressed on leukocytes [1, 2], and there are further chemokines and receptors whose function is yet unknown.

Viruses provide further indirect indicators of the importance of chemokines, since several viruses have evolved techniques of subverting immune regulation

Table 1. Chemokines in asthma and COPD

Cell type	Receptor	Ligands	Roles
Eosinophil	CCR1	MIP-1α, RANTES, MCP-3	uncertain: may have a role in eosinophil recruitment or activation
	CCR3	Eotaxin, eotaxin-2, eotaxin-3, MCP-3, MCP-4, RANTES, MCP-2	likely to have major role in eosinophil recruitment and perhaps activation, also a role in eosinophil trafficking to mucosal sites
	CXCR2	MGSA/Gro-α, NAP-2, IL-8, GCP-2	uncertain: may have a role in eosinophil recruitment in atopic individuals
	CCR6	MIP-3α	uncertain: possible role in eosinophil recruitment and activation
T lymphocyte (Th2 subtype)	CCR3, CCR4, CCR8	CCR3: as above CCR4: MDC, TARC CCR8: I-309	probable role in lymphocyte trafficking or recruitment to sites of inflammation
T lymphocyte (Th1 subtype)	CXCR3, CCR5, CCR4	CXCR3: Mig, IP-10, ITAC CCR5: RANTES, MIP-1α, MIP-1β CCR4: as above	probable role in lymphocyte trafficking or recruitment to sites of inflammation
Neutrophil	CXCR1	IL-8, GCP-2	major roles in neutrophil recruitment, and probably in activation
	CXCR2	As above	probable important role in neutrophil recruitment

through the production of viral chemokine receptors, viral chemokines, or chemokine-binding proteins [3, 4].

Chemokines are synthesized by many cell types including leukocytes, endothelial cells, epithelial cells, smooth muscle cells and fibroblasts. These molecules are divided into four structural groups, based on the organization of the first two of their four conserved cysteine amino acids. Two major families exist: CC chemokines, in which the first two cysteines are adjacent, and CXC chemokines, where they are separated by a single amino acid. Two other chemokines have been described: a C chemokine with a single n-terminal cysteine (lymphotactin), and a CX_3C chemokine (fractalkine) with 3 intervening amino acids. Chemokine nomenclature has been a haphazard process based upon considerations of structural homology, function, or more esoteric notions, however a recent international meeting has proposed a more logical nomenclature that may become generally adopted soon. The receptors for these chemokines are expressed in specific patterns on subsets of leukocytes. Each receptor binds selected members of one of the family of chemokines, and are named accordingly as CXCR1 to 5, CCR1 to 11, XCR1 and CX_3CR1 [1, 2] (table 1).

Chemokine receptor expression by leukocytes is not irreversibly fixed, but may vary under certain stimuli by processes including internalization or shedding of receptors (after both homologous and heterologous stimulation) or expression of new receptors. Therefore, chemokine functions on leukocytes in tissues may be different from the more simple experiments examining their roles in vitro using blood-derived cells [5].

Further Roles of Chemokines

In addition to their major roles in local leukocyte recruitment from the microcirculation, chemokines also have distant effects on the bone marrow which enhance leukocyte recruitment. The systemic administration of eotaxin mobilizes eosinophils and their progenitors from the bone marrow [6], whilst IL-8 induces neutrophil release. Additionally, signalling via chemokine receptors may cause leukocyte activation as determined by superoxide generation or degranulation.

Chemokines and Their Receptors in Asthma

The eosinophil may be a central effector cell in asthma. Studies have described eosinophil expression of chemokine receptors including CCR1, CCR3 and CXCR2 [7, 8]. The principal eosinophil chemokine receptor is CCR3, whose ligands include the eotaxin group of chemokines. The eotaxins are unusual in that they only stimulate cells via CCR3 and no other chemokine receptor. Eotaxin causes eosinophil recruitment, superoxide generation and degranulation. CCR3 is also expressed on other cells with specific roles in allergic inflammation, including mast cells and basophils, and is therefore a major drug target. A cautionary note is sounded by research in man showing variations between individuals in eosinophil responses to ligands signalling via CCR1 [8].

Severe asthma is also associated with a marked tissue recruitment of neutrophils, probably mediated by members of the CXC family of chemokines such as IL-8 [9].

Allergic inflammation is regulated by T cells of the Th2 subtype. Much interest has been stimulated by the recent discovery that T cells differentiated to a Th2 phenotype in vitro express CCR3, CCR4 and CCR8 [10–12]. Thus, CCR3 antagonists may modulate the recruitment of Th2 cells and hence the regulation of allergic inflammation in asthma. (CCR4 is also likely to be expressed on Th1 type human T cells [13], and the role of CCR8 in vivo has yet to be addressed.) There is further evidence that the chemokine MCP-1, signalling via the CCR2 receptor, may also play a significant role in the regulation of Th1/Th2 differentiation [14].

Future innovations in asthma therapy may come from the modification of sensitization to allergens. Dendritic cells express selected chemokine receptors that are altered during maturation and are involved in localization of dendritic cells to lymph nodes in order to facilitate antigen presentation to T cells [15].

Chemokines and Their Receptors in COPD

The potential role of chemokines in the slowly progressive inflammation of COPD is less well characterized than that of asthma, although animal models have contributed to our understanding of this condition [16]. Neutrophils may have a major role in the pathology of COPD. These cells express two major receptors, CXCR1 and CXCR2. In vitro evidence suggests that CXCR2 may be more relevant in mediating neutrophil recruitment and CXCR1 in causing neutrophil activation [17]. Neutrophil chemokine receptor phenotype may also be altered in inflammation with the expression of CCR1 and CCR3 [18], suggesting that CC chemokines may play a role in neutrophil function in disease. Other studies have identified roles for macrophages in the pathology of COPD, with an emphasis on their generation of matrix metalloproteinases [19]. In keeping with this, the expression of MCP-1, which acts on the receptor CCR2 and has a major role in monocyte recruitment, is upregulated in COPD [20]. Regulatory lymphocytes, both CD4+ and CD8+, may also play a role in COPD, although the chemokine receptor profile of T cells in COPD has yet to be investigated [21].

Antagonism of Chemokine Function in Human Disease

Since multiple chemokines are active on each receptor, the targeting of single chemokine ligands, by neutralizing humanized antibodies or similar strategies, is unlikely to be effective. In contrast, the selective expression patterns of chemokine receptors suggests that antagonism of these receptors is a feasible therapeutic strategy. These receptors are of the 7-transmembrane, G-protein coupled class, whose historical antagonism (β-blockers, H_2-receptor antagonists) is well established. Small molecule antagonists of CCR1, CCR2, and CXCR2 have been published [22–24], and antagonists of CCR3 have been identified in the patent literature. The plethora of roles of chemokines in the regulation of inflammation suggests that chemokine receptor antagonists may be significant additions to our pharmacological armamentarium.

References

1 Luster AD: Chemokines – chemotactic cytokines that mediate inflammation. N Engl J Med 1998;338:436–445.
2 Homey B, Zlotnik A: Chemokines in allergy. Curr Opin Immunol 1999;11:626–634.
3 Alcamí A, Symons JA, Collins PD, Williams TJ, Smith GL: Blockade of chemokine activity by a soluble chemokine binding protein from a vaccinia virus. J Immunol 1998;160:624–633.
4 Bodaghi B, Jones TR, Zipeto D, Vita C, Sun L, Laurent L, Arenzana-Seisdedos F, Virelizier JL, Michelson S: Chemokine sequestration by viral chemoreceptors as a novel viral escape strategy: Withdrawal of chemokines from the environment of cytomegalovirus-infected cells. J Exp Med 1998;188:855–856.
5 Lukacs NW, Oliveira SH, Hogaboam CM: Chemokines and asthma: Redundancy of function or a coordinated effort? J Clin Invest 1999; 104:995–999.
6 Palframan RT, Collins PD, Williams TJ, Rankin SM: Eotaxin induces a rapid release of eosinophils and their progenitors from the bone marrow. Blood 1998;91:2240–2248.
7 Ponath PD, Qin S, Ringler DJ, Clark-Lewis I, Wang J, Kassam N, Smith H, Shi X, Gonzalo JA, Newman W, Gutierrez-Ramos JC, Mackay CR: Cloning of the human eosinophil chemoattractant, eotaxin. Expression, receptor binding, and functional properties suggest a mechanism for the selective recruitment of eosinophils. J Clin Invest 1996;97:604–612.
8 Sabroe I, Hartnell A, Jopling LA, Bel S, Ponath P, Pease JE, Collins PD, Williams TJ: Differential regulation of eosinophil chemokine signaling via CCR3 and non-CCR3 pathways. J Immunol 1999;162:2946–2955.
9 Wenzel SE, Schwartz LB, Langmack EL, Halliday JL, Trudeau JB, Gibbs RL, Chu EW: Evidence that severe asthma can be divided pathologically into two inflammatory subtypes with distinct physiologic and clinical characteristics. Am J Respir Crit Care Med 1999;160:1001–1008.
10 Gerber BO, Zanni MP, Uguccioni M, Loetscher M, Mackay CR, Pichler WJ, Yawalkar N, Baggiolini M, Moser B: Functional expression of the eotaxin receptor CCR3 in T lymphocytes co-localizing with eosinophils. Curr Biol 1997; 7:836–843.
11 Sallusto F, Mackay CR, Lanzavecchia A: Selective expression of the eotaxin receptor CCR3 by human T helper 2 cells. Science 1997; 277:2005–2007.
12 Bonecchi R, Bianchi G, Bordignon PP, D'Ambrosio D, Lang R, Borsatti A, Sozzani S, Allavena P, Gray PA, Mantovani A, Sinigaglia F: Differential expression of chemokine receptors and chemotactic responsiveness of type 1 T helper cells (Th1s) and Th2s. J Exp Med 1998; 187:129–134.
13 Campbell JJ, Haraldsen G, Pan J, Rottman J, Qin S, Ponath P, Andrew DP, Warnke R, Ruffing N, Kassam N, Wu L, Butcher EC: The chemokine receptor CCR4 in vascular recognition by cutaneous but not intestinal memory T cells. Nature 1999;400:776–780.
14 Gu L, Tseng S, Horner RM, Tam C, Loda M, Rollins BJ: Control of TH2 polarization by the chemokine monocyte chemoattractant protein-1. Nature 2000;404:407–411.
15 Sozzani S, Allavena P, Vecchi A, Mantovani A: The role of chemokines in the regulation of dendritic cell trafficking. J Leukoc Biol 1999; 66:1–9.

16 Shapiro SD: Animal models for chronic obstructive pulmonary disease. Age of klotho and marlboro mice. Am J Respir Cell Mol Biol 2000;22:4–7.
17 Chuntharapai A, Kim KJ: Regulation of the expression of IL-8 receptor A/B by IL-8: Possible functions of each receptor. J Immunol 1995;155:2587–2594.
18 Bonecchi R, Polentarutti N, Luini W, Borsatti A, Bernasconi S, Locati M, Power C, Proudfoot A, Wells TNC, Mackay C, Mantovani A, Sozzani S: Up-regulation of CCR1 and CCR3 and induction of chemotaxis to CC chemokines by IFN-γ in human neutrophils. J Immunol 1999; 162:474–479.
19 Shapiro SD: The macrophage in chronic obstructive pulmonary disease. Am J Respir Crit Care Med 1999;160:S29–S32.
20 de Boer WI, Sont JK, van Schadewijk A, Stolk J, van Krieken JH, Hiemstra PS: Monocyte chemoattractant protein 1, interleukin 8, and chronic airways inflammation in COPD. J Pathol 2000;190:619–626.
21 Kemeny DM, Vyas B, Vukmanovic-Stejic M, Thomas MJ, Noble A, Loh LC, O'Connor BJ: CD8(+) T cell subsets and chronic obstructive pulmonary disease. Am J Respir Crit Care Med 1999;160:S33–S37.
22 Hesselgesser J, Ng HP, Liang M, Zheng W, May K, Bauman JG, Monahan S, Islam I, Wei GP, Ghannam A, Taub DD, Rosser M, Snider RM, Morrissey MM, Perez HD, Horuk R: Identification and characterization of small molecule functional antagonists of the CCR1 chemokine receptor. J Biol Chem 1998;273: 15687–15692.
23 Jones SA, Dewald B, Clark-Lewis I, Baggiolini M: Chemokine antagonists that discriminate between interleukin-8 receptors. Selective blockers of CXCR2. J Biol Chem 1997;272: 16166–16169.
24 White JR, Lee JM, Young PR, Hertzberg RP, Jurewicz AJ, Chaikin MA, Widdowson K, Foley JJ, Martin LD, Griswold DE, Sarau HM: Identification of a potent, selective non-peptide CXCR2 antagonist that inhibits interleukin-8-induced neutrophil migration. J Biol Chem 1998;273:10095–10098.

Dr. Ian Sabroe, Imperial College
Division of Biomedical Sciences
364 Sir Alexander Fleming Building
South Kensington SW7 2AZ (UK)
Tel. +44 171 594 3124, Fax +44 171 594 3119
E-Mail i.sabroe@ic.ac.uk

Chemokine Receptors on Th1 and Th2 Cells

Francesco Sinigaglia[a] Leonardo M. Fabbri[b] Daniele D'Ambrosio[a]

[a]Roche Milano Ricerche, Milan, [b]Section of Respiratory Diseases, University of Modena, Modena, Italy

Summary

CD4+ Th1 and Th2 cells are critical mediators of inflammatory diseases. In the lung, Th1-dominated responses are associated with the presence of a large number of macrophages and neutrophils. By contrast, eosinophilic inflammation associated with mucus hypersecretion is dependent on the presence of Th2 cells. Here we review the traffic signals that enable the differential recruitment of Th1 and Th2 cells for the inflammatory response in the lung.

The four most important chronic inflammatory diseases of the airways are COPD, asthma, cystic fibrosis and bronchiectasis. Although all of them are characterized by a persistent infiltrate of the airway mucosa by mononuclear cells, particularly T cells, the characteristics of T cells and other inflammatory cells are clearly distinct. In COPD, a disease characterized by chronic airway obstruction mainly due to cigarette smoking, the intraluminal airway inflammation is predominantly neutrophilic associated with increased levels of IL-8, and the mononuclear cells infiltrating the airway mucosa are predominantly macrophages and CD8+ T cells [1], possibly of the Tc1 type [2]. The CD8+ T cells correlate with the severity of airflow limitation. In asthma, a disease characterized by reversible airway obstruction mainly due to allergen sensitization in genetically predisposed subjects, the airway inflammation is dominated by eosinophils and mast cells. It is associated with increased levels of IL-4, IL-5, and IL-13, and the mononuclear cells infiltrating the airway mucosa are predominantly CD4+ T cells, of the Th2 type [3]. In addition, unique to asthma is an increased thickness of the reticular layer of the epithelial basement membrane, a phenomenon that might be related to a Th2 pattern of inflammation [4]. In cystic fibrosis, a disease caused by a mutation in a gene located in the long arm of chromosome 7 which encodes for the transmembrane chloride conductance regulatory protein, the chronic airway inflammation is due to chronic bacterial infections and it is dominated by neutrophils and increased levels of IL-8 [5, 6]. The type of mononuclear cells infiltrating the airway mucosa has not been sufficiently characterized. Bronchiectasis is an airway disease characterized by irreversible dilatation of the bronchi and persistent purulent sputum. The chronic airway inflammation is due to chronic bacterial infections and is dominated by neutrophils and, to a lesser extent, eosinophils, and increased levels of IL-8. The mononuclear cells infiltrating the airway mucosa are predominantly CD4+ T cells rather than CD8+ T and macrophages [7].

Mechanisms for Recruitment of Effector T Helper Cells into the Lungs

Localization of inflammatory cells into the lung requires specific interactions with the vascular endothelium and subsequent migration of cells through the vessel wall and within the tissue. Leukocyte extravasation is a multistep process mediated by the interplay of adhesion molecules, chemokines and chemokine receptors which in-

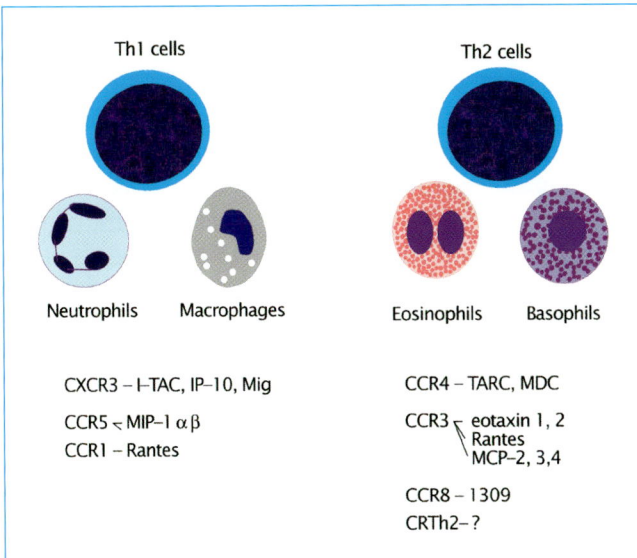

Fig. 1. Coordinated localization of inflammatory cells to the lung. The characteristic leukocytes involved in Th1- or Th2-types immune responses are shown. The major chemokine receptors and their ligands that facilitate the co-localization of these leukocytes are listed below.

volves rolling, firm adhesion, diapedesis and migration within interstitial tissues [8]. Recent studies from our group and others have pointed out that among trafficking signals, chemokines and their receptors provide a central paradigm for understanding the mechanisms that regulate the tissue-specific recruitment of Th1 and Th2 cells [9–11]. Chemokines are members of a large, growing family of small cytokines, which play a key role in the leukocyte recruitment process. There are >40 chemokines identified to date, and these can be classified according to the configuration of cysteine residues near the N-terminus in four major families: CXC, CC, C and CX3C. These molecules exert most of their biological effects by binding to a large family of G-protein-coupled seven-transmembrane receptors (10 CCR, 5 CXCR, 1 CX3CR and 1 CR) leading to activation of multiple intracellular signalling pathways [12]. Given the elevated number of ligands and receptors, the chemokine system is well suited to providing the diversity of signals needed for the exquisite specificity of the recruitment process. As leukocytes roll along blood endothelium, certain chemokine receptors signal a change in integrin conformation and affinity, which leads to firm arrest of the cells. Other chemokines are more important for subsequent steps, such as guiding the leukocytes through the tissue interstitium. Because chemokine receptors are fundamental to leukocyte migration, their expression regulates which subsets of cells are recruited to particular tissues. Blocking chemoattractants or their receptors is thus a logical approach to interfering with harmful inflammatory responses in the lung as well as in other tissues.

Chemokine and Their Receptors for Th1/Th2 Responses

We and others have reported differential expression of several chemokine receptors on either Th1 or Th2 cells [10, 11, 13, 14]. The receptors preferentially expressed on Th1 cells are CCR5 and CXCR3. In addition to these receptors, we have recently shown that CCR1 is also tightly linked to the Th1 program being upregulated in Th1 cells by IL-12 [15, 16]. Selective expression of chemokine receptors results in differential chemotactic responsiveness of Th cells. MIP-1β (CCR5 ligand) and interferon-inducible protein 10 (IP-10) (CXCR3 ligand) preferentially attract Th1 cells. An analysis of lung T cells in sarcoidosis confirmed our in vitro findings. Virtually all the lung T cells expressed CXCR3 [17], thus suggesting that CXCR3 expression may confer on Th1 cells a selective ability to penetrate and localize in the site of granuloma formation. In addition to relying on chemokine receptors, the accumulation of Th1 cells in the lung tissues must also rely on adhesion molecules such as E- and P-selectin ligands [18], as well as on certain integrins which operate for Th1 but not for Th2 cells [15, 19].

In contrast to Th1, Th2 lymphocytes have significantly higher expression of CCR3, CCR4 and CCR8. Interestingly, while levels of CCR3 have been shown to be low and variable in a number of studies, CCR4 is strongly expressed on in-vitro-activated Th2 cells [20]. Furthermore two recent studies have documented CCR4 expression on lung-infiltrating Th2 cells after allergen challenge of asthmatic individuals [M. Mariani et al., in preparation], and an increase of CCR4+ peripheral blood mononuclear cells in atopic dermatitis patients as compared to normal controls [21].

Coordinated Localization of Inflammatory Cells to the Lung: A Central Role for Chemokines?

A fundamental feature of Th1 and Th2 type inflammatory responses is the coordinated involvement of multiple and distinct types of leukocyte subsets, which can be thought of as 'immune functional units' (fig. 1). It is common knowledge that Th1 cells are often found to co-localize with macrophages and neutrophils at peripheral inflammatory sites, whereas eosinophils and basophils are found together with Th2 cells. By producing their mutually exclusive pattern of cytokines, Th1 and Th2 cells influence the activity of other leukocyte subsets as well as that of tissue-resident cells. For instance, bronchial hyperresponsiveness and mucus overproduction in asthma appear to be directly linked to the effects of Th2 cytokines, particularly IL-13, on the resident cells of the lung [22]. Extravascular localization of blood-borne leukocytes requires the expression of currently ill-defined trafficking signals by the target tissue. However, thanks to a series of recent studies, chemokines are emerging as an important means of tissue-specific localization of the Th1 and Th2 'immune functional unit'. Expression of CCR3 by eosinophils, Th2 cells, basophils and even mast cells has been reported and CCR4 expression has been shown on Th2 cells as well as on basophils. The ligands for both receptors, eotaxin for CCR3 and macrophage-derived chemokine (MDC) for CCR4, have been documented in the asthmatic lung and implicated in the pathogenesis of airway hyperactivity. Interestingly, a novel chemokine receptor named CRTH2 has been reported to be highly and selectively expressed on Th2 cells and eosinophils, and even though its ligands are unknown, an agonistic activity appears to be produced by FcγRI-triggered human mast cells [23]. In the case of Th1 cells, CCR1 and CCR5 which are the receptors for several inflammatory chemokines often associated with Th1-type immunity, are shared with monocytes and macrophages. These findings strongly support the theory that certain chemokines may have a critical role in co-localizing several leukocyte subsets to the inflammatory microenvironment. The role of chemokines may not be limited to simply recruiting the right combination of inflammatory cells within the inflammatory microenvironment, but they may also have an active role in determining the morphological characteristics of the inflammatory infiltrate. Indeed, a critical role for certain chemokines in the formation and structural organization of lymphoid organs is already well documented. Thus, it is not difficult to envision a role for chemokines in granuloma formation and in the neogenesis of lymphoid structures that become apparent at sites of chronic inflammation. In asthma, multiple chemokines have been found to participate in orchestrating the different stages of the inflammatory response in the lung, consistent with the idea that these molecules coordinate the migration and the interaction of different leukocyte subsets during an inflammatory response.

Chemokine Receptor Regulation in Th1 and Th2 Cells: A Tool for the Multistep Navigation of Activated T Cells

As discussed in the previous section, a large number of chemokines and their receptors have been involved in regulating the recruitment of the Th1 or Th2 immune functional units. The multiplicity of chemotactic signals acting on a certain type of immune effector cell seems to underline an apparent redundancy in the system. In the case of phagocytes, this redundancy has been proposed as a basis for the required robustness of the inflammatory chemotactic signals. Thus, even though some chemotactic signals may be redundant and dispensable, the overall redundancy of the system may actually be a critical and indispensable feature. Similar considerations may also apply to the Th1 and Th2 immune functional units. However, redundancy in the mechanisms of T cell recruitment may be less than anticipated. Recent findings suggest that distinct chemokine-receptor axes may act at distinct stages of the T cell localization process. For instance, several receptors for inflammatory chemokines, such as CCR1, CCR2, CCR3, CCR5 and CXCR3, are downregulated following TCR triggering of Th1 and Th2 cells. In marked contrast, CCR7, CCR4 and CCR8 are strongly upregulated upon TCR-mediated activation [20]. These changes in chemokine receptor expression may serve to modify the migratory behaviour of activated Th1 and Th2 cells and establish a hierarchy of action among distinct chemokine-receptor axes. Thus, it is conceivable that CCR3, CCR4 and CCR8 may regulate the extravasation of circulating Th2 cells and, upon activation, their re-localization in the tissue microenvironment. On this subject, it is noteworthy that in the study by Gonzalo et al. [24] the MDC-CCR4 axis was shown to act specifically by retaining inflammatory cells within the lung interstitial tissues. In further support of this concept, the reported modulation of chemokine receptor expression in response to a variety of cytokines may be another way to target specialized Th cell subsets to specific microenvironments. Notably, IL-4 upregulates CXCR4 expression on T cells, whereas IL-12 upregulates CCR1 and downregulates CXCR4 expression. Similarly, Th1 and Th2 cytokines have been found to modulate, often in opposite directions, the expression of several chemokine receptors on distinct leukocyte subsets. This extreme plasticity of expression suggests on the one hand, that inhibiting the action of these chemokine receptors may be useful in multiple pathological settings. On the other hand, it also makes these receptors unlikely to serve as selective markers of disease.

References

1 Saetta M, Baraldo S, Corbino L, Turato G, Braccioni F, Rea F, Cavallesco G, Tropeano G, Mapp CE, Maestrelli P, Ciaccia A, Fabbri LM: CD8+ cells in the lungs of smokers with chronic obstructive pulmonary disease. Am J Respir Crit Care Med 1999;160:711–717.

2 Kemeny DM, Vyas B, Vukmanovic-Stejic M, Thomas MJ, Noble A, Loh LC, O'Connor BJ: CD8+ T cell subsets and chronic obstructive pulmonary disease. Am J Respir Crit Care Med 1999;160:S33–S37.

3 Kay AB: Role of T cells in asthma. Chem Immunol 1998;71:178–191.

4 Doucet C, Brouty-Boye D, Pottin-Clemenceau C, Canonica GW, Jasmin C, Azzarone B: Interleukin (IL) 4 and IL-13 act on human lung fibroblasts. Implication in asthma. J Clin Invest 1998;101:2129–2139.

5 Richman-Eisenstat JB, Jorens PG, Hebert CA, Ueki I, Nadel JA: Interleukin-8: An important chemoattractant in sputum of patients with chronic inflammatory airway diseases. Am J Physiol 1993;264:L413–L418.

6 Danel C, Erzurum SC, McElvaney NG, Crystal RG: Quantitative assessment of the epithelial and inflammatory cell populations in large airways of normals and individuals with cystic fibrosis. Am J Respir Crit Care Med 1996;153:362–368.

7 Gaga M, Bentley AM, Humbert M, Barkans J, O'Brien F, Wathen CG, Kay AB, Durham SR: Increases in CD4+ T lymphocytes, macrophages, neutrophils and interleukin 8 positive cells in the airways of patients with bronchiectasis. Thorax 1998;53:685–691.

8 Springer TA: Traffic signals for lymphocyte recirculation and leukocyte emigration: The multistep paradigm. Cell 1994;76:301–314.

9 D'Ambrosio D, Iellem A, Colantonio L, Clissi B, Pardi R, Sinigaglia F: Localization of Th-cell subsets in inflammation: Differential thresholds for extravasation of Th1 and Th2 cells. Immunol Today 2000;21:175–178.

10 Sallusto F, Mackay CR, Lanzavecchia A: Selective expression of the eotaxin receptor CCR3 by human T helper 2 cells. Science 1997;277:2005–2007.

11 Bonecchi R, Bianchi G, Bordignon PP, D'Ambrosio D, Lang R, Borsatti A, Sozzani S, Allavena P, Gray PA, Mantovani A, Sinigaglia F: Differential expression of chemokine receptors and chemotactic responsiveness of type 1 T helper cells (Th1s) and Th2s. J Exp Med 1998;187:129–134.

12 Ward SG, Bacon K, Westwick J: Chemokines and T lymphocytes: More than an attraction. Immunity 1998;9:1–11.

13 Sallusto F, Lenig D, Mackay CR, Lanzavecchia A: Flexible programs of chemokine receptor expression on human polarized T helper 1 and 2 lymphocytes. J Exp Med 1998;187:875–883.

14 Zingoni A, Soto H, Hedrick JA, Stoppacciaro A, Storlazzi CT, Sinigaglia F, D'Ambrosio D, O'Garra A, Robinson D, Rocchi M, Santoni A, Zlotnik A, Napolitano M: The chemokine receptor CCR8 is preferentially expressed in Th2 but not Th1 cells. J Immunol 1998;161:547–551.

15 Colantonio L, Iellem A, Clissi B, Pardi R, Rogge L, Sinigaglia F, D'Ambrosio D: Upregulation of integrin alpha6/beta1 and chemokine receptor CCR1 by interleukin-12 promotes the migration of human type 1 helper T cells. Blood 1999;94:2981–2989.

16 Rogge L, Bianchi E, Biffi M, Bono E, Chang SY, Alexander H, Santini C, Ferrari G, Sinigaglia L, Seiler M, Neeb M, Mous J, Sinigaglia F, Certa U: Transcript imaging of human T helper cell development using oligonucleotide arrays. Nat Genet, in press.

17 Agostini C, Cassatella M, Zambello R, Trentin L, Gasperini S, Perin A, Piazza F, Siviero M, Facco M, Dziejman M, Chilosi M, Qin SX, Luster AD, Semenzato G: Involvement of the IP-10 chemokine in sarcoid granulomatous reactions. J Immunol 1998;161:6413–6420.

18 Austrup F, Vestweber D, Borges E, Lohning M, Brauer R, Herz U, Renz H, Hallmann R, Scheffold A, Radbruch A, Hamann A: P- and E-selectin mediate recruitment of T-helper-1 but not T-helper-2 cells into inflamed tissues. Nature 1997;385:81–83.

19 Clissi B, D'Ambrosio D, Geginat J, Colantonio L, Morrot A, Freshney NW, Downward J, Sinigaglia F, Pardi R: Chemokines fail to up-regulate integrin-dependent adhesion in human Th2 lymphocytes. J Immunol 2000;164:3293–3300.

20 D'Ambrosio D, Iellem A, Bonecchi R, Mazzeo D, Sozzani S, Mantovani A, Sinigaglia F: Selective up-regulation of chemokine receptors CCR4 and CCR8 upon activation of polarized human type 2 Th cells. J Immunol 1998;161:5111–5115.

21 Yamamoto J, Adachi Y, Onoue Y, Okabe Y, Itazawa T, Toyoda M, Seki T, Morohashi M, Matsushima K, Miyawaki T: Differential expression of the chemokine receptors by the Th1- and Th2-type effector populations within circulating CD4+ T cells. J Leukoc Biol, in press.

22 Wills-Karp M: Immunologic basis of antigen-induced airway hyperresponsiveness. Annu Rev Immunol 1999;17:255–281.

23 Nagata K, Tanaka K, Ogawa K, Kemmotsu K, Imai T, Yoshie O, Abe H, Tada K, Nakamura M, Sugamura K, Takano S: Selective expression of a novel surface molecule by human Th2 cells in vivo. J Immunol 1999;162:1278–1286.

24 Gonzalo JA, Pan Y, Lloyd CM, Jia GQ, Yu G, Dussault B, Powers CA, Proudfoot AE, Coyle AJ, Gearing D, Gutierrez-Ramos JC: Mouse monocyte-derived chemokine is involved in airway hyperreactivity and lung inflammation. J Immunol 1999;163:403–411.

Francesco Sinigaglia
Roche Milano Ricerche, Via Olgettina 58
I–20132 Milan (Italy)
Tel. +39 02 2884 803, Fax +39 02 2153 203
E-Mail francesco.sinigaglia@roche.com

CCR-3 Antagonists

Shannon A. Bryan[a]   Paul D. Ponath[b]   Robert S. Wilhelm[c]

[a]National Heart and Lung Institute, Clinical Studies Unit, Imperial College, London, UK,
[b]LeukoSite, Inc., Cambridge, Mass., and Boston, Mass., [c]Inflammatory Diseases Unit, Roche Bioscience, Palo Alto, Calif., USA

Summary

Eosinophils are thought to play a role in many inflammatory diseases, in particular allergy and asthma. Primarily tissue resident cells, eosinophils constitute only about 2–5% of peripheral blood leukocytes. Their selective recruitment into tissues from the blood is largely dependent on chemokines, or 'chemotactic cytokines'. Various functions have been ascribed to chemokines, including many pro-inflammatory activities, such as chemotaxis, integrin activation, and degranulation, which are mediated by receptors differentially expressed on leukocyte subsets. Experimental data from several animal models have demonstrated that the C-C chemokine eotaxin plays an important role in the recruitment of eosinophils into areas of allergic inflammation through its specific interaction with C-C chemokine receptor-3, CCR-3, which is highly expressed on these cells. In addition, accumulating evidence suggests that eotaxin plays a role in the trafficking of other CCR-3-bearing effector cells, such as basophils and alveolar macrophages. It is also implicated in the recruitment of CCR-3-bearing Th2 cells, a key regulator of allergic inflammatory reactions, in part through the allergen driven production of IL-4 and IL-5, which prime and activate basophils and eosinophils. Blockade of CCR-3, therefore, may reduce the level of both effector and regulatory cell infiltrates at sites of allergic inflammation and hence, CCR-3 has recently emerged as an exciting new therapeutic target for allergy and asthma.

Table 1. Sites of CCR-3 expression and ligand production

Cellular expression of CCR-3	CCR-3 ligands	Known sites of CCR-3 ligand production
Eosinophils	Eotaxin	Airway epithelium
Th2 cells		Airway smooth muscle cells
Basophils		Alveolar macrophages
Alveolar macrophages		Vascular endothelium
		Nasal polyp epithelium
		Eosinophils
		T cells
	Eotaxin-2	Airway epithelium
	Eotaxin-3	Vascular endothelium
	MCP-2	Monocytes
		Osteosarcoma cells
	MCP-3	Osteosarcoma cells
	MCP-4	Airway epithelial cells
	RANTES	T cells
		Eosinophils
		Macrophages
		Fibroblasts
		Airway epithelium
		Airway smooth muscle cells
		Renal epithelium
		Mesangial cells

Molecular Mechanisms of Action

CCR-3 is a seven-transmembrane-spanning, pertussis toxin-sensitive G-protein coupled receptor (GPCR) [1, 2] which binds several chemokine ligands (functional receptor agonists) including eotaxin, eotaxin-2, eotaxin-3, RANTES, MCP-3, and MCP-4 among others (table 1). While the eotaxins appear to utilize CCR-3 exclusively, RANTES, MCP-3, and MCP-4 have a more promiscuous binding nature and are ligands for additional chemokine receptors [3]. Ligand binding and activation of chemokine receptors stimulates the release of GDP from the α-subunit of the heterotrimeric G protein, and its subsequent replacement with GTP results in dissociation of the monomeric Gα subunit from the Gβγ heterodimer. The free Gβγ subunit activates phospholipase C that in turn leads to the activation of protein kinase C via diacylglycerol and to the release of intracellular calcium stores via inositol triphosphate. The subsequent activation of MAP

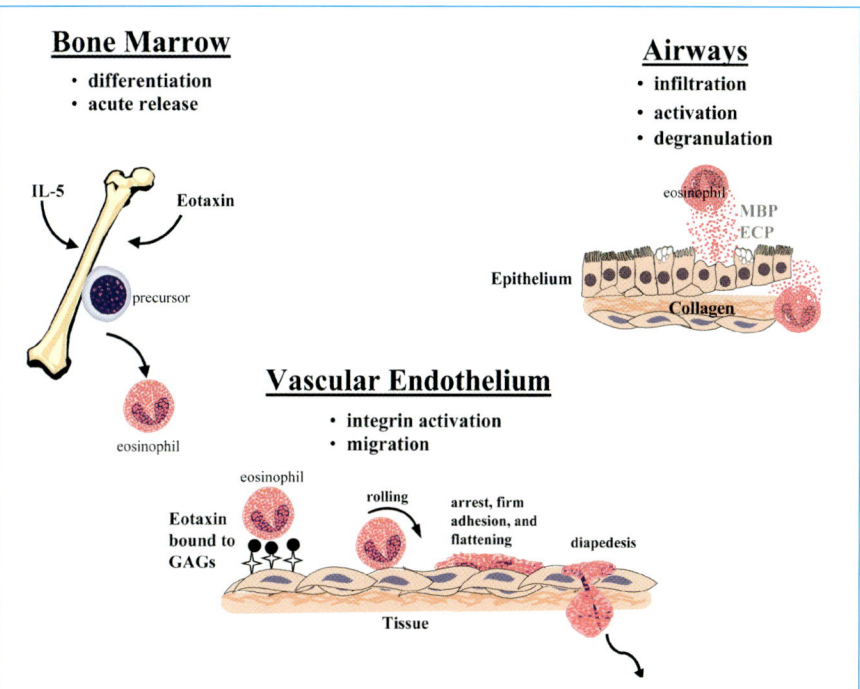

Fig. 1. Sites of eotaxin activity during eosinophil migration: eotaxin synergizes with IL-5 to release eosinophils and their precursors from the bone marrow into the circulation. Chemotactic gradients set up by chemokines bound to glycosaminoglycans (GAGs) on the endothelial surface direct the migration of eosinophils into the tissues to areas of inflammation. Once in the tissues, eosinophils release their granules containing major basic protein (MBP) and eosinophil cationic protein (ECP) resulting in fibrosis and epithelial denudation.

kinases via tyrosine kinase is required for cytoskeletal reorganization, chemotaxis and degranulation [4, 5]. The small GTP-binding proteins, Rac and Rho, are also activated and play a role in actin polymerization, leading to membrane ruffling and pseudopod formation [5]. Chemokine receptor activation is followed by internalization of the receptor via an endocytic pathway, which is shared with the receptor for transferrin [6].

Cellular Mechanisms of Action (fig. 1)

CCR-3 is predominately expressed on eosinophils (40,000–60,000 receptors per cell [4]) and has been shown to be the principal chemokine receptor on these cells [7]. Th2 cells [8], basophils [9], and alveolar macrophages [10] have also been shown to express CCR-3, although these cells express several other additional chemokine receptors. Under the influence of IL-5 and eotaxin [11], eosinophils migrate from the bone marrow into the peripheral circulation where they tether and roll along the vascular endothelium sampling for chemokine via a selectin dependent process. CCR-3 engagement of eotaxin (or other CCR-3 ligands) bound to glycosaminoglycans present on the endothelium, triggers integrin activation, resulting in arrest and firm adhesion of the eosinophil followed by diapedesis and migration within tissue along a chemokine gradient. Upon activation or stimulation by various factors in the tissues, eosinophils may release cytoplasmic components such as cytotoxic granule proteins, lipid mediators and cytokines that cause tissue destruction and recruit additional inflammatory cells to the site [12]. Incubation of Th2 cells with TGF-β or IFN-γ causes a downregulation of CCR-3 expression [13, 14]. This suggests that chemokines and their receptors may also play a role in T cell inflammatory response.

CCR-3 Inhibition

The rationale for targeting of CCR-3 is supported by both human and rodent studies. Both CCR-3 and eotaxin are elevated in the bronchial mucosa of atopic asthmatics, and this elevation seems to correlate with disease severity [15]. Neutralization of murine chemokine ligands, such as eotaxin, RANTES, MCP-3, MCP-5, and MIP-1α (murine MIP-1α is a potent ligand for murine MIP-1α, however, human MIP-1α does not bind to human CCR-3) with monoclonal or polyclonal antibodies has proven efficacious in several rodent models of inflammatory disease including antigen-specific airway inflammation [16]. Because these chemokines bind multiple receptors, however, it remains unclear which receptor/ligand pair play key roles in the disease process. In contrast, a neutralizing antibody to murine eotaxin that binds CCR-3 only has been reported to reduce the accumulation of lung eosinophils in an ovalbumin-challenged mouse by 60–70% as well as reducing antigen-induced airway hyperreactivity

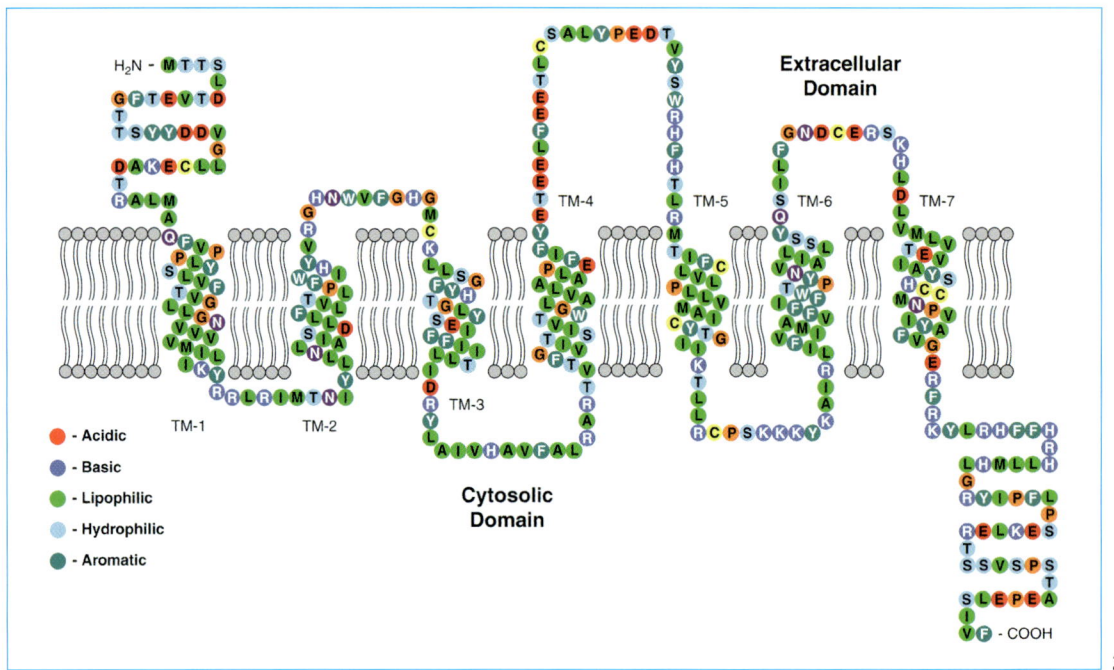
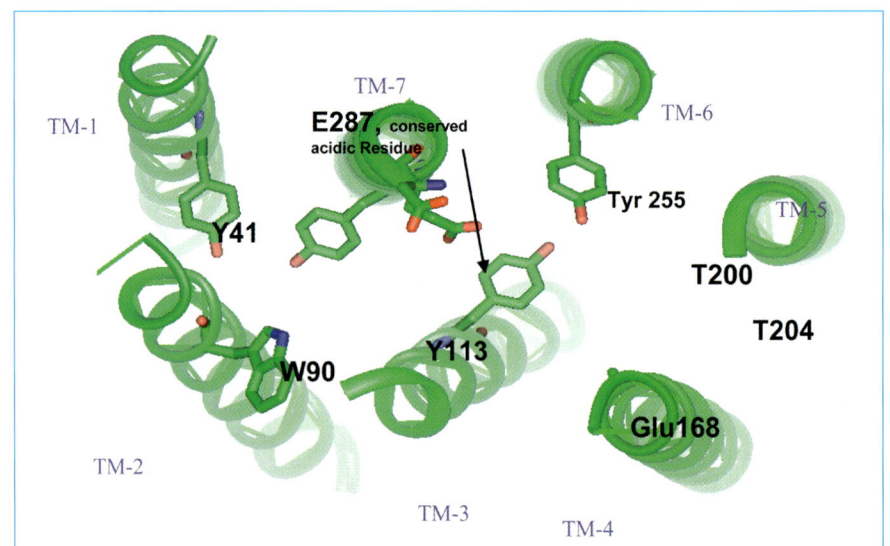

Fig. 2. Snake-plot of the CCR-3 receptor showing the presumed transmembrane regions (TM).

Fig. 3. Structure of the CCR-3 receptor showing 7-transmembrane helical bundles.

by 50% [17]. In addition, depletion of eotaxin using targeted gene disruption in mice has been shown to decrease eosinophil numbers in the BAL fluid 18 h after inhaled allergen challenge when compared to eotaxin +/+ mice, although eotaxin –/– mice still mounted an eosinophil response when compared to unsensitized control mice [18]. Together, these studies indicate that eotaxin, and thus CCR-3, plays a role in eosinophil recruitment, but that additional chemokines or other chemoattractants are able to recruit eosinophils in the absence of eotaxin. To address this issue further and to examine the role of CCR-3, receptor-blocking monoclonal antibodies have been developed against guinea pig and mouse CCR-3 [19, 20], and these have been shown to inhibit infiltration of eosinophils into guinea pig and mouse lungs, respectively. Furthermore, a monoclonal antibody specific for human CCR-3 has been developed (7B11, Leukosite Inc.) [7] and in vitro antagonism of the receptor was demonstrated with this antibody [21] on both eosinophils and basophils [9], resulting in decreased chemotaxis and a decrease in histamine release from basophils.

Receptor Structure (fig. 2, 3)

The chemokine receptors share identity with other GPCRs as evidenced by conservation of amino acids at particular loci within the transmembrane helices. Common residues in the GPCR family are the glycine (G) and asparagine (N) in TM-1, aspartic acid (D) in TM-2, tryptophan (W) in TM-4, and tyrosine (Y) in TM-5. The signature region for all chemokine receptors is found in TM-7 where the glutamic acid is separated by six amino acids from a cystein/cystein motif (CC), which in turn, is spaced one amino acid distant from an asparagine/proline motif (NP). It is interesting to consider that these conserved amino acids may be critical for ligand binding and receptor activation, and depending on accessibility, may also serve as potential recognition sites for designed antagonists. Whereas the biogenic amine receptors are typically characterised by a glutamic acid or aspartic acid in TM-3, this site is a tyrosine in CCR-3; a glutamic acid is found instead in TM-7. The 7-transmembrane-spanning helical bundle of CCR-3 forms a channel that presumably plays a role in coordinating the chemokine for activation of the receptor.

CCR-3 Antagonists

Inspection of the general chemokine patent literature suggests a pharmacophore similar to antagonists of biogenic amine receptors. A basic nitrogen within the framework of the antagonist seems to be an important element, which upon protonation at physiologic pH, probably binds to an anionic residue within the receptor. This seems to hold true for CCR-3 antagonists as well. Several companies have filed patents on CCR-3 small molecule antagonists [22]. Unfortunately, very little information is provided in terms of intrinsic potency, selectivity, or efficacy within an animal model.

Compound 1 (fig. 4) was reported by LeukoSite as having dual activity for CCR-3 (100% inhibition at 3 μM with eotaxin-stimulated chemotaxis of eosinophils) and CCR-1 (66% inhibition at 10 μM with RANTES-induced chemotaxis of HL60 cells). Compound 2 was described in a Banyu Pharmaceutical patent as having very impressive intrinsic activity on both CCR-3 (IC_{50} = 0.74 nM) and CCR-1 (IC_{50} = 1.8 nM). However, the ethyl quat salt probably imparts vulnerability in terms of variable absorption and therefore, it is not a likely drug candidate via the oral route. Piperazine analogues have also been described by Roche Bioscience and Merck. Compound 3 is reported to inhibit CCR-3 (IC_{50} = 400 nM). Compound 4 was described in a Merck patent that made broad claims as antagonists of multiple chemokine receptors.

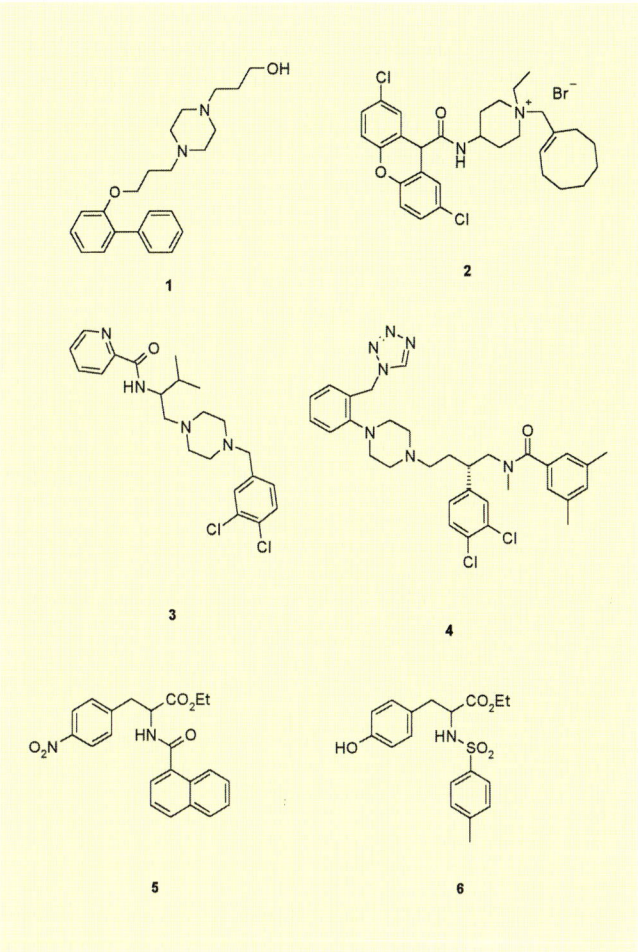

Fig. 4. Chemical structures of CCR-3 antagonists: 1: Leukosite Inc.; 2: Banyu Pharmaceuticals; 3: Roche Bioscience; 4: Merck; 5, 6: SmithKline Beecham.

More recently, SmithKline Beecham claimed the utility of compounds 5 and 6 as CCR-3 antagonists. These compounds are notable due to the absence of a basic nitrogen, and it remains to be seen what activity they demonstrate and whether they antagonize in some unique way.

Outside of the patent literature, efficacy in a murine model of asthma has been reported [23] for a putative CCR-3 antagonist (structure not revealed). The compound was reported to have an effect in an ovalbumin-challenged mouse, reducing BAL eosinophils to baseline at 30 mg/kg when administered subcutaneously.

Conclusions

Although there are few data as yet that support the use of CCR-3 antagonists in allergic diseases, this therapeutic approach seems a reasonable means to deplete the selective migration of inflammatory cells (eosinophils, basophils and Th2 cells). Since this is a selective inhibition, there may be fewer side effects such as those seen with broad-spectrum anti-inflammatory drugs like corticosteroids. Since chemokines may bind to more than one chemokine receptor, blocking cell-specific receptors appears to be a more useful target.

References

1 Combadiere C, Ahuja SK, Murphy PM: Cloning and functional expression of a human eosinophil CC chemokine receptor. J Biol Chem 1995;270:16491–16494.
2 Ponath PD, Qin S, Ringler DJ, Clark-Lewis I, Wang J, Kassam N, Smith H, Shi X, Gonzalo J-A, Newman W, Gutierrez-Ramos J-C, Mackay CR: Cloning of the human eosinophil chemoattractant, eotaxin. Expression, receptor binding, and functional properties suggest a mechanism for the selective recruitment of eosinophils. J Clin Invest 1996;97:604–612.
3 Murphy PM, Baggiolini M, Charo IF, Hebert CA, Horuk R, Matsushima K, Miller LH, Oppenheim JJ, Power CA: International union of pharmacology.XXII. Nomenclature for chemokine receptors. Pharmacol Rev 2000;52:145–176.
4 Alam R: Chemokines in allergic inflammation. J Allergy Clin Immunol 1997;99:273–277.
5 Premack BA, Schall TJ: Chemokine receptors: gateways to inflammation and infection. Nat Med 1996;2:1174–1178.
6 Zimmerman N, Conkright JJ, Rothenberg ME: CC chemokine receptor-3 undergoes prolonged ligand-induced internalisation. J Biol Chem 1999;274:12611–12618.
7 Heath H, Qin S, Rao P, Wu L, LaRosa G, Kassam N, Ponath PD, Mackay CR: Chemokine receptor usage by human eosinophils The importance of CCR3 demonstrated using an antagonistic monoclonal antibody. J Clin Invest 1997;99:178–184.
8 Sallusto F, Mackay CR, Lanzavecchia A: Selective expression of the eotaxin receptor CCR3 by human T helper 2 cells. Science 1997; 277:2005–2007.
9 Uguccioni M, Mackay CR, Ochensberger B, Loetscher P, Rhis S, LaRosa GJ, Rao P, Ponath PD, Baggiolini M, Dahinden CA: High expression of the chemokine receptor CCR3 in human blood basophils. Role in activation by eotaxin, MCP-4, and other chemokines. J Clin Invest 1997;100:1137–1143.
10 Park IW, Koziel H, Hatch W, Li X, Du B, Groopman JE: CD4 receptor-dependent entry of human immunodeficiency virus type-1 env-pseudotypes into CCR5-, CCR3-, and CXCR4-expressing human alveolar macrophages is preferentially mediated by the CCR5 coreceptor. Am J Respir Cell Mol Biol 1999;20:864–871.
11 Palframan RT, Collins PD, Williams TJ, Rankin SM: Eotaxin induces a rapid release of eosinophils and their progenitors from the bone marrow. Blood 1998;91:2240–2248.
12 Rothenberg ME: Eotaxin: An essential mediator of eosinophil trafficking into mucosal tissues. Am J Respir Cell Mol Biol 1999;21:291–295.
13 D'Ambrosio D, Iellem A, Bonecchi R, Mantovani A, Sinigaglia F: Selective upregulation of chemokine receptors CCR4 and CCR8 upon activation of polarised human type 2 Th cells. J Immunol 1998;161:5111–5115.
14 Sallusto F, Lenig D, Mackay CR, Lanzavecchia A: Flexible programs of chemokine receptor expression on human polarised T helper 1 and 2 lymphocytes. J Exp Med 1998;187:875–883.
15 Ying S, Robinson DS, Meng Q, Rottman J, Kennedy R, Ringler DJ, Mackay CR, Daugherty BL, Springer MS, Durham SR, Williams TJ, Kay AB: Enhanced expression of eotaxin and CCR3 mRNA and protein in atopic asthma. Association with airway hyperresponsiveness and predominant co-localization of eotaxin mRNA to bronchial epithelial and endothelial cells. Eur J Immunol 1997;27:3507–3516.
16 Gonzalo JA, Lloyd CM, Wen D, Wells TN, Martinez AC, Dorf M, Bjerke T, Coyle AJ, Gutierrez-Ramos JC: The coordinated action of CC chemokines in the lung orchestrates allergic inflammation and airway hyperresponsiveness. J Exp Med 1998;188:157–167.
17 Gonzalo JA, Lloyd CM, Kremer L, Finger E, Martinez AC, Siegelman MH, Cybulsky M, Gutierrez-Ramos JC: Eosinophil recruitment to the lung in a murine model of allergic inflammation. The role of T cells, chemokines, and adhesion receptors. J Clin Invest 1996;98:2332–2345.
18 Rothenberg ME, MacLean JA, Pearlman E, Luster AD, Leder P: Targeted disruption of the chemokine eotaxin partially reduces antigen-induced tissue eosinophilia. J Exp Med 1997; 185:785–790.
19 Sabroe I, Conroy DM, Gerard NP, Li Y, Collins PD, Post TW, Jose PJ, Williams TJ, Ponath PD: Cloning and characterization of the guinea pig eosinophil eotaxin receptor, C-C chemokine receptor-3: Blockade using a monoclonal antibody in vivo. J Immunol 1998;161: 6139–6147.
20 Grimaldi JC, Grunig G, Seymour BW, Cottrez F, Robinson DS, Hosken N, Ferlin WG, Wu X, O'Garra A, Coffman RL: Depletion of eosinophils in mice through the use of antibodies specific for C-C chemokine receptor 3 (CCR3). J Leukoc Biol 1999;65:846–853.
21 Elsner J, Petering H, Kluthe C, Kimmig D, Smolarski R, Ponath PD, Kapp A: Eotaxin-2 activates chemotaxis-related events and release of reactive oxygen species via pertussis toxin-sensitive G proteins in human eosinophils. Eur J Immunol 1998;28:2152–2158.
22 Patent literature for CCR3 Antagonists: Leukosite (1998) WO Patent 98/14480; Banyu (1997) WO Patent 97/24325; Roche (1998) DE 19837386-A; Merck (1998) WO Patent 98/25617; SKB (1999) WO Patent 99/55324; SKB (1999) WO Patent 99/55330.
23 Bertrand C: CC chemokine receptor blockade as a new therapy for asthma. From the Laboratory to the Clinic, Oxford, Sept 25–29, 1999.

Dr. Robert Wilhelm
Roche Bioscience, 3401 Hillview Avenue
Palo Alto, CA 94304 (USA)
Tel. +1 650 855 5213, Fax +1 650 354 2442
E-Mail robert-s.wilhelm@roche.com

Interleukin-8 Receptor (CXCR2) Antagonists

Henry M. Sarau   Katherine L. Widdowson   Michael R. Palovich   John R. White
David C. Underwood   Don E. Griswold

Departments of Pulmonary Biology, Medicinal Chemistry and Immunology,
SmithKline Beecham Pharmaceuticals, King of Prussia, Pa., USA

Summary

There is general agreement for a key role of airway inflammation in the establishment and progression of several lung diseases. In many of these diseases, neutrophils and their products may play an important role in the pathophysiology. Neutrophils migrate into the lung in response to various chemoattractants, including the CXC chemokine, IL-8. The majority of these chemotactic agents interact with cell surface 7-transmembrane receptors, such as IL-8 activating CXCR1 and CXCR2 on neutrophils. There is evidence for a role of IL-8 in lung disease, including COPD. We have recently identified a class of compounds that are selective CXCR2 antagonists. In the present study the in vitro and in vivo pharmacology of SB 265610, a prototype compound from this series, is described. The results indicate that antagonists, like SB 265610, may be useful for defining the role of neutrophils and CXCR2 in lung inflammation.

Inflammation of the airways is a feature of a variety of lung diseases, including COPD [1], acute respiratory distress syndrome [2], asthma [1, 3], chronic bronchitis [4], pulmonary fibrosis [5] and cystic fibrosis [6]. The inflammatory process is complex involving the release of many mediators, including chemoattractants that recruit inflammatory cells into the site of tissue damage. This is a normal physiological response to fight infection, but excessive recruitment and activation of these cells mediate tissue damage and slow healing. Therefore, inhibition of inflammatory cell recruitment may be an appropriate therapeutic strategy for several pulmonary diseases.

A key event in many lung diseases is the recruitment of neutrophils from the blood stream to the site of inflammation with the subsequent release of degradative enzymes and pro-inflammatory mediators. Neutrophils are present in large numbers in the lungs of patients with chronic airway disease, including COPD [1]. The increased percentage of neutrophils in sputum of COPD patients correlates negatively with a measure of pulmonary function, forced expiratory volume in 1s (FEV_1). The concentration of the CXC chemokine, IL-8, was also increased and correlated with neutrophil numbers, suggesting a direct cause and effect relationship [1].

Recruitment of neutrophils depends on their attachment to the endothelium through upregulation of ICAM-1/E-selectin on endothelial cells and CD11b/CD18 on PMNs. The regulation of CD11b/CD18 may be mediated via IL-8 interaction with cell surface receptors. In human neutrophils, IL-8 binds to two distinct receptors with similar affinity (CXCR1 and CXCR2). Several closely related chemokines containing a common amino terminal Glu^4-Leu^5-Arg^6 (ELR) sequence, including GRO-α, GRO-β, GRO-γ, NAP-2 and ENA-78, bind only to CXCR2 [7]. It remains unclear whether human neutrophil chemotaxis in vivo is mediated by one or both receptors, but in vitro studies with a selective CXCR2 antagonist, SB 225002, indicate the importance of this receptor for chemotactic activity [8].

In this report we describe evidence for a role of IL-8 in lung disease and the in vitro and in vivo characterization of SB 265610 (fig. 1), a potent and selective CXCR2 antagonist. The results demonstrate that inhibition of CXCR2 alone is sufficient to inhibit human neutrophil chemotaxis in vitro, and that oral administration of SB 265610 inhibits neutrophil recruitment in a rabbit model of lung inflammation.

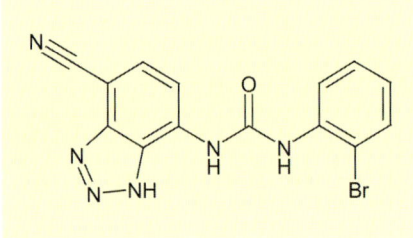

Fig. 1. Structure of SB 265610.

Role of IL-8 and Its Receptors in Lung Inflammation

IL-8 is a member of the large proinflammatory chemokine family that affects immune and inflammatory cells. IL-8, a CXC chemokine, is a 72-amino-acid protein that is produced by many cells including neutrophils, monocytes, stromal cells, epithelial cells, dermal fibroblasts, keratinocytes, vascular endothelial cells, large granular lymphocytes and human gastric cancer cells [9, 10]. IL-8 activates human neutrophils, T cells, B cells, basophils, IL-2 activated natural killer cells and IL-3- or GM-CSF-stimulated eosinophils [11, 12]. IL-8 and GRO-α upregulate functional responses for other chemoattractants, e.g., fMLP receptor expression on human neutrophils [13]. There is growing evidence that IL-8 is a major player in neutrophil trafficking [9].

CXCR1 and CXCR2 share 77% amino acid identity [14, 15]. CXCR1 and CXCR2 are present on human neutrophils with different distribution patterns [16]. CXCR2 is expressed on subsets of T cells, including CD4+, CD8+ and CD56+NK, and it is this receptor, rather than CXCR1, which is key for chemotaxis of these cells [8, 17, 18]. Thus, CXCR2 is strategically positioned to regulate the entry of neutrophils and T cells into sites of inflammation.

In chronic inflammatory diseases, including COPD, several immune and inflammatory cells, including neutrophils, T cells and macrophages are believed to contribute to the underlying pathophysiology [19, 20]. Neutrophil activation results in the release of a number of inflammatory mediators and proteinases, including elastase and matrix metalloproteinases which may contribute to progressive fibrosis, airway stenosis and destruction of lung parenchyma, leading to an accelerated decline in airway function [21]. In animal models of acute lung injury, administration of neutralizing monoclonal antibodies to IL-8 reduces neutrophil infiltration and tissue damage [22]. In the present study we demonstrate the inhibition of neutrophil recruitment into the inflamed lung with a small molecule antagonist of CXCR2, providing additional evidence for a pathophysiological role for IL-8 in lung inflammation.

SB 265610: In vitro Pharmacology

A series of diphenylureas were identified using a high throughput screen as selective inhibitors of CXCR2 [23]. A prototype, SB 225002, was recently reported [8], but the utility of the compound was limited by its lack of oral activity in animal models. Affinity for the IL-8 receptors was determined using [^{125}I]-IL-8 binding to membranes of CHO cells stably expressing either CXCR1 (CHO-CXCR1) or CXCR2 (CHO-CXCR2). SB 265610 was evaluated in this assay and competed for IL-8 binding to CHO-CXCR2 membranes with an IC_{50} = 39.1 ± 11.0 nM (n = 3) and CHO-CXCR1 with an IC_{50} = 7,400 ± 2,400 nM (n = 3) (fig. 2A). When tested for functional activity in human neutrophils, which express both CXCR1 and CXCR2, SB 265610 inhibited GRO-α-induced Ca^{2+} mobilization (CXCR2 mediated) with an IC_{50} of 5.2 ± 1.5 nM (n = 10). The compound was considerably weaker as an inhibitor of IL-8-induced Ca^{2+} mobilization (CXCR1- and CXCR2-mediated) with an IC_{50} of 426 nM (n = 2) (fig. 2B). Additionally, the compound inhibited IL-8-induced Ca^{2+} mobilization in RBL 2H3 cells stably expressing CXCR1 with an IC_{50} of 453 ± 177 nM (n = 3), confirming its lower affinity for this receptor (data not shown).

SB 265610 was evaluated for inhibition of human neutrophil chemotaxis in response to maximally effective concentrations of GRO-α, IL-8 and C5a. Using freshly isolated peripheral blood neutrophils from 3 individuals, SB 265610 inhibited GRO-α or IL-8-induced chemotaxis with similar IC_{50}s of 4.5 nM and 7.6 nM (n = 3), respectively (fig. 3). There was no inhibition by SB 265610 of C5a-induced chemotaxis in concentrations up to 330 nM, suggesting the activity against IL-8- or GRO-α-induced chemotaxis was specific and not the result of effects on general cell mobility. These data indicate that inhibition of CXCR2 alone is sufficient to inhibit IL-8-induced chemotaxis of human neutrophils, at least in vitro.

Effects of SB 265610 of LPS-Induced Airway Neutrophilia

To assess the activity of SB 265610 in an animal model, rabbits were chosen because they, like humans, express both CXCR1 and CXCR2 on peripheral blood neutrophils [24]. Aerosol LPS administration to rabbits pro-

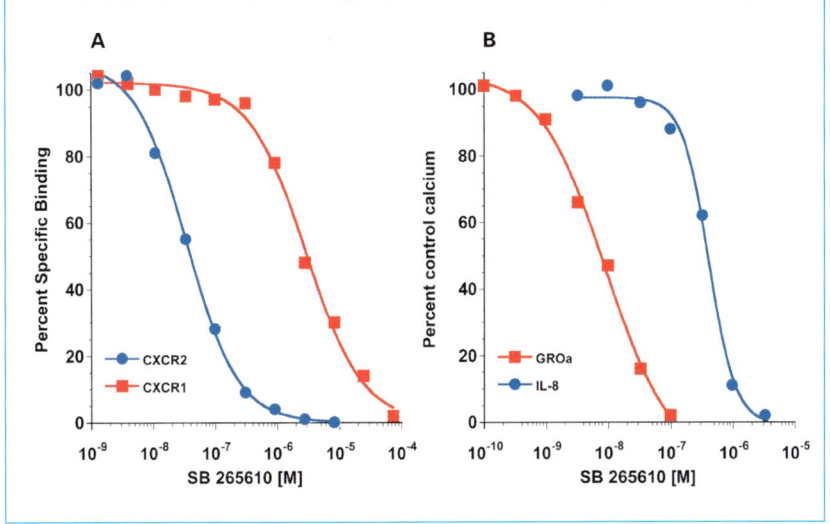

Fig. 2. A Inhibition of 250 pM [^{125}I]-IL-8 binding in CXCR1-CHO and CXCR2-CHO cell membranes by SB 265610. Results are expressed as percent inhibition of specific binding defined in the presence of 1 µM cold IL-8. **B** Inhibition of IL-8- and GRO-α-induced Ca^{2+} mobilization in human PMNs by SB 265610. Results are expressed as percent inhibition of 1 nM IL-8 or GRO-α-induced Ca^{2+} mobilization in vehicle treated controls. Values are the mean of 3 individual experiments.

Fig. 3. Inhibition by SB 265610 of IL-8-, GRO-α- and C5a-induced chemotaxis of human PMNs. Results are presented as percent inhibition of vehicle-treated control cells. Values are the mean of 3 individual experiments.

duced profound airway neutrophilia, assessed by BAL. In this rabbit model of airway inflammation, SB 265610 (5–25 mg/kg, p.o., 1 h before and 4 h after aerosol LPS challenge), produced significant inhibition of neutrophilia induced by 30 µg/ml LPS with an ID$_{50}$ of 10.5 mg/kg, (fig. 4).

Conclusions

There is accumulating evidence for a role of IL-8 and inflammatory cells, including neutrophils and T cells in lung diseases. SB 265610 is a potent, competitive and reversible CXCR2 antagonist. The in vitro evaluation of SB 265610 demonstrates that it has 100-fold lower affinity for CXCR1 relative to CXCR2 but inhibits both IL-8- and GRO-α-induced human neutrophil chemotaxis with similar potency, suggesting that CXCR2 is the relevant receptor for this activity. Additionally, the compound demonstrated oral activity in a rabbit airway neutrophilia model, supporting a role for CXCR2 in neutrophil trafficking in vivo. The pathophysiological significance of IL-8 and CXCR2 in lung diseases awaits clinical evaluation with CXCR2 antagonists like SB 265610.

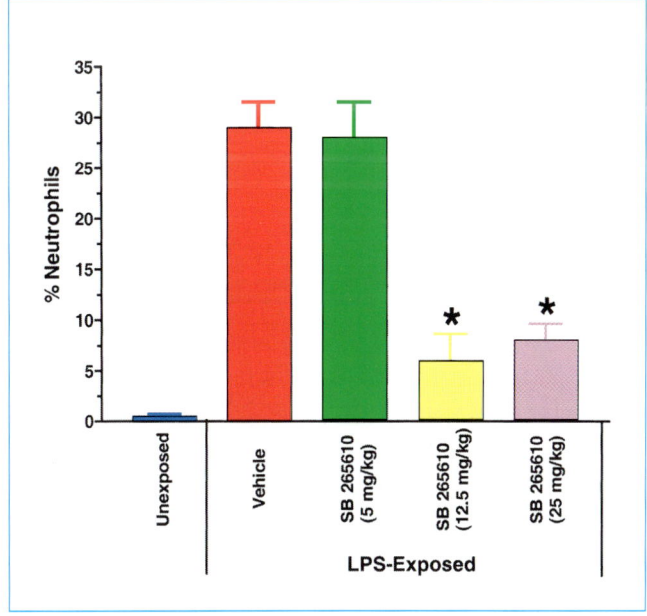

Fig. 4. Effect of SB 265610 on LPS-induced lung neutrophil infiltration in rabbits. SB 265610 (5–25 mg/kg or vehicle, 20 ml of PEG 400/H$_2$O: 50/50) was administered to conscious rabbits 1 h prior to and 4 h after challenge with an aerosol of LPS (30 µg/ml for 15 min). At 24 h after challenge, rabbits underwent BAL, cells were stained and neutrophils counted. Data are expressed as percent of at least 100 leukocytes counted; * $p < 0.05$ versus vehicle-treated group.

References

1 Keatings VM, Collins PD, Scott DM, Barnes PJ: Differences in interleukin-8 and tumor necrosis factor-α in induced sputum from patients with chronic obstructive pulmonary disease or asthma. Am J Respir Crit Care Med 1996;153:530–534.

2 Aggarwal A, Baker CS, Evans TW Haslam PL: G-CSF and IL-8 but not GMCSF correlate with severity of pulmonary neutrophilia in acute respiratory distress syndrome. Eur Respir J 2000;15:895–901.

3 Ordonez CL, Shaughnessy TE, Matthay MA, Fahy JV: Increased neutrophil numbers and IL-8 levels in airway secretions in acute severe asthma. Am J Respir Crit Care Med 2000;161:1185–1190.

4 Saetta M, Turato G, Facchini FM, Corbino L, Lucchini RE, Casoni G, Maestrelli P, Mapp CE, Ciaccia A, Fabbri LM: Inflammatory cells in the bronchial glands of smokers with chronic bronchitis. Am J Respir Crit Care Med 1997;156:1633–1639.

5 Yamanouchi H, Fujitu J, Hojo S, Yoshinouchi t, Kamei T, Yamadori I, Ohtsuki Y, Ueda N, Takahara J: Neutrophil elastase: alpha-1-proteinase inhibitor complex in serum and bronchoalveolar lavage fluid in patients with pulmonary fibrosis. Eur Respir J 1998;11:120–125.

6 Koller DY, Nething I, Otto J, Urbanek R, Eichler I: Cytokine concentrations in sputum from patients with cystic fibrosis and their relation to eosinophil activity. Am J Respir Crit Care Med 1997;155:1050–1054.

7 Ceretti DP, Kozlosky CJ, VandenBos T, Nelson N, Gearing DP, Beckmann MP: Molecular characterization of receptors for human interleukin-8, GRO/melanoma growth-stimulatory activity and neutrophil activating peptide-2. Mol Immunol 1993;30:359–367.

8 White JR, Lee JM, Young PR, Hertzberg RP, Jurewicz AJ, Chaikin MA, Widdowson K, Foley JJ, Martin LD, Griswold DE, Sarau HM: Identification of a potent, selective non-peptide CXCR2 antagonist that inhibits interleukin-8-induced neutrophil migration. J Biol Chem 1998;273:10095–10098.

9 Baggiolini M: Chemotactic and inflammatory cytokines; CXC and CC proteins. Adv Exp Med Biol 1993;351:1–11.

10 Schroder JM: Chemotactic cytokines in the epidermis. Exp Derm 1992;1:12–19.

11 Baggiolini M, Dewald B, Moser B: Interleukin-8 and related chemotactic cytokines; CXC and CC chemokines. Adv Immunol 1994;55:97–179.

12 Mukaida N, Harada A, Matsushima K: A novel leukocyte chemotactic and activating cytokine, interleukin-8 (IL-8). Cancer Treat Res 1995;80:261–286.

13 Metzner B, Barbisch M, Parlow F, Kownatzki E, Schraufstatter I, Norgauer J: Interleukin-8 and GRO alpha prime human neutrophils for superoxide anion production and induce up-regulation of N-formyl peptide receptors. J Invest Dermatol 1995;104:789–791.

14 Holmes WE, Lee J, Kuang WJ, Rice GC, Wood WI: Structure and functional expression of a human interleukin-8 receptor. Science 1991;253:1278–1280.

15 Murphy PM, Tiffany HL: Cloning of complementary DNA encoding a functional human interleukin-8 receptor. Science 1991;253:1280–1283.

16 Chuntharapai A, Lee J, Hebert CA, Kim KJ: Monoclonal antibodies detect different distribution patterns of IL-8 receptor A and IL-8 receptor B on human peripheral blood leukocytes. J Immunol 1994;153:5682–5688.

17 Tanaka J, Nomiyama H, Yamamoto T, Hamada F, Kambara T: T-cell chemotactic activity of cytokine LD78 – A comparative study with interleukin-8, a chemotactic factor for the T-cell CD45RA+ phenotype. Int Arch Allergy Immunol 1993;100:201–208.

18 Xu LL, Kelvin DJ, Ye GQ, Taub DD, Benbaruch A, Oppenheim JJ, Wang JM: Modulation of IL-8 receptor expression on purified human T lymphocytes is associated with changed chemotactic responses to IL-8. J Leukoc Biol 1995;57:335–342.

19 Thompson BP, Daughton D, Robbins GA, Ghafouki MA, Oehlerking M, Rennard SI: Intramural airway inflammation in chronic bronchitis. Characterization and correlation with clinical parameters. Am Rev Respir Dis 1989;140:1527–1537.

20 Jeffery P K: Structural and inflammatory changes in COPD: A comparison with asthma. Thorax 1998;53:129–136.

21 Stockley RA: Neutrophils and protease/antiprotease imbalance. Am J Respir Crit Care Med 1999;160:S49–S52.

22 Braddus VC, Boylan AM, Hoeffel JM, Kim KJ, Sadick M, Chuntharapai A, Hebert CA: Neutralization of IL-8 inhibits neutrophil influx in a rabbit model of endotoxin-induced pleurisy. J Immunol 1994;152:2960–2967.

23 Widdowson, K, Veber DF, Jurewicz AJ, Nie H, Hertzberg RP, Holl W, Sarau HM, Foley JJ, Lee JM, White JR: Discovery and characterization of potent, small molecule interleukin-8 receptor antagonists; in Ramage R, Epton R (eds): Peptides 1996. Leiden, Escom, 1998, pp 87–90.

24 Prado GN, Thomas KM, Suzuki H, LaRosa GJ, Wilkinson N, Folco E, Navarro J: Molecular characterization of a novel rabbit interleukin-8 receptor isotype. J Biol Chem 1994;269:12391–12394.

Henry M. Sarau, PhD, Associate Director
Department of Pulmonary Biology, UW 2531
SmithKline Beecham Pharmaceuticals
709 Swedeland Road
King of Prussia, PA 19406 (USA)
Tel. +1 610 270 4930, Fax +1 610 270 5381
E-Mail skip_sarau-1@sbphrd.com

Adhesion Molecule Inhibitors

Adhesion Molecule Antagonism: An Overview

Bruce S. Bochner

Department of Medicine, Division of Clinical Immunology, The Johns Hopkins University School of Medicine, Johns Hopkins Asthma and Allergy Center, Baltimore, Md., USA

Summary

Leukocyte subtypes express different sets of cell adhesion molecules. They interact with various combinations of counterligands on vascular endothelium, respiratory epithelium, matrix proteins and other tissue structures at distinct steps of the inflammatory cascade. Not only are these molecules necessary for recruitment into sites of inflammation, but the pattern and level of expression on a given cell will determine which leukocytes get recruited. Because these critical events occur locally at a site of inflammation, a variety of strategies are being used to generate pharmacologic antagonists of adhesion molecules. Many are entering clinical trials, and some may prove useful for local or systemic treatment of diseases including asthma, allergy and COPD.

Leukocyte Adhesion Molecules

Leukocytes constitutively express many different types of adhesion molecules (fig. 1, 2). The patterns and levels of expression vary widely. L-selectin is found exclusively on leukocytes. It functions as an adhesion molecule for lymph node and vascular endothelium, especially under conditions of blood flow [1]. The N-terminal lectin region is directly responsible for adhesion. Leukocytes also express a variety of glycosylated selectin ligands. The levels and patterns of selectin ligand expression also differ among leukocyte subtypes [1, 2]. Biosynthesis of many selectin ligands results from the sequential activity of specific sialyl- and fucosyl-transferases [3].

Several ligands for selectins have been identified [1] (fig. 1). Virtually all leukocytes constitutively express P-selectin glycoprotein ligand-1 (PSGL-1). Murine leukocytes express E-selectin ligand-1 (ESL-1), a molecule with as yet no human homologue. Memory skin-homing lymphocytes express the cutaneous lymphocyte antigen (CLA) [4]. Glycolipid ligands for E-selectin, termed myeloglycans, have been described on neutrophils.

Integrins are molecules with α and β subunits [5]. Subunits combine to form approximately 25 different heterodimers [1]. Integrin expression on leukocytes is quite varied. For example, β1 and β3 integrins are expressed on leukocytes, endothelium, and epithelium, while β2 integrin expression is restricted to leukocytes. Within the α subunit, there is often an inserted or 'I' domain, that mediates adhesion. Also, conformational changes in integrins regulate integrin avidity [5].

Endothelial and Epithelial Adhesion Molecules

Endothelial cells express many types of adhesion molecules. P-selectin exists preformed and is expressed within minutes of stimulation with agents such as histamine or LTC_4 [1]. Unlike P-selectin, E-selectin expression requires new mRNA and protein synthesis initiated in response to cytokines (table 1). Expression is transient, declining over 24–48 h towards undetectable levels.

Two members of the immunoglobulin superfamily, the intracellular adhesion molecules ICAM-1 and ICAM-2, are implicated in leukocyte-endothelial interactions. Both are constitutively expressed on endothelial cells, but cytokines can enhance ICAM-1 expression (table 1). Ligands include the integrins αLβ2 (LFA-1) and αMβ2 (Mac-1) (fig. 1). Another important immunoglobulin superfamily molecule is vascular cell adhesion molecule-1 (VCAM-1) [1]. Like E-selectin, its expression is induced de novo by interleukin-1 (IL-1) or tumor necrosis factor (TNF). Unlike E-selectin, expression is maximal by 24–48 h, and VCAM-1 can be selectively upregulated by IL-4 or IL-13 [6]. The combination of IL-4 or IL-13 with TNF or IL-1 is

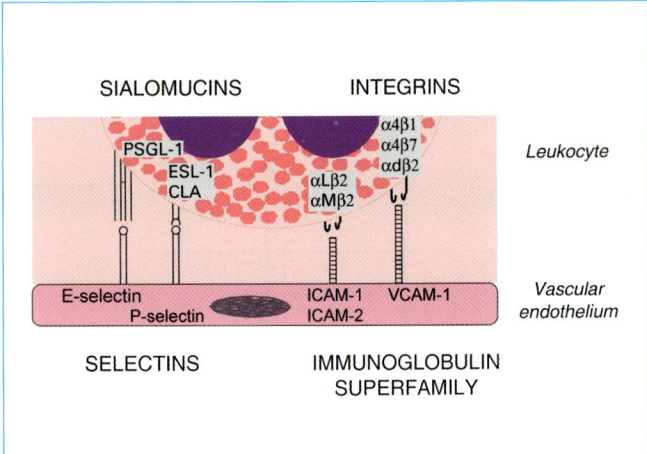

Fig. 1. Examples of families of adhesion molecule ligands on leukocytes and endothelial cells. Note that some adhesion molecules are missing (e.g., L-selectin) and that no single leukocyte expresses all of these structures (e.g., CLA is found on memory T cells, while α4 integrins are not expressed by neutrophils).

Fig. 2. Adhesion molecules on leukocytes and endothelium and their role during various steps in cell recruitment. Integrins are designated using common names for their α and β subunits. PSGL-1 = P-selectin glycoprotein-1; ESL-1 = E-selectin ligand-1; CLA = cutaneous lymphocyte antigen; PECAM = platelet endothelial cell adhesion molecule; VCAM = vascular cell adhesion molecule; ICAM = intercellular adhesion molecule.

Table 1. Regulation of endothelial and epithelial adhesion molecule expression by cytokines[1]

Stimulus	ICAM-1		VCAM-1		E-selectin	
	endothelial	epithelial	endothelial	epithelial	endothelial	epithelial
None	3+	3+	0	0	0	0
IL-1 or TNF	4+	4+	3+	2+	4+	4+
IL-4 or IL-13	3+	3+	2+	1+	0	0
IFN-γ	4+	4+	0	0	0	0
IL-1 or TNF[2] and IL-4 or IL-13	3+	3+	4+	4+	0	0

[1] Based on data using human umbilical vein endothelium and respiratory epithelial cell lines.
[2] Concentrations just below those that by themselves will induce adhesion molecule expression.

particularly synergistic (table 1). Ligands for VCAM-1 include the integrins α4β1 (or VLA-4), α4β7 and αdβ2 (fig. 1) [1, 7].

One additional member of the immunoglobulin superfamily implicated in leukocyte recruitment is platelet-endothelial cell adhesion molecule-1 (PECAM-1). It is constitutively expressed on endothelial cells and most leukocytes. PECAM-1 may function during transendothelial migration [8], but because its intracellular portion contains immunoreceptor tyrosine-based inhibitory motifs (ITIMs), its primary function may instead be cell signaling [9].

Epithelial cells resemble endothelial cells in their expression of ICAM-1, but are not capable of expressing any of the selectins. Induction of both ICAM-1 and VCAM-1 in epithelial cell lines by cytokines has been reported (table 1) [10]. Additionally, epithelial and endothelial cells express their own unique patterns of integrins that they use primarily for interactions with tissue matrix [11, 12].

Due to their prominent expression on eosinophils, basophils, and T lymphocytes, and their absence on neutrophils, α4β1 and its ligands are believed to play a prominent role in allergic inflammation. They recognize the amino acid sequence IDS in VCAM-1 and a related amino acid sequence, LDV, in fibronectin [4]. Like α4β1, α4β7 binds to fibronectin and VCAM-1, but it also binds mucosal addressin cell adhesion molecule-1 (MAdCAM-1) found in the gut [4]. The β7 subunit can pair with another subunit, αE, on lymphocytes where it functions as a ligand for E-cadherin found on the basolateral surface of epithelial cells [13].

Endothelial and Epithelial Interactions

Leukocyte emigration from the intravascular compartment into extravascular sites is a multistep process, divided into distinct but overlapping stages (fig. 2). Under the forces of blood flow, cells initially undergo the process of tethering and rolling. This is mediated primarily by selectins and their counterligands [14], although the integrins α4β1 and αdβ2, via interactions with VCAM-1, can also participate [15, 16]. The next step involves firm leukocyte adhesion to the endothelial surface. This integrin-dependent event probably requires leukocyte activation, resulting from exposure of leukocytes to factors produced by and/or displayed on the surface of endothelial cells [14]. This rapid activation increases the avidity and expression of integrins on the leukocyte surface, leading to enhanced binding to immunoglobulin superfamily molecules such as ICAM-1, ICAM-2 and VCAM-1. Together, these first two steps are termed 'margination'. Subsequent transendothelial migration is mediated primarily by ICAM-1 and β2 integrins, but VCAM-1, PECAM-1 and their ligands also can participate [8, 17]. Pathways regulating the ensuing migration through the tissue matrix, and transepithelial migration into the epithelium and airway lumens, are less well understood. In vitro and in vivo, transepithelial leukocyte migration, like transendothelial migration, appears to be primarily mediated by ICAM-1 and β2 integrins [18], but this cannot explain the entire pathway [11, 17]. Studies with knockout or hypomorphic mice also implicate ICAM-2 [19], VCAM-1 [18], CD34 (a ligand for L-selectin) [20] and αEβ7 [21] in this process.

Selective Leukocyte Accumulation

Models of selective leukocyte recruitment suggest that adhesion molecules work in concert with cytokines, chemokines, and other activating factors, to influence leukocyte migration [14]. For instance, tissue accumulation of subsets of leukocytes, especially eosinophils, basophils, and Th2 lymphocytes, is a hallmark of chronic allergic inflammation. One such paradigm by which adhesion molecules might facilitate allergic cell recruitment is shown in figure 3. A variety of studies in both animals and humans provide support for this paradigm [1].

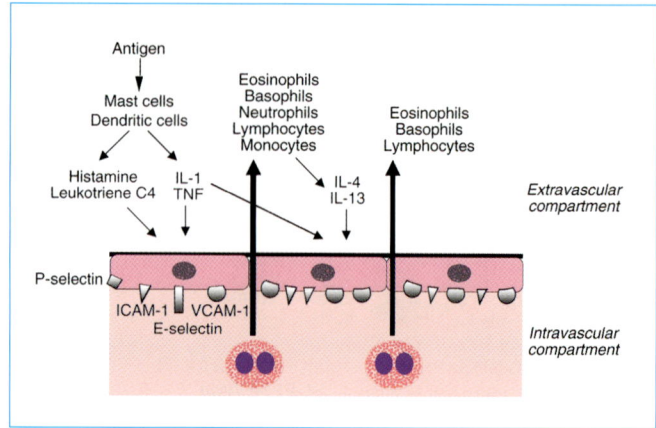

Fig. 3. Proposed sequence of cytokine production and endothelial adhesion molecule induction during allergic inflammation. Initial antigen exposure leads to the local release of IL-1 and TNF from mast cells and dendritic cells, resulting in endothelial expression of ICAM-1, E-selectin, and VCAM-1. Other more rapidly acting mediators, such as histamine and sulfidopeptide leukotrienes, induce P-selectin. This pattern of endothelial cell activation facilitates the early adhesion and transendothelial migration of many different leukocyte types. The subsequent production of IL-4 and IL-13 by lymphocytes, basophils and other cells, either alone or in synergy with IL-1 and TNF, may lead to augmented preferential VCAM-1 expression, favoring further recruitment of cells bearing α4β1 integrins, such as eosinophils, basophils and lymphocytes.

Table 2. Therapeutic strategies for antagonizing adhesion molecules

Block cell surface expression
   Cytokine and cytokine receptor antagonists
   Antisense nucleotides
   Fucosyl- or sialyl-transferase inhibitors
   Metalloprotease inhibitors
Block function
   Low molecular weight competitive antagonists
   Oligosaccharides and glycomimetics
   Linear and cyclic peptides
   Monoclonal antibodies
   Soluble adhesion molecule constructs
   Integrin 'activation' inhibitors

From Bochner [22] with permission.

Blocking Cell Adhesion Molecules

Novel therapies that target adhesion molecules (table 2) [3, 22] may soon provide not only the pharmacologic verification of their importance in inflammatory diseases but also an alternative approach to the treatment of airway diseases.

References

1 Bochner BS: Cellular adhesion in inflammation; in Middleton JE, Reed C, Ellis E, Adkinson NF, Yunginger J, Busse W (eds): Allergy Principles and Practice, ed 5. St. Louis, Mosby, 1998, pp 94–107.
2 Varki A: Selectin ligands: Will the real ones please stand up? J Clin Invest 1997;99:158–162.
3 Lowe JB, Ward PA: Therapeutic inhibition of carbohydrate-protein interactions in vivo. J Clin Invest 1997;99:822–826.
4 Briskin M: Pathways of cell recruitment to mucosal surfaces; in Bochner BS (ed): Cell Adhesion Molecules in Allergic Diseases. New York, Dekker, 1997, pp 105–128.
5 Hunt SW III, Kellermann S-A, Shimizu Y: Integrins, integrin regulators and the extracellular matrix: The role of signal transduction and leukocyte migration; in Bochner BS (ed): Cell Adhesion Molecules in Allergic Disease. New York, Dekker, 1997, pp 73–104.
6 Bochner BS, Klunk DA, Sterbinsky SA, Coffman RL, Schleimer RP: Interleukin-13 selectively induces vascular cell adhesion molecule-1 (VCAM-1) expression in human endothelial cells. J Immunol 1995;154:799–803.
7 Grayson MH, Van der Vieren M, Sterbinsky SA, Gallatin WM, Hoffman PA, Staunton DE, Bochner BS: αdβ2 Integrin is expressed on human eosinophils and functions as an alternative ligand for VCAM-1. J Exp Med 1998;188:2187–2191.
8 Vaporciyan AA, DeLisser HM, Yan H-C, Mendiguren II, Thom SR, Jones ML, Ward PA, Albelda SM: Involvement of platelet-endothelial cell adhesion molecule-1 in neutrophil recruitment in vivo. Science 1993;262:1580–1582.
9 Newman PJ: Switched at birth: A new family for PECAM-1. J Clin Invest 1999;103:5–9.
10 Atsuta J, Sterbinsky SA, Plitt J, Schweibert LM, Bochner BS, Schleimer RP: Phenotyping and cytokine regulation of the BEAS-2B human bronchial epithelial cell: Demonstration of inducible expression of the adhesion molecules VCAM-1 and ICAM-1. Am J Respir Cell Mol Biol 1997;17:571–582.
11 Polito AJ, Proud D: Epithelial cells: Phenotype, substratum and mediator production; in Bochner BS (ed): Cell Adhesion Molecules in Allergic Disease. New York, Dekker, 1997, pp 43–72.
12 Bochner BS, Klunk D, Sterbinsky SA, Schleimer RP: Phenotyping of cultured human umbilical vein endothelial cells using the workshop blind panel mAb; in: Schlossman S, Boumsell L, Gilks W, Harlan J, Kishimoto T, Morimoto C, Ritz J, Shaw S, Silverstein R, Springer T, Tedder T, Todd R (eds): Leukocyte Typing V: White Cell Differentiation Antigens. New York, Oxford University Press, 1995, pp 1773–1776.
13 Cepek KL, Shaw SK, Parker CM, Russell GJ, Morrow JS, Rimm DL, Brenner MB: Adhesion between epithelial cells and T lymphocytes mediated by E-cadherin and the αEβ7 integrin. Nature 1994;372:190–193.
14 Springer TA: Traffic signals on endothelium for lymphocyte recirculation and leukocyte emigration. Annu Rev Physiol 1995;57:827–872.
15 Sriramarao P, von Andrian UH, Butcher EC, Bourdon MA, Broide DH: L-selectin and very late antigen-4 integrin promote eosinophil rolling at physiological shear rates in vivo. J Immunol 1994;153:4238–4246.
16 Van der Vieren M, Crowe DT, Hoekstra D, Adams L, Vazeux R, Grayson MH, Bochner BS, Staunton DE: The leukocyte integrin adb2 binds VCAM-1: Evidence for a binding interface between I domain and VCAM-1. J Immunol 1999;163:1984–1990.
17 Ebisawa M, Bochner BS, Schleimer RP: Eosinophil-endothelial interactions and transendothelial migration. in Bochner BS (ed): Cell Adhesion Molecules in Allergic Diseases. New York, Dekker, 1997, pp 173–186.
18 Gonzalo JA, Lloyd CM, Kremer L, Finger E, Martinez C, Siegelman MH, Cybulsky M, Gutierrez-Ramos JC: Eosinophil recruitment to the lung in a murine model of allergic inflammation – the role of T cells, chemokines, and adhesion receptors. J Clin Invest 1996;98:2332–2345.
19 Gerwin N, Gonzalo JA, Lloyd C, Coyle AJ, Reiss Y, Banu N, Wang BP, Xu H, Avraham H, Engelhardt B, Springer TA, Gutierrez-Ramos JC: Prolonged eosinophil accumulation in allergic lung interstitium of ICAM-2-deficient mice results in extended hyperresponsiveness. Immunity 1999;10:9–19.
20 Suzuki A, Andrew DP, Gonzalo JA, Fukumoto M, Spellberg J, Hashiyama M, Takimoto H, Gerwin N, Webb I, Molineux G, Amakawa R, Tada Y, Wakeham A, Brown J, McNiece I, Ley K, Butcher EC, Suda T, Gutierrez-Ramos JC, Mak TW: CD34-deficient mice have reduced eosinophil accumulation after allergen exposure and show a novel crossreactive 90-kD protein. Blood 1996;87:3550–3562.
21 Schon MP, Arya A, Murphy EA, Adams CM, Strauch UG, Agace WW, Marsal J, Donohue JP, Her H, Beier DR, Olson S, Lefrancois L, Brenner MB, Wakeham A, Grusby MJ, Parker CM: Mucosal T lymphocyte numbers are selectively reduced in integrin alpha E (CD103)-deficient mice. J Immunol 1999;162:6641–6649.
22 Bochner BS: Cellular adhesion and its antagonism. J Allergy Clin Immunol 1997;100:581–585.

Bruce S. Bochner, MD, Professor of Medicine
Department of Medicine
Division of Clinical Immunology
The Johns Hopkins University
School of Medicine
Johns Hopkins Asthma and Allergy Center
5501 Hopkins Bayview Circle
Baltimore, MD 21224-6801 (USA)
Tel. +1 410 550 2131, Fax +1 410 550 2130
E-Mail bbochner@jhmi.edu

Small-Molecule VLA-4 Antagonists

Steven P. Adams Roy R. Lobb

Biogen Inc., Cambridge Mass., USA

Summary

The α4 integrins, α4β1 (VLA-4) and α4β7, are heterodimeric cell-surface proteins involved in both cell-cell and cell-matrix interactions. Widely expressed on leukocytes, these integrins are critical regulators of pathophysiologic responses in inflammation and autoimmune disease. The central role of integrin α4β1 in animal models of inflammatory disease has been extensively documented using α4-specific monoclonal antibodies (mAbs). Important advances have been made in identifying potent and selective small-molecule inhibitors for further development, strongly suggesting that α4β1 should be an accessible small-molecule target. Moreover, biological evaluation of advanced compounds suggests that efficacy comparable to that achieved with mAbs is possible which, based on clinical results with an mAb, augurs well for eventual success with this target. Here we summarize recent advances in α4β1 research with particular emphasis on the chemistry of small molecule antagonists, and on asthma as a clinical target.

Molecular and Cellular Mechanisms of Action

The α4β1 integrin is expressed at high levels on mononuclear leukocytes, mast cells, macrophages, basophils, and eosinophils [1–3]. Although originally thought not to be expressed on neutrophils (PMNs), recent studies suggest α4β1 can also be expressed on this cell type at low but functionally significant levels [4].

Vascular cell adhesion molecule-1 (VCAM-1) and the alternatively spliced type III connecting segment-1 (CS-1) of fibronectin are the only ligands for α4β1 well characterized to date. Recent work suggests α4β1 also binds another matrix ligand, osteopontin, a secreted phosphoprotein with multiple functions [5]. The possible role of osteopontin as an α4β1 ligand is intriguing as it is strongly upregulated in many disease states, including the inflamed lung [6].

Numerous studies have demonstrated a critical role for α4β1 in leukocyte recruitment, and in particular the role of this integrin in eosinophil function has been well documented [1, 2]. More recently, it has become clear that the interaction of α4β1 and other leukocyte integrins on emigrated cells with matrix molecules within the inflamed tissue plays a critical role in their priming, activation and survival [2, 7]. In this light, extensive in vitro studies show that α4 may play a particularly important role in PMN function following emigration into tissues [4]. The pathophysiological significance of these results in human asthma requires further study, since PMNs are recruited into the lung in animal models of allergic lung disease and in human asthma [8, 9]. However, the critical ability of this integrin to modulate the function of the multiple leukocyte cell types involved in allergic responses has made it a particularly attractive intervention point for drug development.

α4 Integrins and Asthma: In vivo Data

The role of α4 integrins in allergic lung inflammation has been extensively studied using mAbs. The in vitro and in vivo effects of these mAbs have been reviewed recently [2, 4] and can be summarized as follows (table 1). In five animal species sensitized to one of three different antigens, three distinct blocking mAbs to α4 profoundly inhibit allergic lung inflammation. Importantly, in three of three models tested, local delivery to the lung is efficacious. In one murine model, systemic and local delivery were carefully compared. While both delivery modes fully blocked eosinophil recruitment into the lung, only local delivery blocked cytokine release in the lung, mucus secretion, and airway hyperresponsiveness. Other recent

Table 1. Validation of integrin α4β1 in animal models of airway disease

Species	Antigen	mAb	Route of administration	Reference
Mouse	ovalbumin	PS/2	i.n.	10
Rat	ovalbumin	TA-2	i.v.	11
Guinea pig	ovalbumin	HP1/2	i.v., i.p.	12
Rabbit	dust mite	PS/2	Aerosol	13
Sheep	*Ascaris suum*	HP1/2	i.v., aerosol	14

studies implicate α4 integrins in mast cell function and extend their role in the recruitment of leukocyte subsets to the lung, particularly eosinophils [15]. Taken jointly, these data strongly suggest that α4 integrins expressed on cells within the inflamed lung are the therapeutic target. Finally, support for a role for α4 integrins in other allergic conditions, such as allergic conjunctivitis, continues to emerge [16].

Biochemical Properties of α4β1

On resting cells, integrin α4β1 binds soluble ligands with low affinity. However, a continuum of high affinity states is observed when cells, or purified receptor, are exposed to different divalent metal ion conditions or activating mAbs specific to the β1 subunit [17]. Additionally, receptor activation leads to increased avidity in static cell adhesion assays and causes immediate firm arrest of Jurkat cells rolling on VCAM-1 under flow [18]. While high-affinity states have not been observed directly in vivo, α4β1 inhibitors that bind selectively to the high-affinity receptor prevent arrest and firm adhesion of cells under flow conditions without inhibiting initial tethering and rolling, a function dependent on low affinity receptor [19]. These results suggest that the detailed interplay between low and high receptor affinity states may orchestrate key cell adhesion phenomena essential for cell trafficking in vivo. To the extent that α4β1-mediated pathology is induced by discrete activation states of the receptor, it may be desirable to identify therapeutic agents selective for these receptor forms.

Therapeutic Approaches

Monoclonal Antibodies. As noted above, mAbs to α4 that block ligand binding have been employed extensively to validate the role of α4 in animal disease models. These mAbs bind to complex epitopes adjacent to the ligand binding site and prevent macromolecular ligands from binding to resting as well as activated receptor forms. On the other hand, they do not inhibit the binding of small molecule ligand mimics [17]. A humanized mAb based on the IgG4 framework has been developed through phase II clinical trials in multiple sclerosis (table 2) [21].

Peptide Analogs. Several groups have developed peptide inhibitors of α4β1 based on the Leu-Asp-Val sequence from CS-1 recognized by the receptor [28]. These peptides competitively inhibit the binding of natural ligands and stimulate the appearance of ligand-induced epitopes, properties consistent with ligand mimics. Generally, these peptide analogs bind preferentially to activated receptor, and to varying degrees they exhibit selectivity for α4β1 compared to α4β7 [22]. BIO-1211, an α4β1-selective tight-binding peptide analog selective for activated receptor, inhibits early and late airway responses following antigen exposure in a sheep model of allergic airway disease, and it also reverses established antigen-induced hyper-responsiveness [23]. Additionally, administration of the compound for several days prior to antigen exposure blocks infiltration of α4β1-bearing cells, including eosinophils, suggesting that α4β1 inhibition may provide an important anti-inflammatory profile in allergic disease. An aerosol formulation of BIO-1211 has progressed to phase II clinical trials in patients with mild to moderately severe asthma.

A cyclic peptide inhibitor, ZD-7349, administered by minipump, inhibits murine collagen-induced arthritis as well as other lymphocyte-mediated allergic pathologies [25]. Development of a slow-release depot formulation of this compound for treatment of autoimmune and allergic diseases has begun.

Small-Molecule Inhibitors. Encouraging medicinal chemistry efforts, apparent in the recent patent literature, have independently identified a number of related chemical series. Some of these compounds appear to exhibit desirable pharmaceutical properties; however, the relative lack of detailed information from peer-reviewed sources prevents any firm conclusions on the overall attractiveness of these series. An early orally bioavailable agent, TR-14035, which binds to both α4 integrins, has entered phase I trials slated for inflammatory bowel disease.

Overall, results obtained to date testify to the power of medicinal chemistry coupled with modern target-based screening methods in the discovery of potent integrin antagonists. While the conversion of peptide lead molecules to viable, orally bioavailable mimetics is a frequently difficult challenge, it is increasingly apparent that inte-

Table 2. Advanced inhibitors of integrin α4β1

Structure	Company	Properties and activity	Development stage	Reference
Humanized mAb (IgG4) Natalizumab, Antegren™	Elan	two doses of drug 4 weeks apart ↓ new active and gadolinium enhancing lesions by 50% over 12 weeks; MRI assessment; no effect on clinical relapse rate	phase II MS	20, 21
BIO-1211	Biogen	binding: $K_D = 0.07$ nM adhesion: $IC_{50} = 1$ nM sheep airways model: effective at 0.1 mg/kg (aer)	phase II asthma	22, 23
TR-14035	Tanabe	binding: $IC_{50} = 1$ nM adhesion (α4β1): $IC_{50} = 46$ nM (α4β7): $IC_{50} = 5$ nM oral bioavailability: 60% (rat), 20% (dog) DNFB-induced DTH: $ED_{50} = 30$ mg/kg (oral) DSS colitis: $ED_{50} = 10$ mg/kg (oral)	phase I IBD	24
Cyclo(MePhe-Leu-Asp-Val-D-Arg-D-Arg) ZD-7349	Zeneca	adhesion: $IC_{50} = 0.3$ μM OVA-induced DTH: $ED_{50} = 0.1$ mg/kg CIA: effective at 10 mg/kg/day by minipump	development	25
	Roche	binding: $IC_{50} = 0.2$ nM adhesion: $IC_{50} = 9$ nM	preclinical	26
	Genentech	adhesion: $IC_{50} = 0.5$ nM	preclinical	27

grin targets are accessible by this approach. The results bode well for the eventual identification of effective therapeutic agents against α4 integrins.

Clinical Experience with Monoclonal Antibodies: Multiple Sclerosis

One humanized anti-α4 integrin antibody (natalizumab; Antegren™) is currently in clinical trials and published data are available [21]. Following an initial safety and pharmacokinetic study, the effect of Antegren on lesion activity was assessed by magnetic resonance imaging (MRI) in a randomized, double-blind, placebo-controlled trial in 72 patients with active relapsing-remitting and secondary progressive MS. Patients received two intravenous infusions of mAb or placebo 4 weeks apart, and they were monitored over 24 weeks with serial MRI and clinical assessment. The treated group exhibited significantly fewer new active lesions (mean 1.8 versus 3.6 per patient) and new enhancing lesions (mean 1.6 versus 3.3 per patient) than the placebo group over the first 12 weeks, while there was no significant difference in the number of new active or enhancing lesions in the second 12 weeks of the study. The treatment showed that mAb against α4 integrin results in a significant reduction in the number of new active lesions on MRI. Importantly, these data suggest that α4 integrin blockade in man is safe, at least for a period of about 2 months, and may have anti-inflammatory potential.

Conclusions

Small molecule antagonists of α4 integrins are not particularly difficult to generate, and orally active inhibitors with suitable pharmacokinetic and pharmacodynamic properties should soon follow. The role of receptor activation in disease settings and the importance of compartmentalization of the α4β1 target remain as major open questions that may require clinical evaluation of parenteral and orally active agents with a spectrum of properties to achieve satisfactory answers.

References

1 Lobb RR, Hemler ME: The pathophysiologic role of alpha 4 integrins in vivo. J Clin Invest 1994;94:1722–1728.
2 Lobb RR: Adhesion molecule antagonists in animal models of asthma; in Bochner B (ed): Adhesion Molecules in Allergic Disease. New York, Marcel Dekker, 1997, pp 393–405.
3 Lobb RR, Adams SP: Small molecule antagonists of α4 integrins: Novel drugs for asthma. Exp Opin Invest Drugs 1999;8:935–945.
4 Johnston B, Kubes P: The alpha4-integrin: An alternative pathway for neutrophil recruitment? Immunol Today 1999;20:545–550.
5 Bayless KJ, Meininger GA, Scholtz JM, Davis GE: Osteopontin is a ligand for the α4β1 integrin. J Cell Sci 1998;111:1165–1174.
6 Murry CE, Giachelli CM, Schwartz SM, Vracko R: Macrophages express osteopontin during repair of myocardial necrosis. Amer J Pathol 1994;145:1450–1462.
7 de Fougerolles AR, Sprague AG, Nickerson-Nutter CL, Chi-Rosso G, Rennert PD, Gardner H, Gotwals PJ, Lobb RR, Koteliansky VE: Regulation of inflammation by collagen-binding integrins alpha1beta1 and alpha2beta1 in models of hypersensitivity and arthritis. J Clin Invest 2000;105:721–729.
8 Wenzel SE, Szefler SJ, Leung DY, Sloan SI, Rex MD, Martin RJ: Bronchoscopic evaluation of severe asthma. Persistent inflammation associated with high dose glucocorticoids. Am J Respir Crit Care Med 1997;156:737–743.
9 Fahy JV, Kim KW, Liu J, Boushey HA: Prominent neutrophilic inflammation in sputum from subjects with asthma exacerbation. J Allergy Clin Immunol 1995;95:843–852.
10 Henderson WR Jr, Chi EY, Albert RK: Blockade of CD49d (α4 integrin) on intrapulmonary but not circulating leukocytes inhibits airway inflammation and hyperresponsiveness in a mouse model of asthma. J Clin Invest 1997; 100:3083–3092.
11 Hojo M, Maghni K, Issekutz TB, Martin JG: Involvement of α-4 integrins in allergic airway responses and mast cell degranulation in vivo. Am J Respir Crit Care Med 1998;158:1127–1133.

12 Pretolani M, Ruffie C, Lapa e Silva JR, Joseph D, Lobb RR, Vargaftig BB: Antibody to very late activation antigen 4 prevents antigen-induced bronchial hyperreactivity and cellular infiltration in the guinea pig airways. J Exp Med 1994;180:795–805.
13 Metzger WJ: Therapeutic approaches to asthma based on VLA-4 integrin and its counter receptors. Springer Semin Immunopathol 1995;16:467–478.
14 Abraham WM, Sielczak MW, Ahmed A, Cortes A, Lauredo IT, Kim J, Pepinsky B, Benjamin CD, Leone DR, Lobb RR, Weller PF: Alpha 4-integrins mediate antigen-induced late bronchial responses and prolonged airway hyperresponsiveness in sheep. J Clin Invest 1994; 93:776–787.
15 Hisada T, Hellewell PG, Teixeira MM, Malm MG, Salmon M, Huang TJ, Chung KF: Alpha4 integrin-dependent eotaxin induction of bronchial hyperresponsiveness and eosinophil migration in interleukin-5 transgenic mice. Am J Respir Cell Mol Biol 1999;20:992–1000.
16 Ebihara N, Yokoyama T, Kimura T, Nakayasu K, Okumura K, Kanai A, Ra C: Anti VLA-4 monoclonal antibody inhibits eosinophil infiltration in allergic conjunctivitis model of guinea pig. Curr Eye Res 1999;19:20–25.
17 Chen LL, Whitty A, Lobb RR, Adams SP, Pepinsky RB: Multiple activation states of integrin alpha 4 beta 1 detected through their different affinities for a small molecule ligand. J Biol Chem 1999;274:13167–13175.
18 Alon R, Kassner PD, Carr MW, Finger EB, Hemler ME, Springer TA: The integrin VLA-4 supports tethering and rolling in flow on VCAM-1. J Cell Biol 1995;128:1243–1253.
19 Chen C, Mobley JL, Dwir O, Shimron F, Grabovsky V, Lobb RR, Shimizu Y, Alon R: High affinity very late antigen-4 subsets expressed on T cells are mandatory for adhesion strengthening but not for rolling on VCAM-1 in shear flow. J Immunol 1999;162:1084–1095.
20 Leger OJ, Yednock TA, Tanner L, Horner HC, Hines DK, Keen S, Saldanha J, Jones ST, Fritz LC, Bendig MM: Humanization of a mouse antibody against human alpha-4 integrin: A potential therapeutic for the treatment of multiple sclerosis. Hum Antibodies 1997;8:3–16.

21 Tubridy N, Behan PO, Capildeo R, Chaudhuri A, Forbes R, Hawkins CP, Hughes RA, Palace J, Sharrack B, Swingler R, Young C, Moseley IF, MacManus DG, Donoghue S, Miller DH: The effect of anti-alpha4 integrin antibody on brain lesion activity in MS. Neurology 1999; 53:466–472.
22 Lin KC, Ateeq HS, Hsiung SH, Chong LT, Zimmerman CN, Castro A, Lee WC, Hammond CE, Kalkunte S, Chen LL, Pepinsky RB, Leone DR, Sprague AG, Abraham WM, Gill A, Lobb RR, Adams SP: Selective, tight-binding inhibitors of integrin alpha4beta1 that inhibit allergic airway responses. J Med Chem 1999; 42:920–994.
23 Abraham WM, Gill A, Ahmed A, Sielczak MW, Lauredo IT, Botvinnikova Y, Lin KC, Pepinsky B, Leone DR, Lobb RR, Adams SP: A small molecule tight-binding inhibitor of the integrin α4β1 blocks antigen-induced airway responses and inflammation in experimental asthma in sheep. Am J Respir Crit Care Med 2000;162:603–611.
24 Sircar I, Gudmundsson KS, Martin R: Inhibitors of α4 mediated cell adhesion. Patent application No WO9936393, 1999.
25 Dutta AS: Cell Adhesion Inhibiting Compounds. Patent application No WO9749731, 1997.
26 Chen L, Guthrie RW, Huang TN, Hull K, Sidduri A, Tilley JW: N-alkanoyl phenylalanine derivatives. Patent application No WO9910312, 1999.
27 Jackson DY, Quan C, Artis DR, Rawson T, Blackburn B, Struble M, Fitzgerald G, Chan K, Mullins S, Burnier JP, Fairbrother WJ, Clark K, Berisini M, Chui H, Renz M, Jones S, Fong S: Potent alpha 4 beta 1 peptide antagonists as potential anti-inflammatory agents. J Med Chem 1997;40:3359–3368.
28 Adams SP, Lobb RR: Inhibitors of integrin alpha 4 beta 1 (VLA4). Ann Reports Med Chem 1999;34:179–188.

Steven P. Adams, Biogen, Inc.
12 Cambridge Center
Cambridge, MA 02142 (USA)
Tel. +1 617 679 2012, Fax +1 617 679 2616
E-Mail Steve_Adams@Biogen.com

Selectin Antagonists

Therapeutics for Airway Inflammation

Kurt L. Berens   Peter Vanderslice   Brian Dupré   Richard A.F. Dixon

Texas Biotechnology Corporation, Houston, Tex., USA

Summary

The role of adhesion molecules in the maintenance of persistent inflammation in asthma and chronic obstructive pulmonary disease is accepted, albeit incompletely understood. The selectin family of adhesion molecules mediates primary events in a complex cascade leading to the tissue localization and activation of inflammatory cells in many diseases. Blockade of selectins represents a novel therapeutic approach to interrupt the inflammatory cycle by inhibiting the extravasation of leukocytes at the earliest opportunity in the recruitment process.

The Selectin Family

The selectin (CD62) family of adhesion molecules is comprised of three members and their nomenclature is based on their original source of identification and their primary biologic localization. E-selectin (endothelial), P-selectin (platelet) and L-selectin (leukocyte) are structurally similar with high homology in humans and structural conservation across species [1]. The selectins are proteins with an N-terminal C-type lectin domain, an epidermal-growth-factor-like domain, a variable number of consensus repeats similar to complement-receptor-binding regions, with a membrane spanning component and a short cytoplasmic tail [2]. The selectins interact with various counter-ligands to mediate leukocyte cell rolling and these are summarized in table 1.

Role of Selectins in Inflammation

The selectins interact with their counter-ligands to initiate cell rolling along the vascular endothelium. The rolling of leukocytes allows for subsequent interaction with the integrin family of adhesion molecules, the latter mediating capture and firm adhesion (fig. 1). Selectins are either constitutively expressed and/or inducible by various stimuli. P-selectin is preformed in platelets and stored for rapid mobilization in the Weibel-Palade bodies. E-selectin expression can be induced by tumor necrosis factor-α (TNF-α), interleukin-1 (IL-1) and lipopolysaccharide, with maximal expression approximately 4 h after stimulation. L-selectin is constitutively expressed on the surface of most leukocytes and is rapidly shed in response to an inflammatory stimulus. The biologic consequence of L-selectin shedding is unknown, although it may be related to downstream cell signaling events [2].

Table 1. Selectins and their counter-ligands

Selectin	Localization	Ligands
E-selectin (CD62E)	Activated endothelium	ESL-1 PSGL-1 (CD162) sialyl Lewis^x (CD15s) sialyl Lewis ^{a} L-selectin
P-selectin (CD62P)	Platelets, endothelium	PSGL-1 (CD162) sialyl Lewis^x (CD15s) sialyl Lewis^a L-selectin
L-selectin (CD62L)	Most unactivated leukocytes	E- and P-selectin sialyl Lewis^x (CD15s) PSGL-1 (CD162)

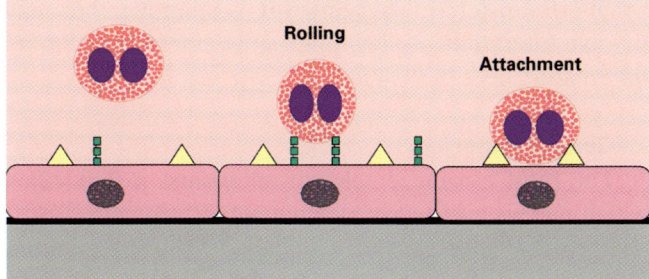

Fig. 1. Leukocyte rolling-adhesion paradigm.

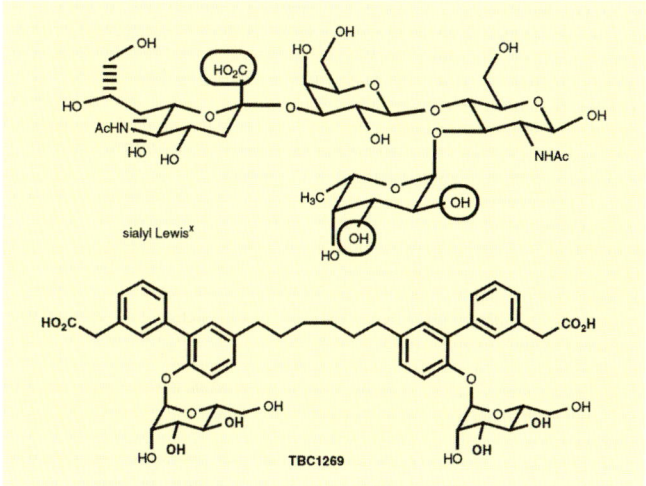

Fig. 2. Structural comparison of sLe^x and TBC1269.

Rationale for Selectin Antagonist Development

All three selectins have been implicated in the development of airway inflammation in animal models of asthma [3–5]. In a primate model of asthma, administration of a monoclonal antibody to E-selectin significantly improved airway mechanics during the late-phase response and reduced the number of neutrophils in bronchoalveolar lavage (BAL) fluid [3]. Upon allergen challenge, P-selectin-deficient mice contained far fewer eosinophils in BAL fluid and demonstrated a significantly reduced airway hyperresponsiveness (AHR) as compared to wild-type mice [4]. In a sheep model of allergic asthma, pretreatment with an L-selectin monoclonal antibody significantly reduced both the early and late airway response (EAR, LAR) and eliminated 24-hour AHR [5]. These data would suggest that selectin blockade may prove a viable treatment for inflammatory diseases of the airways.

Consequence of Selectin Inhibition

Immunosuppression is a potential side effect of chronic blockade of selectins. A human example has been identified in an extremely rare human syndrome known as leukocyte adhesion deficiency type II (LAD II) [6]. A defect in fucose metabolism in these patients results in improper biosynthesis of selectin ligands and presents biologically as a unique immunosupression. LAD II patients have chronic opportunistic infections of the mucosa and gingiva. Mice made deficient in various selectins by targeted gene deletion have yielded some useful information regarding the anticipated effects of chronic selectin blockade in humans. Deficiency in a single selectin is generally well tolerated. Mice deficient in both E- and P-selectin are associated with more deleterious effects. Mice deficient in all three selectins show a more severe phenotype compared to mice with a single selectin deficiency or a combined deficiency of two selectins [7]. The significance of this remains unclear since the relevance of these models to the scenario of chronic selectin blockade in humans has not yet been established.

Therapeutic Approaches

Glycomimetics, recombinant soluble ligands and small-molecule inhibitors are in various stages of development as potential therapeutic agents. Examples of each class are given below.

Cylexin®. Cylexin is a complex carbohydrate with structural similarity to sialyl Lewis x (sLe^x), a natural carbohydrate ligand for the selectins. Cylexin® has been shown to significantly reduce the degree of injury in a canine myocardial ischemia-reperfusion model [8] and to be effective as an adjunct therapy to tissue plasminogen activator in reducing myocardial infarct size in an electrolytic canine model [9]. Cylexin® has also proved effective in reducing the degree of restenosis following ballon injury in New Zealand White rabbits [10]. Other sLe^x mimetics have been reported in the literature, although these compounds are still early in development [11, 12].

Recombinant Soluble P-Selectin Glycoprotein Ligand-1. As with Cylexin, recombinant soluble P-selectin glycoprotein ligand-1 (rsPSGL-1) has been determined to be efficacious in models of ischemia-reperfusion injury [13, 14] and as an adjunct to tissue plasminogen activator in a porcine thrombosis model [15]. rsPSGL-1 has also demonstrated striking synergistic effects with low doses of cyclosporine in prolonging kidney allograft survival in a rat model [16].

TBC1269. TBC1269 is a small molecule selectin antagonist that inhibits all three selectins in vitro [17]. A dimeric form of sLe^x, sialyl di-Lewis x, inspired the design of TBC1269 (fig. 2).

Although proven effective in animal models of ischemia-reperfusion injury [18], TBC1269 is perhaps unique in that it has been evaluated in several animal models of asthma and lung injury as well [5, 19]. To date, the compound has proven efficacious in mouse, rat, rabbit, guinea pig and sheep models of allergic asthma. In the sheep model, pretreatment with aerosolized TBC1269 at 0.3 mg/kg resulted in a reduction of the EAR and elimination of the LAR and AHR [5]. The reduction in EAR was associated with an inhibition of histamine release from mast cells suggesting the compound may be disrupting key signal transduction pathways of the inflammatory response. Consistent with the mechanism of a selectin antagonist, the blockade in LAR and AHR was associated with a significant reduction in neutrophils in BAL. TBC1269 was also effective in preventing the LAR and AHR if dosed 90 min, but not 4 h, following antigen challenge [5]. This result was consistent with the predicted time course of selectin involvement in the inflammation cascade.

Route of Administration

In the sheep model discussed above, TBC1269 had similar effects on EAR, LAR, and AHR when dosed either by aerosol or intravenously although a higher dose was required intravenously [5]. Classically, selectin antagonists would be anticipated to work in the vascular compartment since this is the site where their function is most prolific. Interestingly, recent studies have demonstrated that cell adhesion antagonists may offer greater protection in an asthma setting when administered locally as opposed to systemically [20]. The mechanism of action when administered via the airway is unknown, but may involve alteration of signaling pathways of resident inflammatory cells in the lung.

Clinical Experience

The most advanced selectin antagonist is TBC1269, which has been tested intravenously in asthmatics in an allergen challenge phase II clinical trial. In this randomized, double-blind, placebo-controlled study, a single 30 mg/kg intravenous dose significantly reduced the airway recruitment of eosinophils compared to placebo controls [21]. Trends toward improvements in airway mechanics (FEV$_1$) were observed in the per-protocol group of TBC1269-treated patients, but the differences were not statistically significant in this pilot study of 21 patients. Another selectin antagonist to reach clinical development, Cylexin, has not been tested in humans with asthma. Cylexin showed no benefit over placebo in a 138-patient trial for the treatment of reperfusion injury in infants undergoing cardiopulmonary bypass to facilitate the surgical repair of life threatening heart defects. Based on the results from this and another phase III trial which did not meet the primary endpoint, the development of Cylexin has been halted [22].

Conclusions

Selectin antagonists represent an opportunity to mitigate inflammation at one of the earliest points in the inflammatory cycle [23]. By blocking the activity of the selectins, leukocyte rolling is significantly impaired and subsequent tissue extravasation is markedly diminished. Diseases such as asthma and COPD manifest an inflammatory component which is substantial and persistent, and these diseases may be ideally managed with a selectin antagonist in combination with bronchodilator therapy.

References

1 Vestweber D (ed): The Selectins: Initiators of Leukocyte Endothelial Adhesion. Harwood, 1997, pp 1–2.
2 Kansas GS: Selectins and their ligands: Current concepts and controversies. Blood 1996;88: 3259–3287.
3 Gundel RH, Wegner CD, Torcellini CA, Clarke CC, Haynes N, Rothlein R, Smith CW, Letts LG: Endothelial leukocyte adhesion molecule-1 mediates antigen-induced acute airway inflammation and late-phase airway obstruction in monkeys. J Clin Invest 1991;88:1407–1411.
4 DeSanctis GT, Wolyniec WW, Green FH, Qin S, Jiao A, Finn PW, Noonan AA, Joetham AA, Gelfand E, Doerschuk CM, Drazen JM: Reduction of allergic airway responses in P-selectin-deficient mice. J Appl Physiol 1997; 83:681–687.
5 Abraham WM, Ahmed A, Sabater JR, Lauredo IT, Botvinnokova Y, Bjercke RJ, Hu X, Revelle MB, Kogan TP, Scott IL, Dixon RAF, Yeh ETH, Beck PJ: Selectin blockade prevents antigen-induced late bronchial responses and airway hyperresponsivess in allergic sheep. Am J Respir Crit Care Med 1999;159:1205–1214.
6 Becker DJ, Lowe JB: Leukocyte adhesion deficiency type II. Biochim Biophys Acta 1999; 1455:193–204.
7 Jung U, Ley K: Mice lacking two or all three selectins demonstrate overlapping and distinct functions for each selectin. J Immunol 1999; 162:6755–6762.
8 Lefer DJ, Flynn DM, Phillips ML, Ratcliffe M, Buda AJ: A novel sialyl Lewis^x analog attenuates neutrophil accumulation and myocardial necrosis after ischemia and reperfusion. Circulation 1994;90:2390–2401.
9 Silver MJ, Sutton JM, Hook S, Lee P, Malycky JL, Phillips ML, Ellis SG, Topol EJ, Nicolini FA: Adjunctive selectin blockade successfully reduces infarct size beyond thrombolysis in the electrolytic canine coronary artery model. Circulation 1995;92:492–499.

10 Barron MK, Lake RS, Buda AJ, Tenaglia AN: Intimal hyperplasia after balloon injury is attenuated by blocking selectins. Circulation 1997;96:3587–3592.
11 Norman KE, Anderson GP, Kolb HC, Ley K, Ernst B, Sialyl Lewis (x) (sLe(x)) and an sLe(x) mimetic, CGP69669A, disrupt E-selectin-dependent leukocyte rolling in vivo. Blood 1999; 91:475–483.
12 Todderud G, Nair X, Lee D, Alford J, Davern L, Stanley P, Bachand C, Lapointe P, Marinier A, Martel A, Menard M, Wright JJ, Bajorath J, Hollenbaugh D, Aruffo A, Tramposch KM: BMS-190394, a selectin inhibitor, prevents rat cutaneous inflammatory reactions. J Pharmacol Exp Ther 1997;282:1298–1304.
13 Dulkanchainun TS, Goss JA, Imagawa DK, Shaw, GD, Anselmo DM, Kaldas F, Wang T, Zhao D, Busuttil AA, Kato H, Murray NG, Kupiec-Weglinski, Busuttil RW: Reduction of hepatic ischemia/reperfusion injury by a soluble P-selectin glycoprotein ligand-1. Ann Surg 1998;227:832–840.
14 Hayward R, Campbell B, Shin YK, Scalia R, Lefer AM: Recombinant Soluble P-selectin glycoprotein ligand-1 protects against myocardial ischemia reperfusion injury in cats. Cardiovasc Res 1999;41:65–76.
15 Kumar A, Villani MP, Patel UK, Keith JC Jr, Schaub RG: Recombinant soluble form of PSGL-1 accelerates thrombolysis and prevents reocclusion in a porcine model. Circulation 1999;99:1363–1369.
16 Kusaka M, Zandi-Nejad K, Kato S, Beato F, Nagano H, Shaw GD, Tilney NL: Exploitation of the continuum between early ischemia/reperfusion injury and host alloresponsiveness: Indefinite kidney allograft survival by treatment with a soluble P-selectin ligand and low-dose cyclosporine in combination. Transplantation 1999;67:1255–1261.
17 Kogan TP, Dupré B, Bui H, McAbee KL, Kassir JM, Scott IL, Hu X, Vanderslice P, Beck PJ, Dixon RAF: Novel synthetic inhibitors of selectin-mediated cell adhesion: Synthesis of 1,6-bis[3-(3-carboxymethylphenyl)-4-(2-α-D-mannopyranosyloxy)-phenyl]hexane (TBC1269). J Med Chem 1998;41:1099–1111.
18 Palma Vargas JM, Toledo-Pereyra L, Dean RE, Harkema JM, Dixon RAF, Kogan TP: Small molecule selectin inhibitor protects against liver inflammatory response after ischemia and reperfusion. J Am Coll Surg 1997;185:365–372.
19 Ramos-Kelly JR, Toledo-Pereyra LH, Jordan JA, Rivera-Chavez FA, Dixon RAF, Ward PA: Upregulation of lung chemokines associated with hemorrhage is reversed with a small molecule multiple selectin inhibitor. J Am Coll Surg 1999;189:546–553.
20 Henderson WR Jr, Chi EY, Albert RK, Chu SJ, Lamm WJ, Rochon Y, Jonas M, Christie PE, Harlan JM: Blockade of CD49d (alpha4 integrin) on intrapulmonary but not circulating leukocytes inhibits airway inflammation and hyperresponsiveness in a mouse model of asthma. J Clin Invest 1997;100:3083–3092.
21 Texas Biotechnology Corporation press release, September 9, 1998.
22 Cytel Corporation press release, March 30, 1999.
23 Montefort S, Holgate ST, Howarth PH: Leukocyte-endothelial adhesion molecules and their role in bronchial asthma and allergic rhinitis. Eur Respir J 1993;6:1044–1054.

Richard A.F. Dixon, PhD
Texas Biotechnology Corporation
20th Floor, 7000 Fannin
Houston, TX 77030 (USA)
Tel. +1 713 796 8822, Fax +1 713 796 8928
E-Mail rdixon@tbc.com

ICAM-1 and VCAM-1 Antagonists

Ivan M. Richards   Vandana Khare Slatter

Pharmacia Corporation, Kalamazoo, Mich., USA

Summary

The accumulation and activation of inflammatory cells in the respiratory tract in asthma and COPD is critically dependent on the ordered expression of specific adhesion molecules on subsets of leukocytes, and the expression of counter-receptors, such as intercellular adhesion molecule-1 (ICAM-1; CD54) and vascular cell adhesion molecule-1 (VCAM-1; CD106) on endothelial cells. ICAM-1 and VCAM-1 can also be selectively expressed on other cell types in the lungs, e.g. epithelial cells (ICAM-1), fibroblasts (ICAM-1 and VCAM-1) and T lymphocytes (ICAM-1). Products of activated eosinophils and neutrophils within the airway wall cause epithelial damage which results in airway hyperresponsiveness. Some known anti-inflammatory agents such as glucocorticoids have been shown to inhibit the expression of VCAM-1 and ICAM-1 in the lungs and respiratory tract. Novel agents directed towards blocking VCAM-1 or ICAM-1 specifically, and currently in preclinical and clinical development, have been described and include monoclonal antibodies, soluble forms of ICAM-1 and VCAM-1, oligonucleotides (antisense) and small molecules. However, to date none of these approaches have yielded an agent in late stage clinical development.

Rationale

Inhibition of VCAM-1 and/or ICAM-1 will prevent the accumulation of inflammatory cells within the airway wall and reduce their capacity to damage airway epithelium and promote nonspecific airway hyperresponsiveness (AHR), a characteristic feature of both asthma and COPD.

Role of ICAM-1 and VCAM-1

Nonspecific AHR is a hallmark of asthma in man [1] and can also be demonstrated in patients with COPD [2]. AHR is believed by many investigators to be caused by epithelial damage arising from the accumulation of activated leukocytes in the airway wall. Although inflammation is a characteristic of both diseases, inflammation in the peripheral airways predominates in COPD, and inflammation in the central airways predominates in asthma. Changes in lung mechanics correspond to the anatomical sites of inflammation; COPD is characterized by reduced maximum expiratory flow and slow forced emptying of the lungs whilst asthma is characterized by variable and reversible airflow limitation. There are also major differences in the nature of the inflammatory cell populations involved in the two diseases and these can be closely correlated with appropriate differences in adhesion molecule expression. Asthma is associated with an eosinophil and lymphocyte-rich airway inflammation whilst in COPD neutrophils predominate [3]. Although inflammatory leukocytes are the primary effector cells which cause epithelial damage, their recruitment, activation and survival in the airways are thought to be orchestrated by cytokines released by subsets of T cells. In asthma, CD4+ T cells predominate while in COPD CD8+ T cells play a more significant role [4]. The recruitment of inflammatory cells into the airway wall is critically dependent on the ordered expression of adhesion molecules on the leukocyte surface and the expression of counter-receptors on endothelial cells or in tissues. Cytokines play a critical role in upregulating adhesion molecules on leukocytes or endothelial cells. An essential first step in the recruitment of leukocytes from the circulation into the tissues is adhesion to the blood vessel wall. A rolling phenomenon mediated by the selectin family of molecules (reviewed by Dixon and McKinney [5] in this volume) precedes firm adhesion and transmigration of leukocytes. Firm adhesion occurs via binding of $\beta 2$ integrins on neutrophils with ICAM-1 on endothelial cells, while binding of VLA-4 on the surface of eosinophils and lymphocytes with upregulated VCAM-1 on endothelial cells is critically important for adhesion of the latter cell types in allergic tissue injury (fig. 1). The targeted disruption of the interaction between VCAM-1 and the β1 integrin, VLA-4, or ICAM-1 and β2 integrins, is an attractive approach for preventing the accumulation of eosinophils or neutrophils, respectively, into the lungs and respiratory tract.

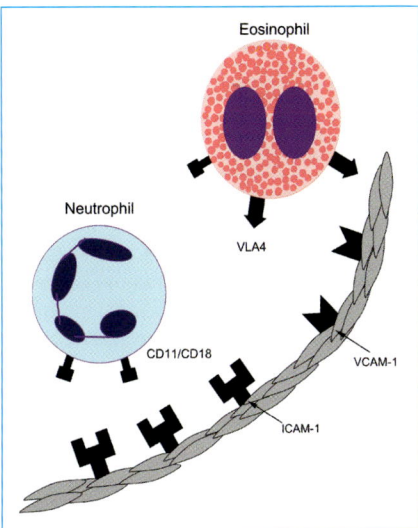

Fig. 1. VCAM-1 and ICAM-1 are expressed on activated endothelial cells. VLA-4 (CD49d), a ligand for VCAM-1 is expressed on eosinophils, monocytes, T and B lymphocytes but not neutrophils allowing for the selective recruitment of granulocytes during allergic tissue injury. β2 integrins (CD11a/CD18 and CD11b/CD18) expressed on neutrophils are responsible for firm adhesion of neutrophils to ICAM-1 in COPD.

Concept Testing

VCAM-1. A much greater emphasis has been placed on the discovery of inhibitors of VLA-4 (CD49d; reviewed by Lobb and Adams [6] in this volume) rather than its counter-receptor, VCAM-1. However, studies in animal models of allergic tissue injury and in man strongly support a role for VCAM-1 in asthma. Upregulated expression of VCAM-1 has been shown in disease, and increased levels of soluble VCAM-1 have been shown following segmental allergen challenge in asthmatics [7, 8]. Upregulated VCAM-1 has also been demonstrated following antigen-challenge in sensitized mice (fig. 2), and eosinophilic airway inflammation in these mice was prevented by treatment with anti-VCAM-1 monoclonal antibody [7]. Currently, there is no specific anti-rat VCAM-1 antibody to test the concept that eosinophil recruitment is dependent on VCAM-1 in this species although antibodies to VLA-4, the major counter-receptor for VCAM-1, have demonstrated efficacy in rat eosinophilic lung inflammation [10]. VLA-4 is also upregulated on lymphocytes migrating into lung tissue following antigen challenge [11]. There is no evidence that VCAM-1 is responsible for the recruitment of neutrophils in COPD.

ICAM-1. Convincing evidence implicating ICAM-1 in asthma has arisen from in situ evidence from tissues, bronchoalveolar lavage cells and bronchoalveolar lavage fluid from asthmatics [12–14] and a wealth of evidence from allergen-induced lung tissue inflammation in animals [15–17]. In contrast, there have been few reports of

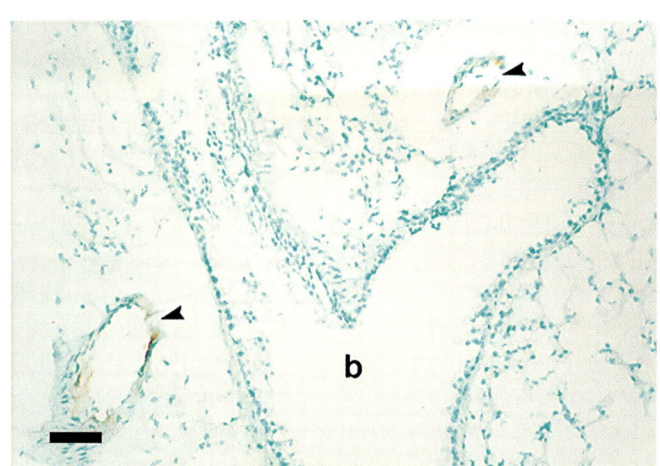
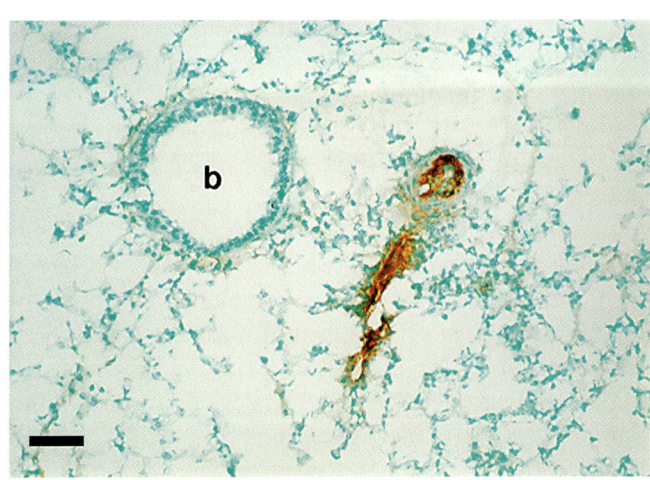

Fig. 2. Immunohistochemical staining of lung tissue obtained 72 h after ovalbumin challenge in oralbumin-sensitized mice. Tissues were stained with anti-vascular cell adhesion molecule (VCAM-1) monoclonal antibody M/K-2.7. Weak staining of VCAM-1 in 2 arterioles (arrows) in the lung was observed in vehicle-sensitized, ovalbumin-challenged mice (**A**), and very strong staining in lung arterioles but not in bronchioles (b) was seen in ovalbumin-sensitized, ovalbumin-challenged mice (**B**). Bar = 50 μm.

Table 1. Antisense compounds in development targeting VCAM-1 or ICAM-1

Compound	Company	Development status	VCAM-1	ICAM-1	Comments
ISIS 2302	ISIS	asthma – preclinical (US); Psoriasis- PhII (US, Europe)		√	antisense oligonucleotide ISIS 2302 is not currently being pursued for Crohn's disease and rheumatoid arthritis
ISIS compounds (2nd generation class; earlier class included ISIS 5876)	Isis	inflammation – preclinical (US)		√	antisense oligonucleotide
AGI 1067	AtheroGenics/ Schering Plough	atherosclerosis; restenosis – phase II (US)	√		composite vascular protectant reported to be a gene expression inhibitor, to block production of VCAM-1 and MCP-1 inflammatory genes and to reduce arterial inflammation leading to atherosclerosis

the role of ICAM-1 in COPD. In one study [18], the levels of lymphocyte function associated antigen (LFA-1) and MAC-1, counter receptors on circulating neutrophils were measured in addition to circulating levels of soluble ICAM-1 (sICAM-1). During disease exacerbation, the expression of LFA-1, MAC-1 and the levels of sICAM-1 decreased although this might not reflect the expression of these molecules in the lungs. However, higher levels of sICAM-1 have been described in smokers than in non-smokers [19]. Rhinovirus infections are a major cause of asthma exacerbation, and ICAM-1 is not only the cellular receptor for 90% of rhinoviruses but has been shown to be inducible by the virus itself, thereby promoting infection and increased inflammatory cell recruitment to the airway wall [20,21]. ICAM-1 is therefore an attractive target for the development of novel drugs which inhibit virus-induced asthma exacerbations.

Clinical Approaches

ICAM-1 and VCAM-1 clearly make valid targets for the discovery of novel treatments for asthma and COPD, although it is our opinion, after reviewing the literature, that the difficulties associated with developing novel compounds designed to block these molecules may have been underestimated, and we discovered an extraordinary number of failures. Although the formal title of this chapter is 'ICAM-1 and VCAM-1 Antagonists', we did not restrict this review of current agents in discovery or development to traditional small-molecule pharmacological antagonists of these molecules. Indeed, this approach may be untenable given that a small-molecule antagonist would be required to block a critically important binding site, or sites, within large and complex proteins. Monoclonal antibodies, antisense molecules, soluble ICAM-1 and soluble VCAM-1, and small-molecule inhibitors may all offer alternative opportunities for the discovery of novel therapies which prevent the expression of these molecules or block the expressed molecule. Extensive efforts have been made using monoclonal antibodies to validate the role of ICAM-1 in allergic tissue injury [11, 15–17] and exploring clinical applications. However, to our knowledge, efforts to pursue anti-ICAM-1 monoclonal antibodies in the clinic for the treatment of asthma or COPD have stalled, and most current activity appears to be in exploring antisense molecules primarily for other indications (table 1). Isis is working on an antisense molecule, ISIS-2302 to block ICAM-1 and has pursued inflammatory bowel disease (Crohn's disease, ulcerative colitis), psoriasis, renal transplant rejection, and rheumatoid arthritis as initial disease targets. [22, 23]. However, several indications are currently not being envisaged. Due to a limited clinical response, development of ISIS-2302 for the rheumatoid arthritis indication has been discontinued [24]. Also, following the unexpected failure of the company's pivotal clinical trial of ISIS-2302 in Crohn's disease, Isis has not yet determined whether it will continue to investigate ISIS-2302 for this indication [25]. Antisense oligonucleotides to block

VCAM-1 in inflammation (a second-generation class) are in preclinical development at Isis [C. Frank Bennett, PhD, Isis Pharmaceuticals, June 5, 2000, pers. commun.]. AtheroGenics is working in concert with Schering Plough on a composite vascular protectant, AGI 1067, claimed to be a gene expression inhibitor which blocks production of VCAM-1 and MCP-1 inflammatory genes. It is reported to be in phase II development for the treatment of atherosclerosis [26].

Although there is a wealth of evidence indicating that ICAM-1 and VCAM-1 make attractive targets for novel therapeutics for treating COPD and asthma, validation of these targets awaits systematic clinical trials of the novel agents currently in development.

References

1 Hargreave FE, Ryan G, Thomson NC, O'Byrne PM, Latimer K, Juniper EF, Dolovich J: Bronchial responsiveness to histamine or methacholine in asthma: Measurement and clinical significance. J Allergy Clin Immunol 1981; 68: 347–355.
2 Brand PL, Postma DS, Kerstjens HA, Koeter GH: Relationship of airway hyperresponsiveness to respiratory symptoms and diurnal peak flow variation in patients with obstructive lung disease. The Dutch CNSLD Study Group. Am Rev Resp Dis 1991;143:916–921.
3 Peleman RA, Rytila PH, Kips JC, Joos GF, Pauwels RA: The cellular composition of induced sputum in chronic obstructive pulmonary disease. Eur Respir J 1999;13:839–843.
4 Jeffery PK: Differences and similarities between chronic lung disease and asthma. Clin Exp Allergy 1999;29:14–26.
5 Berens KL, Vanderslice P, Dupré B, Dixon RAF: Selectin antagonists. Therapeutics for airway inflammation. Prog Respir Res. Basel, Karger, 2001, vol 31, pp 306–309.
6 Adams SP, Lobb RR: Small-molecule VLA-4 antagonists. Prog Respir Res. Basel, Karger, 2001, vol 31, pp 302–305.
7 Ohkawara Y, Yamauchi K, Maruyama N, Hoshi H, Ohno I, Honma M, Tanno Y, Tamura G, Shirato K, Ohtani H: In situ expression of the cell adhesion molecules in bronchial tissues from asthmatics with airflow limitation: In vivo evidence of VCAM-1/VLA-4 interaction in selective eosinophil infiltration. Am J Respir Cell Mol Biol 1995;12:4–12.
8 Zangrilli JG, Shaver JR, Cirelli RA, Cho SK, Garlisi CG, Falcone A, Cuss FM, Fish JE, Peters SP: VCAM-1 levels after segmental challenge correlate with eosinophil influx and IL-4 and IL-5 production, and the late phase response. Am J Respir Crit Care Med 1995;151:1346–1353.
9 Chin JE, Hatfield CA, Winterrowd GE, Brashler JR, Vonderfecht SL, Fidler SF, Griffin RL, Kolbasa KP, Krzesicki RF, Sly LM, Staite ND, Richards IM: Airway recruitment of leukocytes is dependent on α4-integrins and vascular cell adhesion molecule-1. Am J Physiol 1997;272:L219–L229.
10 Richards IM, Kolbasa KP, Hatfield CA, Winterrowd GE, Vonderfecht SL, Fidler SF, Griffin RL, Brashler JR, Krzesicki RF, Sly LM, Ready KR, Staite ND, Chin JE: Role of very late activation antigen-4 in the antigen-induced accumulation of eosinophils and lymphocytes in the lungs and airway lumen of sensitized brown Norway rats. Am J Respir Cell Mol Biol 1996;15:172–183.
11 Kennedy JD, Hatfield CA, Fidler SF, Winterrowd GE, Chin JE, Richards IM: Phenotypic characteristics of T lymphocytes emigrating into lung tissue and the airway lumen following antigen inhalation in sensitized mice. Am J Respir Cell Mol Biol 1995;12:613–623.
12 Bentley AM, Durham SR, Robinson DS, Menz G, Storz C, Cromwell O, Kay AB, Wardlaw AJ: Expression of endothelial and leukocyte adhesion molecules intercellular adhesion molecule-1, E-selectin, and vascular cell adhesion molecule-1 in the bronchial mucosa in steady state and allergen-induced asthma. J Allergy Exp Immunol 1993;92:857–868.
13 Takahashi N, Liu MC, Proud D, Yu X-Y, Hasegawa S, Spannhake EW: Soluble intercellular adhesion molecule-1 in bronchoalveolar lavage fluid of allergic subjects following segmental allergen challenge. Am J Respir Crit Care Med 1994;150:704–709.
14 Montefort S, Lai CKW, Kapahi P, Leung J, Lai KN, Chan HS, Haskard DO, Howarth PS, Holgate ST: Circulating adhesion molecules in asthma. Am J Resp Crit Care Med 1994;149:1149–1152.
15 Richards IM, Kolbasa KP, Winterrowd GE, Hatfield CA, Vonderfecht SL, Fidler SF, Griffin RL, Brashler JR, Krzesicki RF, Lane CL, Anderson DC, Sly LM, Staite ND, Chin JE: Role of intercellular adhesion molecule-1 in antigen-induced lung inflammation in brown Norway rats. Am J Physiol 1996;271:L267–L276.
16 Gundel RH, Wegner CD, Torcellini CA, Letts GL: The role of intercellular adhesion molecule-1 in chronic airway inflammation. Clin Exp Allergy 1992;22:569–575.
17 Hatfield CA, Brashler JR, Winterrowd GE, Bell FP, Griffin RL, Fidler SF, Kolbasa KP, Mobley JM, Shull KL, Richards IM, Chin JE: Intercellular adhesion molecule-1 deficient mice have antibody responses but impaired leukocyte recruitment. Am J Physiol 1997;273:L513–L523.
18 Noguera A, Busquets X, Sauleda J, Villaverde JM, Macnee W, Agusti AG: Expression of adhesion molecules and G Proteins in circulating neutrophils in chronic obstructive pulmonary disease. Am J Respir Crit Care Med 1998;158:1664–1668.
19 Bergmann S, Siekmeier R, Mix C, Jaross W: Even moderate cigarette smoking influences the pattern of circulating monocytes and the concentration of sICAM-1. Respir Physiol 1998;114:269–275.
20 Papi A, Johnston SL: Rhinovirus infection induces expression of its own receptor intercellular adhesion molecule 1 (ICAM-1) via increased NF-kappa B-mediated transcription. J Biol Chem 1999;274:9707–9720.
21 Yamaya M, Sekizawa K, Suzuki T, Yamada N, Furukawa M, Ishizuka S, Nakayama K, Terajima M, Numazaki Y, Sasaki H: Infection of human respiratory submucosal glands with rhinovirus: Effects on cytokine and ICAM-1 production. Am J Physiol 1999;277:L362–L371.
22 Bennett CF: Antisense oligonucleotide therapeutics. Exp Opin Invest Drugs 1999;8(3).
23 Yacyshyn BR, Bowen-Yacyshyn MB, Jewell L, Tami JA, Bennett CF, Kisner DL, Shanahan WR Jr: A placebo-controlled trial of ICAM-1 antisense oligonucleotide in the treatment of Crohn's disease. Gastroenterology 1998;114:1133–1142.
24 Isis presents data from phase II trial of Isis 2302 in rheumatoid arthritis Press Release. Isis Pharmaceuticals, Inc. Iddb (http://www.iddb.com), 15 November 1999.
25 Isis Pharmaceuticals Inc announces restructuring and expense reduction plan; company has approximately 3 years of cash under the new operating plan Press Release. Isis Pharmaceuticals, Inc. Iddb (http://www.iddb.com), 18 January 2000.
26 AtheroGenics announces launch of phase II clinical trial for post-angioplasty restenosis Press Release. AtheroGenics Inc. IDdb (http://www.iddb.com), 1999 October 12.

Ivan M. Richards, PhD
Pharmacia Corporation
301, Henrietta Street
Kalamazoo, MI 49001 (USA)
Tel. +1 616 833 1040, Fax +1 616 833 9763
E-Mail ivan.m.richards@am.pnu.com

Inhibition of Cell Signalling

Eosinophil G-Protein-Coupled Receptor Signalling: An Overview

Mark A. Lindsay   Patricia M. De Souza   Oonagh T. Lynch   Mark A. Giembycz

Thoracic Medicine, National Heart and Lung Institute, Imperial College School of Medicine, London, UK

Summary

There are approximately 140,000 genes in the human genome. This figure is significantly higher than conventional estimates and indicates that the genome is far more complex than originally appreciated. Clearly, this revised number of genes has implications for those that encode G-protein-coupled receptors (GPCR), which are believed to account for up to 5% of the total genome in some species. In this short article, we briefly describe the BLT receptor as a model system for understanding GPCR signalling in eosinophils. However, it is possible that approximately 7,000 genes encode GPCRs, with additional complexity arising from alternative mRNA splicing and different promoter usage. Thus, despite significant advances in our understanding of GPCRs in general and their expression on eosinophils in particular, we have only begun to understand what is probably the largest cell surface receptor family known. The potential for therapeutic intervention with small molecule inhibitors is, therefore, potentially enormous.

Eosinophils are potent effector cells that are important in parasitic/immune surveillance of mucosal-epithelial surfaces, including those of the gut, skin and airways. However, in addition to these tissue-preserving functions, eosinophils have been implicated in inflammatory responses associated with a number of non-parasitic disorders including atopic dermatitis and asthma [1]. In these situations, the inappropriate migration and activation of eosinophils is thought to lead to the release of a host of inflammatory lipid and protein mediators, as well as the production of toxic oxygen radicals following the activation of the NADPH oxidase [1].

A two-step process has been advanced to explain the translocation of eosinophils from the circulation into tissue. In this paradigm, circulating eosinophils initially are primed by cytokines including IL-3, IL-5 and GM-CSF and then migrate into tissue where they are activated, the latter processes being dependent upon agonists that act via G-protein-coupled receptors (GPCRs) [2]. Consistent with this idea is the knowledge that agonism of CCR3 by chemokines such as eotaxin is associated with mobilization of eosinophils from the bone marrow [3]. Thus, the identification and characterization of GPCRs may allow the development of new therapeutic agents that could impact on eosinophil maturation, survival and activation thereby suppressing eosinophilic inflammation.

Expression of GPCRs on Eosinophils

GPCRs are characterized by an extracellular N-terminal sequence followed by seven transmembrane spanning domains, with three extracellular and three intracellular loops, and an intracellular C-terminus. Conserved cysteine residues within the N-terminal sequence and in the third extracellular loop are thought to form a disulphide bond that is required for ligand binding whilst a second disulphide bond is probably formed between conserved cysteine residues with the first and second extracellular loops. The functional responses to ligand binding are transduced by G-proteins, which are heterotrimeric molecules consisting of α-, β- and γ- subunits. Multiple isoforms of each subunit are present in mammalian cells and approximately 20 different α-isoforms, five β-isoforms and 10 γ-isoforms have been identified. A number of these subunits have been found in human and guinea pig eosinophils including G_{α_s}, $G_{\alpha_{i3}}$, G_{α_o}, $G_{\alpha_{q/11}}$ and G_β [4].

Table 1. GPCRs expressed by eosinophils

GPCRs	Natural ligand(s)	Species	G-Protein
PAF-R	C_{16}-PAF, C_{18}-PAF	human	G_i/G_o
		guinea pig	?
BLT-R	LTB_4	human	?
		guinea pig	?
Cys-LT-R[1]	LTC_4, LTD_4, LTE_4	human	G_i/G_o
		guinea pig	G_q/G_{11}
LXA_4-R	LXA_4	human	G_i/G_o
		mouse	G_i/G_o
DP-R	PGD_2	human	?
?	5-HETE, 5-oxo-ETE	human	G_i/G_o
CCR1	MIP-1α, RANTES, MCP-2, MCP-3, MCP-5, leukotactin-1	human	?
		guinea pig	?
CCR3	eotaxin-1, 2, 3, leukotactin-1, MCP-3, MCP-4, RANTES	human	G_i/G_o
		guinea pig	G_i/G_o
		mouse	G_i/G_o
CCR6	MIP-3α	human	G_i/G_o
CXCR3	γIP-10, Mig	human	?
CXCR4	SDF-1α	human	G_i/G_o
C3a-R	C3a	human	G_i/G_o
C5a-R	C5a	human	G_i/G_o
		guinea pig	G_i/G_o
FRP[1]	fMLP	human	G_i/G_o
NK_1-R	SP, NKA, NKB	human	?
CGRP-R[1]	CGRP, amylin, calcitonin, adrenomedullin	human	G_q/G_{11}
$VPAC_1$-R	VIP, secretin	human	?
P2Y-R[1]	ATP, UTP	human	G_i/G_o
A2-R	adenosine	human	?
A3-R	adenosine	human	?
$EP_{2/4}$-R	PGE_2	human	G_s
		guinea pig	G_s
$β_2$-AR	adrenaline, noradrenaline	human	G_s
H_1-R	histamine	human	?
H_2-R	histamine	human	?
H_3-R	histamine	human	?

5-Oxo-ETE = 5-oxo-eicosatetraenoate.
[1] Receptor subtype unknown.

Only 20 GPCRs have, thus far, been unequivocally identified on eosinophils [1] (table 1). However, this number is likely to grow rapidly given that the sequences of around 850 GPRCs are now known.

Activation and Inhibition of Eosinophils by Agonists of GPCRs

GPCRs are linked to a vast array of signal transduction pathways that ultimately promote or suppress many functional responses (table 2). With the exception of the receptors for cysteinyl-leukotrienes and calcitonin gene-related peptide, which are believed to act through $G_{q/11}$, most ligands that activate and inhibit eosinophils are thought to signal through receptors coupled to $G_{i/o}$ and G_s, respectively. In this article, we briefly review GPCRs in general with emphasis on the BLT receptor, which has been studied in some detail. Readers interested in other GPRCs including those that act via G_s are directed to a recent review of this subject [1].

Human Eosinophils. Little is known of the intracellular mechanism(s) by which agonism of GPCRs activates human eosinophils. Agonists that activate receptors coupled through $G_{i/o}$ such as PAF, RANTES, C3a, C5a, eotaxin, 5-oxo-eicosatetraenoate and MIP-3α evoke rapid and transient increases in the cytosolic free Ca^{2+} concentration ($[Ca^{2+}]_c$) and activate extracellular signal-regulated protein kinase (ERK)-1/2, phosphatidylinositol 3-kinase (PtdIns 3-kinase) and protein kinase B [5–9]. In addition, the CCR3 agonist, eotaxin, also promotes the phosphorylation and activation of p38 MAP kinase (fig. 1) [6]. While the functional responses that result from activation of these pathways are for the most part unknown, small-molecule inhibitors, such as PD 098059 and SB 203580, have implicated ERK-1/2 and p38 MAP kinase in eotaxin-induced chemotaxis and degranulation in vitro and rolling in vivo [6, 7].

Guinea Pig Eosinophils. Guinea pig peritoneal eosinophils can be obtained in large numbers and this has allowed detailed biochemical studies to be performed that are not currently possible with human eosinophils. Perhaps the most studied GPCR expressed by guinea pig eosinophils is the BLT receptor at which LTB_4 is a natural agonist, and we have used this receptor as a model system (fig. 2).

The human BLT receptor was cloned in 1997 from retinoic acid-differentiated HL-60 cells and is composed of 352 amino acids encoded by the *LTB4R* gene that has been localized to the q11.2–12 region of chromosome 14 [10]. Depending on species and, possibly tissue within the same species, the BLT receptor couples through either $G_{i/o}$ or G_{16} [10, 11]. An analysis of [^{3}H]LTB_4 binding to membrane fractions prepared from CHO cells and retinoic acid-differentiated HL-60 and COS-7 cells transfected with the cDNA for the human and murine BLT receptor showed similar binding characteristics with K_ds of 0.14 and 0.15 nM, respectively [10]. Binding studies have also identified and partially characterized receptors for LTB_4 on guinea pig eosinophils [12–14] using [^{3}H]LTB_4 as radioligand. However, notable differences are apparent between studies. Using intact peritoneal eosinophils from guinea pigs, Ng et al. [13] reported that [^{3}H]LTB_4 interacts with an apparently homogeneous population of binding sites with a B_{max} of 40,000 sites per cell and a K_d of 2.8 nM, which is approximately 10-fold lower than that reported in the transfection experiments described by

Table 2. Eosinophil responses at a glance

Function	BLT	Cys-LT¹	fMLP	PAF	CCR1	CC	CCR6	CXCR1/2²	CXCR4	VP-AC₁	C3a	C5a	P2Y¹	A₂	A₃	NK₁	β₂³	DP	EP₂	H₁	H₂	H₃
NADPH oxidase	↑		↑	↑	↑	↑					↑	↑	↑	↓(?)	↓(?)	↑	↓	↓		↑(?)		
Degranulation	↑		↑	↑		↑					↑	↑			↓	↑	↓	↓	↓			
Chemotaxis	↑	↑	↔	↑	↔	↑	↑				↑	↑	↑		↓	↑	↓	↑				
Chemokinesis	↑		↔					↑	↑							↓	↑			↑(?)	↑(?)	
Actin polymerization			↔	↑	↑		↑					↑										
Adhesion			↑	↑	↑	↑					↑					↓				↑(?)		
Homotypic aggregation	↑			↑							↑					↓			↓			
LTB₄ release				↑																		
LTC₄/D₄ release			↑	↑							↑					↓						
PAF release				↑							↑											
TXB₂ release	↑		↑	↑							↑											
PGE₂ release	↑			↑																		
PGI₂ release	↑			↑																		
PGD₂ release				↑																		
FGF₂α release				↑																		
Lipid body formation				↑																		
CR1 expression	↑																					
CR3 expression			↑	↑		↑						↑				↓	↓					
FcεR expression	↑			↑																		
IgE binding				↑											↑							
Apoptosis	↓	↓																	↓			
Shedding of L-selectin			↑	↑												↓			↓			
ICAM-1 expression				↑																		
Oestrogen binding											↑											
IL-8 release			↑	↑	↑						↑											
MCP-1 release			↑																			
Hypodensity			↑																			
Priming			↑												↑							
MIF release											↑											
Ca²⁺ mobilization	↑		↑	↑	↑	↑	↑	↑	↑		↑	↑	↑		↑			↑	↓			↑(?)

↑ = Response augmented; ↓ = response inhibited; ↔ = Weak stimulatory effect; (?) = response and/or receptor subtype requires conformation.
¹ Receptor subtype unknown.
² Expression of receptor equivocal.
³ Subtype unclear.

Yokomizo et al. [10]. The sites labelled in eosinophils probably represent functional receptors since various compounds related structurally to LTB₄ compete with the radioligand with affinities that correlate closely with their ability to induce chemotaxis and to evoke the formation of superoxide anions [13]. The rank order of potency of ligands for the displacement of [³H]LTB₄ from intact peritoneal eosinophils differs from the rank order obtained using membranes from COS-7 cells transfected with the BLT receptor which might indicate species difference, BLT receptor heterogeneity (see below) and/or the existence of different conformations of a single BLT receptor. With respect to the latter possibilities, Maghni et al. [12] reported that [³H]LTB₄ labels a heterogeneous population of binding sites on guinea pig alveolar eosinophils; approximately 1,000 sites per cell are labelled with high affinity ($K_D = 1$ nM) whereas the remainder (5,500 sites per cell) are labelled with low affinity ($K_D = 63$ nM). Similar results have been obtained with guinea pig peritoneal eosinophils [14]. Thus, a small population ($B_{max} = 900$

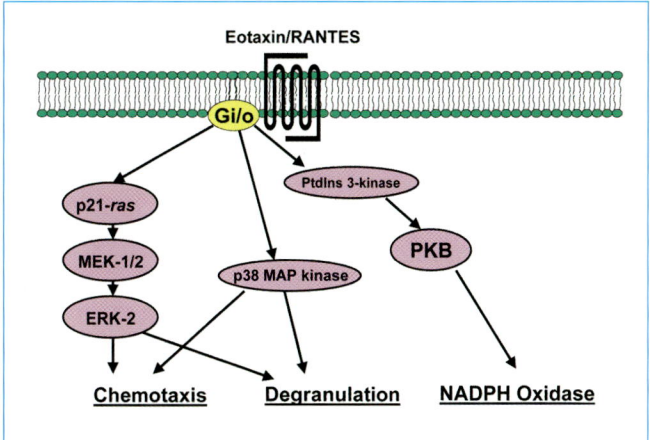

Fig. 1. CCR3-mediated signalling in human eosinophils. AA = Arachidonic acid.

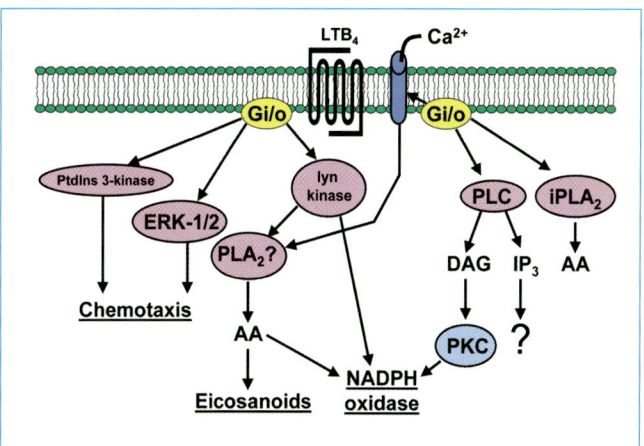

Fig. 2. Signalling pathways activated by LTB$_4$ in guinea pig eosinophils.

sites per cell) of receptors for which LTB$_4$ has high affinity (K$_D$ = 0.3 nM) was identified by radioligand binding together with a large number of sites (60,000 per cell) at which LTB$_4$ has relatively low affinity (K$_D$ = 140 nM). Again, the finding that various metabolites of LTB$_4$ competed with [^{3}H]LTB$_4$ for binding to alveolar eosinophils with a rank order of potency in good agreement with their ability to induce chemotaxis [12] supports the belief that the high-affinity sites represent bona fide receptors. Of considerable interest is the role of the two populations of receptor expressed by these cells. Maghni et al. [12] have considered the hypothesis, posed originally by Goldman and Goetzl [15], that they mediate different functional responses: the receptor for which LTB$_4$ has high affinity subserving chemokinesis and chemotaxis; the receptor for which LTB$_4$ has low affinity, mediating respiratory burst and prostanoid generation. This contention derives from the finding that the affinity of U-75302, a BLT receptor antagonist, determined from binding studies differs (~ 17-fold) between the two populations of receptor [12]. Collectively, the available data suggest that peritoneal eosinophils express the same BLT receptor that is labelled with high affinity by [^{3}H]LTB$_4$ on guinea pig alveolar eosinophils (albeit at a much higher [~ 40-fold] density). A reason for the inability of Ng et al. [13] to identify receptors on guinea pig peritoneal eosinophils for which LTB$_4$ has low affinity may relate to the fact that in those studies [^{3}H]LTB$_4$ was not used at concentrations that would detect low-affinity sites.

LTB$_4$ exerts a number of effects on eosinophils (table 2), and progress in understanding the second messenger pathways underlying LTB$_4$ receptor signal transduction has been made. In guinea pig eosinophils LTB$_4$ induces a rapid and transient accumulation of Ins(1,4,5)P_3 and elevates [Ca^{2+}]$_c$ via a pertussis-toxin (PTX)-sensitive pathway [16–19]. However, Ca^{2+} mobilization appears to be mediated independently of Ins(1,4,5)P_3 as the maximum increase in [Ca^{2+}]$_c$ (EC$_{50}$ = 0.6 nM) occurs in the absence of a detectable rise in Ins(1,4,5)P_3 mass (EC$_{50}$ = 200 nM). Consistent with this conclusion is that the rise in [Ca^{2+}]$_c$ is extracellular in origin and enters the cell via a PTX-sensitive, receptor-operated Ca^{2+} channel [17–19]. In addition to coupling to PLC, LTB$_4$ also promotes the extracellular release of [^{3}H]arachidonic acid [19, 20]. This effect is likely to be due to the direct coupling of the LTB$_4$ receptor to a PLA$_2$ since it is preserved under conditions where signalling through PLC is prevented [19]. The elaboration of [^{3}H]arachidonic acid is biphasic [19], implying the existence of two PLA$_2$s, one of which is activated via a Ca^{2+}- and PTX-dependent pathway while activation of the other is Ca^{2+}-independent and insensitive to PTX [19, 20]. LTB$_4$ also causes a rapid activation of the *src*-related tyrosine kinases, p53 and p56^{lyn} [20] and the subsequent activation of ERK-1 and ERK-2 [21, 22]. Interestingly, the ability of LTB$_4$ to activate the NADPH oxidase and Ca^{2+}-dependent PLA$_2$ is mediated via a lyn kinase-dependent mechanism that is divorced from the activation of ERK1 and ERK2, which regulate LTB$_4$-induced chemotaxis [20, 22].

A comparison of the concentration-response relationships which describe a number of biochemical responses evoked by LTB$_4$ implies that the increase in [Ca^{2+}]$_c$ and the subsequent activation of the Ca^{2+}-dependent PLA_2 is mediated via the BLT receptor for which LTB_4 has high affinity. In contrast, $Ins(1,4,5)P_3$ accumulation (an index of PLC activity) and the activation of Ca^{2+}-independent PLA_2 is mediated by the BLT receptor for which LTB_4 has low affinity. In agreement with Maghni et al. [12], those data support the idea that the two populations of the LTB_4 receptor mediate chemotaxis and activation of NADPH oxidase, respectively.

References

1 Giembycz, MA, Lindsay MA: Pharmacology of the eosinophil. Pharmacol Rev 1999;51:213–340.
2 Collins PD, Marleau S, Griffiths-Johnson DA, Jose PJ, Williams TJ: Cooperation between interleukin-5 and the chemokine eotaxin to induce eosinophil accumulation in vivo. J Exp Med 1995;182:1169–1174.
3 Palframan RT, Collins PD, Williams TJ, Rankin SM: Eotaxin induces a rapid release of eosinophils and their progenitors from the bone marrow. Blood 1998;91:2240–2248.
4 Lacy P, Thompson N, Tian M, Solari R, Hide I, Newman TM, Gomperts BD: A survey of GTP-binding proteins and other potential key regulators of exocytotic secretion in eosinophils. Apparent absence of rab3 and vesicle fusion protein homologues. J Cell Sci 1995;108:3547–3556.
5 Coffer PJ, Schweizer RC, Dubois GR, Maikoe T, Lammers JW, Koenderman L: Analysis of signal transduction pathways in human eosinophils activated by chemoattractants and the T-helper 2-derived cytokines interleukin-4 and interleukin-5. Blood 1998;91:2547–2557.
6 Kampen GT, Stafford S, Adachi T, Jinquan T, Quan S, Grant JA, Skov PS, Poulsen LK, Alam R: Eotaxin induces degranulation and chemotaxis of eosinophils through the activation of ERK2 and p38 mitogen-activated protein kinases. Blood 2000;95:1911–1917.
7 Boehme SA, Sullivan SK, Crowe PD, Santos M, Conlon PJ, Sriramarao P, Bacon KB: Activation of mitogen-activated protein kinase regulates eotaxin-induced eosinophil migration. J Immunol 1999;163:1611–1618.
8 Sullivan SK, McGrath DA, Liao F, Boehme SA, Farber JM, Bacon KB: MIP-3α induces human eosinophil migration and activation of the mitogen-activated protein kinases (p42/p44 MAPK). J Leuk Biol 1999;66:674–682.
9 O'Flaherty JT, Kuroki M, Nixon AB, Wijkander J, Yee E, Lee SL, Smitherman PK, Wykle RL, Daniel LW: 5-Oxo-eicosatetraenoate is a broadly active, eosinophil-selective stimulus for human granulocytes. J Immunol 1996;157:336–342.
10 Yokomizo T, Izumi T, Chang K, Shimizu, T: A G-protein-coupled receptor for leukotriene B_4 that mediates chemotaxis. Nature 1997;387:620–624.
11 Gaudreau R, Le Gouill C, Metaoui S, Lemire S, Stankova J, Rola-Pleszczynski M: Signalling through the leukotriene B_4 receptor involves both α_i and α_{16}, but not α_q or α_{11} G-protein subunits. Biochem J 1998;335:15–18.
12 Maghni, K, de Brum-Fernandes AJ, Foldes-Filep E, Gaudry M, Borgeat P, Sirois P: Leukotriene B_4 receptors on guinea pig alveolar eosinophils. J Pharmacol Exp Ther 1991;258:784–789.
13 Ng CF, Sun FF, Taylor BM, Wolin MS, Wong PY: Functional properties of guinea pig eosinophil leukotriene B_4 receptor. J Immunol 1991;147:3096–3103.
14 Sehmi R, Rossi AG, Kay AB, Cromwell O: Identification of receptors for leukotriene B_4 expressed on guinea-pig peritoneal eosinophils. Immunology 1992;77:129–135.
15 Goldman DW, Goetzl EJ: Heterogeneity of human polymorphonuclear leukocyte receptors for leukotriene B_4. Identification of a subset of high affinity receptors that transduce the chemotactic response. J Exp Med 1984;159:1027–1041.
16 Teixeira MM, Giembycz MA, Lindsay MA, Hellewell PG: Pertussis toxin shows distinct early signalling events in platelet-activating factor-, leukotriene B_4-, and C5a-induced eosinophil homotypic aggregation in vitro and recruitment in vivo. Blood 1997;89:4566–4573.
17 Subramanian N: Leukotriene B_4 induced steady state calcium rise and superoxide anion generation in guinea pig eosinophils are not related events. Biochem Biophys Res Commun 1992;187:670–676.
18 Perkins RS, Lindsay MA, Barnes PJ, Giembycz MA: Early signalling events implicated in leukotriene B_4-induced activation of the NADPH oxidase in eosinophils: Role of Ca^{2+}, protein kinase C and phospholipases C and D. Biochem J 1995;310:795–806.
19 Lindsay MA, Perkins RS, Barnes PJ, Giembycz MA: Leukotriene B_4 activates the NADPH oxidase in eosinophils by a pertussis toxin-sensitive mechanism that is largely independent of arachidonic acid mobilization. J Immunol 1998;160:4526–4534.
20 Lynch OT, Giembycz MA, Daniels I, Barnes PJ, Lindsay MA: Pleiotropic role of lyn kinase in leukotriene B_4-induced eosinophil activation. Blood 2000;95:3541–3547.
21 Araki R, Komada T, Nakatani K, Naka M, Shima T, Tanaka T: Protein kinase C-independent activation of Raf-1 and mitogen-activated protein kinase by leukotriene B_4 in guinea pig eosinophils. Biochem Biophys Res Commun 1995;210:837–843.
22 Lindsay MA, Haddad EB, Rousell J, Teixeira MM, Hellewell PG, Barnes PJ, Giembycz MA: Role of the mitogen-activated protein kinases and tyrosine kinases during leukotriene B_4-induced eosinophil activation. J Leuk Biol 1998;64:555–562.

Dr. Mark A. Linsday
Thoracic Medicine
National Heart and Lung Institute
Imperial College School of Medicine
Dovehouse Street
London SW3 6LY (UK)
Tel. +44 207 352 8121 (ext 3061)
Fax +44 207 351 5675
E-Mail m.lindsay@ic.ac.uk

Phosphodiesterase 4 Inhibitors

Theodore J. Torphy[a] Christopher H. Compton[b] Meretta J. Marks[c]
Graham Sturton[d]

SmithKline Beecham Pharmaceuticals, [a]King of Prussia, Pa., USA, [b]Harlow, UK, and
[c]Collegeville, Pa., USA, and [d]Bayer plc Pharma Research, Stoke Poges, Slough, UK

Summary

PDE4 is a major cAMP-metabolizing enzyme in immune and inflammatory cells, airway smooth muscle and pulmonary nerves. Hence PDE4 inhibitors produce a wide range of pharmacological actions that, if replicated in the clinic, may be beneficial in the therapy of asthma and COPD. These include anti-inflammatory effects, bronchodilation, and modulation of pulmonary nerves. Indeed, initial clinical data on these agents are encouraging, and suggest that PDE4 inhibitors may have broad utility in the treatment of pulmonary disease. However, full knowledge of the therapeutic value of this novel compound class awaits the outcome of long-term clinical trials.

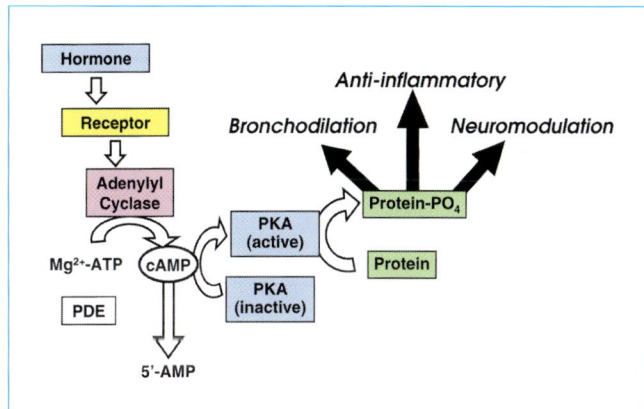

Fig. 1. Beneficial role of cAMP in pulmonary diseases. Illustrated is the standard second-messenger cascade whereby cAMP activates protein kinase A (PKA). PKA phosphorylates key cellular proteins, which leads to a broad suppression of inflammatory cell activity, bronchodilation, and modulation of pulmonary neuronal activity. This cascade can be activated by stimulating adenylyl cyclase, the enzyme that produces cAMP, or inhibiting phosphodiesterase, a superfamily of enzymes that inactivate cAMP.

Background

Among its myriad of biological actions, the second messenger cAMP relaxes airway smooth muscle, suppresses the actions of immune and inflammatory cells, and modulates pulmonary nerve activity [1, 2]. Thus, as illustrated in figure 1, increasing cAMP content in these tissues should be of substantial benefit in the treatment of pulmonary disorders such as asthma and COPD [2, 3].

One pharmacological approach toward elevating the concentration of cAMP in target tissues is by inhibiting its metabolism by cyclic nucleotide phosphodiesterases (PDEs), enzymes that hydrolyze cAMP to its inactive 5'-nucleotide product. Indeed, theophylline is a prototypical nonselective PDE inhibitor that has been used in the treatment of airway diseases for over 60 years. The therapeutic utility of theophylline, however, is limited by its marked gastrointestinal, cardiovascular and central nervous system side effects. These side effects stem primarily from the ability of theophylline to inhibit PDE activity nonselectively in all tissues of the body.

A breakthrough in the design of new PDE inhibitors with the potential of radically improved clinical utility emerged with the recognition that PDEs are an eleven-membered superfamily of genetically distinct enzymes

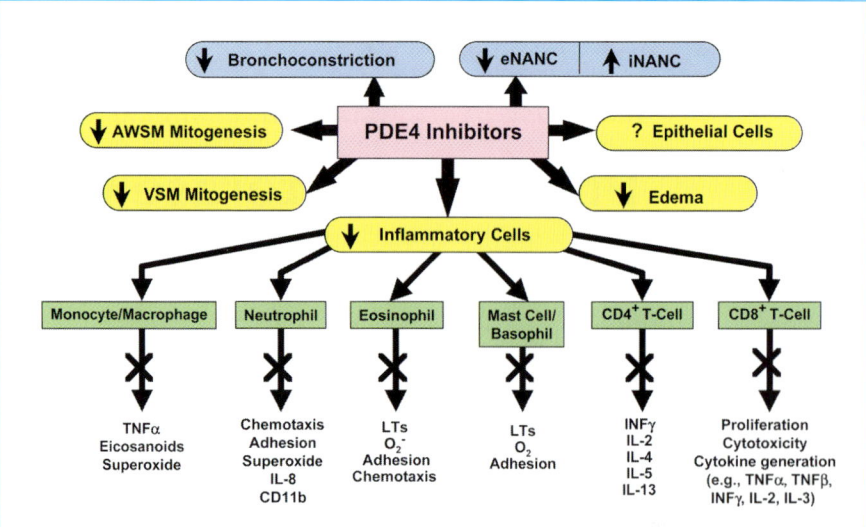

Fig. 2. Potential therapeutic actions of PDE4 inhibitors in pulmonary disease. Preclinical studies indicate that PDE4 inhibitors produce a broad spectrum of functional effects that provide a compelling rationale for the use of these agents in the treatment of pulmonary disease. These effects include a wide range of inhibitory actions on inflammatory cell trafficking and activation, suppression of pulmonary edema, inhibition of smooth muscle mitogenesis, and modulation of nonadrenergic, noncholinergic neuronal activity.

[4]. Two key characteristics make PDEs particularly attractive as drug targets. Firstly, the complement of PDE isozymes, and therefore their functional roles, varies among tissues and cell types. Secondly, highly potent and isozyme-selective inhibitors have been synthesized for a number of the PDE families. With regard to asthma and COPD, PDE4 has been identified as the predominant cAMP-metabolizing isozyme in immune and inflammatory cells, airway smooth muscle, and pulmonary nerves [1–3]. Hence the concept emerged that specifically targeting PDE4 with a new generation of isozyme-selective inhibitors would yield compounds with markedly improved efficacy and side effect profiles compared with older, nonselective agents.

Therapeutic Rationale

Asthma. As illustrated in figure 2, there are strong therapeutic rationales for the use of PDE4 inhibitors in both asthma [1, 2] and COPD [3]. As alluded to earlier, PDE4 inhibitors are pluripotent anti-inflammatory agents, with actions against eosinophils, T lymphocytes, monocytes and macrophages, and neutrophils. These agents also suppress pulmonary edema and have the unique capacity to inhibit the activity of excitatory (contractile) nonadrenergic non-cholinergic nerves, while simultaneously potentiating inhibitory (relaxant) nonadrenergic noncholinergic nerves. Their ability to suppress airway smooth muscle mitogenesis [5] hints that PDE4 inhibitors may impact the airway remodeling that occurs in severe, long-standing asthma.

COPD. While a number of therapeutic alternatives are available for asthma, COPD represents a huge unmet medical need. Like asthma, COPD is associated with airway inflammation [6]. However, whereas the inflammatory process in asthma can be described simplistically as a CD4+ T-cell-driven eosinophilia, COPD is marked by an increase in the numbers or activity of CD8+ T cells, macrophages and neutrophils. Importantly, the inflammation of the lung associated with COPD is reported to be insensitive to steroids [7], thus highlighting the need for novel anti-inflammatory therapies. The reported effects of PDE4 inhibitors in vitro and in animal models suggest that, in addition to short-term effects on bronchomotor tone, they may find utility in reducing the protease burden associated with neutrophilic inflammation, as well as modulating the activity of CD8+ T cells and macrophages. Such effects have the potential of slowing the accelerated decline in lung function seen in patients with COPD.

Biological Actions of PDE4 Inhibitors

Cellular Effects. Elevation of cAMP by PDE4 inhibitors down regulates functional responses (i.e., chemotaxis, cytokine and chemokine production, mediator release, adhesion molecule expression) of most cells involved in the inflammatory processes associated with asthma and COPD [1–3]. The efficacy of PDE4 inhibitors varies with the cell type and function being examined. Thus, inhibition of PDE4 alone is sufficient to reduce the function of neutrophils, eosinophils, monocytes and basophils substantially, while dual PDE3/4 inhibition is required for optimum efficacy against macrophage activation and for relaxation of airway smooth muscle. Effects on lymphocyte, endothelial, epithelial, neuronal cells and smooth muscle proliferation may further influence the in vivo and clinical profile of PDE4 inhibitors.

The identification of subtypes of genetically distinct PDE4s (A–D) offers the opportunity to evaluate the role of subtype specific PDE4 inhibitors in suppression of inflammatory cell function [8]. The selectivity of such compounds to date has been limited. However, two recent reports suggest such an approach may be successful. Selective inhibition of the D subtype appears to be a successful strategy for inhibition of eosinophil function in vitro [9], while inhibition of the A and B subtypes correlates better with suppression of monocyte TNF-α production [8].

Activity in Animal Models. As might be expected from this cellular profile, PDE4 inhibitors are effective against a number of features of the pulmonary response to antigen in animal models. These agents inhibit bronchoconstriction and eosinophilic inflammation in rodents and small mammals, as well as microvascular leakage induced by a number of inflammatory mediators [1, 2]. Studies in primates have extended the profile of activity to include inhibition of the late asthmatic response in squirrel monkeys [10] and antigen-induced hyperresponsiveness in acute and/or subchronic protocols in cynomolgus monkeys [11, 12]. The protection against antigen-induced hyperresponsiveness may be particularly important in view of its association with both the clinical manifestations of asthma and its response to therapy.

There is less information on the effects of PDE4 inhibitors in animal models of COPD. In part this is because such models are less well developed and understood than is true for asthma. One characteristic of COPD is a neutrophilic lung inflammation. PDE4 inhibitors suppress neutrophilic lung inflammation induced by lipopolysaccharide in rats and guinea pigs [13, 14]. To date, there are no reports documenting activity of PDE4 inhibitors in models of tobacco-smoke-induced inflammation or lung damage. Expanding our knowledge of the activity of PDE4 inhibitors in models that reflect characteristics of COPD is fertile ground for future studies.

Toxicology

The principal toxicological observation with both selective PDE4 and nonselective PDE inhibitors is a focal, necrotizing vasculitis in rodents [15]. The relationship between this and the testicular and thymic atrophy also observed in rats [16] is currently under investigation. The suggestion that the toxicological risk of PDE4 inhibitors to humans is low is based on the following arguments:
- The therapeutic window in rodents is large
- This toxicological profile is not observed in other species such as the rabbit or monkey
- The nonselective PDE inhibitor, theophylline, has been used extensively in man without associated clinical hazard.

Class-Associated Side Effects

The promise that PDE4 inhibitors will have an improved side effect profile over non-selective compounds has largely been borne out in early clinical trials, particularly with regard to cardiovascular and most central nervous system side effects. Nonetheless, gastrointestinal side effects, including nausea, vomiting and dyspepsia, limit the dosages of these compounds that can be administered to humans [17–20]. Apart from gastrointestinal adverse effects and headache, no tolerability issues have been reported with this class of compound in man, and gastrointestinal adverse experiences observed in patients treated with SB 207499 (Ariflo®) have generally been mild to moderate, transient and self-limiting [21, 24–26, 29]. Longer-term data from a 12-month study with SB 207499 in patients with mild to moderate asthma [26] revealed no new tolerability issues, and no drug-related effects on vital signs, ECG or clinical laboratory parameters were observed. Side effects appear to be an extension of the pharmacology of PDE4 inhibitors, i.e., inhibition of PDE4 in nontarget tissues [20]. A path forward in improving, although not eliminating this side effect profile was illuminated by research indicating that PDE4 isozymes exist in two distinct structural conformations that differentially recognize various classes of inhibitors [20]. Inhibition of one of the conformers, termed 'HPDE4', is associated with side effects of PDE4 inhibitors, whereas inhibition of the second conformer, 'LPDE4', is associated with many albeit not all of the therapeutic effects of this compound class. A second generation of PDE4 inhibitors, typified by SB 207499, has been designed to take advantage of this unique observation and is currently in clinical development [3].

Drugs in Clinical Development

Not surprisingly, pharmaceutical companies have expended substantial effort in exploiting the therapeutic potential of PDE4 inhibitors in a range of inflammatory diseases. At least 25 companies are active in the area. Compounds that are reported to be in clinical development are listed in table 1.

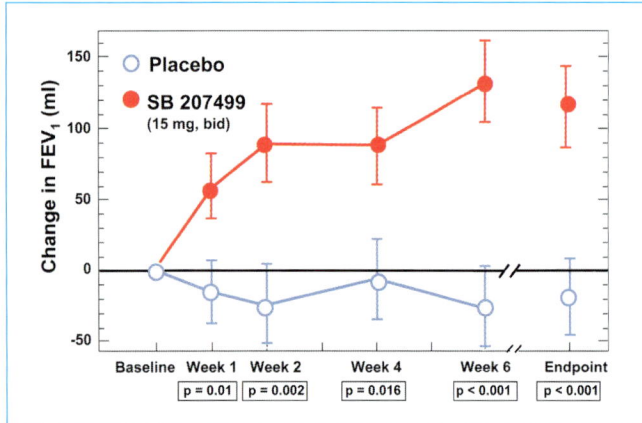

Fig. 3. SB 207499 (Ariflo®) improves pulmonary function in patients with COPD. In a 6-week double-blind study, SB 207499 produced significant and sustained improvements in trough FEV_1. By week 6 the improvement versus placebo averaged 160 ml or 11%. This compares to an average improvement of 5.4% produced by two puffs of salbutamol given at the initiation of the study just prior to administering the first dose of SB 207499 [29].

Table 1. PDE4 inhibitors in clinical development

Compound	Company	Indication	Route	Status
Ariflo® (SB 207499)	SmithKline Beecham	COPD	oral	phase III
		asthma		phase II
Arofylline (LAS-31025)	Almirall-Prodesfarma	asthma	oral	phase III
		asthma	inhaled	phase I
Atizoram (CP-80633)	Pfizer	atopic dermatitis	topical	phase II
		psoriasis	topical	phase II
BAY-19-8004	Bayer	asthma	oral	phase II
		COPD	oral	phase II
CC-3052	Celgene	asthma	oral	Phase I
CDC-801	Celgene	Crohn's disease	oral	phase II
Cipamfylline (BRL 61063)	Leo	atopic dermatitis	topical	phase II
LAS-33774	Almirall-Prodesfarma	atopic dermatitis	topical	phase I
Roflumilast (B9302–107)	Byk-Gulden	asthma	oral	phase III
		COPD	oral	phase II
SCH-351591	Celltech/Schering Plough	asthma	oral	phase I
SH-636	Schering AG	multiple sclerosis	oral	phase I
V-11294A	Napp	asthma	oral	phase II
YM-976	Yamanouchi	asthma	oral	phase I

Clinical Experience

Asthma. In keeping with preclinical experience, PDE4 inhibitors attenuate the late asthmatic response to inhaled allergen in patients with mild asthma [21, 22]. In addition, both SB 207499 and roflumilast have produced clinically relevant activity in patients with exercise induced asthma [23, 24].

In a 6-week double-blind study with SB 207499 in patients with mild to moderate asthma who were receiving concomitant treatment with inhaled corticosteroids and as-needed salbutamol, SB 207499 improved trough pulmonary function test parameters from week one in addition to having a first dose bronchodilator effect [25]. Improvements in pulmonary function were not observed in a study reported with CDP840 exploring first dose bronchodilator effects [21]. Sustained improvements in pulmonary function associated with a reduction in the cardinal symptoms of asthma were reported in a twelve-month study with SB 207499, suggesting tolerance does not occur with continued dosing of PDE4 inhibitors [26, 27].

COPD. In a 6-week double-blind study SB 207499 produced robust, clinically relevant improvements in trough pulmonary function measurements in patients with moderately severe COPD [28, 29]. The effect of SB 207499 on FEV_1 in this study is illustrated in figure 3. The improvement in pulmonary function was associated with beneficial effects on health status, exertional dyspnea, rescue bronchodilator use, and resting and post-exercise SaO_2 [28, 29]. Long-term clinical efficacy data with SB 207499 and other PDE4 inhibitors in patients with COPD are awaited.

Conclusions

The preclinical data supporting the potential utility of PDE4 inhibitors in asthma and COPD are compelling. A particularly appealing aspect of this compound class is its potential to have multiple therapeutic effects, including anti-inflammatory, bronchodilator and neuromodulatory activities. Notwithstanding the strength of the preclinical rationale, the spectrum of therapeutic activities and the side effect profile of PDE4 inhibitors await definition in long term clinical trials. Considering the intense development activity directed at this compound class, such information should not be long in coming.

References

1 Teixeira MM, Gristwood RW, Cooper N, Hellewell PG: Phosphodiesterase (PDE)4 inhibitors: anti-inflammatory drugs of the future? Trends Pharmacol Sci 1997;18:164–170.
2 Torphy TJ: Phosphodiesterase isozymes: Molecular targets for novel antiasthma agents. Am J Respir Crit Care Med 1998;157:351–370.
3 Torphy TJ, Barnette MS, Underwood DC, Griswold DE, Christensen SB, Murdoch RD, Nieman RB, Compton CH: Ariflo (SB 207499), a second generation phosphodiesterase 4 inhibitor for the treatment of asthma and COPD: From concept to clinic. Pulm Pharmacol Ther 1999;12:131–135.
4 Soderling SH, Beavo JA: Regulation of cAMP and cGMP signaling: New phosphodiesterases and new functions. Curr Opin Cell Biol 2000;12:174–179.
5 Panettieri RA, Eszterhas A, Cieslinski LB, Torphy TJ: Ariflo® (SB 207499) modulates human airway smooth muscle cell proliferation induced by mitogens. Am J Respir Crit Care Med 2000;161:A697.
6 Jeffrey PK: Structural and inflammatory changes in COPD: A comparison with asthma. Thorax 1998;53:129–136.
7 Barnes PJ: Inhaled corticosteroids are not beneficial in chronic obstructive pulmonary disease. Am J Respir Crit Care Med 2000;161:342–344.
8 Manning CD, Burman M, Christensen BC, Cieslinski LB, Essayan DM, Grous M, Torphy TJ, Barnette MS: Suppression of human inflammatory cell function by subtype-selective PDE4 inhibitors correlates with inhibition of PDE4A and PDE4B. Brit J Pharmacol 1999;128:1393–1398.
9 Nicotinamide derivatives as selective inhibitors of PDE4. Exp Opin Ther Patents 1999;9:481 485.
10 Turner CR, Anderson CJ, Smith WB, Watson JW: Effect of rolipram on responses to acute and chronic antigen exposure in monkeys. Am J Respir Crit Care Med 1994;149:1153–1159.
11 Jones TR, McAuliffe M, McFarlane CS, Piechuta H, Macdonald D, Rodger IW: Effects of a selective phosphodiesterase IV inhibitor (CDP-840) in a leukotriene-dependent non-human primate model of allergic asthma. Can J Physiol Pharmacol 1998;76:210–217.
12 Fitch N, Freeman MS, Sturton RG, Harris P, Lindell D, Gundel R: The effect of an oral phosphodiesterase (PDE)4 inhibitor, BAY 19-8004, in primate asthma models. Am J Respir Crit Care Med 2000;161:A201.
13 Underwood DC, Osborn RR, Bochnowicz S, Hay DWP, Torphy TJ: The therapeutic activity of SB 207499 (Ariflo®), a second generation phosphodiesterase 4 (PDE4) inhibitor, is equivalent to that of prednisolone in models of pulmonary inflammation. Am J Respir Crit Care Med 1998;157:A827.
14 Spicer D, Clark E, Bowyer N, Fitzgerald MF: Efficacy of the selective phosphodiesterase (PDE) 4 inhibitor, BAY 19-8004, in a rat model of neutrophilic lung inflammation. Am J Respir Crit Care Med 2000;161:A578.
15 Larson JL, Pino MV, Geiger LE, Simeone CR: The toxicity of repeated exposures to rolipram, a type IV phosphodiesterase inhibitor, in rats. Pharmacol Toxicol 1996;78:44–49.
16 Weinberger MA, Friedman L, Farber TM, Moreland FM, Peters EL, Gilmore CE, Khan MA: Testicular atrophy and impaired spermatogenesis in rats fed high levels of the methylxanthines caffeine, theobromine, or theophylline. J Environ Pathol Toxicol 1978;1:669–688.
17 Horowski R, Sastre-Y-Hernandez: Clinical effects of the neurotropic selective cyclic AMP phosphodiesterase inhibitor rolipram in depressed patients: Global evaluation of the preliminary reports. Curr Ther Res 1985;38:23–29.
18 Murdoch RD, Cowley H, Upward J, Webber D, Wyld P: The safety and tolerability of Ariflo® (SB 207499), a novel selective phosphodiesterase 4 inhibitor, in healthy male volunteers. Am J Respir Crit Care Med 1998;157:A409.
19 Duplantier AJ, Biggers MS, Chambers RJ, Cheng JB, Cooper K, Damon DB, Eggler JF, Kraus KG, Marfat A, Masamune H, Pillar JS, Shirley TJ, Umland JP, Watson JW: Biarycarboxylic acids and amides: Inhibition of phosphodiesterase type IV versus [^{3}H]rolipram binding activity ant their relationship to emetic behavior in the ferret. J Med Chem 1996;39:120–125.
20 Barnette MS, Christensen SB, Underwood DC, Torphy TJ: Phosphodiesterase 4: Biological underpinnings for the design of improved inhibitors. Pharmacol Rev Commun 1997;8:65–73.
21 Harbinson PL, MacLeod D, Hawksworth R, O'Toole S, Sullivan PJ, Heath P, Kilfeather S, Page CP, Costello J, Holgate ST, Lee TH: The effect of a novel orally active selective PDE4 isozyme inhibitor (CDP 840) on allergen-induced responses in asthmatic subjects. Eur Respir J 1997;10:1008–1014.
22 Nell H, Leichtl S, Rathgeb M, Neuhauser M, Bardin PG, Louw C: Acute anti-inflammatory effect of the novel phosphodiesterase inhibitor Roflumilast on allergen challenge in asthmatics after a single dose. Am J Respir Crit Care Med 2000;161:A200.
23 Nieman RB, Fisher BD, Amit O, Dockhorn RJ: SB 207499 (Ariflo), a second-generation, selective oral phosphodiesterase type 4 (PDE4) inhibitor, attenuates exercise induced bronchoconstriction in patients with asthma. Am J Respir Crit Care Med 1998;157:A413.
24 Timmer W, Leclerc G, Birraux G, Neuhauser M, Hatzelman A, Bethke T, Wurst W: Safety and efficacy of the new PDE4 inhibitor roflumilast administered to patients with exercise-induced asthma over 4 weeks. Am J Respir Crit Care Med 2000;161:A505.
25 Compton C, Cedar E, Nieman RB, Amit O, Langley SJ, Sapene M: Ariflo improves pulmonary function in patients with asthma: Results of a study in patients taking inhaled corticosteroids. Am J Respir Crit Care Med 1999;195:A624.
26 Compton C, Duggan M, Cedar E, Nieman RB, Amit O, Tabona MV, Bernebau L: Safety of Ariflo in a 12 month study of patients with asthma. Am J Respir Crit Care Med 2000;161:A200.
27 Compton C, Duggan M, Cedar E, Nieman RB, Amit O, Tabona MV, Bernebau L: Ariflo Efficacy in a 12 month study of patients with asthma. Am J Respir Crit Care Med 2000;161:A505.
28 Compton CH, Gubb J, Cedar E, Bakst A, Nieman RB, Amit O, Ayres J, Brambilla C: Ariflo (SB 207499), a second generation, oral PDE4 inhibitor, improves quality of life in patients with COPD. Am J Respir Crit Care Med 1999;195:A522
29 Compton CH, Gubb J, Cedar E, Nieman RB, Amit O, Brambilla C, Ayres J: The efficacy of Ariflo (SB 207499), a second generation, oral PDE4 inhibitor, in patients with COPD. Am J Respir Crit Care Med 1999;195:A806.

Theodore J. Torphy
SmithKline Beecham Pharmaceuticals
709 Swedeland Road, UW2523
King of Prussia, PA 19406-0939 (USA)
Tel. +1 610 270 6821, Fax +1 610 270 4114
E-Mail theodore_j_torphy@sbphrd.com

Therapies Acting on Transcription

Therapies Acting on Transcription: An Overview

G. Caramori   I.M. Adcock

Thoracic Medicine, National Heart and Lung Institute, Imperial College of Science, Technology and Medicine, London, UK

Summary

In the future, the role of transcriptions factors and the genetic regulation of their expression in asthma and COPD may be an increasingly important aspect of research, as this may be one of the critical mechanisms regulating the expression of clinical phenotype and their responsiveness to therapy. Despite recent advances in the knowledge of the pathogenesis of asthma and COPD, much more research on their molecular mechanisms are needed to aid the logical development of new therapies for these common and important diseases, particularly in COPD were no effective treatments currently exist.

Inflammation is a central feature of many lung diseases, including asthma and COPD. The specific characteristics of the inflammatory response and the site of inflammation differ between these diseases, but all involve the recruitment and activation of inflammatory cells and changes in the structural cells of the lung [1]. These diseases are characterized by an increased expression of many proteins involved in the complex inflammatory cascade. These inflammatory proteins include cytokines, chemokines, growth factors, enzymes, receptors and adhesion molecules. The increased expression of most of these proteins is the result of enhanced gene transcription since many of the genes are not expressed in normal cells under resting conditions but are induced in a cell-specific manner. Changes in gene transcription are regulated by transcription factors [2].

Transcription factors may amplify and perpetuate the inflammatory process. Abnormal functioning of transcription factors may determine disease severity and responsiveness to treatment. The increased understanding of the role of transcription factors in the pathogenesis of asthma and COPD has also opened an opportunity for the development of new potential anti-inflammatory drugs. Several new compounds based on interacting with specific transcription factors or their activation pathways are now in development for the treatment of asthma and COPD and some drugs already in clinical use (such as glucocorticoids) work via transcription factors.

Glucocorticoids are the most effective therapy in the long-term control of asthma and appear to reduce inflammation in asthmatic airways largely by inhibiting the action of transcription factors that regulate abnormal gene expression [3]. Glucocorticoids are less effective in COPD than in asthma, indicating that different genes and transcription factors are involved and also emphasizing the importance of cell-specific transcription factors. One concern about this approach is the specificity of such drugs, but it is clear that transcription factors have selective effects on the expression of certain genes and this may make it possible to be more selective.

In addition, there are cell-specific transcription factors that may be targeted for inhibition, which could provide selectivity of drug action. One such example is GATA-3, which has a restricted cellular distribution [4]. In asthma, it may be possible to target drugs to the airways by inhalation, as is currently done for inhaled glucocorticoids to avoid any systemic effects.

Despite the discovery of numerous transcription factors, there is still relatively little information about the regulation of transcription factors in diseases such as asthma and COPD. Here we briefly overview the physiological function of transcription factors in normal cells and their potential role in the pathogenesis of asthma and COPD.

Table 1. Transcription factor families involved in asthma pathogenesis

GR	STATs
NF-κB	NF-AT
AP-1	GATA
CREB	

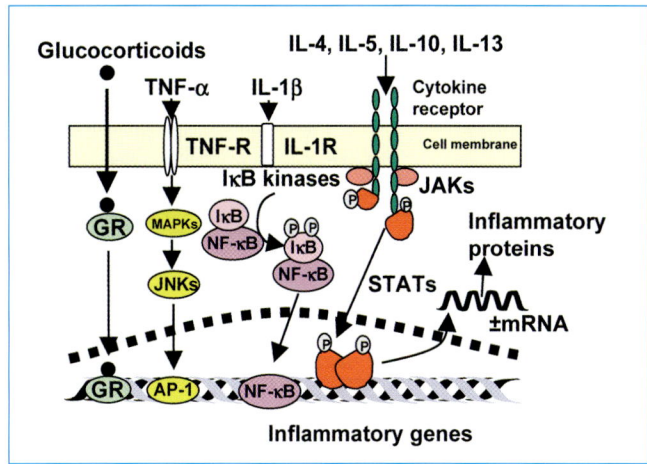

Fig. 1. Multiple pathways mediate transcription factor modulation of inflammatory genes.

Transcription Factors

Transcription factors are proteins that bind to DNA-regulatory sequences of target genes to modify the rate of gene transcription. This may result in increased or decreased protein synthesis and subsequently altered cellular function [5].

Many transcription factors are common to several cell types (ubiquitous) and may play a general role in the regulation of inflammatory genes, whereas others are cell specific and may determine the phenotypic characteristics of a cell.

Transcription factor activation is complex and may involve multiple intracellular signal transduction pathways, including kinases (such as MAPKs, JAKs and PKC) stimulated by cell-surface receptors. Activation of MAPK pathways by inflammatory stimuli leads to activation of a number of ubiquitous transcription factors such Elk-1, c-Myc, c-Jun, c-Fos, SRF and C/EBPβ [6]. Transcription factors may also be directly activated by ligands (e.g. glucocorticoids) or be activated within the cytoplasm, resulting in exposure of nuclear localization signals and targeting to the nucleus. Transcription factors may therefore convert transient environmental signals at the cell surface into long-term changes in gene transcription, thus acting as 'nuclear messengers' (fig. 1).

One of the most important concepts to have emerged is the demonstration that maximal transcription factor activation is associated with coincident activation of several intracellular pathways and transcription factors. This may explain how transcription factors that are ubiquitous may regulate particular genes in certain cell types. The complexity of the activation pathways and their ability to engage in cross-talk enable cells to overcome inhibition of one pathway and retain a capacity to activate specific transcription factors.

Binding of transcription factors to their specific binding motifs in the promoter region may alter transcription by interacting directly with components of the basal transcription apparatus or via cofactors that link the specific transcription factor to the basal transcription apparatus.

Large proteins that bind to the basal transcription apparatus may bind many transcription factors and thus act as integrators of gene transcription. These coactivator molecules include CREB-binding protein (CBP), and the related p300, thus allowing complex interactions between different signalling pathways. DNA is wound around histone proteins to form nucleosomes and the chromatin fibre in chromosomes. It has long been recognized at a microscopic level that chromatin may become dense or opaque due to the winding or unwinding of DNA around the histone core. CBP and p300 have HAT activity which is activated by transcription factors, such as AP-1, NF-B and STATs [7].

Acetylation of histone residues results in unwinding of DNA coiled around the histone core, thus opening up the chromatin structure allowing transcription factors to bind more readily and increase transcription. Deacetylation of histone, increases the winding of DNA round histone residues, resulting in dense chromatin structure and reduced access of transcription factors to their binding sites, thereby leading to repressed transcription of genes [8] (fig. 2).

Role of the Transcription Factors in the Pathogenesis of Bronchial Asthma

The chronic airway inflammation of asthma is unique in that the airway wall is infiltrated by T-lymphocytes of the Th2 phenotype, eosinophils, macrophages/monocytes and mast cells. In addition, an 'acute-on-chronic' inflammation may be observed during exacerbations, with an increase in eosinophils and sometimes neutrophils [1].

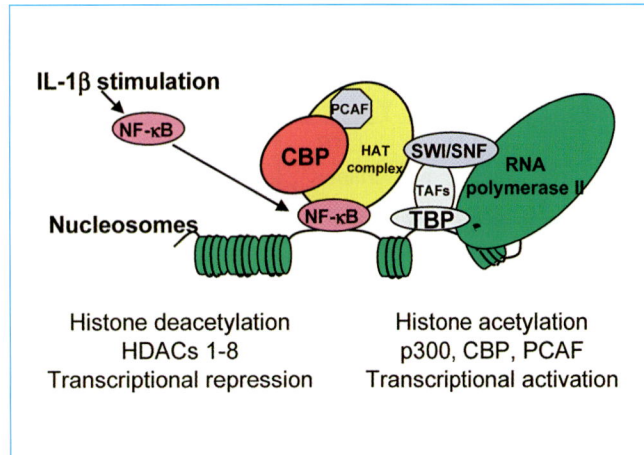

Fig. 2. Transcription factors influence gene expression through modulation of histone acetylation and recruitment of RNA polymerase II.

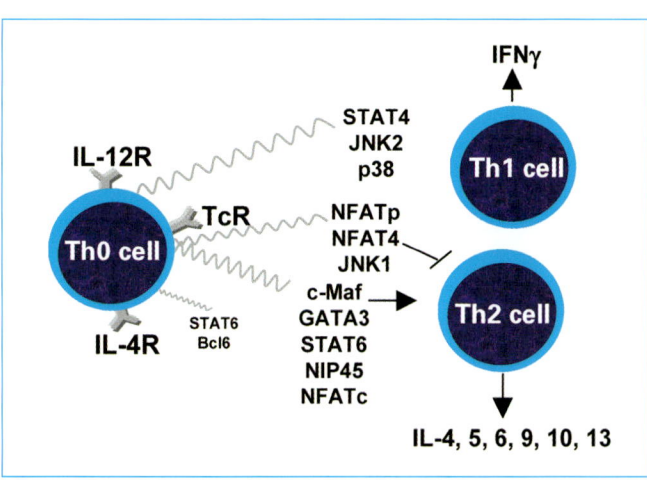

Fig. 3. Differentiation of T cell subtypes depends upon the action of a number of cell-specific transcription factors.

Transcription Factors May Modulate the Severity of Airway Inflammation in Asthma. Activation of NF-κB leads to the coordinated induction of multiple genes that are expressed in inflammatory and immune cells. While NF-κB is not the only transcription factor involved in regulation of the expression of these genes it often appears to have a decisive regulatory role. NF-κB often functions in cooperation with other transcription factors, such as AP-1 and C/EBP, that are also involved in regulation of inflammatory and immune genes. [See Bennett et al., 9, this volume].

NF-κB is activated by many of the stimuli that exacerbate asthmatic inflammation. There is also evidence for activation of NF-κB in the bronchial epithelial cells of patients with asthma [10]. The role of NF-κB should be seen as an amplifying and perpetuating mechanism that exaggerates the inflammatory process through the coordinated activation of multiple inflammatory genes. AP-1 is predominantly a Fos/Jun heterodimer which is activated by various cytokines, including TNF-α and IL-1β via several tyrosine kinases and MAPKs [6]. AP-1, like NF-κB, regulates many of the inflammatory and immune genes that are overexpressed in asthma. Indeed, maximal activation of these genes often requires the simultaneous activation of both transcription factors. There is evidence for increased expression of c-Fos in bronchial epithelial cells in asthmatic airways [11].

STAT6 knockout mice have no response to IL-4, do not develop Th2 cells in response to IL-4, fail to produce IgE and BHR and BAL eosinophilia after allergen sensitization indicating the critical role of STAT6 in allergic responses [12, and see Schaefer et al., 13, this volume].

Transcription Factors May Modulate the Differentiation of Th1/Th2. CD4+ Th cells can be divided into three major subsets termed Th1, Th2, and Th0 based on the pattern of cytokines they produce [14]. Th1 cells produce predominantly IL-2 and IFN-γ and predominantly promote cell-mediated immune responses. Th2 cells produce mainly IL-4, IL-5 and IL-13 and increase IgE production, thereby playing a crucial role in allergic reaction. Th0 cells produce both Th1 and Th2 cytokines and differentiate into Th1 and Th2 cells.

Th1 and Th2 cell differentiation and cytokine release involves several transcription factors. For example, Th2 cell differentiation requires GATA-3 [see Ray and Ray, 15, this volume] and STAT6 [see Schaefer et al., 13, this volume] (fig. 3). Identification of the critical intracellular signalling mechanisms involved in Th2 cell differentiation and activation could provide new anti-asthma targets [see Koulis and Robinson, 16, this volume].

Transcription Factors May Modulate Anti-Asthma Drug Responses. Glucocorticoids are the most effective therapy used to treat asthmatic inflammation [see Dahl and Nielsen, 17, this volume]. They act by binding to a specific cytoplasmic receptor (GR) which is able to translocate to the nucleus and act as a transcription factor. GR can either switch on the expression of anti-inflammatory genes, such as SLPI and lipocortin-1, or more importantly switch off inflammatory gene expression by targeting pro-inflammatory transcription factors such as AP-1 and NF-κB or members of the MAPK pathways [18].

Role of Transcription Factors in the Pathogenesis of COPD

In contrast to the enormous increase in our understanding of the pathogenesis of asthma, knowledge of the molecular pathogenesis of COPD is extremely limited.

Transcription Factors May Modulate the Clinical Manifestations of COPD. The chronic airflow obstruction in COPD results from a combination of small airway disease and loss of lung elasticity due to destruction of the lung parenchyma. The mechanisms of the chronic lower airway inflammation, lung parenchyma destruction and mucus hypersecretion in COPD are not certain. However, it is likely that cigarette smoke (and/or other irritants) activate alveolar macrophages (and possibly epithelial cells and CD8+ T lymphocytes) in the lower respiratory tract that release chemotactic factors to attract neutrophils. All these cells then can release many inflammatory mediators, and current research in COPD is focused on the balance proteases/antiproteases, oxidants/antioxidants, pro- and anti-inflammatory cytokines [19].

The modulation of the inflammatory response in COPD by genetic factors associated to transcription factors may be in part the cause of the different clinical phenotypes of the patients with COPD. Interestingly, only a fraction of all the patients with severe COPD develop a chronic pulmonary hypertension and this is associated with a worst prognosis. In these patients, there is structural remodelling of the arterial walls and it is tempting to speculate that structural remodelling of the pulmonary arterial walls could be linked to the induction or repression of transcription factors, such as hypoxia-inducible factor-1, in these cells.

References

1 Barnes PJ, Chung KF, Page CP: Inflammatory mediators of asthma: An update. Pharmacol Rev 1998;50:515–596.
2 Buratowski S: Mechanisms of gene activation. Science 1995;270:1773–1774.
3 Barnes PJ: Anti-inflammatory actions of glucocorticoids: Molecular mechanisms. Clin Sci (Colch) 1998;94:557–572.
4 Zheng W, Flavell RA: The transcription factor GATA-3 is necessary and sufficient for Th2 cytokine gene expression in CD4 T cells. Cell 1997;89:587–596.
5 Calkhoven CF, Ab G: Multiple steps in the regulation of transcription-factor level and activity. Biochem J 1996;317:329–342.
6 Karin M: Mitogen-activated protein kinase cascades as regulators of stress responses. Ann NY Acad Sci 1998;851:139–146.
7 Kadonaga JT: Eukaryotic transcription: An interlaced network of transcription factors and chromatin-modifying machines. Cell 1998;92:307–313.
8 Struhl K, Moqtaderi Z: The TAFs in the HAT. Cell 1998;94:1–4.
9 Bennett BL, Manning AM: Activator protein-1 and nuclear factor-kappa B. Prog Respir Res. Basel, Karger, 2001, vol 31, pp 337–341.
10 Hart LA, Krishnan VL, Adcock IM, Barnes PJ, Chung KF: Activation and localization of transcription factor, nuclear factor-kappaB, in asthma. Am J Respir Crit Care Med 1998;158:1585–1592.
11 Demoly P, Chanez P, Pujol JL, Gauthier RC, Michel FB, Godard P, Bousquet J: Fos immunoreactivity assessment on human normal and pathological bronchial biopsies. Respir Med 1995;89:329–335.
12 Barnes PJ: Chronic obstructive pulmonary disease: New opportunities for drug development. Trends Pharmacol Sci 1998;19:415–423.
13 Schaefer G, Venkataraman C, Schindler U: STAT6: Role in IL-4-mediated signalling. Prog Respir Res. Basel, Karger, 2001, vol 31, pp 346–349.
14 Romagnani S: The Th1/Th2 paradigm. Immunol Today 1997;18:263–266.
15 Ray A, Ray P: GATA-3: A Th2-selective target. Prog Respir Res. Basel, Karger, 2001, vol 31, pp 222–225.
16 Koulis A, Robinson DS: T cell immunomodulation: An overview. Prog Respir Res. Basel, Karger, 2001, vol 31, pp 212–216.
17 Dahl R, Nielsen LP: Steroids: An overview. Prog Respir Res. Basel, Karger, 2001, vol 31, pp 86–90.
18 Karin M: New twists in gene regulation by glucocorticoid receptor: Is DNA binding dispensable? Cell 1998;93:487–490.
19 Barnes PJ: Chronic obstructive pulmonary disease. N Eng J Med 2000;343:269–280.

Dr. Gaetano Caramori
Centro di Ricerca su Asma e BPCO
Università di Ferrara
Via Savonarola 9
I-44100 Ferrara (Italy)
Tel. +39 0532 210420, Fax +39 0532 210297
E-Mail crm@unife.it

Chromatin Modification

Fyodor D. Urnov   Alan P. Wolffe

Sangamo Biosciences, Richmond, Calif., USA

Summary

The targeting of chromatin modification is an integral part of every gene regulatory pathway in eukaryotes, and the reversible acetylation of lysine residues in the NH_2-terminal tails of the core histones is one of the major such modifications observed in vivo. We summarize existing evidence that connects the action of histone acetyltransferases and deacetylases to transcriptional control, describe currently available pharmacological agents that regulate their activity, highlight recent discoveries of chromatin modification pathways involved in the regulation of genes relevant to the etiology of allergy and asthma, and conclude by offering a basic scientists' perspective on the practice, promise, and pitfalls of using histone tail acetylation and deacetylation to regulate genes in vivo.

An integral component of every gene regulatory pathway in metazoa, chromatin represents a marvel of seeming contradictions by both packaging and revealing the genome. The textbook image of chromatin as a monotonously repetitive entity obscures its potential for undergoing dynamic structural transitions: the 40 million nucleosomes compacting DNA in each one of our cells are tended to by complexes that assemble, destroy, move, and chemically modify them – all these functions are exploited by transcriptional regulators to effect gene control [1]. This review focuses on a particular class of covalent modification – the reversible acetylation of lysine residues in the NH_2-terminal tails of the core histones (fig. 1a). Discovered by V. Allfrey and D. Mirsky in 1964, the humble ε-acetyl group became the focus of an extraordinary research effort after the identification in 1996 by D. Allis, S. Roth, and their colleagues of the histone acetyltransferase (HAT) Gcn5p as a transcriptional activator in yeast and in ciliates, and the concomitant discovery by S. Schreiber and coworkers that the histone deacetylase (HDAC) Rpd3p is a transcriptional repressor in yeast and in mammals. In the 5 years since, a great number of HATs and their functional antagonists, the HDACs, have been characterized and connected to every aspect of genomic function in eukaryotes [3, 4]. The HAT/HDAC pathway of gene control operates in all cells and provides investigators with an efficient lever to regulate gene expression in vivo [5, 6]; it thus represents an attractive target for designing therapeutic intervention strategies in clinical practice.

This review summarizes existing evidence that connects the HAT/HDAC pathway to transcriptional control, describes currently available pharmacological agents that regulate its activity, highlights recent discoveries of its involvement in gene regulatory pathways relevant to the etiology of allergy and asthma, and concludes by offering a basic scientists' perspective on the practice, promise, and pitfalls of using histone tail acetylation and deacetylation to regulate genes in vivo.

Histone Tail Modification in Transcriptional Control

The nucleosome is a compact union between 8 molecules of core histones and approximately 146 bp of DNA [1]. Quite unlike the 'featureless cylinder' cartoon nucleosome common in schematics, it is enveloped in a web of long, positively charged tentacles (fig. 1b): the NH_2-terminal lysine-rich tails of the core histones that are the targets for acetylation and deacetylation. While we do not currently know their structure [7], robust genetic evidence points to the NH_2-terminal histone tails' essential role in gene control and genomic function in general: it is known,

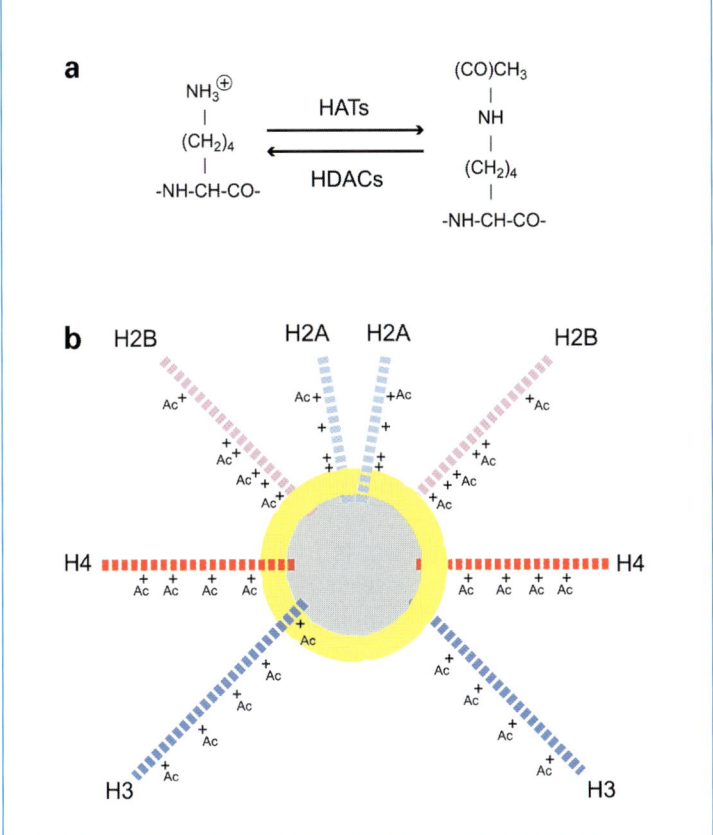

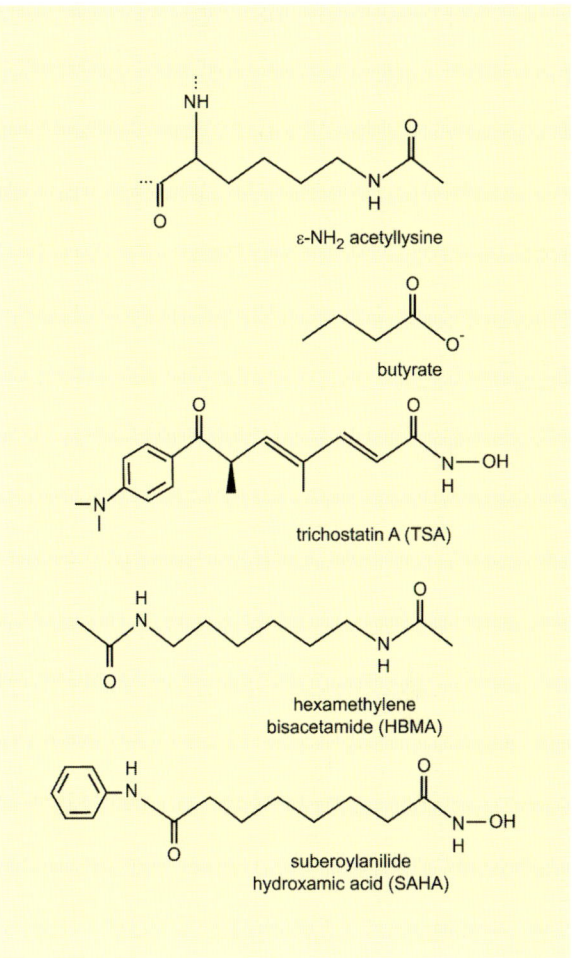

Fig. 1. a Chemical equation of core histone NH_2-terminal tail acetylation on the ε-NH_2 group of lysine residues. **b** Schematic representation of a nucleosome [based on data in ref. 2]; histone octamer core is shown in light grey, DNA superhelix – in dark grey, the histone tails – as black dashed lines (each dash corresponds to one amino acid). The location of the lysine residues in the tails is indicated by a '+' sign, and of those residues that are the targets of acetylation in vivo, by 'Ac'. The length of the tails as shown is approximately to scale with the size of the core histone octamer.

Fig. 2. Chemical formulas for the HDACs' natural substrate and for some currently used HDAC inhibitors. Detailed descriptions of the hybrid-polar compounds HMBA, SAHA, and others, can be found in reference 16.

for instance, that the tails are required for cell viability, as well as both transcriptional repression and activation in vivo [8].

While it is at present unclear how histone tail acetylation affects the structure of chromatin in vivo – available evidence suggests that it promotes the unfolding of chromatin [8], transcription factor access to DNA [1], and transcriptional elongation [9] – a wide variety of data point to its use as a regulatory mechanism. For instance, a large number of HATs and HDACs are involved in transcriptional regulation [10]. In addition, the level of histone acetylation at particular loci in the genome is positively correlated with their transcriptional activity [11], and the lysine residues in the histone tails assembled at gene promoters are bona fide targets of acetylation by HATs [12]. HATs are also known to have nonhistone targets, e.g., various transcription factors and components of the basal transcription machinery [10]. Both HATs and HDACs are found in large multiprotein complexes that are targeted to particular loci in the genome by various transcriptional activators and repressors [13, 14], and in many cases, a nice correlation exists between the capacity of such regulators to target HATs/HDACs and their ability to control gene expression [4, 14, 15].

Pharmacological Intervention with HATs and HDACs

Studies of HAT and HDAC function in gene regulation have reaped great benefit from the availability of small molecules that inhibit HDAC activity (fig. 2); these range from simple organic molecules, such as sodium butyrate, to more complex fungal-derived trichostin A (TSA) and trapoxin [6] and synthetic 'hybrid polar compounds' [16]. Nanomolar doses of TSA have been shown to relieve repression exerted by unliganded nuclear hormone receptors [14], the methylated DNA-binding protein MeCP2 [15], and many other transcriptional repressors [3].

While HDAC inhibitors are useful reagents, they need to be applied with caution, in large part because they exert pan-cellular effects, and very likely alter the transcriptional program of a significant number of genes (see below). Importantly, many transcriptional repressors [see ref. 18 and references therein] can continue to exert some silencing action even in the presence of concentrations of TSA that are known to inhibit 100% of all HDAC activity in the cell. It has been hypothesized that these regulators exploit pathways for repression auxiliary to HDAC targeting, and that direct interactions with the basal transcription machinery underlie these pathways; there are at present no in vivo data illuminating the mechanism of such action.

The importance of such observations for clinical practice is illustrated by evidence for the role of HDAC targeting in mediating repression of loci located within hypermethylated DNA stretches: symmetrical methylation of cytosines within CpG dinucleotides is an important regulatory phenomenon in vertebrate genomes [13] which contributes to host genome defence and stability, epigenetic phenomena such as imprinting [19], and possibly tissue-specific gene regulation. Biochemical approaches revealed the existence of a protein with high selectivity for methylated DNA termed MeCP2; it acts as a potent transcriptional repressor and exploits HDAC targeting for action [13]. Remarkably, while TSA robustly relieved methylation-driven repression in noncancerous cells [17], this agent alone proved incapable of reactivating a promoter whose activity was silenced by the mistargeting of DNA methylation in transformed cells [20], and required the abetting action of a DNA demethylating agent, 5-azacytidine.

However the HDAC inhibitors do act, for clinical purposes their most significant property is a well-characterized capacity to effect cell cycle arrest and promote differentiation of a great variety of normal and transformed cells in culture, as well as their known anti-oncogenic action in humans [21, 22] (see below). It is unclear how this action occurs, but the disrupted balance between cell proliferation and differentiation in transformed cells is thought to be influenced by the failure to activate differentiation-specific genes either by the use of transcriptional repressors, through the failure to recruit coactivators, or through interference with coactivator function. In line with this notion, the etiology of a number of leukemias has been traced to aberrant recruitment of histone acetyltransferases and deacetylases to gene promoters [23]. For instance, in acute promyelocytic leukemia (APL), the gene for the retinoic acid receptor-α (RAR-α) has been shown to be fused to the gene for the promyelocytic leukemia zinc finger protein (PLZF) or the gene for the promyelocytic leukemia protein (PML) – the latter two proteins are sequence-specific DNA-binding factors; the resulting fusion proteins recruit histone deacetylase via the RAR ligand-binding domain moiety to silence transcription [23]. Up to 80% of patients with APL achieve significant improvement following treatment which includes all-*trans* retinoic acid – the ligand for RAR-α – that acts to release HDAC from the fusion protein [24]. A related example involves action by the oncoprotein v-ErbA: it is a mutated version of the chicken thyroid hormone receptor-α, and is thought to constitutively silence TR-regulated genes that are required for cell cycle arrest and differentiation in immature haematopoietic progenitors [25]. As a result, the avian erythroblastosis virus that carries v-ErbA causes fatal erythroleukaemia in chickens; importantly, TSA both efficiently relieves v-ErbA-mediated repression [18, 26] and promotes differentiation of normal as well as transformed erythroid progenitors.

The current literature contains an extensive collection of studies in which the phenotypes of particular transformed cells and the activity of particular oncogenesis-related promoters in their genomes are shown to be responsive to the action of HDAC inhibitors. In 1998, Warrell et al. [22] described the clinical application of the HDAC inhibitor sodium butyrate to the treatment of a patient with a severe case of APL that was resistant to all-*trans* retinoic acid. According to that study, ~3 weeks after the administration of the HDAC inhibitor in conjunction with retinoic acid, virtually complete clinical and cytological remission was achieved. This observation offers promise for the future of pharmacologically targeting the HAT/HDAC pathway for therapeutic purposes.

Chromatin in Gene-Regulatory Pathways Relevant to the Aetiology of Allergy and Asthma

Given their ubiquity in the nucleus, it is exceedingly likely that targeting of particular HATs and HDACs is exploited in the regulation – and the pathological misregulation – of most genes implicated in the progression of pulmonary disorders. Thus, the potential exists for the development of judicious intervention strategies into disease progression using the modulation of chromatin and non-histone protein acetylation states.

One conspicuous example is the known anti-inflammatory action of ligands for the glucocorticoid receptor (GR), which has been effectively used in the clinical management of asthma (see relevant articles elsewhere in this volume). As all members of the nuclear hormone receptor superfamily, liganded GR exploits the targeting of various chromatin modification complexes, including the HATs CBP/p300 and SRC-1 [27]. Overexpression of CBP/p300 increases the transcription activation potential of liganded GR [28], as well as its capacity to overcome the transrepressive action of NF-κB [29]. Many current models suggest that such coactivators as CBP and p300 are limiting in the nucleus, and that competition for the small amounts of these essential coactivators between various transcription factors is an important regulatory mechanism in specifying cell phenotype [30]. It is likely, therefore, that the anti-inflammatory action of glucocorticoids could be potentiated by the concomitant application of HDAC inhibitors; it is useful to note in this connection that transcriptional activation by GR is initiated with a nucleosome-scale chromatin disruption phenomenon discovered by K. Zaret and K. Yamamoto in 1984, which as of itself is most likely not HAT-dependent [1]. The coactivators CBP/p300 activate transcription at a step subsequent to this chromatin disruption [31], and it is quite possible that the presence of an HDAC inhibitor will, to some extent, mimic the targeting of HATs by liganded GR. In several cases, TSA was shown to stimulate the basal activity of particular promoters in the absence of targeting of a HAT [for instance ref. 18, 32]; such action likely reflects the fact that the nucleus contains a considerable number of 'philandering' HATs and HDACs, and abrogating HDAC activity allows the HATs to act promiscuously. On GR-regulated promoters, however, such action by HATs would be more conspicuous due to the large-scale chromatin remodelling already exerted by the liganded receptor. It is important to note that a complicating circumstance in the application of HDAC inhibitors to potentiate GR action is the known role for transrepression in the antiinflammatory effects of glucocorticoids (see relevant articles in this volume).

A second example concerns recent observations of chromatin-remodelling phenomena at promoters for various cytokines involved in immune system function, such as IL-12 [33], and IL-4/5/13 [34]. These promoters appear to undergo classical two-stage activation in which an initial STAT-mediated large-scale nucleosome disruption event potentiates binding to promoters by such regulators as GATA-3 [35]; recent evidence also suggests a STAT6-independent role for GATA-3 per se in the initial remodelling event [36]. Whatever the precise sequence of action of various factors at these promoters, some of them appear to undergo DNA demethylation concomitant with activation [37]. The initial establishment and maintenance of the methylation-induced repressed state are both intimately connected to the targeting of HDACs [17, 38], and it is possible, therefore, that the action of HDAC inhibitors will stimulate some of these promoters, although the caveat discussed above with regards to the study by Cameron et al. [20] applies in this case as well.

Conclusion

Successful targeting of HATs and HDACs in clinical practice awaits a more profound understanding of the structural and mechanistic underpinnings of this pathway in vivo. For example, as discussed above, it is still unclear, how histone hyperacetylation upregulates transcription. This gap in our knowledge creates a problem because it precludes a better understanding of the mechanisms and effects of action by HDAC inhibitors such as TSA. Robustly effective at nanomolar concentrations, it is clearly a very potent agent; the phenotypes observed as a consequence of its action, however, must be interpreted with great caution, since it is very likely that it changes the transcriptional program of much of the nucleus. New methodologies for genome-wide expression profiling [39] should prove very useful in this sense. Finally, new techniques exist that offer the promise of targeting of chromatin modifying activities to specific loci in the genome [40]. It is possible that the use of such methods to effect regulation of specific genes – rather than the genome-wide application of pharmacological agents – may be an effective means to parsimoniously alter cell phenotype.

References

1 Wolffe AP, Guschin D: Chromatin structural features and targets that regulate transcription. J Struct Biol 2000;129:102–122.
2 Wolffe AP, Hayes JJ: Chromatin disruption and modification. Nucleic Acids Res 1999;27: 711–720.
3 Cheung WL, Briggs SD, Allis CD: Acetylation and chromosomal functions. Curr Opin Cell Biol 2000;12:326–333.
4 Ng HH, Bird A: Histone deacetylases: Silencers for hire. Trends Biochem Sci 2000;25:121–126.
5 Lau OD, Kundu TK, Soccio RE, Ait-Si-Ali S, Khalil EM, Vassilev A, Wolffe AP, Nakatani Y, Roeder RG, Cole PA: HATs off: Selective synthetic inhibitors of the histone acetyltransferases p300 and PCAF. Mol Cell 2000;5:589–595.
6 Yoshida M, Horinouchi S, Beppu T: Trichostatin A and trapoxin: novel chemical probes for the role of histone acetylation in chromatin structure and function. Bioessays 1995;17: 423–430.
7 Luger K, Mader AW, Richmond RK, Sargent DF, Richmond TJ: Crystal structure of the nucleosome core particle at 2.8 A resolution. Nature 1997;389:251–260.
8 Hansen JC, Tse C, Wolffe AP: Structure and function of the core histone N-termini: More than meets the eye. Biochemistry 1998;37: 17637–17641.
9 Wittschieben BO, Fellows J, Du W, Stillman DJ, Svejstrup JQ: Overlapping roles for the histone acetyltransferase activities of SAGA and Elongator in vivo. Embo J 2000;19:3060–3068.
10 Sterner DE, Berger SL: Acetylation of histones and transcription-related factors. Microbiol Mol Biol Rev 2000;64:435–459.
11 Grunstein M: Histone acetylation in chromatin structure and transcription. Nature 1997;389: 349–352.
12 Zhang W, Bone JR, Edmondson DG, Turner BM, Roth SY: Essential and redundant functions of histone acetylation revealed by mutation of target lysines and loss of the Gcn5p acetyltransferase. Embo J 1998;17:3155–3167.
13 Bird AP, Wolffe AP: Methylation-induced repression – belts, braces, and chromatin. Cell 1999;99:451–454.
14 Collingwood TN, Urnov FD, Wolffe AP: Nuclear receptors: coactivators, corepressors and chromatin remodeling in the control of transcription. J Mol Endocrinol 1999;23:255–275.
15 Magnaghi-Jaulin L, Ait-Si-Ali S, Harel-Bellan A: Histone acetylation and the control of the cell cycle. Prog Cell Cycle Res 2000;4:41–47.
16 Richon VM, Emiliani S, Verdin E, Webb Y, Breslow R, Rifkind RA, Marks PA: A class of hybrid polar inducers of transformed cell differentiation inhibits histone deacetylases. Proc Natl Acad Sci U S A 1998;95:3003–3007.
17 Jones PL, Veenstra GJ, Wade PA, Vermaak D, Kass SU, Landsberger N, Strouboulis J, Wolffe AP: Methylated DNA and MeCP2 recruit histone deacetylase to repress transcription. Nat Genet 1998;19:187–191.
18 Urnov FD, Yee J, Sachs L, Bauer A, Beug H, Shi YB, Wolffe AP: Targeting of N-CoR and histone deacetylase 3 by the oncoprotein v-ErbA yields a chromatin infrastructure-dependent transcriptional repression pathway. EMBO J 2000;15:1–17.
19 Wolffe AP, Matzke MA: Epigenetics: Regulation through repression. Science 1999;286: 481–486.
20 Cameron EE, Bachman KE, Myohanen S, Herman JG, Baylin SB: Synergy of demethylation and histone deacetylase inhibition in the re-expression of genes silenced in cancer. Nat Genet 1999;21:103–107.
21 Archer SY, Hodin RA: Histone acetylation and cancer. Curr Opin Genet Dev 1999;9:171–174.
22 Warrell RP Jr, He LZ, Richon V, Calleja E, Pandolfi PP: Therapeutic targeting of transcription in acute promyelocytic leukemia by use of an inhibitor of histone deacetylase. J Natl Cancer Inst 1998;90:1621–1625.
23 Lin RJ, Egan DA, Evans RM: Molecular genetics of acute promyelocytic leukemia. Trends Genet 1999;15:179–184.
24 Slack JL, Rusiniak ME: Current issues in the management of acute promyelocytic leukemia. Ann Hematol 2000;79:227–238.
25 Stunnenberg HG, Garcia-Jimenez C, Betz JL: Leukemia: The sophisticated subversion of hematopoiesis by nuclear receptor oncoproteins. Biochim Biophys Acta 1999;1423:F15–F33.
26 Ciana P, Braliou GG, Demay FG, von Lindern M, Barettino D, Beug H, Stunnenberg HG: Leukemic transformation by the v-ErbA oncoprotein entails constitutive binding to and repression of an erythroid enhancer in vivo. Embo J 1999;17:7382–7394.
27 Adcock IM, Nasuhari Y, Barnes PJ: Role of CBP in glucocorticoid-induced gene repression. Biochem Soc Trans 1998;26:S255.
28 Chen H, Lin RJ, Schiltz RL, Chakravarti D, Nash A, Nagy L, Privalsky ML, Nakatani Y, Evans RM: Nuclear receptor coactivator ACTR is a novel histone acetyltransferase and forms a multimeric activation complex with P/CAF and CBP/p300. Cell 1997;90:569–580.
29 Sheppard KA, Phelps KM, Williams AJ, Thanos D, Glass CK, Rosenfeld MG, Gerritsen ME, Collins T: Nuclear integration of glucocorticoid receptor and nuclear factor-kappaB signaling by CREB-binding protein and steroid receptor coactivator-1. J Biol Chem 1998;273: 29291–29294.
30 Goodman RH, Smolik S: CBP/p300 in cell growth, transformation, and development. Genes Dev 2000;14:1553–1577.
31 Li Q, Imhof A, Collingwood TN, Urnov FD, Wolffe AP: p300 stimulates transcription instigated by ligand-bound thyroid hormone receptor at a step subsequent to chromatin disruption. Embo J 1999;18:5634–5652.
32 Nagy L, Kao HY, Chakravarti D, Lin RJ, Hassig CA, Ayer DE, Schreiber SL, Evans RM: Nuclear receptor repression mediated by a complex containing SMRT, mSin3A, and histone deacetylase. Cell 1997;89:373–380.
33 Weinmann AS, Plevy SE, Smale ST: Rapid and selective remodeling of a positioned nucleosome during the induction of IL-12 p40 transcription. Immunity 1999;11:665–675.
34 Agarwal S, Viola JP, Rao A: Chromatin-based regulatory mechanisms governing cytokine gene transcription. J Allergy Clin Immunol 1999;103:990–999.
35 Ray A, Cohn L: Th2 cells and GATA-3 in asthma: New insights into the regulation of airway inflammation. J Clin Invest 1999;104:985–993.
36 Ouyang W, Lohning M, Gao Z, Assenmacher M, Ranganath S, Radbruch A, Murphy KM: Stat6-independent GATA-3 autoactivation directs IL-4-independent Th2 development and commitment. Immunity 2000;12:27–37.
37 Agarwal S, Rao A: Modulation of chromatin structure regulates cytokine gene expression during T cell differentiation. Immunity 1998;9: 765–775.
38 Robertson KD, Ait-Si-Ali S, Yokochi T, Wade PA, Jones PL, Wolffe AP: DNMT1 forms a complex with rb, E2F1 and HDAC1 and represses transcription from E2F-responsive promoters. Nat Genet 2000;25:338–342.
39 Young RA: Biomedical discovery with DNA arrays. Cell 2000;102:9–15.
40 Kim JS, Pabo CO: Getting a handhold on DNA: Design of poly-zinc finger proteins with femtomolar dissociation constants. Proc Natl Acad Sci U S A 1998;95:2812–2817.

Alan P. Wolffe, PhD
Sangamo Biosciences
Pt. Richmond Tech. Centre
501 Canal Blvd., Suite A100
Richmond, CA 94804 (USA)
Tel. +1 510 970 6000 (ext. 216)
Fax +1 510 236 8951
E-Mail awolffe@sangamo.com

Activator Protein-1 and Nuclear Factor-Kappa B

Brydon L. Bennett   Anthony M. Manning

Signal Pharmaceuticals, Inc., San Diego, Calif., USA

Summary

This review describes the role of the nuclear transcription factors activator protein-1 (AP-1) and nuclear factor-kappa B (NF-κB) in asthma and COPD. Specifically, we present the opportunities for modulating these factors with novel pharmaceuticals by targeting proteins that regulate the activity of AP-1 and NF-κB.

Signal transduction is the mechanism whereby cells relay information received from the external environment to multiple intracellular sites, resulting in a variety of molecular 'responses' that may either change the cell itself (i.e. differentiation) or cause it to release factors back to the external environment to induce changes elsewhere (i.e. activation). Transcription factors are components of the signal transduction machinery that act in the nucleus to promote the transcription of genes, leading to the de novo production of proteins. The transcription factors, activator protein-1 (AP-1) [1] and nuclear factor-kappa B (NF-κB) [2] are expressed in multiple cell types and play a dominant role in the transcription of many immune-related genes. For this reason, inhibition of AP-1 and/or NF-κB may provide a powerful means for down-regulating many of the molecular events that culminate in inflammation and structural damage of the lung. To date, there are no clinically available drugs that specifically target either of these transcription factors, although anti-inflammatory drugs such as glucocorticoids may exert part of their therapeutic benefit through inhibition of these factors.

Activator Protein-1 and Nuclear Factor-Kappa B in the Lung

The inflamed asthmatic lung contains a milieu of chemical mediators, cytokines, chemokines, and proteolytic enzymes secreted by a range of resident and infiltrating cell types (fig. 1). AP-1 and NF-κB have been shown to be activated in almost all cells of the asthmatic lung including bronchial epithelium, vascular endothelium, alveolar fibroblasts, mast cells, and leukocytes [3]. Immunostaining of inflamed lung shows high levels of nuclear NF-κB in lung epithelium and leukocytes [4, 5]. Staining of rat lung immediately following antigen challenge shows activated NF-κB in the endothelial lining of the capillaries [Manning, unpubl. obs.]. Similarly, electrophoretic mobility shift assays (EMSA) of bronchoalveolar lavage (BAL) fluid cells or lung tissue show high levels of AP-1 and NF-κB DNA-binding activity [6]. Furthermore, a significant portion of the genes activated in the asthmatic lung are known to be regulated by AP-1 and/or NF-κB. Therefore, activated AP-1 and NF-κB are unifying molecular entities that characterize asthma. Expression and activation of NF-κB and AP-1 in the setting of COPD have not been reported, and therefore the potential role for these factors in this disease remains unknown.

Table 1 lists a number of asthma-related genes whose transcription is dependent on the activity of AP-1 and NF-κB. Many of these genes are regulated by both AP-1 and NF-κB. Note that the matrix metalloproteinases may be preferentially regulated by AP-1, so that AP-1 inhibitors may provide more selective drugs for COPD [7].

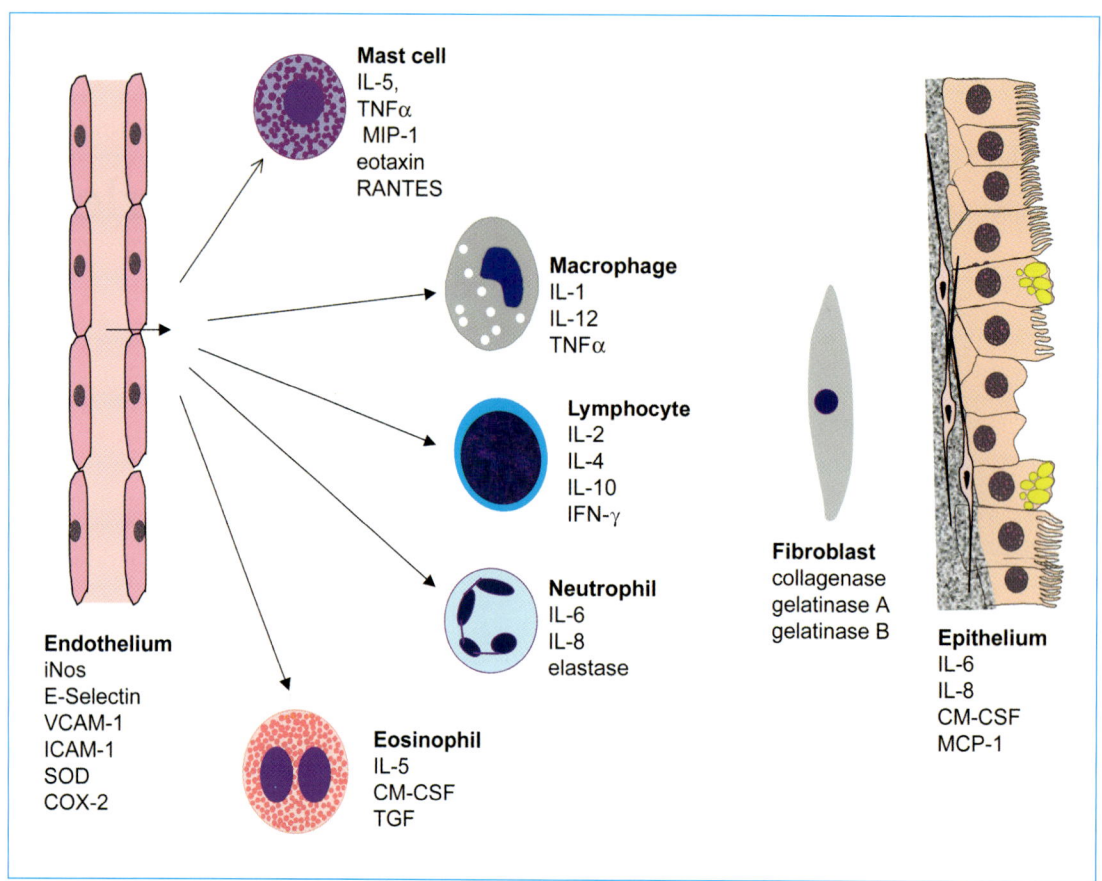

Fig. 1. Schematic representation of leukocyte infiltration and inducible gene expression in the inflamed lung. Lung inflammation is a dynamic process involving multiple cell types and signaling mediators, of which a few are shown here. Many of these inducible genes are regulated by AP-1 and NF-κB. The diagram shows representative leukocytes adhering to, and migrating through the endothelial lining of an alveolar capillary. Leukocytes migrate up the concentration gradient (arrow) formed by diffusion of specific leukocyte chemoattractant molecules released from the site of inflammation, e.g. activated mast cell. Activated fibroblasts release a range of matrix-degrading and -remodeling enzymes that may alter the parenchyma and epithelial lining of the lung. Inflamed and damaged epithelium becomes permeable to both cytokines and infiltrating leukocytes, which collect with mucus secretions in the airways as asthmatic lavage fluid.

Table 1. AP-1 and NF-κB-inducible genes identified in asthma and COPD

Cell surface receptors	*Chemokines and cytokines*	*Enzymes*	IkBα
E-Selectin	Eotaxin	Cyclooxygenase-2 (COX-2)	c-*myc*
Intercellular adhesion molecule 1 (ICAM-1)	Interleukin-1	12-Lipoxygenase	c-*jun*
	Interleukin-2	Lysozyme	p53
Mucosal adressin cell... ...adhesion molecule (MadCAM-1)	Interleukin-3	NADPH quinone oxidoreductase	
	Interleukin-6	Nitric oxide synthase (iNOS)	*Other proteins*
Vascular cell adhesion molecule 1 (VCAM-1)	Interleukin-8	Phospholipase A2	A20
	Interleukin-12	Superoxide dismutase (SOD)	C-reactive protein
CD11b (MAC-1 subunit)	GM-CSF	Collagenase-1 (MMP-1)	Laminin
CD25 (IL-2 receptor)	G-CSF	Gelatinase B (MMP-9)	Peptide transporter (TAP-1)
CD48	M-CSF	Stromelysin (MMP-3)	Proteasome subunit LMP2
CD69	Macrophage inflammatory protein-1 (MIP-1α)		Tissue inhibitor of metallo- proteinase 1 (TIMP-1)
Immunoglobulin kappa light chain		*Transcription factors*	
MHC class I	Macrophage inflammatory protein-2	Interferon regulatory factors-1, -2	
MHC class II invariant chain (Ii)	Monocyte chemotactic protein 1 (MCP-1)	NF-κB precursor p100	Vimentin
Tissue factor	RANTES	NF-κB precursor p105	
	Tumor necrosis factor (TNF-α)	c-*rel*	

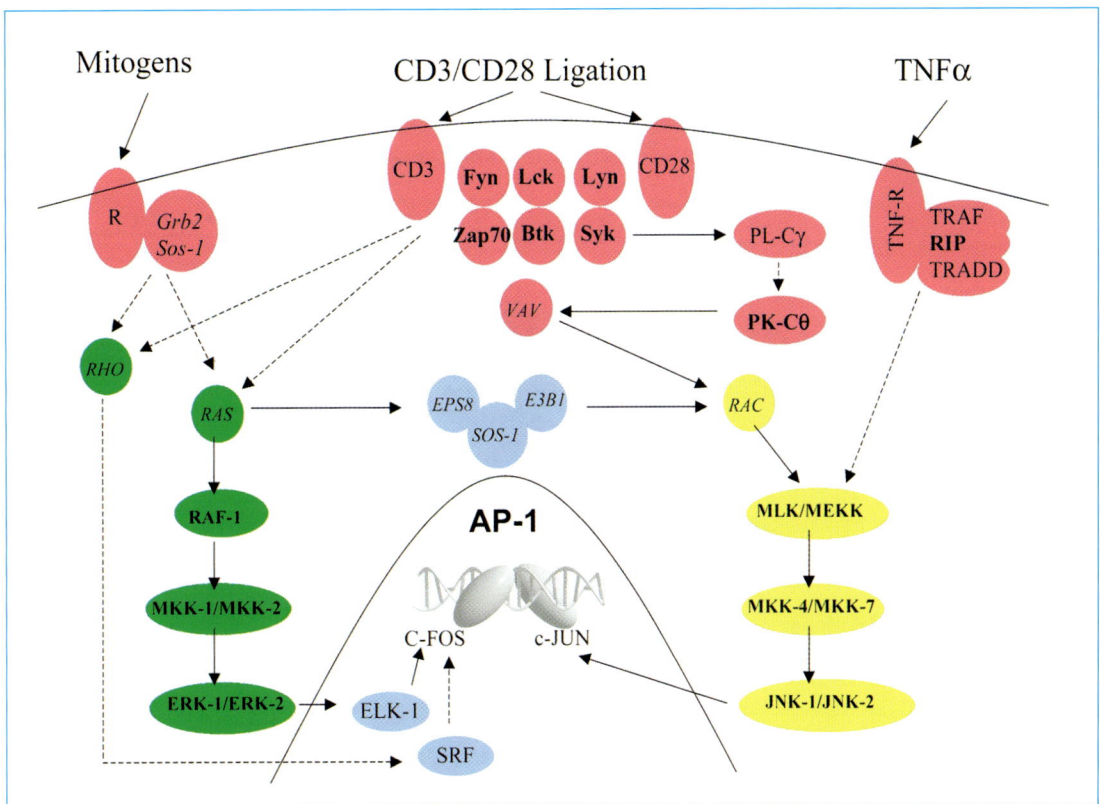

Fig. 2. AP-1 signaling pathway. The transcription factor AP-1 can be activated by diverse stimuli including mitogens, pro-inflammatory stimuli, antigen presentation, cell stress, and osmotic shock. Activated AP-1 (c-Fos/c-Jun) can be regulated by mitogen-activated protein kinase (MAPK) pathways. For example, activated Ras leads to activation of a kinase cascade through raf, MKK-1, -2, and ERK-1, -2 and subsequent phosphorylation of the transcription factor, Elk-1. Activated Elk-1 upregulates transcription of the c-*Fos* gene resulting in increased levels of c-Fos protein. In the second pathway, activated Rac-1 leads to activation of a kinase cascade through MLK/MEKK, MKK-4,-7 and JNK-1, -2. Activated JNK transduces the signal from the cytoplasm to the nucleus where it phosphorylates c-Jun resulting in enhanced transcriptional activity of AP-1. GTP-binding proteins are shown in italics, and protein kinases are shown in bold. Dotted lines represent pathways in which intermediate proteins are either poorly understood or not shown. SRF = Serum response factor.

Signaling Pathways: Targets for Therapeutic Intervention

Transcription factor activation is a result of a signaling cascade involving successive tiers of signaling proteins. This cascade network allows for both amplification of the signal, and specificity of the response arising from different stimuli [8]. The AP-1 and NF-κB signaling pathways are comprised of multiple kinases that serially phosphorylate downstream substrate kinases and transcription factors (fig. 2, 3). Following receptor activation by ligand, a variety of receptor-associated factors, GTP-binding proteins, tyrosine and serine/threonine kinases are activated. The precise composition and order of activation of these receptor-associated factors are highly dependent upon the cell type and the activated receptor complex. For example, while TNF receptor activation results in a receptor complex comprised of TRAF, RIP and death domain proteins [9], antigen presenting cell interaction with the T cell receptor (CD3) and costimulatory molecules (e.g. CD28) results in an activation complex comprised of tyrosine kinases (e.g. Fyn, Lck, Zap70) and GTPases (e.g. grb2, sos) [10]. The complexity and variety of these upstream signaling intermediates have provided a host of potential therapeutic targets that may provide enhanced cell type and stimulus specificity. However, it is clear that many of these pathways exhibit significant redundancy, so that deletion of one component does not exert a dominant inhibitory effect. Nevertheless, all of these stimuli and intermediates propagate signals that ultimately lead to strong activation of AP-1 and NF-κB. In figures 2 and 3 we have shown in detail the downstream portion of the signaling cascades leading to activation of both AP-1 and

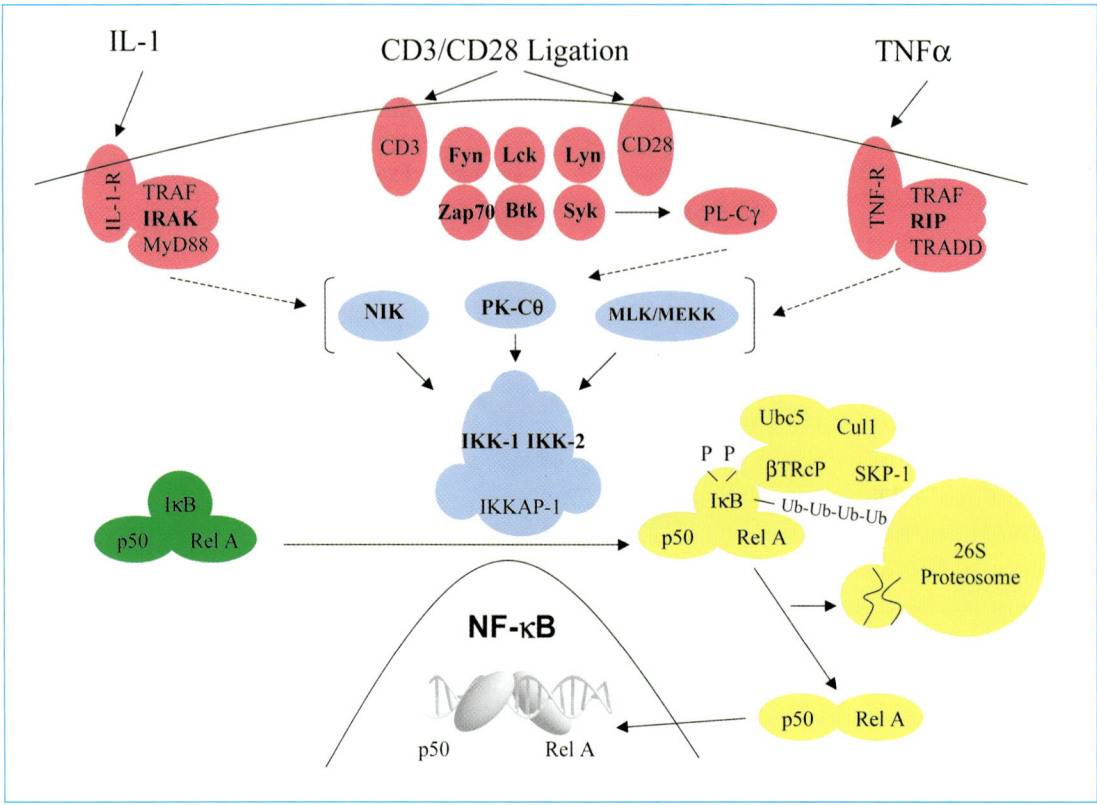

Fig. 3. NF-κB signaling pathway. The transcription factor NF-κB, can be activated by diverse stimuli including pro-inflammatory cytokines, antigen presentation, bacterial endotoxin, viral infection, UV, and reactive oxygen species. Stimulatory signals are transduced by receptor-protein complexes via at least one of four serine threonine kinases; NIK, protein kinase Cθ, MLK-3, and MEKK-1, to activate the IKK 'signalsome', a 900-kD multiprotein complex. Cytoplasmic NF-κB is recruited to the signalsome where the inhibitor molecule, IκB, is phosphorylated on two serine residues. Phosphorylated IκB becomes a substrate for the IκB-ligase complex that covalently attaches multiple ubiquitin polypeptides to IκB, thereby targeting it for degradation by the 26S proteasome. NF-κB is then translocated to the nucleus where it binds to specific elements in gene promoters. (Protein kinases are printed in bold).

NF-κB. These final signaling steps appear to be remarkably consistent regardless of cell type and stimulus. Furthermore, overexpression of inactive versions (dominant negative mutants) of any of these proteins significantly block transcription factor activation in a stimulus independent manner [11].

Prototypical AP-1 is a heterodimer comprised of two proteins, c-fos and c-jun. Related AP-1 transcription factors may be dimers of Fos, JunB, c-Jun, JunD, Fra-1 and Fra-2 [1]. c-Fos and c-Jun are regulated independently by separate mitogen-activated protein kinase (MAPK) cascades. For example, p21 Ras activates the MAPKKK, raf-1, which phosphorylates the MAPKK, MEK, which in turn phosphorylates the MAPK, ERK, which phosphorylates and activates the transcription factor Elk-1. Elk-1 binds to and promotes transcription of the c-*fos* gene leading to increase levels of c-fos protein. Additional transcription factors, such as serum response factor (SRF), may augment transcription of the c-*fos* gene. In another pathway, the small GTPases Rac-1 and cdc42 may be activated by Ras or other upstream pathways. Rac-1 activates an MAPKKK (e.g. MLK, MEKK) that phosphorylates an MAPKK, MKK, which in turn phosphorylates JNK. Nuclear JNK then phosphorylates c-jun, significantly enhancing the transcriptional activity of AP-1 [12].

NF-κB is a heterodimer of p50 (NF-κB1) and p65 (RelA) [2]. NF-κB-like transcription factors are dimers of p50, p52, RelA, RelB and c-rel. NF-κB is retained in the cytoplasm by an inhibitory protein, IκB, which masks the nuclear localization signal present on NF-κB. Upstream signaling pathways converge at a 900-kD multiprotein complex called the 'signalsome', which contains at least three proteins, IKK-1, IKK-2 and IKKAP-1/NEMO [13]. The IκB kinase, IKK-2 is believed to play a central role in pro-inflammatory signaling leading to phosphorylation of IκB and targeting it for ubiquitination and subsequent degradation by the 20S proteasome. This releases NF-κB for transport to the nucleus where it promotes the transcription of multiple genes (table 1).

Current and Future Therapies

At present, there are no prescribed drugs for asthma and COPD that target AP-1 or NF-κB. Aspirin, which has been shown to inhibit IKK-2 at high concentrations [14], is not effective in treating asthma. The most effective treatment for asthma, corticosteroids, exhibits striking suppression of the same inflammatory genes that are regulated by NF-κB and AP-1. This correlate has driven the search for mechanisms that explain the connection between glucocorticoid receptor activity and suppression of AP-1 and NF-κB gene regulation. One reported mechanism is that levels of the endogenous inhibitor of NF-κB, IκB, are upregulated following administration of glucocorticoids [15, 16], thereby suppressing NF-κB transcriptional activity. A second proposed mechanism for glucocorticoid action is the inhibition of histone acetylation and chromatin remodeling that is required for the transcription of transiently expressed (e.g. inflammatory) genes [17, 18]. Although this mechanism does not involve inhibition of the NF-κB signaling pathway per se, it does reinforce the potential efficacy of drugs blocking the signaling pathways leading to AP-1 and NF-κB activation.

Targets for drug discovery include all the signaling enzymes of these pathways (fig. 2, 3). The IκB kinase, IKK-2 appears to be a central regulator of NF-κB for all inflammatory stimuli and thus represents a target with significant modulating potential. More selective inhibitors may be found by targeting stimulus-dependent, or cell-specific enzymes such as NIK, MEKK-1, PK-Cθ, p56Lck, and Zap70. Additional targets include the ubiquitin ligase and proteosome machinery that targets IκB for proteolytic degradation. In the AP-1 pathway, all the MAPK family members are candidate drug targets including raf-1, MEK, ERK, MEKK, MLK, MKK and JNK. Indeed, SP600125, an ATP- competitive inhibitor of JNK, inhibits the infiltration of leukocytes into the lung in both acute and chronic models of antigen-induced lung inflammation in the rat [Bennett, unpubl. obs.]. Inhibition of other signaling intermediates, such as Ras, EPS8, Rac-1, Grb2 and Sos-1, may also provide anti-inflammatory effects, although the multiple signaling activities of some of these molecules may prove to be a liability.

References

1 Karin M, Zg L, Zandi E: AP-1 function and regulation. Curr Opin Cell Biol 1997;9:240–246.
2 Karin M: The beginning of the end: IκB kinase (IKK) and NF-κB activation. J Biol Chem 1999;274:27339–27342.
3 Barnes PJ, Adcock IM: Transcription factors and asthma. Eur Respir J 1998;12:221–234.
4 Adcock IM: Transcription factors as activators of gene transcription: AP-1 and NF-κB. Monaldi Arch Chest Dis 1997;52:178–186.
5 Yang l, Cohn L, Zhang DH, Homer R, Ray A, Ray P: Essential role of NF-κB in the induction of eosinophilia in allergic airway inflammation. J Exp Med 1998;188:1739–1750.
6 Manning AM, Bell FP, Rosenbloom CL, Chosay JG, Simmons CA, Northrup JL, Shebuski RJ, Dunn CJ, Anderson DC: NF-κB is activated during acute inflammation in vivo in association with elevated endothelial cell adhesion molecule gene expression and leukocyte recruitment. J Inflamm 1995;45:283–296.
7 Segura-Valdez L, Pardo A, Gaxiola M, Uhal BD, Becerril C, Selman M: Upregulation of gelatinases A and B, collagenases 1 and 2, and increased parenchymal cell death in COPD. Chest 2000;117:684–694.
8 Huang C-Y, Ferrell JE: Ultrasensitivity in the mitogen-activated protein kinase cascade. Proc Natl Acad Sci USA 1996;93:10078–10083.
9 Nagata S: Apoptosis by death factor. Cell 1997; 88:355–365.
10 Raab M, Cai YC, Bunnell SC, Heyeck SD, Berg LJ, Rudd CE: p56Lck and p59Lyn regulate CD28 binding to phosphatidylinositol 3-kinase, growth factor receptor-bound protein GRB-2, and T cell-specific protein-tyrosine kinase ITK: Implications for T-cell costimulation. Proc Natl Acad Sci USA 1995;92:8891–8895.
11 Chen BK, Kung HC, Tsai TY, Chang WC: Essential role of mitogen-activated protein kinase pathway and c-Jun induction in epidermal growth factor-induced gene expression of human 12-lipoxygenase. Mol Pharmacol 2000;57: 153–161.
12 Davis RJ: Signal transduction by the c-Jun N-terminal kinase. Biochem Soc Symp 1999;64: 1–12.
13 Mercurio F, Murray BW, Shevchenko A, Bennett BL, Young DB, Li JW, Pascual G, Motiwala A, Zhu H, Mann M, Manning AM: IκB kinase (IKK)-associated protein 1, a common component of the heterogeneous IKK complex. Mol Cell Biol 1999;19:1526–1538.
14 Yin MJ, Yamamoto Y, Gaynor RB: The anti-inflammatory agents aspirin and salicylate inhibit the activity of IκB kinase-beta. Nature 1998;396:77–80.
15 Scheinman RI, Cogswell PC, Lofquist AK, Baldwin Jr AS: Role of transcriptional activation of IκBα in mediation of immunosuppression by glucocorticoids. Science 1995;270:283–286.
16 Auphan N, DiDonato JA, Rosette C, Helmberg A, Karin M: Immunosuppression by glucocorticoids: Inhibition of NF-κB activity through induction of IκB synthesis. Science 1995;270: 286–290.
17 Ghosh S: Regulation of inducible gene expression by the transcription factor NF-κB. Immunol Res 1999;19:183–189.
18 Barnes PJ: Anti-inflammatory actions of glucocorticoids: Molecular mechanisms. Clin Sci (Colch) 1998;94:557–572.

Brydon L. Bennett, PhD
Pre-clinical Development
Signal Pharmaceuticals, Inc.
5555 Oberlin Drive
San Diego, CA 92121 (USA)
Tel. +1 858 558 7500, ext. 8214
Fax +1 858 623 0870
E-Mail bbennett@signalpharm.com

Inhibition of p38 MAP Kinase

David C. Underwood   Don E. Griswold

Department of Pulmonary Biology, SmithKline Beecham Pharmaceuticals, King of Prussia, Pa., USA

Summary

The discovery of the p38 mitogen-activated protein kinase (MAPK) signal transduction pathway and identification of specific inhibitors has ushered in a growing area of research into the role of p38 MAPK in pulmonary pathophysiology. Both in vitro and in vivo studies have elucidated the expression of isoforms of p38 MAPK and suggested an important role in the production and action of inflammatory cytokines. Further work in this area promises to give rise to a deeper understanding of these pathways as well as a potential insight into advances in therapy for both asthma and COPD.

Molecular Mechanisms

The mitogen-activated protein kinase (MAPK) network represents at least twelve cloned highly conserved, proline-directed serine-threonine protein kinases which, when activated by cell stresses (DNA damage, heat or osmotic shock), exogenous agents (anisomycin, Na arsenite, lipopolysaccharide, LPS) or pro-inflammatory cytokines, TNF-α and IL-1β, can phosphorylate and activate other kinases or nuclear proteins such as transcription factors in either the cytoplasm or the nucleus (fig. 1) [for reviews, see ref. 1–3]. The ubiquitous stress-activated protein kinase, p38 MAPK, is represented by at least 4 isoforms (α, β, γ, δ), several of which are considered important in processes critical to the inflammatory response and tissue remodeling [3]. The predominant kinases in monocytes and macrophages, p38α and p38β, appear more widely expressed compared to p38γ (skeletal muscle) or p38δ (testes, pancreas, prostate, small intestine, and in salivary, pituitary and adrenal glands) [3–5]. A number of substrates of p38 MAP kinase have been identified including other kinases (MAPKAP K2/3, PRAK, MNK1/2, MSK1/RLPK, RSK-B), transcription factors (ATF2/6, myocyte enhancer factor 2, nuclear transcription factor-β, CHOP/GADD153, Elk1 and SAP-1A1) and cytosolic proteins (stathmin), many of which are important physiologically [1, 3]. A part of the signaling process in the nucleus includes the phosphorylation of various factors, such as activating transcription factor-2 (ATF2), at sites that increase their transcriptional activity [6–8]. Along with subunits of nuclear factor (NF)-B, ATF2 is thought to bind to the AP-1 site as a heterodimer and positively regulate the expression of the promoters of several cytokine genes [9]. In alveolar macrophages, it has been shown that inhibition of p38 kinases with SB 203580 reduces cytokine gene products [10]. These observations suggest mechanisms by which the p38 kinases might regulate transcription. Through the use of specific inhibitors, the potential role of this stress-induced kinase in airway disease has begun to be studied. Although the phosphorylation of transcription factors appears to parallel or overlap p38 activation, the extent of their contribution to the anti-inflammatory activity of p38 MAPK inhibition is unclear.

Of equal or greater importance is the contribution of p38 to inducible gene expression by stabilizing mRNA through an MAPKAPK-2 and 3′ UTR AU-rich motif-targeted mechanism [3, 11, 12]. In addition, when MAPKAPK-2 is phosphorylated by p38, the complex formed appears to be translocated to the cytoplasm providing post-transcriptional regulation of cytokine expression [13].

The complex process of lung inflammation in asthma, COPD and acute respiratory distress syndrome (ARDS) reflect coordinated intercellular communication among infiltrating leukocytes, vascular endothelium, airway epithelium, smooth muscle cells and alveolar macrophages (fig. 2) [14, 15]. The lung inflammatory response is thought to be orchestrated by macrophage- and epithelial-derived cytokines, such as TNF-α and IL-1β which en-

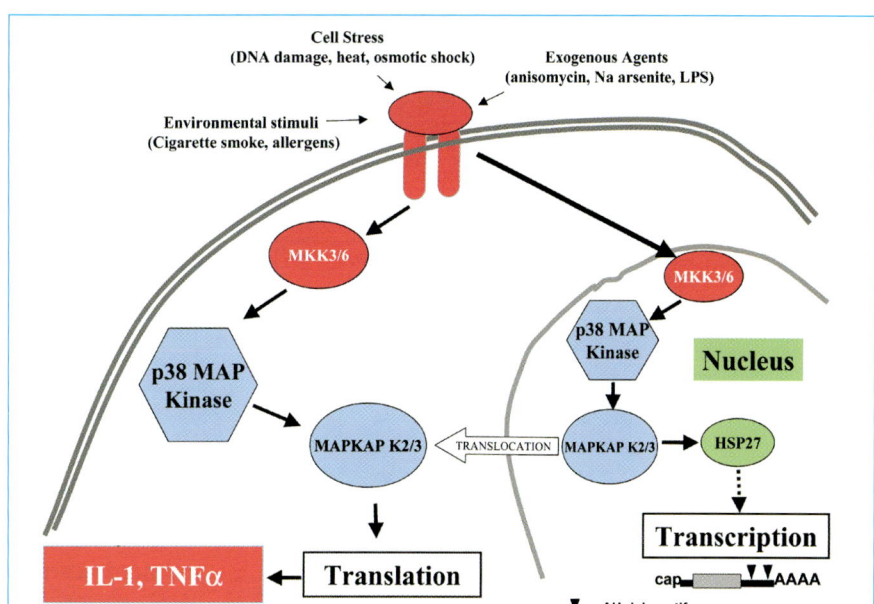

Fig. 1. Schematic representation of the p38 MAPK signaling cascade. A variety of inflammatory mediators activate p38 MAPK which may phosphorylate other downstream kinases or nuclear proteins, such as transcription factors, in either the cytoplasm or the nucleus, thus creating the potential for an amplified inflammatory process in the lung.

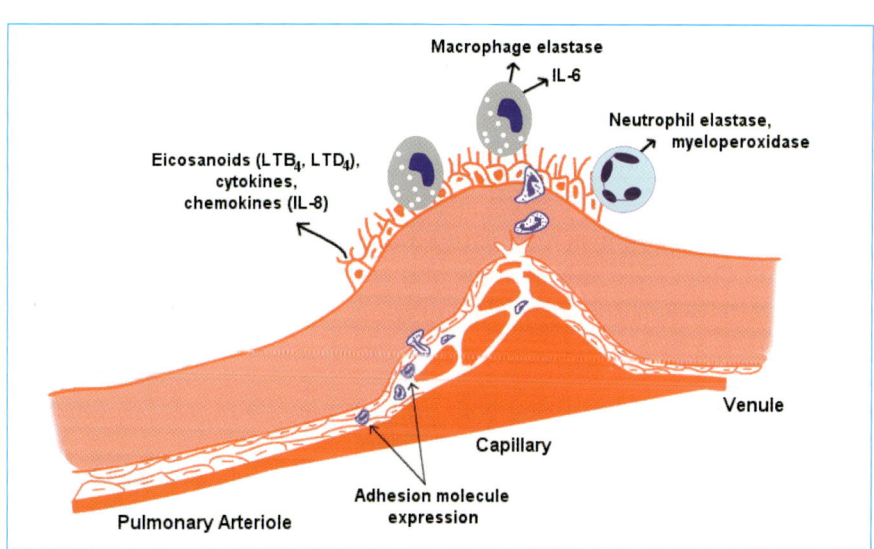

Fig. 2. Schematic representation of p38-mediated inflammatory cell chemotaxis and activation in the lung.

hance the expression of vascular adhesion molecules (ICAM-1, E-selectin) and neutrophil chemotaxins or chemokines, such as IL-8, to generate the release of destructive oxidants and proteases [15].

Although a role for p38 kinase inhibitors in the treatment of pulmonary disease has only recently been postulated [3, 16, 17], it is well known that inflammatory cytokines (TNF-α, IFN-γ, IL-4, IL-5) and chemokines (IL-8, RANTES, eotaxin) are capable of regulating or supporting chronic airway inflammation [18]. The production and action of many of the potential mediators of airway inflammation have been shown to be dependent upon the stress-induced MAP kinase or p38 kinase cascade (table 1). Activation of the p38 kinase pathway by numerous environmental stimuli results in the elaboration of recognized inflammatory mediators whose production is considered to be translationally regulated. In addition, a variety of inflammatory mediators activate p38 MAPK which may then activate downstream targets of the MAPK system including other kinases or transcription factors, thus creating the potential for an amplified inflammatory process in the lung. Several reports support the association of p38 kinase activation to a plethora of pulmonary events: LPS- and TNFα-induced ICAM-1 expression on pulmonary microvascular endothelial cells [21, 22], MMP-9 activation [23], hypoxia-induced stimulation of pulmo-

Table 1. List of representative activities of p38 MAP kinase in the lung

Cell	Activity	Reference
Eosinophil	chemotaxis (airway; guinea pig, mouse)	Underwood et al. [16]
	apoptosis (peripheral; human)	Kankaanranta et al. [19]
	apoptosis, persistence (airway; guinea pig)	Underwood et al. [16]
Neutrophil	chemotaxis (airway; guinea pig)	Underwood et al. [17]
Alveolar macrophage	IL-6 production (airway; guinea pig)	Underwood et al. [17]
	PMA-induced matrix metalloproteinase activity (airway; human)	Simon et al. [20]
	matrix metalloproteinase activity (airway; guinea pig)	Underwood et al. [17]
Endothelial cells (in vivo)	expression of ICAM-1 (human; pulmonary vascular)	Mulligan et al. [21]
Endothelial cells (in vitro)	adhesion molecule upregulation (human pulmonary)	Tamura et al. [22]
Epithelium and subepithelium	fibrosis (airway; rat)	Underwood et al. [17]
Pulmonary arterial smooth muscle cells	hypoxia-induced activation	Scott et al. [23]
Heart	right ventricular hypertrophy (rat)	Underwood et al. [17]

nary artery cells [20], hyperosmolarity-induced IL-8 expression in bronchial epithelial cells [24] and enhanced eosinophil trafficking and survival [16, 19].

Asthma

Although multiple cell types, both inflammatory and structural, have been postulated to be involved in the pathology of asthma, clearly the eosinophil has received the most attention [25]. In airways disease, especially asthma, the accumulation and activation of eosinophils appear as a marker of the disease, and are postulated to contribute to the development and maintenance of airway inflammation by releasing proinflammatory cytokines, lipid mediators, cytotoxic cationic proteins and oxygen radicals [18, 25]. In addition, while over 50 different mediators have been implicated in asthma, the eicosanoids (e.g. LTB_4, LTD_4), cytokines (TNF-α, IL-5, etc.) and chemokines (RANTES, eotaxin and IL-8) have received recent focus because of the availability of appropriate detection antibodies and the demonstrated efficacy of selective antagonists and inhibitors [18]. The ability of the p38 MAP kinase inhibitor, SB 239063, to inhibit antigen-induced accumulation of eosinophils in the airways of both mice and guinea pigs demonstrates inhibition of chemotaxis of this granulocyte [16]. In addition, chemokines such as RANTES and eotaxin have been recognized as potential contributors to the pathophysiology of asthma, and demonstrated inhibition of these cytokines as well as IgE synthesis via inhibition of CD23 expression by the p38 MAPK inhibitor, SB 203580, provide further evidence for the importance of this pathway in allergic disease [3].

Only recently has the persistence and maintenance of lung eosinophilia been evaluated. SB 239063 substantially reduced persistent airway eosinophilia, suggesting a more complex activity additional to simple inhibition of chemotaxis into the airways [16]. The demonstration of enhanced apoptosis which may signal for phagic capture by alveolar macrophages [26] provides an additional unique mechanism by which p38 kinase inhibitors may provide a therapeutic benefit in chronic airway inflammation. It has been consistently demonstrated that human cultured eosinophils purified from peripheral blood undergo rapid apoptosis when placed into primary culture [19, 25, 26]; this phenomenon is diminished with IL-5 supplementation [19, 25, 26]. Enhanced in vitro apoptosis was clearly shown in the presence of the earlier generation p38 MAP kinase inhibitors, SB 203580 and SB 202190 [19]. Furthermore, SB 239063 enhanced the apoptosis of a persistent population of guinea pig eosinophils isolated from the lung in the presence of IL-5 [16].

The recent demonstration of activated p38 MAPK in the lung where cell-cell interactions may play an equally important role in not only the survival of inflammatory cells, but also the activation state of these cells is evidence of the potential to enhance a naturally occurring neutralization of the pathogenesis of this granulocyte [16].

COPD

COPD is characterized by a chronic inflammatory process in the lung with features including: (1) increased inflammatory cells (neutrophils, macrophages and CD8+ T cells) in airway and parenchyma; (2) increased inflammatory cytokine and chemokine expression, and (3) increased proteases (elastases, cathepsins and matrix metalloproteinases) [15]. Trafficking and activation of the neutrophil, believed to play a central role in the pathophysiology of COPD, results in the release of a number of inflammatory mediators and proteinases, most importantly neutrophil elastase which contributes to the progressive fibrosis, airway stenosis and destruction of the lung parenchyma, leading to an accelerated decline in airway function and presentation of cor pulmonale [15, 27]. Neutrophil elastase is also a powerful mucus secretagogue and thus may contribute to the characteristic mucus hypersecretion that characterizes lung inflammation [15]. Several reports support the involvement of p38 kinase activation to events which may be associated with COPD: LPS- and TNF-α-induced ICAM-1 expression on pulmonary microvascular endothelial cells [21, 22], hypoxia-induced stimulation of pulmonary artery cells [23], MMP-9 activation [20], hyperosmolarity-induced IL-8 expression in bronchial epithelial cells [24]. Airway neutrophil infiltration, IL-6 levels and MMP-9 activity, assessed by bronchoalveolar lavage after LPS inhalation, were markedly inhibited by the p38 MAPK inhibitor, SB 239063 [17]. In guinea pig cultured alveolar macrophages, SB 239063 inhibited LPS-induced IL-6 production [17]. In addition, treatment with SB 239063 attenuated bleomycin-induced pulmonary fibrosis model in rats, significantly inhibiting right ventricular hypertrophy (indicative of secondary pulmonary hypertension) and increases in lung hydroxyproline synthesis (indicative of collagen synthesis and fibrosis) [17].

Therefore, p38 MAP kinase inhibitors, such as SB 239063 demonstrate activity against a range of sequelae commonly associated with asthma and COPD, providing support for the therapeutic potential of this class of kinase inhibitors in chronic airway disease.

References

1 Cohen P: The search for physiological substrates of MAP and SAP kinases in mammalian cells. Trends Cell Biol 1997;7:353–361.
2 Herlaar E, Brown Z: p38 MAPK signalling cascades in inflammatory disease. Molec Med Today 1999;5:439–447.
3 Lee JC, Kumar S, Griswold DE, Underwood DC, Votta BJ, Adams JL: Inhibition of p38 MAP kinase as a therapeutic strategy. Immunopharmacology 2000;47:185–201.
4 Kumar S, McDonnell PC, Gum RJ, Hand AT, Lee JC, Young PR: Novel homologues of CSBP/p38 MAP kinase: Activation, substrate specificity and sensitivity to inhibition by pyridinyl imidazoles. Biochem Biophys Res Commun 1997; 235:533–538.
5 Wang XS, Diener K, Manthey CL, Wang S, Rosenzweig B, Bray J, Delaney J, Cole CN, Chan-Hui PY, Mantlo N, Lichenstein HS, Zukowski M, Yao Z: Molecular cloning and characterization of a novel p38 mitogen-activated protein kinase. J Biol Chem 1997;272:23668–23674.
6 Nick, JA, Avdi NJ, Gerwins P, Johnson GL, Worthen GS: Activation of a p38 mitogen-activated protein kinase in human neutrophils by lipopolysaccharide. J Immunol 1996;156:4867–4875.
7 Cuenda A, Cohen P, Buee-Scherrer V, Goedert M: Activation of stress-activated protein kinase-3 (SAPK3) by cytokines and cellular stresses is mediated via SAPKK3 (MKK6): Comparison of the specificities of SAPK3 and SAPK2 (RK/p38). EMBO J 1997;16:295–305.
8 Raingeaud JS, Gupta S, Rogers JS, Dickens M, Han J, Ulevitch RJ, Davis RJ: Pro-inflammatory cytokines and environmental stress cause p38 mitogen-activated protein kinase activation by dual phosphorylation on tyrosine and threonine. J Biol Chem 1995;270:7420–7426.
9 Stein B, Baldwin AS Jr., Ballard DW, Greene WC, Angel P, Herrlich P: Cross-coupling of the NF-kappa B p65 and Fos/Jun transcription factors produces potentiated biological function. EMBO J 1993;12:3879–3891.
10 Carter AB, Monick MM, Hunninghake GW: Both Erk and p38 kinases are necessary for cytokine gene transcription. Am J Respir Cell Mol Biol 1999;20:751–758.
11 Winzen R, Kracht M, Ritter B, Wilhelm A, Chen C-YA, Shyu A-B, Muller M, Gaestel M, Resch K, Holtmann H: The p38 MAP kinase pathway signals for cytokine-induced mRNA stabilization via MAP kinase-activated protein kinase 2 and an AU-rich region-targeted mechanism. EMBO J 1999;18:4969–4980.
12 Kontoyiannis D, Pasparakis M, Pizarro TT, Cominelli F, Kollias G: Impaired on/off regulation of TNF biosynthesis in mice lacking TNF AU-rich elements: Implications for joint and gut-associated immunopathologies. Immunity 1999;10:387–398.
13 Ben-Levy R, Hooper S, Wilson R, Paterson HF, Marshall CJ: Nuclear export of the stress-activated protein kinase p38 mediated by its substrate MAPKAP kinase-2. Curr Biol 1998; 8:1049–1057.
14 Hunninghake GW, Crystal RG: Cigarette smoking and lung destruction: Accumulation of neutrophils in the lungs of cigarette smokers. Am Rev Respir Dis 1983;128:833–838.
15 Wanner A, Boushey H, Lee TH, Perruchoud AP: Inflammation in chronic obstructive pulmonary disease. Proceedings from the Transatlantic Airway Conference. Am J Respir Crit Care Med 1999;160:S1–S79.
16 Underwood DC, Osborn RR, Kotzer C, Adams J, Lee JC, Carpenter DC, Bochnowicz S, Thomas H, Hay DWP, Griswold DE: SB 239063, a potent p38 MAP kinase inhibitor reduces inflammatory cytokine production, airways eosinophil infiltration and persistence. J Pharmacol Exp Ther 2000;293:281–288.
17 Underwood DC, Osborn RR, Bochnowicz S, Webb EF, Rieman DJ, Lee JC, Romanic AM, Adams JL, Hay DWP, Griswold DE: Reduction of airway neutrophilia, inflammatory cytokine production, matrix metalloproteinase activity and fibrosis by the p38 MAP kinase inhibitor, SB 239063. Am J Physiol, in press.
18 Barnes PJ, Chung KF, Page CP: Inflammatory mediators of asthma: An update. Pharmacol Rev 1998;50:515–596.
19 Kankaanranta H, De Souza PM, Barnes PJ, Salmon M, Giembycz MA, Lindsay MA: SB 203580, an inhibitor of p38 mitogen-activated protein kinase, enhances constitutive apoptosis of cytokine-deprived human eosinophils. J Pharmacol Exp Ther 1999;290:621–628.
20 Simon C, Goepfert H, Boyd D: Inhibition of the p38 mitogen-activated protein kinase by SB 203580 blocks PMA-induced M_r 92,000 type IV collagenase secretion and in vitro invasion. Cancer Res 1988;58:1135–1139.
21 Mulligan MS, Vaporciyan AA, Miyaasaka M, Tamatani T, Ward PA: Tumor necrosis factor alpha regulates in vivo intrapulmonary expression of ICAM-1. Am J Pathol 1993;142:1739–1749.
22 Tamura DY, Moore EE, Johnson JL, Zallen G, Aiboshi J, Silliman CC: p38 mitogen-activated protein kinase inhibition attenuates intercellular adhesion molecule-1 up-regulation on human pulmonary microvascular endothelial cells. Surgery 1998;124:403–407.
23 Scott PH, Paul A, Belham CM, Peacock AJ, Wadsworth RM, Gould GW, Welsh D, Plevin R: Hypoxic stimulation of the stress-activated protein kinases in pulmonary artery fibroblasts. Am J Respir Crit Care Med 1998;158:958–962.
24 Hashimoto S, Matsumoto M, Gon Y, Nakayama T, Takeshita I, Horie T: Hyperosmolarity-induced interleukin-8 expression in human bronchial epithelial cells through p38 mitogen-activated protein kinase. Am J Respir Crit Care Med 1999;159:634–640.
25 Giembycz MA, Lindsay MA: Pharmacology of the eosinophil. Pharmacol Rev 1999;51:213–339.
26 Stern M, Meagher L, Savill J, Haslett C: Apoptosis in human eosinophils. Programmed cell death in the eosinophil leads to phagocytosis by macrophages and is modulated by IL-5. J Immunol 1992;148:3543–3549.
27 MacNee W: Pathophysiology of cor pulmonale in chronic obstructive pulmonary disease, state-of-the-art: Pt 1, 2. Am J Respir Crit Care Med 1994;150:833–852; 1158–1168.

David C. Underwood, PhD
SmithKline Beecham Pharmaceuticals
Department of Pulmonary Biology, UW2532
709 Swedeland Road
King of Prussia, PA 19406 (USA)
Tel. +1 610 270 6751, Fax +1 610 270 5381
E-Mail David_C_Underwood@sbphrd.com

STAT6

Role in IL-4-Mediated Signaling

Gabriele Schaefer   Chandrasekar Venkataraman   Ulrike Schindler

Tularik, Inc., South San Francisco, Calif., USA

Summary

STAT6 is a transcription factor that plays a central role in both IL-4 and IL-13 signaling. This report summarizes the function of STAT6 in Th2 cell development and illustrates its implications in asthma and atopic diseases. Based on the data derived from STAT6-deficient mice, we postulate that STAT6 is an excellent therapeutic target for various allergic conditions.

Functional Domains of STAT Proteins

STAT6 belongs to a family of transcription factors known as signal transducer and activator of transcription (STAT). STAT proteins play a fundamental role in transmitting intracellular signals elicited by cytokines and growth factors [1, 2]. The overall structure of a STAT protein is shown in figure 1. The amino-terminal domain mediates protein:protein interactions either with other transcription factors or among individual STAT proteins. STAT:STAT interaction leads to tetramer formation and cooperative DNA binding. Recently, the crystal structures of two different STAT dimers bound to its DNA recognition site were solved [3, 4]. The DNA binding domain located in the center of the molecule mediates interaction with specific DNA elements. A linker region separates the DNA binding and the src homology 2 (SH2) domain. The SH2 domain is essential for the recognition of phosphorylated tyrosine residues in the intracellular domain of the cognate cytokine receptor. The tyrosine residue that becomes phosphorylated upon activation is located downstream of the SH2 domain. The carboxy-terminal end bears the transcription activation domain.

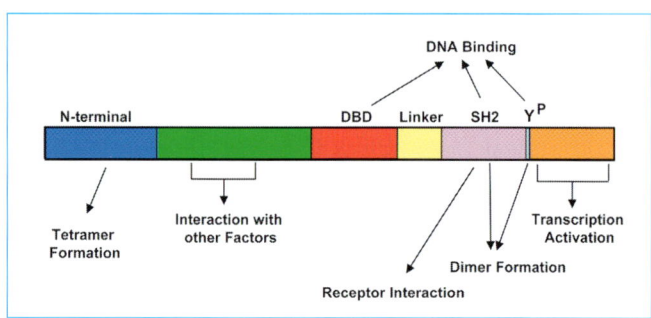

Fig. 1. Functional domains of STAT proteins. DBD = DNA-binding domain.

Activation of STAT6 by IL-4 and IL-13

STAT6 is activated by two cytokines, IL-4 and IL-13. The activation cycle is illustrated in figure 2. Both cytokines mediate their effect through the IL-4 receptor alpha chain, which heterodimerizes upon ligand binding with an additional receptor chain that is distinct for the two cytokines [5]. Receptor ligation leads to activation of the associated kinases, Jak-1 and Jak-3, which in turn phosphorylate specific tyrosine residues in the intracellular domain of the receptor. STAT6 is recruited to the receptor and interacts with these phosphotyrosine residues via its SH2 domain. The specificity of this interaction is dictated by the nature of the amino acids following the phosphotyrosine residues. Subsequently, STAT6 itself becomes phosphorylated, is released from the receptor, dimerizes and translocates to the nucleus where it binds specific DNA sequences located in the promotor of

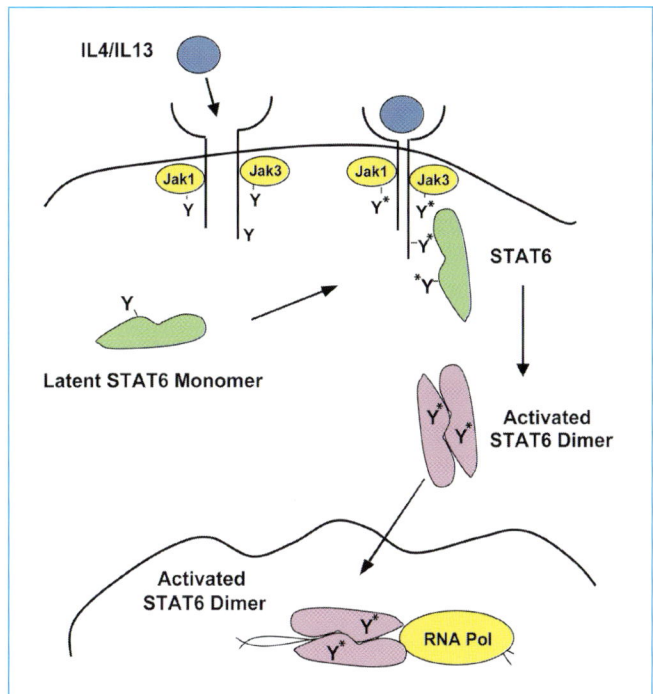
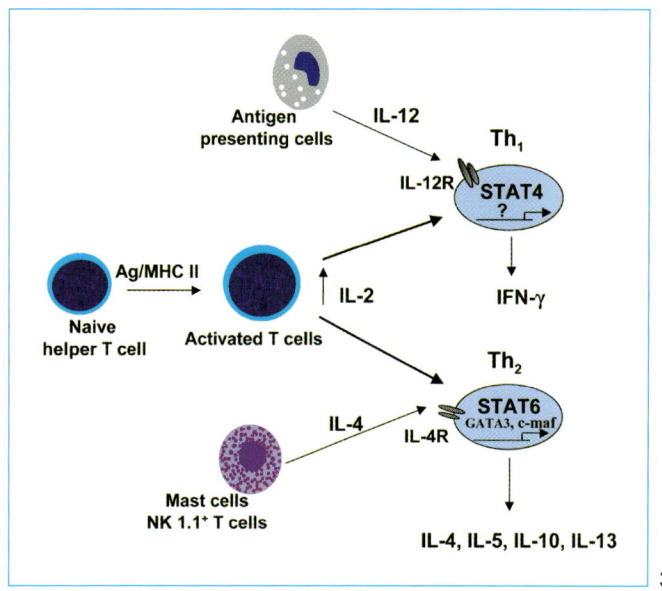

Fig. 2. Activation of STAT6-signaling pathway.
Fig. 3. Development of T-helper cell subsets.

IL-4/IL-13-responsive genes. STAT6 has unique DNA-binding properties in that it recognizes an N4 site (TTCN4GAA) in addition to the general N3 (TTCN3GAA) site which is bound by all STAT proteins [6]. IL-4-responsive elements that are bound by STAT6 have been identified in a number of genes including CD23, MHCcII, the IL-4 receptor alpha chain and the germline epsilon promoter. Transcriptional activation of the germline epsilon promoter is required for class switching to the IgE isotype. IL-4-induced expression of the untranslated germline transcript requires integrity of the STAT6-binding site as well as of the adjacent C/EBP-binding site. Hence, in some cases STAT6 needs to cooperate with other transcription factors to drive IL-4-induced gene expression.

Role of STAT6 in Th2 Differentiation

Naive CD4+ T cells can develop into two distinct T-helper cell subpopulations, Th1 or Th2, depending on the nature and dose of the antigen and the cytokine milieu during the initial immune response. The two subsets are defined by their unique cytokine expression profiles. Th1 cells produce IFN-γ and lymphotoxin and are important for cell-mediated immunity. Th2 cells produce IL-4, IL-5, IL-10 and IL-13 and are required for humoral immune response (fig. 3). The presence of IL-12 during the initial priming drives the polarization process towards the Th1 lineage, whereas the presence of IL-4 promotes Th2 development. Differentiation towards a specific T-helper cell subset is not only dependent on the presence of the key cytokine but also depends on the integrity of the corresponding downstream signaling pathway. The importance of STAT6 in Th2 differentiation has been established using STAT6-deficient mice. In the absence of STAT6, T-lymphocytes fail to differentiate into Th2 cells in response to either IL-4 or IL-13, and B-cells do not produce IgE [7–9]. Activation of STAT6 occurs very rapidly, whereas the development of Th2 cells requires several days. Hence, it is controversial whether STAT6 is directly involved in the induction of Th2-associated cytokine expression. Recently, it has been shown that ectopic expression of activated STAT6 in developing Th1 cells induces Th2-specific cytokines and suppresses the expression of IFN-γ, presumably by upregulating two other Th2-specific transcription factors, GATA3 and c-*maf* [10]. GATA3 strongly activates the IL-5 promoter and to some extent the IL-4 promotor, whereas c-*maf* acts at the IL-4 promotor site [11–13]. Thus, STAT6 may not directly induce the Th2 cytokines but may instead be the gatekeeper for the expression of other downstream transcription factors that are directly involved in cytokine production.

STAT6 as a Drug Target for Asthma

Allergic asthma is a complex inflammatory disease characterized by airway hyperresponsiveness, increased serum IgE levels, and elevated eosinophil infiltration. The pathology associated with asthma is mainly attributed to the hyperactivity of Th2 lymphocytes. These cells release IL-4, IL-5, IL-10, and IL-13, which are major players in a variety of different inflammatory processes.

The role of IL-5 in asthma has been studied using IL-5-deficient mice. IL-5 contributes to the growth, differentiation and activation of eosinophils. In a mouse model of allergic inflammation, IL-5-deficient mice are severely impaired in the induction of eosinophil differentiation and maturation, whereas IgE serum levels are not affected [14].

In contrast, IL-4-deficient mice do not produce IgE, but show somewhat normal eosinophilic inflammation. Interestingly, IL-4-receptor-deficient mice reveal a much stronger defect in inflammatory responses when compared to IL-4-deficient mice. This effect can be explained by the fact that the IL-4 receptor alpha chain is also shared by IL-13. IL-13 shares many biological functions with IL-4, such as enhanced CD23 expression on B cells and IgE isotype switching [15]. However, IL-13 also has unique functions and appears to be a central mediator of allergic asthma [16].

STAT6 is the common signal transducer of IL-4 receptor alpha and mediates IL-4- and IL-13-induced responses. The pivotal role of STAT6 in asthma was demonstrated in murine model systems. STAT6-deficient mice do not develop antigen-induced airway hyperresponsiveness and they do not show mucus-containing cells in the airway epithelium following antigen exposure. More importantly, antigen treatment of STAT6-deficient mice does not lead to an increase of Th2 cytokines. Consequently, IL-4-induced serum IgE levels are abrogated and IL-5-dependent induction of eosinophil differentiation is severely defective [17, 18].

A downstream target of STAT6 is the transcription factor GATA3, which is also essential in Th2 development. Overexpression of a dominant-negative mutant of GATA3 in mice demonstrates the important role of GATA3 in allergic asthma. These transgenic mice show reduced Th2 cytokine levels and a reduction in airway eosinophilia, mucus production and IgE synthesis [19]. Similar observations have been made in STAT6-deficient mice. Recently, it was shown that GATA3 is upregulated upon STAT6 activation [10], suggesting that STAT6 inhibition would also eliminate GATA3 function.

Taken together, these studies demonstrate that STAT6 inhibition affects the functions of all Th2 cytokines, IL-4, IL-5, and IL-13, which are involved in the establishment of asthma. Hence, STAT6 is a superb drug target for the treatment of asthma and atopic diseases.

Mutations in the IL-4-Signaling Pathway in Humans

It remains to be determined whether the observations made in murine models also apply to humans. However, clinical data suggest that IL-4 signaling is clearly involved in human asthma. For example, expression of a mutant form of the IL-4 receptor alpha chain in allergic patients is associated with increased IL-4 signaling [20]. Furthermore, a significant increase of GATA3 expression was seen in asthmatic patients [21]. Collectively, these data indicate that inappropriate regulation of the genes involved in IL-4 production or IL-4 signaling may account for the clinical symptoms of asthma in humans.

Concluding Remarks

STAT6 is a central regulator of both IL-4 and IL-13 signal transduction, and genetic studies have demonstrated that STAT6 is an excellent therapeutic target for the treatment of various allergic conditions. Based on the knowledge of STAT6 activation, agents which disrupt docking of STAT6 to the IL-4 receptor and prevent subsequent dimerization should be useful in the treatment of a broad range of allergic and atopic diseases. If administered prophylactically, such agents should inhibit STAT6 function and prevent the development of antigen-specific Th2 cells. Abrogation of STAT6 function can also favor the selective expansion of Th1 cells leading to IFN-γ production, which can in turn suppress ongoing damage by Th2 cytokines. An ideal STAT6 inhibitor should block all Th2-mediated deleterious effects such as IgE production, mucus accumulation in inflamed airways and eosinophilic recruitment. Finally, STAT6 inhibitors have an unequivocal advantage of being selective in preventing Th2 effects without causing general immunosuppression. The therapeutic value of STAT6 inhibitors needs to be rigorously tested in various model systems in order to develop better drugs to treat asthmatic patients.

References

1 Heim M H: The Jak-STAT pathway: Cytokine signalling from the receptor to the nucleus. J Recept Signal Transduct Res 1999;19:75–120.
2 Darnell JE Jr: STATs and gene regulation. Science 1997;277:1630–1635.
3 Becker S, Groner B, Muller CW: Three-dimensional structure of the Stat3beta homodimer bound to DNA. Nature 1998;394:145–151.
4 Chen X, Vinkemeier U, Zhao Y, Jeruzalmi D, Darnell JEJ, Kuriyan J: Crystal structure of a tyrosine phosphorylated STAT-1 dimer bound to DNA. Cell 1998;93:827–839.
5 Chomarat P, Banchereau J: Interleukin-4 and interleukin-13: Their similarities and discrepancies. Int Rev Immunol 1998;17:1–52.
6 Schindler U, Hoey T, McKnight SL: Differentiation of T-helper lymphocytes: Selective regulation by members of the STAT family of transcription factors. Genes Cells 1996;1:507–515.
7 Kaplan MH, Schindler U, Smiley ST, Grusby MJ: Stat6 is required for mediating responses to IL-4 and for development of Th2 cells. Immunity 1996;4:313–319.
8 Shimoda K, van Deursen J, Sangster MY, Sarawar SR, Carson RT, Tripp RA, Chu C, Quelle FW, Nosaka T, Vignali DA, Doherty PC, Grosveld G, Paul WE, Ihle JN: Lack of IL-4-induced Th2 response and IgE class switching in mice with disrupted Stat6 gene. Nature 1996;380:630–633.
9 Takeda K, Tanaka T, Shi W, Matsumoto M, Minami M, Kashiwamura S, Nakanishi K, Yoshida N, Kishimoto T, Akira S: Essential role of Stat6 in IL-4 signalling. Nature 1996;380:627–630.
10 Kurata H, Lee HJ, O'Garra A, and Arai N: Ectopic expression of activated Stat6 induces the expression of Th2-specific cytokines and transcription factors in developing Th1 cells. Immunity 1999;11:677–688.
11 Zhang, DH, Yang L, Ray A: Differential responsiveness of the IL-5 and IL-4 genes to transcription factor GATA-3. J Immunol 1998; 161:3817–3821.
12 Ranganath S, Ouyang W, Bhattarcharya D, Sha WC, Grupe A, Peltz G, Murphy KM: GATA-3-dependent enhancer activity in IL-4 gene regulation. J Immunol 1998;161:3822–3826.
13 Ho IC, Hodge MR, Rooney JW, Glimcher LH: The proto-oncogene c-*maf* is responsible for tissue-specific expression of interleukin-4. Cell 1996;85:973–983.
14 Foster PS, Hogan SP, Ramsay AJ, Matthaei KI, Young IG: Interleukin 5 deficiency abolishes eosinophilia, airways hyperreactivity, and lung damage in a mouse asthma model. J Exp Med 1996;183:195–201.
15 Punnonen J, Aversa G, Cocks BG, McKenzie AN, Menon S, Zurawski G, de Waal Malefyt R, de Vries JE: Interleukin 13 induces interleukin 4-independent IgG4 and IgE synthesis and CD23 expression by human B cells. Proc Natl Acad Sci USA 1993;90:3730–3734.
16 Wills-Karp M, Luyimbazi J, Xu X, Schofield B, Neben TY, Karp CL, Donaldson DD: Interleukin-13: Central mediator of allergic asthma. Science 1998;282:2258–2261.
17 Kuperman D, Schofield B, Wills-Karp M, Grusby MJ: Signal transducer and activator of transcription factor 6 (Stat6)-deficient mice are protected from antigen-induced airway hyperresponsiveness and mucus production. J Exp Med 1998;187:939–948.
18 Akimoto T, Numata F, Tamura M, Takata Y, Higashida N, Takashi T, Takeda K, Akira S: Abrogation of bronchial eosinophilic inflammation and airway hyperreactivity in signal transducers and activators of transcription (STAT)6-deficient mice. J Exp Med 1998;187: 1537–1542.
19 Zhang D-H, Yang L, Cohn L, Parkyn L, Homer R, Ray P, Ray A: Inhibition of allergic inflammation in a murine model of asthma by expression of a dominant-negative mutant of GATA-3. Immunity 1999;11:473–482.
20 Hershey GK, Friedrich MF, Esswein LA, Thomas ML, Chatila TA: The association of atopy with a gain-of-function mutation in the alpha subunit of the interleukin-4 receptor (see comments). N Engl J Med 1997;337:1720–1725.
21 Nakamura Y, Ghaffar O, Olivenstein R, Taha RA, Soussi-Gounni A, Zhang DH, Ray A, Hamid Q: Gene expression of the GATA-3 transcription factor is increased in atopic asthma. J Allergy Clin Immunol 1999;103:215–222.

G. Schaefer
Tularik, Inc.
Two Corporate Drive
South San Francisco, CA 94080 (USA)
Tel. +1 650 825 7482, Fax +1 650 825 7400
E-Mail gschaefer@tularik.com

Retinoids

Paula N. Belloni

Roche Bioscience, Palo Alto, Calif., USA

Summary

Retinoic acid receptor (RAR) agonists (vitamin A analogues) have been developed clinically to treat a variety of inflammatory skin disorders and to promote the repair of UV-induced skin damage. Epidemiological studies have established an inverse relationship between plasma retinol status and the degree of airway obstruction associated with COPD. Current treatment of moderate to severe emphysema is palliative at best. Recent preclinical studies suggest that an analogue of vitamin A, all-*trans* retinoic acid (ATRA) may promote the repair and/or re-alveolarization of parenchymal lesions associated with emphysema. RAR agonists have the potential to be used as anabolic therapy that could not only slow progression, but reverse the disease process, leading to improved lung function and quality of life. Clinical proof-of-concept studies are merited, but identification of most appropriate patient populations and clinical surrogates of improvement represent significant challenges in this potential novel therapy.

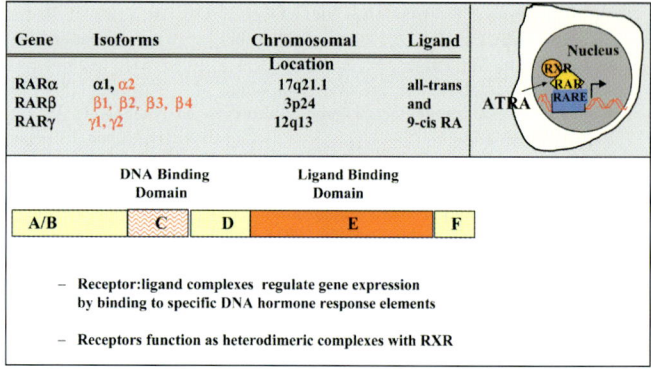

Fig. 1. Mechanism of action RA nuclear hormone receptors.

Molecular Basis of Action

Retinoids are a class of compounds structurally related to vitamin A, comprising natural and synthetic compounds. Retinoic acid (RA) and its other naturally occurring retinoid analogs (9-*cis*-RA, 13-*cis*-RA, all-*trans* 3,4-didehydro-RA, 4-oxo RA and retinol) are pleiotropic regulatory compounds that modulate the structure and function of a wide variety of inflammatory, immune and structural cells. Retinoids exert their biological effects through a series of nuclear receptors that are ligand-inducible transcription factors belonging to the steroid/thyroid nuclear hormone receptor superfamily [1]. The ligand bound heterodimer binds to RA response elements (RARE) in the noncoding region target genes to repress or enhance expression (fig. 1). Retinoids can also modulate gene expression by binding directly to specific transcription factors such as AP-1, interfering with the protein-protein interactions, analogous to glucocorticoids [2].

The retinoid receptors are classified into two families, the RA receptors (RARs) and the retinoid X receptors (RXRs), each consisting of three distinct subtypes (α, β, and γ). Within each RAR subtype a variable number of isoforms may be expressed via differential splicing of the primary RNA transcripts. All-*trans* RA (ATRA) is the physiological hormone for the RARs. It binds with approximately equal affinity to all the three RAR subtypes at nanomolar concentrations, but has no significant binding to the RXRs. In contrast, the 9-*cis*-RA isomer is active on both RAR and RXR receptors. ATRA is generated primarily from retinol at the cellular site of action in a highly controlled metabolic pathway [reviewed by Napoli, 3]. Throughout the metabolic processes, retinoid metabolites and ATRA remain complexed to retinoid binding proteins (retinol-binding protein, cellular-retinol-binding protein and cellular RA-binding protein) to protect the cells from hormonal action. Much of the metabolic pathway is autoregulated by local concentrations of ATRA, since excess or inadequate maintenance of ATRA can have significant pathological consequences throughout life.

Cellular Mechanism in Lung Development

RA was initially described as a critical nutrient required for development and maintenance of normal mucociliary function in the lung. In animals depleted of vitamin A, differentiation of airway epithelium was lost and replaced by squamous cell metaplasia [4]. That expression of RARβ2 is associated with suppression of lung neoplasms is well recognized; however, the role of retinoid agonists in chemoprevention or second-line therapy is unclear.

In contrast, the pleiotropic effects induced by ATRA during lung development have been described [5], and may have relevance to potential therapeutic use in emphysema. Lung development involves the formation of primordial lung from the foregut, sequential branching morphogenesis into small airways, followed by three maturation phases: the pseudoglandular, the canalicular and the terminal saccular stage. Epithelium and mesenchyme drive the process by coordinate expression of growth factors, the cognate receptors, and matrix molecules [6]. For example, epithelial cell proliferation and differentiation are driven by peptide growth factors produced by the mesenchyme (EGF, TGF-α, HGF, FGF-7, and TGF-β. Similarly, factors secreted by the epithelium PDGF, IGF, TGF-β2, and matrix deposition promote rapid proliferation of interstitial fibroblasts. In general, peptide growth factors that signal via tyrosine kinase domains promote morphogenesis. In contrast, the cognate receptors with serine/threonine kinase domains, such as the TGF-β receptor family are inhibitory. This extensive process of branching morphogenesis and alveolarization is coupled with angiogenesis and vasculogenesis. RA promotes the temporal and spatial expression of many of these factors and/or receptors by direct interaction with their respective promoters or indirectly by modulating the expression of other transcription factors such as Hox genes, shh, TTF-1, HNF-3 and AP-1.

Expression of the RARs is highly regulated both temporally and spatially at various times during lung development. RARα is associated with instructing epithelial cell differentiation and driving structural changes during the

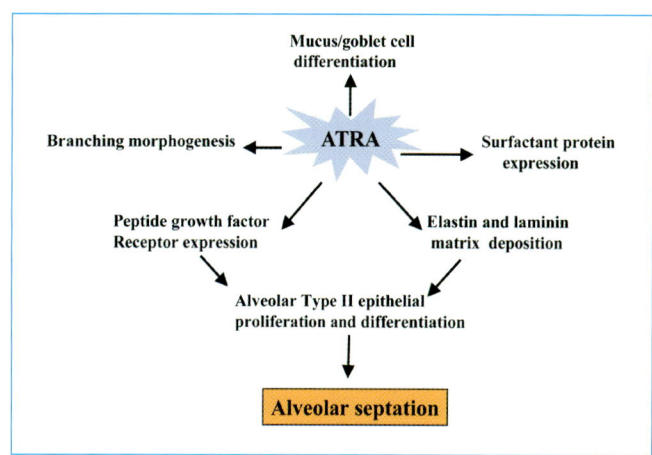

Fig. 2. Effects of ATRA in lung development.

transition from the glandular to the canalicular stage of development. In contrast, RARβ increases significantly in the terminal saccular stage, with the induction of both type II and type I epithelial cells. RARγ tends to be restricted to cells of the mesenchyme throughout this process [7, 8]. Stores of RA granules are abundant in the fibroblastic mesenchyme surrounding alveolar walls, where levels peak just prior to alveolar septation [9]. Deposition of new elastin matrix and septation occurs with subsequent depletion of these retinyl-esters. RA drives these processes by selective and coordinate induction of peptide growth factors, growth factor receptors, and matrix molecules in epithelium and fibroblasts (fig. 2). In neonatal rats fed a vitamin-A-deficient diet or treated with dexamethasone, alveolar septation is significantly reduced. At the molecular level, expression of cellular retinol binding protein and RARβ mRNA is diminished in lungs of vitamin-A-deficient rat pups [10]. In contrast, treatment of neonatal rat pups with ATRA increases lung alveolarization and can reverse the effects of dexamethasone [11]. Additional studies performed ex vivo suggest that terminal branching and type II epithelial cell proliferation require ATRA to modulate the expression of FGF-7 and HGF [12].

Effects in Animal Models of COPD

In adult animals deficient in retinol, the conducting airways undergo reversible squamous metaplasia, transformation of mucociliary epithelium into squamous cells. Conversely, animals supplemented with ATRA given chronic challenges of lipopolysaccharide undergo goblet cell/mucous metaplasia and fibrosis. The airway remodeling mimics that observed in cigarette-smoke-induced

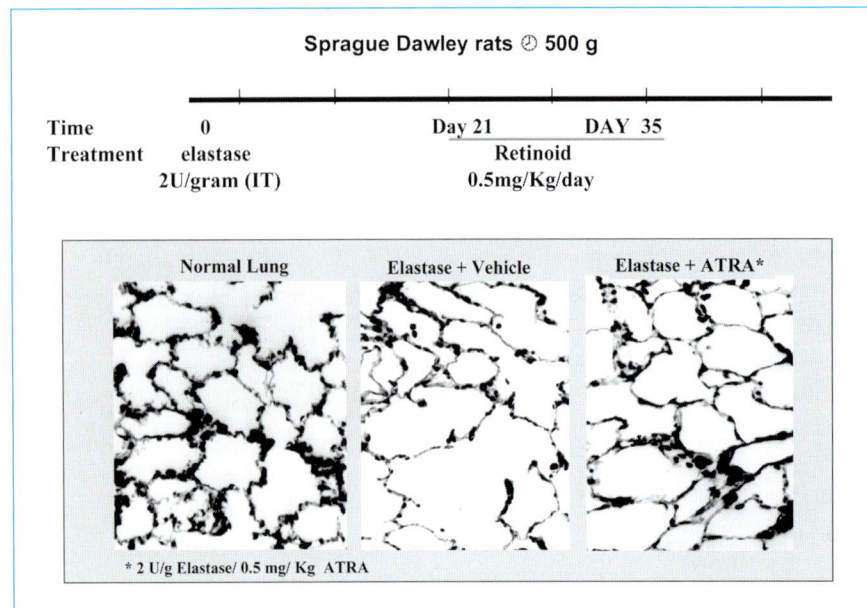
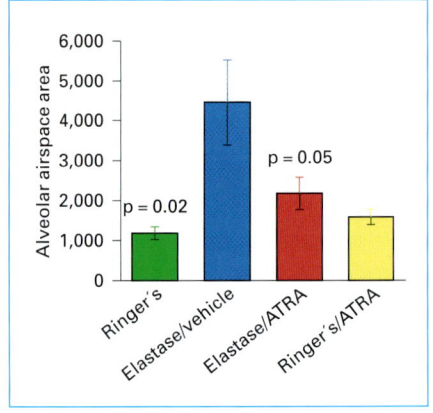

Fig. 3. a Effects of ATRA in repair of elastase-induced alveolar damage. b Effects of ATRA in repair of elastase-induced alveolar damage.

chronic bronchitis, a normal protective/repair response to chronic injury. In contrast to the excessive repair associated with chronic bronchitis, repair is absent or incomplete in preclinical models of emphysema. Elastolytic enzymes (pancreatic and neutrophil elastase, papain, macrophase elastase) instilled into the lungs can induce experimental emphysema. Elastase treatment leads to rapid destruction of the elastin content and permanent disruption of the elastin architecture within the alveolus [13]. Airspace enlargement and partial loss of lung capacity have been measured in the rat. The loss of lung structure and function associated with elastase-induced emphysema is similar to the clinical pathology of mild to moderate human emphysema.

The studies initially reported by Massaro and Massaro [14] and repeated by others suggest that ATRA can reverse the effects of elastase-induced damage in the rat. Emphysema is induced by a single instillation of pancreatic elastase into the lungs. Treatment with RA (0.5 mg/kg) or vehicle is initiated 3 weeks after injury, for 14 days. Changes in alveolar structure (size and number) can be determined by classical or computer-assisted methods of morphometry. Using either method of analysis, treatment of rats with elastase plus vehicle results in a reduction of alveolar number and a 2- to 3-fold increase in alveolar airspace. Treatment with ATRA or 9-cis-RA significantly reverses the damage by more than 50% (fig. 3). ATRA has similar effects on repair of alveolar structures in cigarette-smoke-induced emphysema. Immunolocalization of proliferation-associated antigen suggests that the response to ATRA is limited to alveolar epithelium. Elastase damage also induces loss of lung function in rats. Lung volumes are increased while FEV_1, DL_{CO} and paO_2 are decreased after elastase damage with partial reversal following ATRA treatment.

Toxicology

Retinoid pan agonists have been tested in a variety of preclinical models and clinical pathologies, primarily in dermatology and oncology. The most significant toxicity associated with all retinoids tested to date is teratogenicity since it is a primary mediator of pattern formation in developing fetuses. This toxicity does not represent a significant hurdle for emphysema therapy, since most patients are beyond the child-bearing age, but could be managed if necessary by requiring the use of pharmaceutical birth control agents by all female patients of child-bearing age. ATRA and 13-cis-RA have been tested in several phase I and phase II tirals to assess their potential efficacy in chemoprevention and or chemotherapy. The most common side effect reported from chronic therapy are transient headaches, followed by reactions in skin and mucous membranes, such as, dry skin, itching, flaking cheilitis, and nasal congestion. Bone pain and arthralgia are reported by 20–30% of patients. Significant hyperglycemia and hypercholesterolemia may have clinical importance in emphysema patients if chronic therapy is required.

Therapeutic Approaches

Bronchopulmonary Dysplasia. In adult animals deficient in retinol, the conducting airways undergo squamous metaplasia, transformation of mucociliary epithelium into squamous cells [15]. Similar changes are observed in bronchopulmonary dysplasia, a chronic lung disease encountered in infants after ventilation therapy for respiratory distress. In addition to delayed septation, lung function is impaired in these infants by inadequate levels of surfactant phospholipids which normally line alveoli. Vitamin A deficiency, reduced plasma retinol, is thought to mediate some of the lung pathology in these neonates. Retinol supplementation has been used clinically in these infants. Results from recent clinical studies suggest that supplementation with retinol enhances the survival of these infants [16]. Preclinical studies indicate that supplementation of vitamin-A-deficient rat pups with physiological levels of ATRA not only promotes septation, but also promotes expression of surfactant protein genes [17]. The levels of surfactant protein (A and B) were directly correlated with plasma retinol concentrations. Similar molecular events may contribute to the reduced need for oxygen therapy and improved survival observed in the clinic.

Rationale for Clinical Use in Adult Lung Disease: Acute Respiratory Distress Syndrome and Emphysema. Wound healing occurs in three phases: inflammation, proliferation/granulation, and remodeling [36]. Evidence supporting the capacity for self-renewal or repair in adult lung tissue stems from studies examining the alveolar microenvironment of acute respiratory distress syndrome patients or animals after acute lung injury. After acute lung injury, repair is initiated by an extensive fibroproliferative response, leading to granulation of the alveolar airspaces, a classical wound healing response [18]. PDGF (A and B chain) and TGF-β1 and TGF-β2 are rapidly induced in alveolar epithelial cells in response to injury. PDGF is a potent mitogen for mesenchymal cells whereas, TGF-β retards fibroblasts growth but promotes matrix deposition. PDGFrα expression is markedly enhanced in lung myofibroblasts within 24 h of injury and subsides prior to the deposition of fibrotic matrix proteins [19]. In patients/animals that survive, there is resolution of the granulation tissue with subsequent restoration of the gas exchange apparatus. The reduction in cell mass occurs via apoptosis similar to the final stages of septation in development, as well as in normal wound healing. The effects of RA and PDGF on wound healing in skin are well documented. Additional preclinical studies are required to determine whether similar patterns of gene expression are induced by ATRA in the repair of lung and skin. More importantly, these studies may support potential clinical utility to enhance the rate of repair in acute respiratory distress syndrome as well in emphysema.

Clinical Feasibility Studies in Emphysema. The first clinical assessment of ATRA in the treatment of emphysema was completed in the spring 2000 by UCLA investigators (ATS, May 2000). The study was designed as a 3-month double cross-over to assess the pharmacokinetics, safety and side effect profiles of ATRA, in addition to potential therapeutic benefit. ATRA was tested at 50 mg/m^2/day, 4 days/week in 20 patients with moderate to severe emphysema. Efficacy for treating the physiologic, anatomic and symptomatic manifestations of emphysema was assessed by serial pulmonary function tests, high-resolution computed tomography (HRCT) scans with dynamic spirometry-gated functional imaging using electron beam CT, and quality-of-life questionnaires, respectively, at 0-, 3- and 6-month time intervals. In general, ATRA was well tolerated, with the most common side effects including skin changes, mild headache, hyperlipidemia, mild transaminitis, and mild muscle/bone pain. No global changes in pulmonary function tests were observed; however, preliminary HRCT analysis in the first 12 patients suggests structural improvement in 30% of the regions analyzed in response to drug. In addition, 50% of the patients reported decreased dyspnea and general improvement in quality of life while on ATRA therapy. These early findings suggest that assessment of structural changes by HRCT may be the best surrogate of response to ATRA therapy.

Repair and/or regeneration of lung structure is a novel clinical concept in the context of emphysema. Consequently, there are a number of significant clinical issues to be addressed in future studies. For example, which patient population is most likely to benefit from retinoid anabolic therapy? Patients with severe disease may not have sufficient alveolar structure to repair, while those with mild disease might experience therapeutic benefit that cannot be measured. In addition to identification of optimal retinoid doses, one needs to define the regimen and duration of dosing. The onset of action is rapid and complete within 2 weeks of treatment in preclinical models, however the limited clinical experience with ATRA suggests that more than 3 months of therapy will be required for significant improvement in lung structure or function. Another primary issue is to define the appropriate outcome measures that would reflect improved lung function (FEV_1, DL_{CO}, TLC, paO_2). The National Institute of Health has funded a multicenter trial to assess the feasibility of retinoid treatment on emphysema (FORTE) [20]. The study is scheduled to start late in the year 2000. The objectives of this multicenter trial are to address and perhaps define many of the treatment issues stated above and to identify potential surrogate markers of response to retinoid therapy. The specific goals of the trial include: (1) identify patient populations, drugs and dosing schedules, and noninvasive, clinically applicable outcome measures of emphysema to use in a large-scale trial; (2) evaluate the potential of ATRA and 13-*cis*-RA to reverse anatomic, physiologic and symptomatic manifestations of pulmonary emphysema; (3) evaluate the effects of these retinoids on cellular, molecular and histopathological markers of lung remodeling; (4) determine the safety and side effects of ATRA and 13-*cis*-RA in participants with advanced emphysema. The study design includes assessment of 13-*cis*-RA in addition to ATRA tested at two doses (fig. 4).

Conclusions

ATRA is recognized as a potent embryonic morphogen that has defined roles in the development and postnatal maintenance of most tissues including the lung. While many of the responses to ATRA in vitro and in vivo appear to be contradictory, the effects reflect the capacity of this molecule to 'normalize' rather than specifically stimulate or inhibit cellular behavior.

The current approved clinical uses of ATRA include treatment of promyelocytic leukemia, and treatment and prevention of dermal photoaging. ATRA is thought to reverse epidermal atrophy in photoaging by inducing gene expression profiles similar to those observed earlier in neodevelopment. The remarkable effects of ATRA in experimental models of COPD have stimulated significant hope that ATRA or selective retinoid analogues will bring some benefit to those who suffer with emphysema. Limited epidemiological data have shown an inverse relationship between plasma retinol in smokers and the degree of airway obstruction; therefore it may be reasonable to assume that inadequate levels of RA may contribute to the chronic injury observed in COPD (fig. 5). To achieve significant clinical benefit in moderate to severe disease will likely require chronic therapy, thus development of localized inhaled therapy may be required to achieve a good therapeutic index from a pan retinoid agonist such as ATRA. Alternatively, the oral use of receptor-selective retinoid may promote similar effects in the lung with fewer systemic effects. Either approach merits clinical proof of concept testing with the current lack of disease-modifying therapy.

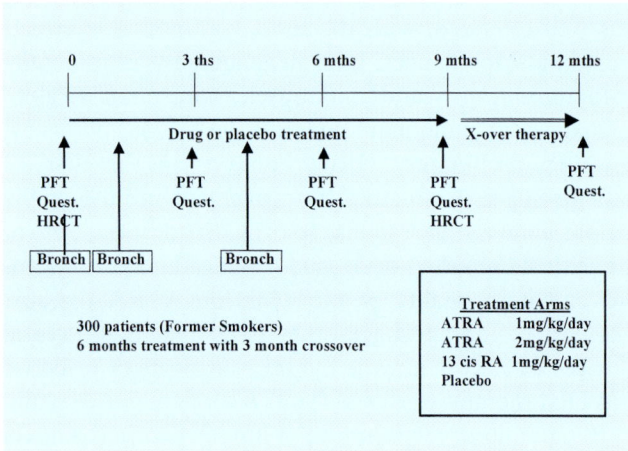

Fig. 4. NIH/FORTE clinical study design for emphysema.

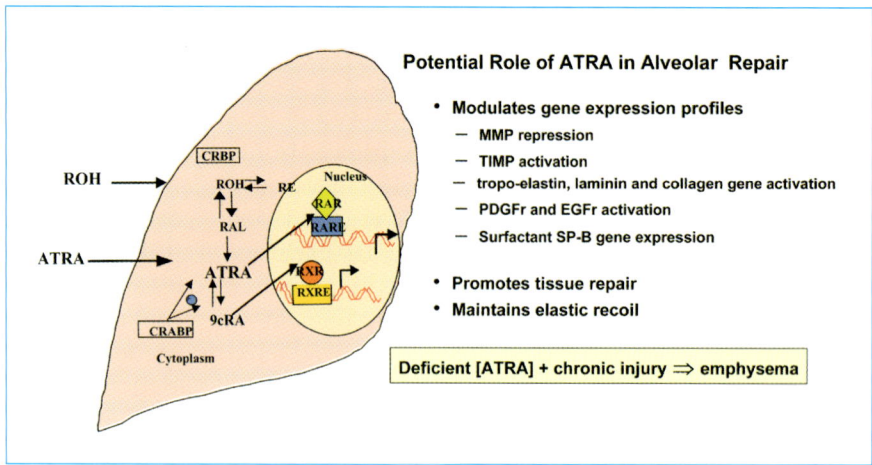

Fig. 5. Potential role of ATRA in emphysema therapy.

References

1 Chambon, P: A decade of molecular biology of retinoic acid receptors. FASEB J 1996;10:940–954.
2 Nagpal S, Athanikar J, Chandraratna RA: Separation of transactivation and AP1 antagonism functions of retinoic acid receptor alpha. J Biol Chem 1995;270:923–927.
3 Napoli JL: Retinoic acid biosynthesis and metabolism. FASEB J 1996;10:993–1001.
4 Chytil F: Retinoids in lung development. FASEB J 1996;10:986–992.
5 Farrell P: Morphological aspects of lung maturation; in Lung Development: Biological and Clinical Perspectives. New York, Academic Press, 1981, vol 1, pp 13–25.
6 Warburton D, Schwartz M, Tefft D, Flores-Delgado G, Anderson KD, Cardoso WV: The molecular basis of lung morphogenesis. Mech Dev 2000;92:55–81.
7 Dolle P, Ruberte E, Leroy P, Morriss-Kay G, Chambon P: Retinoic acid receptors and cellular retinoid binding proteins. I. A systematic study of their differential pattern of transcription during mouse organogenesis. Development 1990;110:1133–1151.
8 Grummer M, Thet LA, Zachman R: Expression of retinoic acid receptors in fetal and newborn rat lung. Pediatr Pulmonol 1994;17:234–238.
9 McGowan SE, Harvey C, Jackson SK: Retinoids, retinoic acid receptors and cytoplasmic retinoid binding proteins in perinatal rat lung fibroblasts. Am J Physiol 1995;269:L463–L472.
10 Grummer MA, Zachman RD: Postnatal rat lung retinoic acid receptor (RAR) mRNA expression and effects of dexamethasone on RARβ mRNA. Pediatr Pulmonol 1995;20:234–240.
11 Massaro G, Massaro D: Postnatal treatment with retinoic acid increases the number of pulmonary alveoli in rats. Am J Physiol 1996;270:L305–L310.
12 Cardoso WV, Williams MC, Mitsialis SA, Joyce-Brady M, Rishi AK, Brody J: Retinoic acid induces changes in the pattern of airway branching and alters epithelial cell differentiation in the developing lung in vitro. Am J Respir Cell Mol Biol 1995;12:464–476.
13 Snider GL: Emphysema: The first two centuries and beyond. Am Rev Respir Dis 1992;146:1615–1622.
14 Massaro GD, Massaro D: Retinoic acid treatment abrogates elastase-induced pulmonary emphysema in rats. Nat Med 1997;3:675–677.
15 Wolbach S, Howe P: Epithelial repair in recovery from vitamin A deficiency. J Exp Med 1933;57:511–517.
16 Tyson JE, Wright LL, Oh W, Kennedy KA, Mele L, Ehrenkranz RA, Stoll BJ, Lemons JA, Stenveson DK, Bauer CR, Korones SB, Fanaroff AA: Vitamin A supplementation for extremely-low-birth-weight infants. National Institute of Child Health and Human Development Neonatal Research Network N Engl J Med 1999;340:1962–1968.
17 Bogue CW, Jacobs HC, Dynia DW, Wilson CM, Gross I: Retinoic acid increases surfactant protein mRNA in fetal rat lung in culture. Am J Physiol 1996;271:L862–L868.
18 Katzenstein A, Myers JL, Mazur MT: Acute interstitial pneumonia: a clinicopathologic, ultrastructural and cell kinetic study. Am J Surg Pathol 1986;10:256–267.
19 Coin PG, Lindroos PM, Bird GS, Osomio-Vargas AR, Roggli VL, Bonner JC: Lipopolysaccharide up-regulates platelet-derived growth factor (PDGF) alpha-receptor expression in rat lung myofibroblasts and enhances response to all PDGF isoforms. J Immunol 1996;156:4797–4806.
20 http://www.nhlbi.nih.gov.nhlbi/rafs/archive/9901cov.htm

Dr. Paula Belloni
Roche Bioscience, 3401 Hillside Avenue
Palo Alto, CA 94304 (USA)
Tel./Fax +1 650 855 6111
E-Mail paula.belloni@roche.com

Genetic Therapy

Asthma and COPD Genetics and Genomics: An Overview

John F.J. Morrison

Global Clinical Genomics, AstraZeneca R&D, Macclesfield, UK

Summary

Therapeutic manipulation of gene expression has started to enter the clinic. The variety of approaches taken by academia and industry are described in this section. These therapies are extremely specific for the target, making detailed understanding of the molecular mechanisms underlying the disease crucial. This overview addresses the strategies that are being used to understand the heterogeneity of asthma and COPD, that are only now becoming apparent with the application of new technologies such as gene arrays.

The application of gene therapy to asthma and COPD is becoming a reality. The technologies that are now available – viral vectors, antisense and ribozymes – are discussed in detail elsewhere in this section. However, for these approaches to be totally successful, a more detailed understanding of the molecular mechanisms underlying the heterogeneity of these diseases is required. This will make the application of gene therapy more logical and produce optimally tailored therapy.

There are three general strategies to dissect these diseases, namely genetic, genomic and proteomic technologies.

Both asthma and COPD have significant heritable components. Asthma in siblings is more likely if one parent has asthma and even more likely if both parents have asthma. For example, an odds ratio of 2.6 and 5.2, respectively, was reported for these inheritance patterns [1].

In New Zealand 1,056 children were followed from birth until the age of 6 years [2]. The risk of developing asthma was increased in children with allergic parents. There was also a higher frequency of asthma in boys than in girls (14.3 versus 6.3%, p < 0.001). For atopy, a clearer pattern of increased risk in offsprings has been shown if the parents had atopy. One study showed a 0–20% risk of atopy if neither parent had atopy, a 30–50% risk with one atopic parent, and 60–100% if both were atopic [3]. Several twin studies studying asthma and atopy have been conducted. For example, a large study of Australian twins (3,808 twin pairs) by Duffy et al. [4] reported a higher concordance for asthma among the monozygotic than dizygotic twins (r = 0.65 and 0.25, respectively, at 95% confidence interval p = 0.05). The genetic factors were found common for both asthma and hay fever with a heritability of 0.60–0.70, and a high correlation between these two traits of 0.52 for males and 0.65 for females.

For COPD, family studies have shown an increased incidence of COPD in relatives of cases as compared to relatives of controls and clustering of COPD in families. A major genetic component to pulmonary function has been shown in twin studies, and there is a significant correlation between the lung function of parents and children. Finally, there is a decreased prevalence of disease with increasing genetic distance [5, 6]. The risk ratio for the disease is approximately 3.

Both diseases have heterogeneous phenotypes, with asthma confounded by the influence of atopy, and COPD by emphysema, and both are influenced by BHR and the ethnic background.

The presence of a significant genetic component prompted two parallel approaches to identify disease genes. In asthma, linkage and association analysis have shown over 700 regions throughout the genome that may contain susceptibility loci to asthma and atopic phenotypes (Cooke database). Many of these will be false positives; however, a more consistent clustering is seen on 5q, 6p, 11q, 12q, 14q and 16p [7–10]. This has led to poly-

Table 1. Asthma candidate genes

IL-4, 9	Esterase D
ADRB2	CD43
Class II MHC	CD19
TNF	ICAM-1
CC10	ACE
FcεRI-β	TCR-β
TCR-αδ	CCR-3
IL4R	IGHG
Mast cell chymase and tryptase	

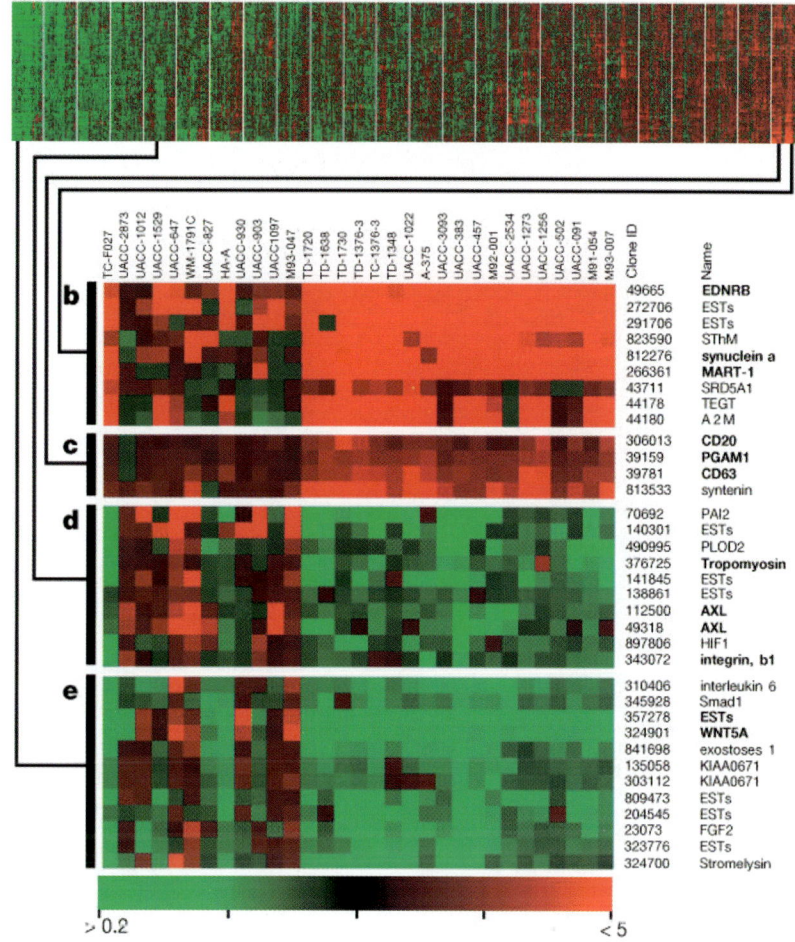

Fig. 1. An example of using microarrays to monitor differential gene expression.

morphism analysis of candidate genes within these regions (table 1). Considerable heterogeneity and ethnic variation are seen in the published associations. The pharmaceutical industry is active in developing antagonists to several of these candidates.

The availability of the human genome sequence and the output of the SNP Consortium will require a change in current gene-hunting strategy. The requirement for large collections of well-characterized families will remain; however, laborious physical mapping will increasingly become unnecessary. Instead, the dense SNP map will be used to generate haplotypes scanning the region of interest, and candidate genes will be identified by association analysis. Not every gene discovered in this way will be a good drug target. In many cases, it will be necessary to 'walk' the signalling pathway using technologies, such as high-throughput Yeast Two-Hybrid screening, until a suitable target is found.

No genome screen for COPD has been published; however, several groups in both academia and the pharmaceutical industry are active in this field. The majority of work in COPD genetics has been the analysis of candidate genes. Reported associations are shown in table 2.

In parallel with genetic analysis, genomic approaches have been applied to understand the molecular basis of these diseases. Publications arising from these technologies are now entering the literature. Syed et al. [11] used high-density grids containing 42,000 unigene clones to analyse CD4+ T-lymphocyte activation in asthma, and Pals et al. [12] and Kilty and Vickers [13] used differential-display PCR to analyse leukocyte and eosinophil activation, respectively.

The advent of gene chips, such as that from Affymetrix, is beginning to revolutionize the analysis of disease (fig. 1). Data from Golub et al. [14] have shown that it is possible to use this technology to classify human leukae-

Table 2. Genetic factors in COPD

α_1-Anti-trypsin	Haem oxygenase-1
α_1-Anti-chymotrypsin	Blood group A
α_2-Macroglobulin	CTFR
Vitamin-D-binding protein	TNF
CYP 1A1	HLA DQ
Immunoglobulin deficiency	Microsomal epoxide hydrolase
Haptoglobin	GST M1

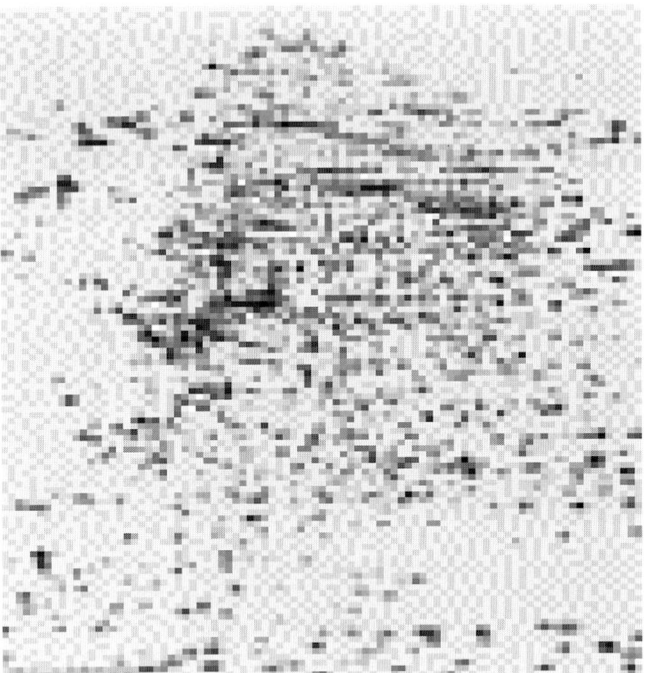

Fig. 2. An example of using 2D gel electrophoresis to analyse tissue protein expression.

mia based solely on gene expression monitoring. They also suggest a strategy for discovering and predicting cancer classes for other types of cancer, independent of previous biological knowledge. An alternative strategy using cluster analysis of the Affymetrix data was applied by Alon et al. [15] to colon cancer. In parallel, Alaiya et al. [16] have used proteomics using two-dimensional gel electrophoresis to classify ovarian cancer (fig. 2).

As technology progresses, the strengths and weaknesses of the different approaches to gene therapy will become apparent. However, with these very specific therapies, the selection of the target becomes critical, and the disease subset to which that therapy is targeted must be clearly defined.

References

1 Dold S, Wjst M, von Mutius E, et al: Genetic risk for asthma, allergic rhinitis and atopic dermatitis. Arch Dis Child 1992;67:1081–1022.
2 Horwood LJ, Fergusson DM, Shannon FT: Social and familial factors in the development of early childhood asthma. Paediatrics 1985;75:859–868.
3 Kaufman HS, Frick OL: The development of allergy in infants of allergic patients: A prospective study concerning the role of heredity. Ann Allergy 1976;37:410–415.
4 Duffy DL, Martin NG, Battistutta D, et al: Genetics of asthma and hay fever in Australian twins. Am Rev Respir Dis 1990;142:1351–1358.
5 Sandford AJ, Weir TD, Pare PD: Genetic risk factors for chronic obstructive disease. Eur Respir J 1997;10:1380–1391.
6 Barnes PJ: Molecular genetics of chronic obstructive pulmonary disease. Thorax 1999;54:245–252.
7 Cookson W: The alliance of genes and environment in asthma and allergy. Nature 1999;402:(suppl):B5–11.
8 Borish L: Genetics of allergy and asthma. Ann Allergy Asthma Immunol 1999;82:413–424.
9 Wiesch DG, Meyers DA, Bleecker ER: Genetics of asthma. J Allergy Clin Immunol 1999;104:895–901.
10 Holgate ST: Genetic and environmental interaction in allergy and asthma. J Allergy Clin Immunol 1999;104:1139–1146.
11 Syed F, Blakemore SJ, Wallace DM et al: CCR7 receptor downregulation in asthma: Differential gene expression in CD4+ T lymphocytes. QJM 1999;92:463–471.
12 Pals CEGM, Verploegen SABW, Raaijmakers JAM et al: Identification of cytokine-induced genes in human leukocytes in vivo. J Allergy Clin Immunol 1999;105:760–768.
13 Kilty IC, Vickers PJ: Studies of differential gene expression in clinically derived eosinophil populations. Clin Exp Allergy 1999;29:1671–1680.
14 Golub TR, Slonim DK, Tamayo P, et al: Molecular classification of cancer: Class discovery and class prediction by gene expression monitoring. Science 1999;286:531–537.
15 Alon U, Barkai N, Notterman DA, et al: Broad patterns of gene expression revealed by clustering analysis of tumor and normal colon tissues probed by oligonucleotide arrays. Proc Natl Acad Sci 1999;96:6745–6750.
16 Alaiya AA, Franzen B, Hagman A, et al: Classification of human ovarian tumours using multivariate data analysis of polypeptide expression patterns. Int J Cancer 2000;86:731–736.

John F.J. Morrison
Global Clinical Genomics
Astra Zeneca R&D, Mereside, Alderley Park
Macclesfield, SK 10 4TG (UK)
Tel. +44 1509 644 109, Fax +44 1509 645 586
E-Mail john.morrison@AstraZeneca.com

Respirable Antisense Oligonucleotides

Jonathan W. Nyce

EpiGenesis Pharmaceuticals, Inc., Princeton, N.J., USA

Summary

Like diseases in other organ systems, virtually every major respiratory disease can be characterized by the discordant expression of one or more genes whose protein products contribute substantially to the underlying pathophysiology. Asthma perhaps exemplifies this process, where evidence has been obtained to support a role for more than 100 different candidate mediators. Respirable antisense oligonucleotides (RASONs) provide a direct means with which to attenuate such discordant gene expression and epigenetically modify disease. The attractiveness of RASONs as a new class of respiratory therapeutics derives from the fact that they can modulate disease at a point more proximal to its cause – the mRNA that will continue the supply of the disease-causing protein – than traditional drugs which target the proteins already participating in the disease. Because they target mRNA, which offers target properties vastly different from proteins, some RASONs can have dramatically longer durations of effect than their traditional pharmaceutical counterparts. Additionally, RASONs can be engineered such that they are virtually entirely metabolized within the lung to a bioinactive form, reducing or eliminating the possibility of the systemic side effects that have been associated with most, if not all, traditional respiratory pharmaceuticals. In general, RASONs can be formulated as liquids or powders, and are thus amenable to delivery by any of the common devices available for respiratory drugs, including nebulizers, metered-dose inhalers, and dry powder inhalers. They are stable for long periods at room temperature, and their synthesis and purification are straightforward. Potentially long durations of effects, and the apparent assistance of pulmonary surfactant in RASON uptake and distribution throughout the lung, combine to improve the pharmacoeconomic characteristics sufficiently to be cost competitive with most currently available respiratory medications.

Antisense Oligonucleotides

Antisense oligonucleotides (ASONs) are short, single-stranded nucleic acids capable of hybridizing very specifically to mRNAs of target genes known or suspected of

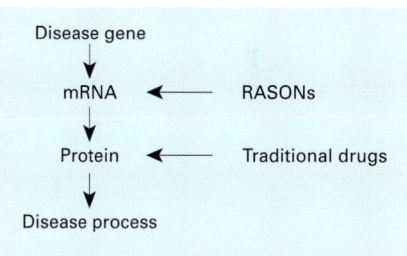

Fig. 1. RASONs interdict at a point more proximal to the disease-associated gene, messenger RNA, than do traditional drugs, which target proteins already participating in the disease process. By interdicting a disease-associated mRNA, RASONs can prevent the actual formation of the disease effector, the protein coded for by the mRNA.

being involved in human disease [1, 2] (fig. 1). ASONs hybridize to target mRNAs via Watson-Crick base pairing, setting in motion a sequence of events which leads to degradation of the mRNA by a poorly defined mechanism, or to direct steric hindrance of mRNA translation (fig. 2). The end result is an epigenetic interference with the production of new protein product from the target gene. At high concentrations, ASONs begin to lose their specificity for target mRNA and, depending on the nature of backbone modifications engineered into them to reduce nuclease degradation, may begin to interact nonspecifically with proteins and other cellular molecules. When applied appropriately, i.e., in concentrations that are effective but low enough to avoid nonspecific interactions, ASONs can be highly selective in their interaction with target mRNA. One solution to successful translation of the therapeutic potential of antisense oligonucleotides

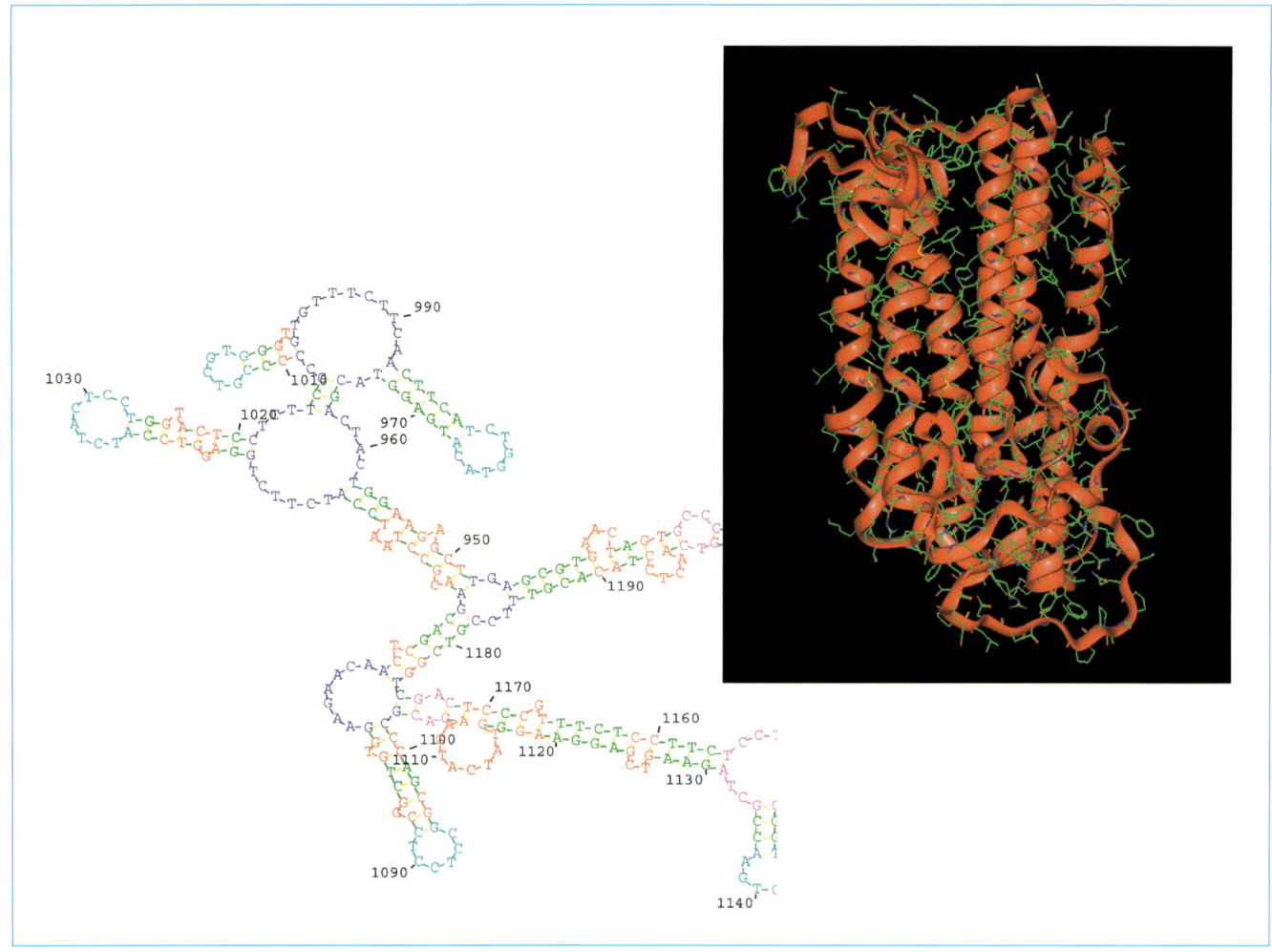

Fig. 2. mRNA (left) vs. protein as a target for therapeutic intervention (mRNA and protein depicted represent the adenosine A_1 receptor).

is local delivery, as illustrated by the nature of the first ASON approved for commercial use, fomivirsen for cytomegalovirus retinitis. Fomivirsen is injected directly into the eye, and offers conclusive validation of the concept that local delivery of ASONs brings to practical fruition the theoretical power of this new class of therapeutics [3, 4].

Ability to Predict Sequence-Related Toxicology in Advance

Antisense technology presents an unusual opportunity to determine whether or not candidate clinical oligonucleotides might interact in a sequence-dependent manner with nontarget mRNAs due to overlapping regions of homology. Statistical considerations indicate that ASONs 14 bases long or longer should be unique in the human genome, unless the target sequence exists within a region conserved within several different genes, e.g., conserved regions within the transmembrane segments of G protein-coupled receptors. Therefore, constructing antisense oligonucleotides longer than 14 bases will generally preclude interaction with non target mRNAs. To be certain that such is the case, northern blots utilizing the candidate antisense as a probe against mRNA isolated from target tissues can confirm hybridization with a single band.

It has been suggested that metabolism of antisense oligonucleotides by exonucleases might generate 'short mers' that could interact with nontarget mRNAs. Several lines of reasoning argue powerfully against this possibility. For example, for most currently available modified antisense oligonucleotides (e.g., phosphorothioates), hybridization capacity diminishes dramatically with the introduction of mismatches between the short mer and nontarget mRNAs. We have shown that a single mismatch is capable of eliminating effective hybridization of a 21-mer phosphorothioate respirable ASON (RASON) to its target [5, 6]. Phosphorothioate modification, while it prevents facile degradation by exonucleases, also destabilizes hybridization potential [7]. Thus, if a 14-mer phosphorothioate product of exonuclease activity had 100% homology to a nontarget mRNA, it would still be unlikely to have enough hybridization potential (because of its short size) to initiate the degradation of that nontarget mRNA. Combined with the fact that only a fraction (about 10%) of potential antisense sequences actually are active, probably due to constraints in targeting certain regions of mRNA molecules, the poor hybridization potential of short phosphorothioate RASONs virtually ensures that properly designed RASONs will not interact in any biologically meaningful way with nontarget mRNA. Finally, the processive nature of most known exonucleases indicates that biologically relevant short mers will not generally be created during exonucleolytic degradation of RASONs, since the exonucleases involved do not release the oligonucleotide until it has been degraded to final products in the three- to five-nucleotide length size.

RASONs for Lung Diseases

The lung represents a unique target for antisense intervention [5, 6]. The lung is lined with a material called surfactant which is primarily composed of zwitterionic lipids that at lung pH are cationic. It is a well-known fact that cationic lipids dramatically improve the uptake of antisense oligonucleotides into cells. Lung surfactant may therefore enhance the miscibility of RASONs, in essence repackaging them to a form more effectively distributed to the target respiratory tissues and cells. In addition, pulmonary surfactant has a high turnover rate and is rapidly interchanged between the surface of the air interface and the deeper tissues of the epithelium (type II pneumocytes). This rapid flux of surfactant may serve to facilitate the transport of RASONs in a manner completely unique as compared to other target organs. EpiGenesis has shown that RASONs are rather uniformly delivered throughout the lung following administration as a nebulized aerosol, reaching deep tissues (e.g., smooth muscle cells).

EPI-2010

EpiGenesis Pharmaceuticals pioneered the field of RASONs, and has several promising RASONs in development. EPI-2010 targets the adenosine A_1 receptor, a receptor involved in both the bronchoconstrictor and inflammatory phases of asthma [8]. Asthma in particular may be associated with a disease-associated upregulation of A_1 receptors. Asthmatic individuals have excess amounts of adenosine in their lungs [9], such that discordantly upregulated A_1 receptor would be constitutively stimulated. Inhaled adenosine causes bronchoconstriction in human asthmatics, and appears to be a more specific differentiator of asthma than the standard methacholine challenge. A_1 receptors are known to be overexpressed in allergic rabbits and rats [10–12]. Bronchial smooth muscle of human asthmatics contracts in an A_1-dependent manner as judged by response to 2-thio-dipropyl-8-cyclopenthylxanthine [13], and allergic non-human primates (e.g., cynomolgus monkeys), respond to inhaled adenosine also in an A_1-dependent manner [8]. In addition, it has been reported recently that the adenosine A_1 receptor is rapidly upregulated in bronchial smooth muscle tissue exposed to human asthmatic serum [14], and that it is also rapidly upregulated in response to oxidative stress by virtue of activation of NF-κB sites in its promoter [15].

Surfactant secretion is known to be regulated by an interplay of adenosine A_1 and A_2 receptors, with A_1 receptors inhibiting surfactant secretion and A_2 receptors enhancing it [16, 17]. Recent evidence indicates that surfactant secretion is diminished in asthma and may contribute significantly to bronchial hyper- responsiveness [18, 19]. The upregulation of the A_1 receptor in asthma may therefore underlie this loss of surfactant, providing a further impetus to develop agents capable of attenuating A_1 receptor function. The role of the neutrophil in moderate to severe asthma, and the established role for the adenosine A_1 receptor in neutrophil adherence to endothelium (and hence neutrophil chemotaxis) [20, 21], offers additional rationale for developing A_1-receptor-specific therapeutics.

Low-dose inhaled EPI-2010 has an unusually long duration of action (6.8 days), and does not appear to escape the lung in bioactive amounts, potentially eliminating the possibility of inducing systemic side effects. These characteristics may relate to certain characteristics of the target mRNA and its protein (e.g., disease-related amounts and half-lives of each).

Conclusions

RASONs represent an exciting new class of respiratory drugs with potential in a number of respiratory diseases mediated by discordant overexpression of targetable mRNAs. While not every discordantly expressed mRNA may represent an optimum target for the RASON approach (for example, due to large amounts or extended half lives of target mRNA or protein), a wide array of targets which have proved challenging for traditional therapeutics may find solution by this technology. Pulmonary surfactant appears to enhance the uptake and delivery of RASONs, making the lung perhaps one of the best possible target organs for oligonucleotide-based therapeutic intervention. RASONs offer the potential to approach respiratory diseases from an entirely fresh point of view, the finely selective targeting of mRNAs to prevent the actual expression of disease-related genes in a way not possible with traditional therapeutics. Such epigene therapy of respiratory diseases opens an exciting new chapter as respiratory medicine advances into the 21st century.

References

1 Crooke ST: An overview of progress in antisense therapeutics. Antisense Nucleic Acid Drug Dev 1998;8:115–122.
2 Agrawal S, Zhao Q: Antisense therapeutics. Curr Opin Chem Biol 1998;2:519–528.
3 Marwick C: First 'antisense' drug will treat CMV retinitis. JAMA 1998;280:871.
4 Leeds JM, Henry SP, Bistner S, Scherrill S, Williams K, Levin AA: Pharmacokinetics of an antisense oligonucleotide injected intravitreally in monkeys. Drug Metab Dispos 1998;26:670–675.
5 Nyce JW, Metzger WJ: DNA antisense therapy for asthma in an animal model. Nature 1997;385:721–725.
6 Nyce JW: Antisense oligonucleotides as emerging drugs. Emerging Drugs: The Prospect for Improved Medicines. London, Asley Publications, 1998, chapt 25, pp 365–375.
7 Stein CA, Tonkinson JL, Yakubov L: Phosphorothioate oligodeoxynucleotides: Antisense inhibitors of gene expression? Pharmacol Ther 1991;52:365–384.
8 Nyce, JW: Insight into adenosine receptor function using antisense and gene-knockout approaches. Trends Pharmacol Sci 1999;20:79–83.
9 Driver AG, Kukoly CA, Ali S, Mustafa SJ: Adenosine in bronchoalveolar lavage fluid in asthma. Am Rev Respir Dis 1993;148:91–97.
10 Ali S, Mustafa SJ, Metzger WJ: Adenosine-induced bronchoconstriction and contraction of airway smooth muscle from allergic rabbits with late-phase airway obstruction: Evidence for an inducible adenosine A_1 receptor. J Pharmacol Exp Ther 1994;268:1328–1334.
11 El-Hashim A, D'Agostino B, Matera MG, Page C: Characterization of adenosine receptors involved in adenosine-induced bronchoconstriction in allergic rabbits. Br J Pharmacol 1996;119:1262–1268.
12 Pauwels RA, Joos GF: Characterization of the adenosine receptors in the airways. Arch Int Pharmacodyn Ther 1995;329:151–160.
13 Bjorck T, Gustafsson LE, Dahlen SE: Isolated bronchi from asthmatics are hyperresponsive to adenosine, which apparently acts by liberation of leukotrienes and histamine Am Rev Resp Dis 1992;145:1087–1090.
14 Hakonarson H, Shanbaky I, Guerra FM, Grunstein MM: Modulation of adenosine A_1, bradykinin B_1, and histamine H_1 receptor expression and function in atopic asthmatic sensitized airway smooth muscle. Proc Am Thoracic Soc Int Congr, Chicago, 1998.
15 Nie G: Oxidative stress increases A_1 adenosine receptor expression by activating nuclear factor kappa B. Mol Pharmacol 1998;53:663–669.
16 Griese M, Gobran LJ, Douglas JS, Rooney SA: Adenosine A_2-receptor-mediated phosphatidylcholine secretion in type II pneumocytes. Am J Physiol 1991;260:L52–L60.
17 Gobran LI, Rooney SA: Adenosine A_1-receptor-mediated inhibition of surfactant secretion in rat type II pneumocytes. Am J Physiol 1990;258:L45–L51.
18 Liu M, Wang L, Holm BA, Enhorning G: Dysfunction of guinea-pig pulmonary surfactant and type II pneumocytes after repetitive challenge with aerosolized ovalbumin. Clin Exp Allergy 1997;27:802–807.
19 Hamm H, Fabel H, Bartsch W: The surfactant system of the adult lung: Physiology and clinical perspectives. Clin Invest 1992;70:637–657.
20 Zahler S, Becker BF, Raschke P, Gerlach E: Stimulation of endothelial adenosine A1 receptors enhances adhesion of neutrophils in the intact guinea pig coronary system. Cardiovasc Res 1994;28:1366–1372.
21 Schwartz LM, Raschke P, Becker BF, Gerlach E: Adenosine contributes to neutrophil-mediated loss of myocardial function in post-ischemic guinea-pig hearts. J Mol Cell Cardiol 1993;25:927–938.

Jonathan W. Nyce, PhD
EpiGenesis Pharmaceuticals, Inc.
Princeton, NJ 08543-7007 (USA)
Tel. +1 609 409 3031, Fax +1 609 409 6126
E-Mail jnyce@epigene.com

Antisense Therapy

C. Frank Bennett

Isis Pharmaceuticals, Inc., Carlsbad, Calif., USA

Summary

Antisense oligonucleotides are short synthetic oligonucleotides designed to bind to RNA by Watson-Crick base pairing rules. Upon binding to the targeted RNA, the oligonucleotides either induce cleavage of the RNA by RNase H, sterically block proteins from interacting with the RNA or disrupt secondary and tertiary structure of the RNA resulting in alterations in its function. The net result from these interactions, provided the RNA encodes a protein product, is inhibition of protein expression. Thus in contrast to conventional drugs, antisense oligonucleotides target the RNA that encodes a protein product. There has been tremendous progress in antisense technology over the last 10 years, with one marketed product, Vitravene™, and approximately 20 antisense drugs in active clinical development. Numerous articles have been published exploring the use of antisense oligonucleotides in inflammation models. This review will focus on the application of the technology for the treatment of pulmonary diseases.

Antisense Chemistry

Natural DNA or RNA are rapidly metabolized by a variety of nucleases present in either serum or cells limiting the utility of unmodified oligonucleotides for antisense therapeutics. Substitution of one of the nonbridging oxygen atoms in the phosphate backbone with sulfur (phosphorothioate modification) dramatically enhances the stability of the oligonucleotide towards nuclease degradation (fig. 1). Phosphorothioate oligodeoxynucleotides, like natural oligodeoxynucleotides support RNase-H-mediated hydrolysis of the targeted RNA, which is the most extensively exploited antisense mechanism of action. Phosphorothioate-modified oligodeoxynucleotides were the first antisense drugs to enter clinical development and the one marketed product, Vitravene™, is a phosphorothioate oligodeoxynucleotide [1, 2]. As a result, extensive information is available regarding their pharmacokinetic and toxicological properties [2–4].

A variety of sugar modified oligonucleotides have been examined in cell culture and animal models. In particular modifications at the 2′-position of the sugar have in particular yielded promising results with the 2′-O-methyl and 2′-O-methoxyethyl modifications being the most advanced (fig. 1). Both types of modifications enhance binding affinity of the oligonucleotide for the target RNA translating to increased potency [5, 6]. Furthermore, the 2′-O-methoxyethyl modification and to a lesser extent the 2′-O-methyl modification increase the resistance of the oligonucleotide to nuclease degradation. Combining the phosphorothioate modification with 2′-O-methyl or 2′-O-methoxyethyl modification can further enhance the tissue half-lives of the oligonucleotides, resulting in more convenient dose schedules for patients. Additionally, 2′-O-methyl- and 2′-O-methoxyethyl-modified oligonucleotides exhibit decreased toxicities compared to phosphorothioate oligodeoxynucleotides [3]. Neither 2′-O-methyl or 2′-O-methoxyethyl oligonucleotides will support RNase H activity, therefore investigators either exploit non-RNase-H-dependent mechanisms [7, 8] or use chimeric oligonucleotides containing 2′-modified sugars and 2′-deoxy sugars to support RNase H activity [6]. A 2′-O-methyl modified chimeric oligonucleotide targeting protein kinase A is currently in clinical trials for the treatment of malignancies. It is anticipated that most of the antisense oligonucleotides entering clinical development in the next few years will be either 2′-O-methyl or 2′-O-methoxyethyl modified.

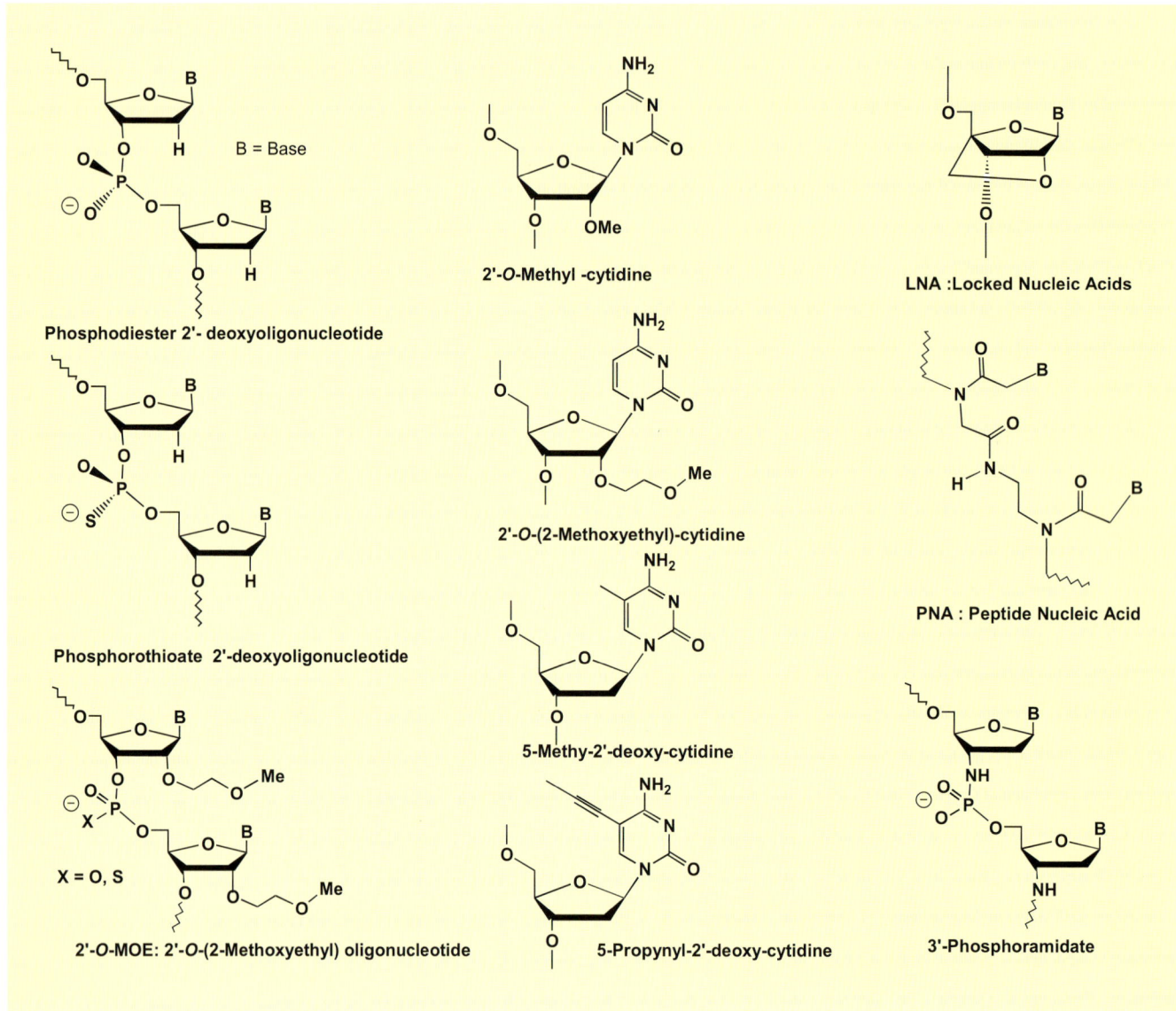

Fig. 1. Examples of oligonucleotide modifications.

Additional modifications which are under evaluation in the laboratory include nucleotides with a 2′-O, 4′-C-methylene bridge (LNA), heterocycle modifications such as the natural 5-methylcytosine modification or 5-propynyl pyrimidine modifications, phosphate modifications such as morpholino or 3′-amidate, phosphate replacements such as methylenemethylimino or thioformacetal, sugar-phosphate replacements such as PNA and oligonucleotide conjugates [9]. All these modifications increase binding affinity to RNA relative to phosphorothioate oligodeoxynucleotides. Relatively little information is available on the pharmacokinetic and toxicological activity of these modifications.

Pharmacokinetics of Oligonucleotides

Phosphorothioate oligodeoxynucleotides are rapidly absorbed from most parenteral sites of administration and exhibit biphasic plasma kinetics with a rapid distribution half-life between 20 min and 1 h. They are highly protein bound and at pharmacologically relevant doses

(1–20 mg/kg) very little intact drug appears in urine. Disappearance out of plasma can largely be accounted for by distribution to tissues, with kidney, liver, spleen bone marrow and lymphoid structures accumulating the highest concentrations of drug. Phosphorothioate oligodeoxynucleotides are eliminated from tissue predominantly through nuclease degradation, exhibiting tissue half-lives between 20 and 48 h. Recent studies have demonstrated that phosphorothioate oligodeoxynucleotides distribute heterogeneously within tissues [10, 11]. Second-generation phosphorothioate modified 2′-O-methyl and 2′-O-methoxyethyl oligonucleotides display similar plasma kinetics and tissue distribution, however they do exhibit prolonged tissue half-lives.

Phosphorothioate oligodeoxynucleotides have limited oral bioavailability ranging from less than 1 to 3% [4, 12]. Second-generation 2′-O-methyl- or 2′-O-methoxyethyl-modified oligonucleotides exhibit significant increases in oral bioavailability, with values up to 40% bioavailability being reported [13, 14]. These values may be further improved with formulations to further enhance absorption. Thus, oral delivery of antisense oligonucleotides may be feasible in the not too distant future.

Antisense oligonucleotides can also be administered topically to skin, colon tissue and lung for local therapy. Preliminary studies by Nicklin et al. [4, 15] examined the disposition of intratracheally administered phosphorothioate oligodeoxynucleotides. They reported dose-dependent systemic bioavailability after intratracheal administration to rats, ranging from 3% bioavailability at a dose of 0.06 mg/kg to 40% at a dose of 6.0 mg/kg. More recently, Templin et al. [submitted] have examined the pharmacokinetics and toxicity of aerosolized phosphorothioate oligodeoxynucleotides. Phosphorothioate oligodeoxynucleotides did not affect the size or behavior of the particles generated from the nebulizer. Immunohistochemical analysis of oligonucleotide disposition in pulmonary tissue demonstrated that the oligonucleotide was found to be associated with bronchiolar epithelial cells, alveolar epithelial cells, endothelial cells and alveolar macrophages. Pharmacologically relevant pulmonary concentrations (3–10 µM) were achieved and maintained for at least 24 h following administration of a 1.2 mg/kg dose. There were no systemic toxicities associated with aerosol administration of phosphorothioate oligodeoxynucleotides. Local effects were seen at the highest dose examined (12 mg/kg) with general compression of alveoli and an increase in the number of pulmonary macrophages. Mice exposed to a dose of 1 mg/kg or below displayed normal lung histology. Thus aerosol delivery of antisense oligonucleotides appears to be a reasonable approach for the treatment of asthma and other pulmonary disorders.

Toxicology of Antisense Oligonucleotides

Clinically, phosphorothioate oligodeoxynucleotides appear to be well tolerated, with transient increases in activated partial thromboplastin time (aPTT) representing the most common side effect [16, 17]. The increase in aPTT appears to be directly related to peak plasma concentration and can be ameliorated by infusing the drug slowly or by decreasing the rate of absorption. Thrombocytopenia has also been reported for some, but not all phosphorothioate oligodeoxynucleotides in clinical trials. In preclinical toxicity studies, most phosphorothioate oligodeoxynucleotides exhibit some degree of immune stimulation in rodents [3]. They do not appear to be antigenic, but are polyclonal activators of B lymphocytes and monocytes. The effects are dose dependent and sequence dependent, with oligodeoxynucleotides containing the CpG motif described by Krieg et al. [18] being especially effective. At high peak plasma concentrations, phosphorothioate oligodeoxynucleotides have also been documented to trigger complement activation in non-human primates [3]. Despite these limited toxicities, much interest has been focused on further improving the profile of phosphorothioate oligodeoxynucleotides. As an example the 2′-O-methyl and 2′-O-methoxyethyl modification reduces the immune stimulatory potential of oligonucleotides.

Pharmacological Effects of Antisense Oligonucleotides in Models of Asthma

Nyce and Metzger [19] demonstrated in a seminal study that antisense phosphorothioate oligodeoxynucleotides designed to inhibit expression of the adenosine A1 receptor (EPI-2010) inhibited adenosine receptor expression in rabbit bronchial smooth muscle when administered by aerosolization. The effects of the oligonucleotide were sequence specific and did not affect expression of the A_2 receptor or bradykinin B_2 receptor. Additionally, the oligonucleotide was shown to inhibit the immediate airway response to dust mite antigen and bronchial hyperresponsiveness to histamine. These results warrant continued exploration of aerosolized adenosine A_1 receptor antisense oligonucleotide for the treatment of asthma.

IL-4 and IL-5 are cytokines predominantly derived from T lymphocytes, which are thought to play an important role in asthma and other allergic disorders. Molet et al. [20] demonstrated that CD4+ cells isolated from ovalbumin-primed rats can transfer late airway response to naïve animals. To address the role of IL-4 and IL-5 in mediating the airway response, they incubated the isolated CD4+ cells ex vivo with IL-4 or IL-5 phosphorothioate oligodeoxynucleotides for 6 h before transfer to naïve animals. The oligonucleotides selectively reduced IL-4 or IL-5 expression in the isolated cells by 30% as assessed by immunocytochemical staining of the cells. The late-phase reaction to ovalbumin was delayed in cells treated with the IL-5 antisense oligonucleotide and significantly inhibited at all time points examined in cells treated with the IL-4 antisense oligonucleotide. Pretreatment of the adoptively transferred T cells with either antisense oligonucleotide failed to significantly reduce the total number of cells in bronchiolar lavage fluid, but the IL-4 antisense oligonucleotide did decrease the number of eosinophils in BAL. More recently, Karras et al. [21] have examined the effects of systemically administered 2′-O-methoxyethyl IL-5 antisense oligonucleotide in an ovalbumin-induced airway hyperreactivity model in mice. They were able to demonstrate that systemic treatment reduced IL-5 protein expression, decreased eosinophil influx into lung and attenuated late-phase airway hyperreactivity in response to ovalbumin challenge. The discrepancies between the two studies may be explained by the different models used for investigation, different oligonucleotide chemistries or duration of exposure to the oligonucleotide. In the later study, chronic treatment with the oligonucleotide was required to produce the desired effect, which suggests that there may be long-lived pools of IL-5 in the lymphocytes or that delivery of oligonucleotide to the lymphocyte was not efficient. Nevertheless, chronic prophylactic treatment of asthmatic patients to achieve effective concentrations in lymphocytes is a viable option, especially with second-generation oligonucleotides.

Recently Hill et al. [22] demonstrated that second-generation 2′-methoxyethyl-modified oligonucleotides targeting STAT6 downregulated germline Cε transcription required for IgE isotype switching in B lymphocytes [22]. Thus STAT6 antisense oligonucleotides may attenuate IL-4 and IL-13 signaling in B lymphocytes. There are many additional genes that could be targeted with antisense oligonucleotides that may offer therapeutic benefit for the treatment of asthma.

Non-Antisense Effects of Oligonucleotides

In addition to desired antisense effects of oligonucleotides, oligonucleotides, like any other drug, are capable of interacting with nontargeted molecules, which may produce pharmacological effects. Several nonantisense effects for phosphorothioate oligodeoxynucleotides have been characterized and often appear to be due to the presence of specific sequence motifs [23]. The CpG motif described above being a pertinent example, as CpG oligonucleotides can alter the immune response to antigens. As described above, phosphorothioate oligodeoxynucleotides with the appropriate CpG motif are potent activators of several immune cell types [18]. CpG oligonucleotides induce secretion of IL-12, IFN-γ and IL-6 from mononuclear cells, which promote T lymphocytes to differentiate into a Th1 phenotype. Several studies have been published demonstrating that CpG oligonucleotides can attenuate airway eosinophilia or airway hyperreactivity in the ovalbumin mouse model [24, 25]. Thus phosphorothioate oligodeoxynucleotides containing the appropriate CpG motif may prove useful for the treatment of asthma.

Conclusion

Antisense oligonucleotides represent a new therapeutic approach for the treatment of asthma. Recent advances in both antisense chemistries and lead identification make antisense technologies a very efficient technology for exploring the role of novel gene products in asthma. First-generation phosphorothioate oligonucleotides can be administered either by parenteral injection or by aerosol. Preliminary studies demonstrate the technical feasibility and safety of aerosolized oligonucleotides. Additional studies are needed to examine the long-term consequences of aerosolized oligonucleotides. Second-generation oligonucleotides offer several advantages over phosphorothioate oligodeoxynucleotides including increased potency, decreased toxicity, and more convenient administration schedules and the option for oral administration. Although the application of this technology for the treatment of asthma has yet to be explored, the preclinical studies are encouraging and with additional time will hopefully lead to products.

References

1 Bennett CF, Condon TP: Use of antisense oligonucleotides to modify inflammatory processes; in Crooke ST (ed): Antisense Research and Application. Berlin, Springer, 1998, pp 371–394.
2 Bennett CF: Antisense oligonucleotide therapeutics. Exp Opin Invest Drugs 1999;8:237–253.
3 Levin AA, Monteith DK, Leeds JM, Nicklin PL, Geary RS, Butler M, Templin MV, Henry SP: Toxicity of oligodeoxynucleotide therapeutic agents; in Crooke ST (ed): Antisense Research and Applications. Heidelberg, Springer, 1998, pp 169–216.
4 Nicklin PL, Craig SJ, Phillips JA: Pharmacokinetic properties of phosphorothioates in animals – absorption, distribution, metabolism and elimination; in Crooke ST (ed): Antisense Research and Application. Berlin, Springer, 1998, pp 141–168.
5 Altmann KH, Dean NM, Fabbro D, Freier SM, Geiger T, Haner R, Husken D, Martin P, Monia BP, Muller M, Natt F, Nicklin P, Phillips J, Pieles U, Sasmor H, Moser HE: Second generation of antisense oligonucleotides: From nuclease resistance to biological efficacy in animals. Chimia 1996;50:168–176.
6 Monia BP, Lesnik EA, Gonzalez C, Lima WF, McGee D, Guinosso CJ, Kawasaki AM, Cook PD, Freier SM: Evaluation of 2′-modified oligonucleotides containing 2′-deoxy gaps as antisense inhibitors of gene expression. J Biol Chem 1993;268:14514–14522.
7 Baker BF, Lot SS, Condon TP, Cheng-Flournoy S, Lesnik EA, Sasmor HM, Bennett CF: 2′-O-(2-Methoxy)ethyl-modified anti-intercellular adhesion molecule 1 (ICAM-1) oligonucleotides selectively increase the ICAM-1 mRNA level and inhibit formation of the ICAM-1 translation initiation complex in human umbilical vein endothelial cells. J Biol Chem 1997;272:1994–2000.
8 Sierakowska H, Sambade MJ, Agrawal S, Kole R: Repair of thalassemic human β-globin mRNA in mammalian cells by antisense oligonucleotides. Proc Natl Acad Sci USA 1996;93:12840–12844.
9 Cook D: Antisense medicinal chemistry; in Crooke ST (ed): Antisense Research and Application. Berlin, Springer, 1998, pp 51–102.
10 Graham MJ, Crooke ST, Monteith DK, Cooper SR, Lemonidis KM, Stecker KK, Martin MJ, Crooke RM: In vivo distribution and metabolism of a phosphorothioate oligonucleotide within rat liver after intravenous administration. J Pharmacol Exp Ther 1998;286:447–458.
11 Butler M, Stecker K, Bennett CF: Cellular distribution of phosphorothioate oligodeoxynucleotides in normal rodent tissues. Lab Invest 1997;77:379–388.
12 Agrawal S, Zhang R: Pharmacokinetics and bioavailability of antisense oligonucleotides following oral and colorectal administration in experimental animals; in Crooke ST (ed): Antisense Research and Application. Berlin, Springer, 1998, pp 525–543.
13 Khatsenko O, Morgan R, Truong L, York-Defalco C, Sasmor H, Conklin B, Geary RS: Absorption of antisense oligonucleotides in rat intestine: Effect of chemistry and length. Antisense Nucleic Acid Drug Dev 2000;10:35–44.
14 Agrawal S, Zhang X, Lu Z, Zhao H, Tamburin JM, Yan J, Cai H, Diasio RB, Habus I, Jiang Z, Iyer RP, Yu D, Zhang R: Absorption, tissue distribution and in vivo stability in rats of a hybrid antisense oligonucleotide following oral administration. Biochem Pharmacol 1995;50:571–576.
15 Nicklin PL, Bayley D, Giddings J, Craig SJ, Cummins LL, Hastewell JG, Phillips JA: Pulmonary bioavailability of a phosphorothioate oligonucleotide (CGP 64128A): Comparison with other delivery routes. Pharm Res 1998;15:583–591.
16 Schechter PJ, Martin RR: Safety and tolerance of phosphorothioates in humans; in Crooke ST (ed): Antisense Research and Application. Berlin, Springer, 1998, pp 233–241.
17 Yacyshyn BR, Bowen-Yacyshyn MB, Jewell L, Tami JA, Bennett CF, Kisner DL, Shanahan WR: A placebo-controlled trial of ICAM-1 antisense oligonucleotide in the treatment of Crohn's disease. Gastroenterology 1998;114:1133–1142.
18 Krieg AM: Mechanisms and applications of immune stimulatory CpG oligodeoxynucleotides. Biochim Biophys Acta 1999;1489:107–116.
19 Nyce JW, Metzger WJ: DNA antisense therapy for asthma in an animal model. Nature 1997;385:721–725.
20 Molet S, Ramos-Barbon D, Martin JG, Hamid Q: Adoptively transferred late allergic response is inhibited by IL-4, but not IL-5, antisense oligonucleotide. J Allergy Clin Immunol 1999;104:205–214.
21 Karras JG, McGraw K, McKay R, Cooper S, Lerner D, Lu T, Walker C, Dean NM, Monia B: Inhibition of antigen-induced eosinophilia and late-phase airway hyperresponsiveness by interleukin-5 antisense oligonucleotide in mouse models of asthma. J Immunol, in press.
22 Hill S, Herlaar E, Le Cardinal AL, van Heeke G, Nicklin P: Homologous human and murine antisense oligonucleotides targeting Stat6. Functional effects on germline Cepsilon transcript. Am J Respir Cell Mol Biol 1999;21:728–737.
23 Stein CA: Phosphorothioate antisense oligodeoxynucleotides: Questions of specificity. Trends Biotechnol 1996;14:147–149.
24 Sur S, Wild JS, Choudhury BK, Sur N, Alam R, Klinman DM: Long-term prevention of allergic lung inflammation in a mouse model of asthma by CpG oligodeoxynucleotides. J Immunol 1999;162:6284–6293.
25 Broide D, Schwarze J, Tighe H, Gifford T, Nguyen MD, Malek S, Van Uden J, Martin-Orozco E, Gelfand EW, Raz E: Immunostimulatory DNA sequences inhibit IL-5, eosinophilic inflammation, and airway hyperresponsiveness in mice. J Immunol 1998;161:7054–7062.

C. Frank Bennett, MD
Isis Pharmaceuticals
Carlsbad Research Center
2292 Faraday Avenue
Carlsbad, CA 92008 (USA)
Tel. +1 760 931 2336
E-Mail fbennett@isisph.com

Ribozyme Therapy

Jennifer A. Sandberg   Patrice A. Lee   Nassim Usman

Ribozyme Pharmaceuticals, Inc., Boulder, Colo., USA

Summary

Ribozymes are catalytic RNA molecules that can cleave targeted RNA in a sequence-specific manner. The ability to target these compounds to a specific molecular target opens up exciting opportunities for rational drug design for the treatment of asthma and COPD. Strategic cleavage of RNA encoding any of the many cytokines and/or their receptors now believed to play a role in the etiology of these diseases could result in effective therapeutics with minimal toxicity. Ribozymes have been demonstrated to be efficacious in vivo, result in minimal toxicity, and are currently in clinical trials. Systemic or pulmonary delivery could be used to deliver ribozymes to their site of action.

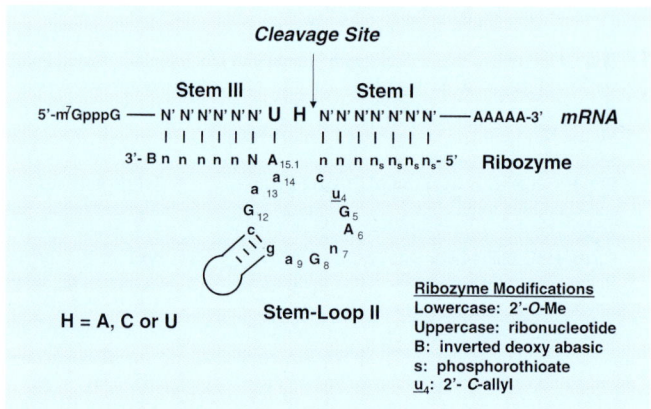

Fig. 1. Structure of a generic, chemically stabilized ribozyme. Nucleotide and backbone chemical modifications to the ribozyme are listed at the right.

Ribozymes

The discovery of ribozymes by Thomas Cech and Sydney Altman [1–3] fundamentally changed the view of the function of RNA in chemistry and biology. Their work unequivocally showed that RNA could act as an enzyme, catalyzing the cleavage and ligation of RNA molecules. Prior to their discovery, RNA had been viewed as a passive molecule responsible for the transmission of information from DNA to proteins (mRNA and tRNA) or for providing structure to RNA-protein complexes. Subsequent studies have shown that RNA can act as an enzyme, capable of catalyzing a diverse number of chemical reactions. Furthermore, these novel activities of RNA now permit the development of enzymatic RNA molecules as therapeutic entities for the treatment of human disease.

There are several naturally occurring ribozyme motifs that have been engineered to produce molecules with improved specificity, stability to nucleases and catalytic turnover [4–6]. Modified hammerhead ribozymes have advanced the furthest in therapeutic applications (fig. 1 and see below). Binding and cleavage of target RNA sequences destroy their ability to direct synthesis of their encoded proteins. After the ribozyme has bound and cleaved its RNA target, it is released from that RNA to search for another target and can repeatedly bind and cleave new targets. The principal advantages offered by these ribozymes are: their specificity, based on the nature of target; the manner in which they bind the target, and the nature of chemical modifications used to stabilize them. The target site is ~15 nucleotides in length, which is statistically expected to be unique in the coding region of the human genome. Since these ribozymes bind their cognate mRNA or viral RNA using two independent binding arms of 6–7 nucleotides in length, interrupted by the nucleotide being cleaved, their binding to the target is weaker than a contiguous sequence of 13–15 nucleotides.

This weaker binding leads to better specificity since mismatches are not tolerated; either the ribozyme falls off or the catalytic core cannot adopt the correct confirmation to cleave the target RNA. Finally, the modifications developed for these stabilized ribozymes consist primarily of 2'-O-methyl nucleotides that are naturally occurring. There are a few minor other modifications (fig. 1) including 3–4 phosphorothioate modifications at the 5'-end. This should be contrasted with large number, 15–20, phosphorothioate DNA linkages in a typical antisense molecule which have been attributed to significant nonspecific interactions with proteins and other biomolecules [7]. Furthermore, since the target is well defined and unique, 15 nucleotides of RNA sequence, ribozymes may have an advantage over small molecules in targeting proteins that are either members of multimember protein families or those that work by large surface protein-protein interactions. All of these attributes of stabilized ribozymes should lead to very specific knockdown of the target RNA and low toxicity. This has been borne out in efficacy and toxicology studies (see below).

Therapeutic Potential of Ribozymes Targeting Mediators of Asthma and COPD

Conserved and accessible sequences within IL-5, TNF-α, ICAM-1 and NF-κB have been identified. Hammerhead and hairpin ribozymes have been designed to target these regions of mRNA [8, unpubl. obs.]. A number of cytokines are involved in the activation of inflammation in asthmatic patients, including platelet activating factor, leukotrienes, IL-1, IL-3, IL-4, IL-5, GM-CSF, TNF-α, γ-interferon, VCAM, ICAM-1, ELAM-1 and NFκB. In addition to these molecules, any cellular receptors that mediate the activities of the cytokines are also good targets for intervention. These targets include, but are not limited to, the IL-1R and TNF-αR on keratinocytes, epithelial and endothelial cells in airways. Similar ribozyme screening efforts are being directed towards identifying appropriate target sequences for IL-4 and TNF-αR. Mediators of chronic pulmonary fibrosis that would be ideal targets for intervention in COPD include, but are not limited to, TNF-α and TGF-β.

Ribozyme Pharmacokinetics

Systemic administration of ribozymes has resulted in uptake into a variety of tissues. In addition to other tissues, intravenous, subcutaneous, or intraperitoneal administration of an antiangiogenic ribozyme (Angiozyme™) in mice resulted in low but detectable levels of the intact ribozyme within the lung up to 1.5 h after dosing [9]. This same ribozyme has also been shown to reduce the number of pulmonary metastases in the Lewis lung carcinoma model after intravenous infusion [10]. Evidence of ribozyme cleavage products has also been observed in the rat lung 48 h after administration of a 2'-O-allyl modified hammerhead anti-P450 ribozyme [11]. Therefore, systemic administration of ribozymes has been shown to result in delivery to and activity in pulmonary tissue.

In addition to systemic delivery, therapy for asthma could also involve direct pulmonary delivery of the ribozyme. To evaluate the potential for pulmonary ribozyme delivery, a preliminary study was conducted to examine the pharmacokinetic behavior of a ribozyme after direct pulmonary administration.

Study Design. Balb/c mice were administered a 10 mg/kg dose supplemented with approximately 5×10^6 cpm of internally labeled [^{32}P]ribozyme as an intravenous infusion (100 μl) in the tail vein or as an intratracheal instillation. Details of the dose solution preparation are described elsewhere [9]. For intratracheal instillation, animals were anesthetized and a 1-cm incision was made to expose the trachea. The ribozyme injection (25 μl) was made with a 28-gauge needle and delivered via a syringe pump at rate of 50 μl/min. The incision was then closed with sutures and the animal allowed to recover on a 37°C warming pad.

Mice were euthanized by CO_2 inhalation at various times after ribozyme administration. On cessation of breathing, the chest cavity was opened, and the animal exsanguinated by cardiac puncture. Collected blood was added to heparinized tubes and centrifuged to separate plasma from cells. Prior to tissue collection, saline was perfused through the heart. Samples of lung were collected and frozen on dry ice until preparation for ribozyme quantitation.

Radioactivity in plasma and tissue was quantitated as previously described [9]. Briefly, total radioactivity was quantitated in prepared samples by liquid scintillation counting and then the percentage of radioactivity associated with intact ribozyme was determined by PAGE and phosphorimage analysis. Noncompartmental analysis was performed on the resulting plasma and tissue concentration data using WinNonlin software (Pharsight Corporation).

Study Results. Plasma and tissue concentrations of ribozyme after intravenous or intratracheal administration of 10 mg/kg ribozyme are shown in figure 2. The rapid elimination of the ribozyme from plasma after intravenous administration is consistent with previous data [9]. However, significant plasma exposure was observed after intratracheal administration long after plasma levels were below detection with intravenous administration. Four hours after intratracheal administration, plasma concentrations were still above 1 μg/ml and over 70% of the ribozyme had been absorbed compared with intravenous administration (table 1). Since intact ribozyme could be detected in only one animal 24 h after intratracheal administration, area under the concentration-time curve

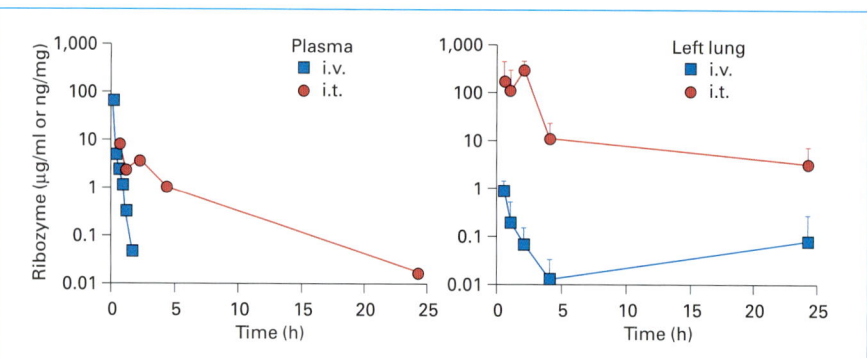

Fig. 2. Concentration of a ribozyme in mouse plasma or lung after intravenous (i.v.) or intratracheal (i.t.) administration of 10 mg/kg. Plasma data are shown as mean and SD with 5 animals per time point.

Table 1. Comparison of exposure (AUC) after intravenous (i.v.) or intratracheal (i.t.) administration of a ribozyme in mice

	AUC i.t. dosing	AUC i.v. dosing	AUC i.t. / AUC i.v.
Plasma, µg·h/ml	14*	19	0.74
Left lung, ng·h/mg	777	1.8	432

Mice received 10 mg/kg as a tail vein injection (100 µl) or direct intratracheal administration under anesthesia (25 µl).
* AUCs for plasma are for 0–4 h since intact ribozyme was only detected in 1 of 5 animals 24 h after intratracheal administration.

(AUC) calculations are only shown for 4 h. However, it is clear that the majority of the dose was absorbed systemically after intratracheal administration compared with intravenous administration.

Intratracheal administration of the ribozyme dramatically increased exposure in the lung. As shown in figure 2 and table 1, lung tissue concentrations were several orders of magnitude higher in animals receiving the intratracheal administration of ribozyme compared with intravenous administration. This resulted in a greater than 400-fold increase in exposure (AUC) in the lung. Therefore, in addition to providing a mode for systemic exposure, pulmonary administration could reduce the dose of ribozyme required for asthma therapy due to the increased exposure over intravenous dosing.

This and previously published studies suggest that systemic as well as direct pulmonary delivery could be utilized for a ribozyme asthma therapy. Recent published data correlate circulating levels of IL-5 in peripheral blood with increased airway eosinophilic inflammation in experimental asthma [12]. Interestingly, a similar correlation with IL-5 levels in resident pulmonary cells could not be established.

Ribozyme Efficacy in vivo

Stabilization chemistries have been developed to render these molecules highly resistant to serum nucleases and thus suitable for therapeutic applications in vivo [6]. Local delivery of ribozymes has been reported to inhibit specifically cytokine-stimulated expression of stromelysin mRNA in a rabbit knee osteoarthritis model [13] and VEGF-stimulated angiogenesis in a rat corneal pocket model [14]. Sioud and Sørensen [15] have shown that a stabilized ribozyme targeting protein kinase C alpha mRNA reduces tumor growth in rats subcutaneously implanted with glioma cells [15]. In additional studies, the Lewis lung carcinoma model in a C57Bl/6 mouse model was used to evaluate anti-tumor and anti-metastatic effects of treatment with ribozymes targeting the VEGF receptors. In this model, both the anti-Flt-1 and the anti-KDR ribozyme inhibited primary tumor growth when administered intravenously by continuous infusion. However, only treatment with the anti-Flt-1 ribozyme resulted in a statistically significant and dose-dependent inhibition of lung metastasis in this model [10]. In further testing of the anti-Flt-1 ribozyme in a model of human colorectal metastasis, the number of liver metastases was also significantly reduced. Hammerhead ribozymes targeting the mRNA of the transcription factor c-*myb* have been shown to inhibit smooth muscle cell proliferation in an animal model of restenosis [16].

Ribozyme Toxicology

Ribozymes have been administered in a variety of animal models with no overt toxicity [10, 17]. A recent study evaluated the toxicity profile of Angiozyme in cynomolgus monkeys [18]. A 4-hour intravenous infusion of 10, 30 or 100 mg/kg or a subcutaneous bolus of 100 mg/kg was well tolerated, with no treatment-related effects observed. No evidence of oligonucleotide-associated toxicity was observed despite peak plasma concentrations up to 400 µg/ml. A similar safety profile has been observed after repeated administration of these compounds [unpubl. obs.]. The favorable toxicology profiles of these ribozymes in experimental animals support the therapeutic potential of ribozymes for the treatment of asthma and other inflammatory diseases.

Ribozyme Clinical Studies

To date, three ribozymes have entered and continue in clinical studies. Two are stabilized synthetic ribozymes based on the structure shown in figure 1. Angiozyme, which targets the *Flt*-1 VEGF receptor, is in several phase II studies and an anti-HCV ribozyme targeting the HCV genome has completed phase I/II studies. A vector-expressed ribozyme targeting the tat and tat/rev regions of the HIV viral genome is in phase II studies. To date, these ribozymes have been well tolerated.

Conclusions

In conclusion, ribozymes are a potentially powerful therapeutic tool, based on their specificity and lack of toxicity, which could be effective and safe for the treatment of asthma and COPD. The ability to deliver these compounds by a variety of routes could also enhance their utility.

References

1 Cech TR, Zaug AJ, Grabowski PJ: In vitro splicing of the ribosomal RNA precursor of Tetrahymena: Involvement of a guanosine nucleotide in the excision of the intervening sequence. Cell 1981;27:487–496.
2 Kruger K, Grabowski PJ, Zaug AJ, Sands J, Gottschling DE, Cech TR: Self-splicing RNA: Autoexcision and autocyclization of the ribosomal RNA intervening sequence of Tetrahymena. Cell 1982;31:147–157.
3 Guerrier-Takada C, Gardiner K, Marsh T, Pace N, Altman S: The RNA moiety of ribonuclease P is the catalytic subunit of the enzyme. Cell 1983;35:849–857.
4 Usman N, McSwiggen JA: Catalytic RNA (ribozymes) as drugs. Annu Rep Med Chem 1995;30:285–294.
5 Usman N, Stinchcomb DT: Design, synthesis and function of therapeutic hammerhead ribozymes. Nucleic Acids Mol Biol 1996;10:243–264.
6 Beigelman L, McSwiggen JA, Draper KG, Gonzalez C, Jensen K, Karpeisky AM, Modak AS, Matulic-Adamic J, DiRenzo AB, Haeberli P, Sweedler D, Tracz D, Grimm S, Wincott FE, Thackray VG, Usman N: Chemical modification of hammerhead ribozymes. Catalytic activity and nuclease resistance. J Biol Chem 1995;270:25702–25708.
7 Henry SP, Monteith D, Levin AA: Antisense oligonucleotide inhibitors for the treatment of cancer. 2. Toxicological properties of phosphorothioate oligodeoxynucleotides. Anti Cancer Drug Des 1997;12:395–408.
8 Sioud M: Ribozyme modulation of lipopolysaccharide-induced tumor necrosis factor-alpha production by peritoneal cells in vitro and in vivo. Eur J Immunol 1996;26:1026–1031.
9 Sandberg JA, Bouhana KS, Gallegos AM, Agrawal AB, Grimm SL, Wincott FE, Reynolds MA, Pavco PA, Parry TJ: Pharmacokinetics of an antiangiogenic ribozyme (Angiozyme™) in the mouse. Antisense Nucleic Acid Drug Dev 1999;9:271–277.
10 Pavco PA, Bouhana KS, Gallegos AM, Agrawal A, Blanchard KS, Grimm SL, Jensen KL, Andrews LE, Wincott FE, Pitot PA, Tressler RJ, Cushman C, Reynolds MA, Parry TJ: Antitumor and antimetastatic activity of ribozymes targeting the mRNA of vascular endothelial growth factor receptors. Clin Cancer Res 2000;6:2094–2103.
11 Desjardins JP, Sproat BS, Beijer B, Blaschke M, Dunkel M, Gerdes W, Ludwig J, Reither V, Rupp T, Iversen PL: Pharmacokinetics of a synthetic, chemically modified hammerhead ribozyme against the rat cytochrome P-450 3A2 mRNA after single iv injections. J Pharmacol Exp Ther 1996;278:1419–1427.
12 Wang J, Palmer K, Lotvall J, Milan S, Lei XF, Matthaei KI, Gauldie J, Inman MD, Jordana M, Xing Z: Circulating, but not local lung, IL-5 is required for the development of antigen-induced airways eosinophilia. J Clin Invest 1998;102:1132–1141.
13 Flory CM, Pavco PA, Jarvis TC, Lesch ME, Wincott FE, Beigelman L, Hunt SW 3rd, Schrier DJ: Nuclease-resistant ribozymes decrease stromelysin mRNA levels in rabbit synovium following exogenous delivery to the knee joint. Proc Natl Acad Sci USA 1996;93:754–758.
14 Parry TJ, Cushman C., Gallegos AM, Agrawal AB, Richardson M, Maloney L, Mokler VR, Wincott FE, Pavco PA: Bioactivity of antiangiogenic ribozymes targeting Flt-1 and KDR mRNA. Nucleic Acids Res 1999;27:2569–2577.
15 Sioud M, Sørensen DR: A nuclease-resistant protein kinase C alpha ribozyme blocks glioma cell growth. Nat Biotechnol 1998;16:556–561.
16 Macejak DG, Lin H, Webb S, Chase J, Jensen K, Jarvis TC, Leiden JM, Couture L: Adenovirus-mediated expression of a ribozyme to c-*myb* mRNA inhibits smooth muscle cell proliferation and neointima formation in vivo. J Virol 1999;73:7745–7751.
17 Lyngstadaas SP, Risnes S, Sproat BS, Thrane PS, Prydz HP: A synthetic, chemically modified ribozyme eliminates amelogenin, the major translation product in developing mouse enamel in vivo. EMBO J 1995;14:5224–5229.
18 Sandberg JA, Sproul CD, Blanchard KS, Bellon L, Powell JA, Caputo FA, Kornbrust DJ, Parker VP, Parry TJ, Blatt LM: Acute toxicology and pharmacokinetic assessment of a ribozyme (Angiozyme™) targeting VEGF receptor mRNA in the cynomolgus monkey. Antisense Nucleic Acid Drug Dev 2000;10:153–162.

Nassim Usman
Ribozyme Pharmaceuticals, Inc.
2950 Wilderness Place
Boulder, CO 80301 (USA)
Tel. +1 303 449 6500, Fax +1 303 449 6995
E-Mail usmann@rpi.com

Gene Therapy

Martin Kolb   Jack Gauldie

Department of Pathology, McMaster University, Hamilton, Canada

Summary

Gene therapy is the newest approach to the treatment of pulmonary disease. It can be defined as the introduction of nucleic acid sequences into cells for the purpose of altering a disease. Cystic fibrosis or α_1-antitrypsin deficiency are diseases associated with single gene defects and represent the obvious rationale for gene therapy in order to replace the defective or absent gene. Chronic acquired respiratory disorders such as COPD, asthma or interstitial lung diseases are considered to be the product of a variety of endogenous (polygenic) and exogenous influences and less obviously associated with gene replacement therapy. These chronic inflammatory conditions likely arise from an imbalance between destructive and protective mechanisms, such that transient gene therapy can be useful to reconstitute the impaired balance by short-term over-expression of protective genes or suppression of damaging genes.

Vectors and Ways of Gene Delivery

Today, different viral and nonviral vector systems are considered useful for lung gene transfer, all with certain advantages and disadvantages (table 1). Currently, the most common vectors for treatment of pulmonary diseases are replication-deficient adenoviruses and synthetic liposome/DNA complexes. Major advantages of adenovectors are their excellent efficiency in gene transfer, demonstrated in numerous systems [1–3]. However, gene expression is transient and if long-term replacement is required, repeated administration is necessary, but this is prevented by the immunogenicity of adenovectors. Immunosuppressive agents can be used to reduce production of neutralizing antiviral antibodies in the host (e.g. corticosteroids or cyclosporin A), procedures that can prolong gene expression but not completely abrogate the antiviral immune response. A second way is to further modify adenovectors by deleting more of the genes encoding for viral proteins and thereby reducing their immunogenicity [1, 4–6]. Liposomes are attractive, because they generate no apparent host immune response and repeated delivery is feasible, but the overall rate of transgene expression is much lower than with viral vectors [1, 4]. It is anticipated that the technical problems in gene delivery will be solved in the foreseeable future.

The lung is an attractive organ for gene transfer because of its accessibility from both airways and vasculature. Transfer of genes via airway with adenovirus vectors or liposomes results in gene expression mainly in lung epithelial cells, and the transgene is compartmentalized to the lung without much in the way of systemic distribution. In contrast, intravenous application of genes transduces predominantly endothelial cells and parenchymal cells of internal organs. Depending on the underlying disease, either route of administration, or even a combination of both might be advantageous to target the lung.

Cystic Fibrosis

Since discovery of the CFTR gene in 1987, cystic fibrosis (CF) has been considered the major lung disease being suited to gene therapy. To date more than 10 clinical trials involving lung gene transfer have been reported, however, none has shown convincing restoration of function [7]. Several reasons can be considered for this failure. (1) The ideal vector system has not yet been developed. Both adenovectors and liposomes have been shown to transfer sufficient amounts of genes to the lung but expression is always transient [2, 7]. The problems associated with repeated administration have already been mentioned. (2) It still must be elucidated, which pulmonary region and which cells are the best target for CF gene therapy. Clinical observations show CF is initially localized in small airways which are likely not within reach of aerosols

Table 1. Currently used vector systems for lung gene transfer [modified from 1 and 3]

Vector	Advantage	Disadvantage
Viral		
Retrovirus	viral genes removed, no viral proteins made, integrates into host DNA, useful for ex vivo cell gene transfer	possible insertional mutagenesis, cell division necessary, low titres
Adenovirus	efficient, transduces non-dividing cells, can be produced in high titres, affinity for epithelial cells, transient expression	prior exposure, immune response, inefficient with repeated application
Adeno-associated virus	virus genes removed, no viral proteins made, transduces non-dividing cells	production labour intensive, small packaging capacity for foreign DNA
Vaccinia virus Canarypox virus Fowlpox virus	can be highly attenuated, large capacity for foreign DNA, efficient transfer to non-dividing cells, host-range restricted, transient expression	pathogenic infection, immune response, inefficient with repeated application
Nonviral		
Naked DNA	simple, non-immunogenic, inexpensive, safe	most inefficient transduction
Cationic liposomes	non-immunogenic, repeated application possible, safe, ease of preparation	gene expression transient and low

currently in use [7]. Mucus plugs and local infections may be real obstacles for gene transfer. The main target tissue for gene transfer is the superficial epithelium, which exhibits all ion transport functions of CFTR and is best accessible via topical administration of vectors. However, the constitutively highest level of CFTR gene expression is localized in bronchial submucosal gland cells. These glands are better accessible by the vasculature and systemic vector application [2, 7]. (3) Replacement of the CFTR gene in the airways alone will probably not compensate for all functional defects in CF patients. Recent data also suggest an impaired ability to clear bacterial airway infections, partly due to non-functional antimicrobial peptides (e.g. human β-defensin 1) [8]. Gene transfer could be used to deliver cytokines to the lung as an adjuvant therapy and thereby support the host response against bacteria. In pneumonia models, survival of animals was improved by transient over-expression of IL-12 and IFN-γ resulting in enhanced clearance of *Klebsiella pneumoniae* and *Pseudomonas aeruginosa* [9]. This fact has important clinical relevance because of increasing antibiotic resistance of *P. aeruginosa*, which persistently colonizes airways in almost all CF patients.

COPD and Emphysema

Although we are not aware of any targeted research in gene therapy for COPD, several possibilities are imaginable. Currently the most accepted theory for the development of COPD is a protease/antiprotease imbalance, similar to emphysema due to hereditary α_1-antitrypsin deficiency. This disease with an underlying single gene defect is by its nature a main target of gene therapy, but most attempts at gene replacement have been limited because of short-term expression and the high concentrations of protein required for therapeutic efficacy [10]. Newer studies show that the pathogenesis of COPD does not only involve elastases but also collagenases and gelatinases [11]. Thus re-establishment of the balance by over-expressing antiprotease genes is theoretically beneficial, and the levels of antiproteases required should be lower than that required for replacement in α_1-antitrypsin deficiency. Experimental models suggest a role for α_1-antitrypsin and secretory leukoprotease inhibitor in COPD [12, 13]. However, there is still need for a convincing study proving the concept of antiprotease treatment for COPD and emphysema. Neutrophils are a major source of proteases and reactive oxygen species, and because of their overabundance in COPD, gene therapy could also target adhesion molecules for neutrophils to reduce the influx of inflammatory cells into the lung parenchyma.

Asthma

Benchmarks for any new intervention in asthma are inhaled corticosteroids and bronchodilators, established therapies for the majority of asthmatic patients [14]. Gene therapy is not likely to provide an alternative in the near future for these therapies, except for the concept of immunomodulation by gene-based vaccines. However, transient gene therapy, such as with anti-inflammatory genes, could bring some benefit for asthmatics with severe disease requiring high doses of systemic corticosteroids, or for patients with corticosteroid-resistant asthma. Another

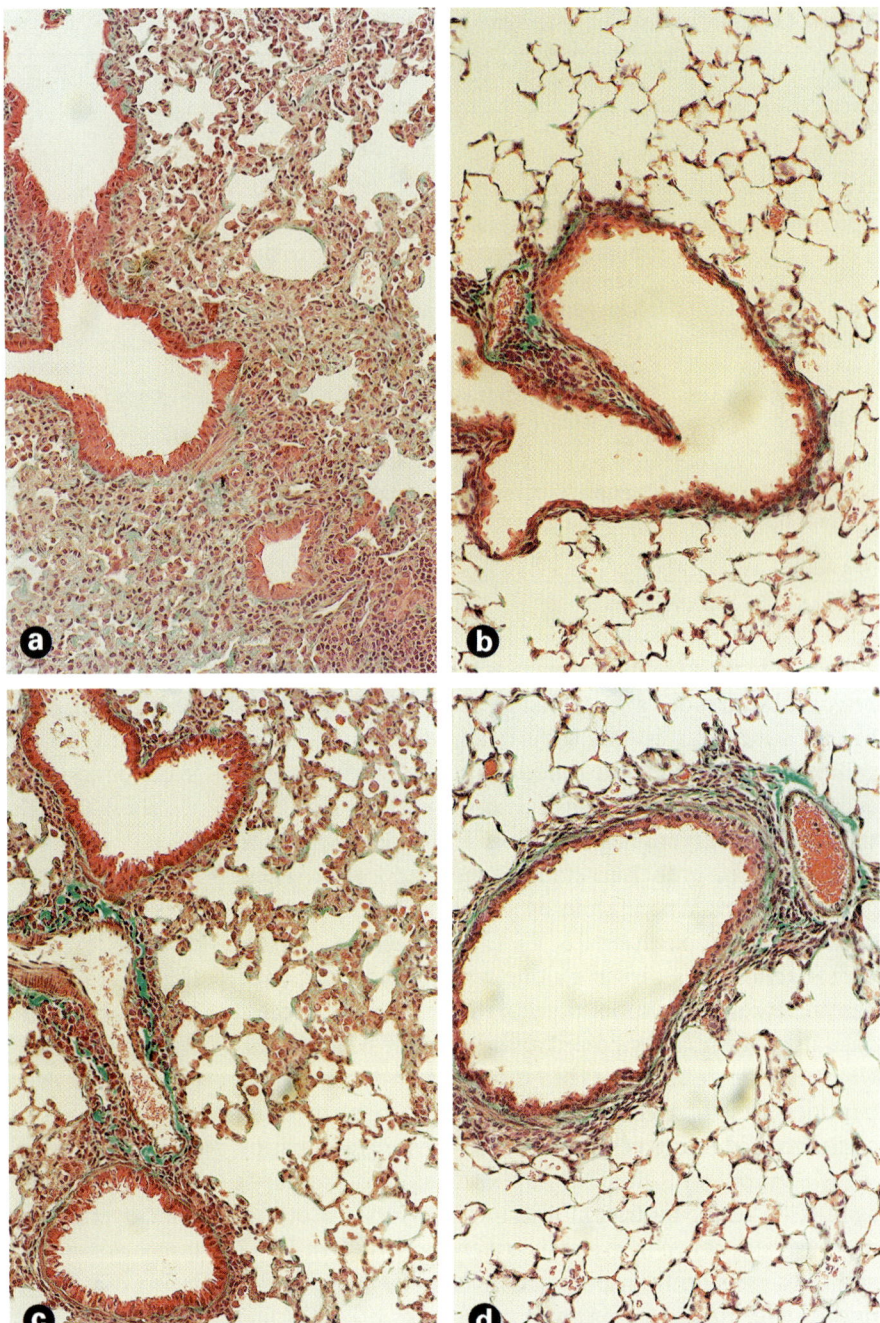

Fig. 1. Morphological appearance of mouse lungs 3 weeks after being exposed to different cytokine genes involved in airway and tissue remodelling. Masson's trichrome. ×200. **a** Airway of a mouse exposed to AdDL70 (control virus without gene insert). **b** Lung of a mouse transfected with a low dose of the TGFβ1 gene shows a subepithelial fibrotic tissue reaction, which is thought to be crucial in the concept of airway remodelling in asthma. **c** TGFβ1 in a 10-fold higher titre induces a more severe and progressive fibrosis of the lung, which is largely abrogated when the gene for decorin, a physiologic opponent of TGF-β is simultaneously administered **d**.

potential target for gene therapy for asthma is airway remodelling, which results in persistent obstruction and likely is not prevented by current anti-inflammatory treatment modalities [15].

Over-Expression of Cytokines. The pathogenesis of asthma involves a large number of different mediators with predominance of Th2 derived cytokines [16]. Transient over-expression of GM-CSF or IL-4 and IL-5 in animal models have been shown to promote asthmatic-like reactions with goblet cell hyperplasia, hypersecretion, eosinophilia, peribronchial myofibroblast proliferation and tissue remodelling [16–18]. Th1 cytokines are able to suppress Th2 reactions and hence over-expression of these mediators could be beneficial in asthma. It has recently been shown that gene transfer of IL-12 inhibits experimental allergic airway disease by suppression of the Th2

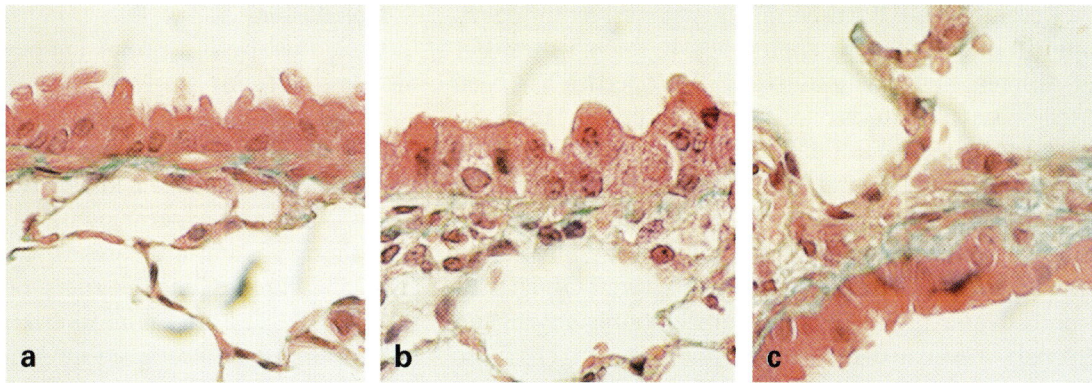

Fig. 2. a Higher magnification (×470) of normal airways. **b** AdDL70 treatment results in a loose peribronchial mononuclear inflammatory reaction without accumulation of collagen. **c** Administration of low level AdTGF-β_1 induces a marked subepithelial fibrosis.

response to aerosolized ovalbumin [19]. Interestingly, over-expression of IL-12 also restored local antiviral immunity, which is impaired in a Th2-dominated environment. This observation has important clinical relevance, considering that obstructive airways disease often exacerbates during viral infections. In similar studies, local or systemic gene transfer of IFNγ significantly inhibited allergen induced airway hyperresponsiveness [20] and IL-10 transfer markedly reduces allergen induced eosinophilia [21].

Over-Expression of Glucocorticoid Receptors and I-κB. Glucocorticoids are used as primary anti-inflammatory agents in asthma. After binding to the glucocorticoid receptor, they repress the expression of pro-inflammatory cytokines via inhibition of transcription factors such as NF-κB, amongst other mechanisms. It has been suggested that patients with corticosteroid-resistant asthma have impaired glucocorticoid receptor activity [22]. A recent study showed that transfer of the glucocorticoid receptor gene in-vitro-mediated inhibition of NF-κB activities, even in the absence of exogenous corticosteroids, and the authors suggested this approach could restore corticosteroid sensitivity in patients [23]. Another possibility to interfere with NF-κB is over-expression of the inhibitory molecule I-κB, which is physiologically bound to NF-κB in the cytoplasm and is degraded during the activation process [14].

Interference with Tissue Remodelling. Airway remodelling is a concept describing processes leading to persistent airflow obstruction and structural changes in the airways of asthmatics [15]. It is speculated that chronic inflammation induces a persistent or recurrent injury-repair response with different growth and repair factors being involved [15, 16].

Table 2. Growth factors implicated in the concept of airway remodelling and possible inhibitory genes

Cytokine/growth factor	Inhibitory genes
TGF-β	Decorin[1], soluble TGF-β receptor[1], Smad7[1]
PDGF	PDGF-β receptor[1]
bFGF	proteoglycans?
IGF	?
EGF	?
GM-CSF	mutant GM-CSF?

[1] Gene transfer successfully demonstrated in animal models.

Immunohistochemistry of human asthmatic airways has shown increased TGF-β presence that correlated with the degree of disease and subepithelial fibrosis [24]. TGF-β has important immunomodulatory properties and its role in tissue remodelling is well known. In lung diseases such as pulmonary fibrosis it is likely that TGF-β is upregulated, because persistent, low degree inflammation demands permanent tissue repair [25]. It is also possible that chronic inflammation in asthma, with recurrent epithelial cell damage, induces a similar pattern of eventually overwhelming tissue repair. Using adenoviral gene transfer we have shown that both TGF-β and GM-CSF induce peribronchial fibrosis and tissue remodelling [17, 26]. The parenchymal fibrotic response exceeds the subepithelial fibrosis seen in chronic asthma by far, due to much higher cytokine levels in tissue and BAL. However, when we administered 5- to 10-fold lower virus doses to mouse lungs, we saw a more subtle peribronchial fibrosis similar to the observations made in human asthmatic airways (fig. 1, 2).

Recently, TGF-β has become a major target for development of gene therapy approaches. In the lung, transfer of different genes with anti-TGF-β properties has been used successfully to reduce fibrotic responses to exogenous fibrogenic stimuli (table 2). The proteoglycan decorin can bind and inhibit TGF-β and is thought to be an endogenous opponent of active TGF-β [27]. Using an adenovirus vector, we have transferred the gene for decorin into lungs of mice treated either with active TGF-β (transiently over-expressed by gene transfer) or bleomycin and strongly modulated the fibrotic response (fig. 1). These experiments show that gene therapy has the potential to efficiently prevent and/or treat chronic lung diseases. The concept of airway remodelling in asthma provides a reasonable basis to further investigate the efficiency of anti-TGF-β gene therapy in appropriate models of chronic obstructive lung disease.

Conclusion

Gene therapy is a promising new treatment for lung diseases. Not only single gene disorders such as CF are potential candidates for gene therapy, but also chronic multigenic and environmental lung diseases, characterized by an imbalance of damaging and protective mechanisms. Numerous experimental models have shown, that gene therapy is not a theoretical concept in a variety of acute and chronic lung disorders, but is a realistic therapeutic goal. The first clinical trials in CF which have started almost 10 years ago have not met expectations, mainly because of 'immature' gene transfer and vector systems. However, it is anticipated that these hurdles will be overcome in the foreseeable future, and make gene therapy a feasible therapeutic alternative in lung disease.

References

1 Kay MA, Liu D, Hoogerbugge PM: Gene therapy. Proc Natl Acad Sci USA 1997;94:12744–12746.
2 Middleton PG, Alton EW: Gene therapy for cystic fibrosis: Which postman, which box? Thorax 1998;53:197–199.
3 Evans CH, Ghivizzani SC, Robbins PD: Blocking cytokines with genes. J Leukoc Biol 1998; 64:55–61.
4 Sallenave JM, Porteous DJ, Haslett C: Gene therapy for lung inflammatory diseases: Not so far away? Thorax 1997;52:742–744.
5 Hitt MM, Parks RJ, Graham FL: Structure and genetic organization of adenovirus vectors; in Friedmann T (ed): The Development of Human Gene Therapy. Cold Spring Harbor, Cold Spring Harbor Laboratory Press, 1999, pp 61–86.
6 Look DC, Brody SL: Engineering viral vectors to subvert the airway defense response. Am J Respir Cell Mol Biol 1999; 20:1103–1106.
7 Boucher RC: Status of gene therapy for cystic fibrosis lung disease. J Clin Invest 1999;103:441–445.
8 Rubin BK: Emerging therapies for cystic fibrosis lung disease. Chest 1999;115:1120–1126.
9 Standiford TJ, Tsai WC, Mehrad B, Moore TA: Cytokines as targets of immunotherapy in bacterial pneumonia. J Lab Clin Med 2000;135:129–138.
10 Song S, Morgan M, Ellis T, Poirier A, Chesnut K, Wang J, Brantly M, Mucyczka N, Byrne BJ, Atkinson M, Flotte TR: Sustained secretion of human alpha-1-antitrypsin from murine muscle transduced with adeno-associated virus vectors. Proc Natl Acad Sci USA 1998;95:14384–14388.
11 Segura-Valdez L, Pardo A, Gaxiola M, Uhal BD, Becerril C, Selman M: Upregulation of gelatinases A and B, collagenases 1 and 2, and increased parenchymal cell death in COPD. Chest 2000;117:684–694.

12 Tomee JF, Koeter GH, Hiemstra PS, Kauffman HF: Secretory leukoprotease inhibitor: A native antimicrobial protein presenting a new therapeutic option? Thorax 1998;53:114–116.
13 Rogers DF, Laurent GJ: New ideas on the pathophysiology and treatment of lung disease. Thorax 1998;53:200–203.
14 Alton EW, Griesenbach U, Geddes DM: Gene therapy for asthma: Inspired research or unnecessary effort? Gene Therapy 1999;6:155–156.
15 Fish JE, Peters SP: Airway remodeling and persistent airway obstruction in asthma. J Allergy Clin Immunol 1999;104:509–516.
16 Chung KF, Barnes PJ: Cytokines in asthma. Thorax 1999;54:825–857.
17 Xing Z, Ohkawara Y, Jordana M, Graham FL, Gauldie J: Transfer of GM-CSF Gene to rat lung induces eosinophilia, monocytosis and fibrotic reactions. J Clin Invest 1996;97:1102–1110.
18 Stämpfli MR, Wiley RE, Neigh GS, Gajewska BU, Lei XF, Snider DP, Xing Z, Jordana M: GM-CSF transgene expression in the airway allows aerolosolized ovalbumin to induce allergic sensitization in mice. J Clin Invest 1998; 102:1704–1714.
19 Hogan SP, Foster PS, Tan X, Ramsay AJ: Mucosal IL-12 gene delivery inhibits allergic airways disease and restores local antiviral immunity. Eur J Immunol 1998;28:413–423.
20 Dow SW, Schwarze J, Heath TD, Potter TA, Gelfand EW: Systemic and local interferon gamma gene delivery to the lungs for treatment of allergen-induced airway hyperresponsiveness in mice. Hum Gene Ther 1999;10:1905–1914.
21 Stämpfli MR, Cwiartka M, Gajewska BU, Alvarez D, Ritz SA, Inman MD, Xing Z, Jordana M: Interleukin-10 gene transfer to the airway regulates allergic mucosal sensitization in mice. Am J Respir Cell Mol Biol 1999;21:586–596.

22 Sher ER, Leung DY, Surs W, Kam JC, Zieg G, Kamada AK, Szefler SJ: Steroid-resistant asthma. Cellular mechanisms contributing to inadequate response to glucocorticoid therapy. J Clin Invest 1994;93:33–39.
23 Mathieu M, Gougat C, Jaffuel D, Danielsen M, Godard P, Bousquet J, Demoly P: The glucocorticoid receptor gene as a candidate for gene therapy in asthma. Gene Ther 1999;6:245–252.
24 Minshall EM, Leung DY, Martin RJ, Song YL, Cameron L, Ernst P, Hamid Q: Eosinophil-associated TGF-beta1 mRNA expression and airways fibrosis in bronchial asthma. Am J Respir Cell Mol Biol 1997;17:326–333.
25 Gauldie J, Sime PJ, Xing Z, Marr B, Tremblay GM: TGFβ gene transfer to the lung induces myofibroblast presence and pulmonary fibrosis; in: Desmoulière A, Tuchweber B (eds): Tissue Repair and Fibrosis. Current topics in Pathology. Berlin, Springer, 1999, vol 13, pp 35–45.
26 Sime PJ, Xing Z, Graham FL, Csaky KG, Gauldie J: Adenovector mediated gene transfer of active TGFβ1 induces prolonged severe fibrosis in rat lung. J Clin Invest 1997;100:768–776.
27 Yamaguchi Y, Mann DM, Ruoslahti E: Negative regulation of TGFβ by the proteoglycan decorin. Nature 1990;346:281–284.

Jack Gauldie, PhD
Department of Pathology
McMaster University
1200 Main Street West
Hamilton, Ont. L8N 3Z5 (Canada)
Tel. +1 905 521 2100, Fax +1 905 577 0198
E-Mail gauldie@mcmaster.ca

Author Index

Abbott, N.N. 247
Adams, S.P. 302
Adcock, I.M. 328
Agosti, J.M. 256
Anderskewitz, R. 121
Anderson, G.P. 54
Axelsson, B. 94

Barnes, P.J. 2, 6, 44, 48
Belloni, P.N. 350
Belvisi, M.G. 98
Bennett, B.L. 337
Bennett, C.F. 365
Berens, K.L. 306
Birke, F. 121
Bochner, B.S. 298
Bolser, D.C. 133
Borish, L. 256
Boushey, H.A. 201
Brattsand, R. 94
Brown, T.J. 98
Bryan, S.A. 274, 288

Caramori, G. 328
Chung, K.F. 242
Cipolla, D. 20
Clark, J.M. 170
Compton, C.H. 141, 321
Conrad, D.H. 206
Corrigan, C.J. 233
Coyle, A.J. 217
Currie, M.G. 156
Cuss, F.M. 133, 269

Dahl, R. 86
Dahlén, S.-E. 115
D'Ambrosio, D. 284

Davies, D.E. 39
Della Cioppa, G. 237
De Souza, P.M. 316
De Vos, C. 128
Dietzel, K. 91
Disse, B. 72
Dixon, R.A.F. 306
Donaldson, D.D. 260
Dougall, I.G. 68
Drazen, J.M. 108
Dupré, B. 306
Durham, S.R. 186

Egan, R.W. 133
Elias, J.A. 260
Engelstätter, R. 91
Evans, R. 165

Fabbri, L.M. 284
Fahy, J.V. 201
Farr, S. 20
Fernandes, D.J. 102
Fick, R. 201
Forssmann, K. 81
Forssmann, W.G. 81
Foster, M.L. 98
Fozard, J.R. 77

Gauldie, J. 374
Giembycz, M.A. 316
Gonda, I. 20
Griswold, D.E. 293, 342
Gutierrez-Ramos, J.-C. 217

Hagan, G.W.E. 60
Hall, I.P. 15
Handley, D.A. 64

Hansel, T.T. 2, 15, 48, 247
Hay, D.W.P. 141, 145
Hersperger, R. 237
Hey, J.A. 133
Hodgson, S.T. 173
Holgate, S.T. 39
Holt, P.R. 68
Hopkin, J.M. 226
Hughes, R.A. 102

Ince, F. 68

Jackson, D.M. 68
Jansen, H.M. 233
Jeffery, P.K. 24
Jennewein, H.M. 121
Johnson, M. 60

Kay, A.B. 182, 191
Keller, A. 91
Keller, T.H. 237
Kharitonov, S.A. 44
Kips, J.C. 247
Kline, J.N. 229
Kobayashi, M. 274
Kolb, M. 374
Koulis, A. 212
Kraft, D. 195
Krieg, A.M. 229
Kurth, M.C. 170

Larché, M. 182, 191
Leckie, M.J. 265
Lee, P.A. 370
Lindsay, M.A. 316
Lobb, R.R. 302
Lynch, O.T. 316

McDonnell, N.D. 247
McLeod, R.L. 133
McMillan, R.M. 111
MacNee, W. 151
Maggi, C.A. 137
Manley, P.W. 77
Manning, A.M. 337
Manning, P.T. 156
Marks, M.J. 321
Martin, R.L. 177
Meade, C.J. 121
Meini, S. 137
Meyer, M. 81
Mohler, K.M. 247
Morley, J. 64
Morrison, J.F.J. 358

Narula, S. 269
Nelson, H.S. 64
Newbold, P. 68
Nielsen, L.P. 86
Nyce, J.W. 361

O'Byrne, P.M. 108
Oldfield, W.L.G. 191
Otulana, B. 20
Out, T.A. 233

Pairet, M. 121
Palovich, M.R. 293
Pater-Huijsen, F.L. de 233
Pauwels, R. 11
Pendergast, W. 165
Ponath, P.D. 288
Pride, N. 30

Rabe, K.F. 54
Ray, A. 222
Ray, P. 222
Richards, I.M. 310
Rihoux, J.P. 128
Robinson, D.S. 212
Rocchiccioli, K.M.S. 68
Rogers, D.F. 160

Sabroe, I. 280
Sandberg, J.A. 370
Sarau, H.M. 293
Schaefer, G. 346
Schindler, U. 346

Shapiro, S.D. 177
Sinigaglia, F. 284
Slatter, V.K. 310
Smith, R.A. 173
Sterk, P.J. 35
Stewart, A.G. 102
Stockley, R.A. 173
Sturton, G. 321
Sur, S. 274

Thompson, J.M. 156
Tong, S.E. 177
Torphy, T.J. 321

Underwood, D.C. 293, 342
Urnov, F.D. 332
Usman, N. 370

Valenta, R. 195
Vanderslice, P. 306
Van Dyke, R.E. 170
Van Wart, H.E. 177
Venkataraman, C. 346
Vlahos, R. 102

Walker, C. 265
White, J.R. 293

Widdowson, K.L. 293
Wilhelm, R.S. 288
Williams, T.J. 280
Williams, W.V. 251
Wills-Karp, M. 260
Wilson, D.R. 186
Witek, T.J., Jr. 72
Wolffe, A.P. 332

Young, A. 68

Subject Index

N-Acetylcysteine, antioxidant therapy in chronic obstructive pulmonary disease 153
Activator protein-1
  levels in lung 337
  lung disease-related gene control 337, 338
  signalling pathway
    overview 339–341
    targeting
      rationale 337
      strategies 341
  structure 340
Acute respiratory distress syndrome, retinoid therapy 353
Adenosine A_1 receptor, antisense targeting 363
Adhesion molecules
  antagonists, see Intercellular adhesion molecule-1, Selectin, Vascular cell adhesion molecule-1, VLA-4
  endothelial cells 298, 299
  endothelial and epithelial interactions 300
  epithelial cells 299, 300
  leukocytes 298
  selective leukocyte accumulation 300
  therapeutic targeting approaches 300
β_2-Adrenoceptor
  airway caliber regulation 55, 56
  genetic polymorphism 16
β_2-Adrenoceptor agonists, see also specific drugs
  disease effects on biochemistry of bronchodilation 56, 57
  dual dopamine D_2 receptor agonist, see Viozan

  long-acting drugs
    clinical use
      asthma 61, 62
      chronic obstructive pulmonary disease 62
    corticosteroid interactions 61
    mechanism of action 60
    non-smooth muscle effects 61
    overview 7
    receptor pharmacology 60, 61
    smooth muscle response 61
  pharmacokinetics 56
  short-acting drugs 7
  side effects 2, 7
  single-isomer drugs
    levalbuterol 66, 67
    mechanism of action 65
    overview 64
    rationale for use 64, 65
Airflow resistance, measurement during tidal breathing 32
Airway hyperreactivity
  airway inflammation relationship 36
  challenge tests 36, 37
  clinical research 37, 38
  disease management 37
  genetics 17, 35
  measurement 36
  mechanisms 35
  pathogenesis 35
  potassium channel openers
    animal studies 79
    clinical studies 80
    rationale for use 78, 79
  rationale for measurement 35

Airway remodeling
  asthma 102
  bronchial epithelium changes 39, 40
  clinical trials of agents 42, 43
  epithelial mesenchymal trophic unit 42
  fibrosis of airway wall 40, 41
  gene therapy interference 377, 378
  glucocorticoid effects 102, 103
  inflammatory cells 39
  2-methoxyestradiol effects 104, 105
  microvasculature changes 41
  nerves 41, 42
  sex differences 103
  smooth muscle 52
  therapeutic targets 42, 102
Albuterol, levalbuterol isomer
  chronic obstructive pulmonary disease studies 66
  cold-induced bronchoconstriction effects 66
  exercise-induced bronchoconstriction effects 66
  mechanism of action 65
  moderate persistent asthma studies 66
  pediatric effectiveness 66
  rationale for use 64, 65
  therapeutic application 66, 67
Allergen immunotherapy, see also Recombinant allergens
  adjuvants 189
  administration routes 188, 189
  allergens and allergoids 183, 189
  subcutaneous immunotherapy
    efficacy 186, 187
    mechanism 187, 188
    safety 187
  T cell response 214

Allergic response, overview 191, 192
α4β1, *see* VLA-4
Antihistamines, *see* specific histamine receptors
Anti-immunoglobulin E, *see* Immunoglobulin E
Antioxidants
   levels in BAL fluid 151, 152
   therapy in chronic obstructive pulmonary disease 153, 154
Antisense oligonucleotides
   administration routes 367, 368
   asthma models, pharmacological effects 367, 368
   mechanism of action 361, 362
   modifications for stability 365, 366
   mucus hypersecretion management 163
   non-antisense effects 368
   pharmacokinetics 366, 367
   respirable oligonucleotides for lung diseases
      EPI-2010 363, 367
      rationale 363
      targets 363, 364
   toxicology
      phosphorothioate oligodeoxynucleotides 367
      sequence-related 362, 363
α_1-Antitrypsin, pulmonary delivery 22
APC 366
   clinical studies 171, 172
   preclinical studies 170
   tryptase inhibition 170
Asthma, *see also* specific treatments
   aims of therapy 6, 7
   airflow limitation 54
   candidate genes 359
   classes of pharmacological therapy 7, 8, 10
   clinical trial design 48–50
   diagnosis 7
   environmental control 7
   gene therapy
      airway remodeling interference 377, 378
      cytokine overexpression 376, 377
      glucocorticoid receptor overexpression 377
      overview 375, 376
   guidelines for treatment
      action plans 10
      mild episodic asthma 9
      mild persistent asthma 9
      moderate persistent asthma 9
      overview 8, 9
      severe persistent asthma 9
      step-down 9, 10
   heredity 358

immunopathology
   chronic bronchiolitis 25, 26
   chronic bronchitis 24, 25
   comparison with chronic obstructive pulmonary disease 27, 28
   inflammation 86
sex differences 103
status of therapies 2–4
ATP-sensitive potassium channel, *see* Potassium channel openers

B7, T cell activation 217–219
BCG, *see* Mycobacterial immunization
BIIL 284 BS, leukotriene B_4 antagonism and effects 124
Breath condensate, exhaled breath analysis 46
Bronchodilation
   compensatory adaptation 57
   disease effects on biochemistry 56, 57
   neuro-humoral regulation of airway caliber 55, 56
   pharmacokinetics of drugs 56
Bronchopulmonary dysplasia, retinoid therapy 352

Carbon monoxide, exhaled breath analysis 45
CD23
   antibody therapy
      immunoglobulin E inhibition 206
      overview 184
   immunoglobulin E interactions 206
   soluble receptor binding of immunoglobulin E 207, 208
   transgenic mouse studies 206, 207
CD28, T cell activation 217, 218
CGS 25019C, leukotriene B_4 antagonism and effects 123
Chemokines
   antagonism in human disease 282
   asthma role 281, 282
   CCR-3
      antagonism
         compounds 291
         rationale 289, 290
      cellular expression 288, 289
      signal transduction 288, 289
      structure 291
   chronic obstructive pulmonary disease 282
   CXCR2
      antagonism with SB 265610
         effects on lipopolysaccharide-induced airway neutrophilia 294, 295
         pharmacology 294
      lung inflammation role 294

      functions 280, 281
   interleukin-8
      functions 293
      lung inflammation role 294, 295
   T helper cells
      chemokine receptors 285, 286
      coordinated localization of inflammatory cells to the lung 285, 286
      mechanisms of lung recruitment 284, 285
      types and receptors 280, 281
Chromatin modification
   corticosteroid effects 335
   cytokine promoters 335
   gene regulatory pathways relevant to allergy and asthma etiology 334, 335
   histone tail modification in transcriptional control 332, 333
   pharmacological intervention with histone acetyltransferases and deacetylases 333, 334
   transcription factors 329
Chronic obstructive pulmonary disease, *see also* specific treatments
   acute exacerbation management 13, 14
   airflow limitation 54
   avoidance of risk factors 11
   candidate genes 359
   chronic disease management guidelines 12, 13
   classes of pharmacological therapy 11, 12
   clinical trial design 50
   epidemiology 4
   gene therapy 375
   genetics 18
   heredity 358
   immunopathology
      chronic bronchiolitis 25, 26
      chronic bronchitis 24, 25
      comparison with asthma 27, 28
      emphysema 26, 27
   oxidative stress
      inflammatory gene induction 152, 153
      systemic oxidative stress 152
      therapeutic options
         anti-inflammatory agents 153
         enhancement of lung antioxidants 153, 154
   oxygen therapy 12
   retinoid therapy 351, 352
   status of therapies 4–6
   surgical treatment 12
Ciclesonide
   activation of prodrug 91
   allergen challenge studies 92, 93
   cortisol levels 92
   dose range finding 92
   receptor affinity 91

Component-resolved diagnosis, recombinant allergens 195
Corticosteroids
 airway remodeling 102, 103
 chromatin modification effects 335
 dose response 87
 glucocorticoid receptor, gene therapy overexpression 377
 inhalation vs oral therapy 3, 8
 leukocyte effects 86
 long-acting β_2-agonist interactions 61
 mechanism of action 88–90
 pharmacokinetic basis of lung selectivity 94
 physiological effects 86, 87
 prodrug, see Ciclesonide
 receptor, see Glucocorticoid receptor
 resistance 3
 side effects 2, 87, 91
 soft steroids
  advantages 97
  inactivation by esterases
   lung esterases 96, 97
   ubiquitous esterases 95
  rationale for development 94, 95
 sparing therapy 8
 T cell effects 212
 time response 87
 transactivation 90, 98, 99
 transrepression 90, 99–101
CP 195543, leukotriene B_4 antagonism and effects 123, 124
CpG oligodeoxynucleotides
 immunostimulatory properties 229
 mechanism of action 229
 preclinical studies 230–232
 rationale for therapy 229
Cromolyn, see Sodium chromoglycate
CTLA-4, T cell activation 217, 218
CXCR2, see Chemokines
Cyclosporin A
 administration routes 238, 239
 animal studies 238
 clinical trials 239, 240
 mechanism of immunosuppression 237, 238
 rationale for asthma treatment 237
Cylexin, selectin antagonism 307, 308
Cystic fibrosis transmembrane conductor, pulmonary delivery of gene therapy vector 22, 374, 375
Cytokines, see also specific cytokines
 antagonists in mucus hypersecretion management 162
 asthma roles
  airway wall remodeling 245
  antigen presentation 244
  eosinophil-associated cytokines 244, 245
  inflammation 243
  Th2-associated cytokines 243, 244
 chronic obstructive pulmonary disease, roles in inflammation 245
 classification of cytokines and receptors 242
 functions 242, 243
 gene therapy overexpression 376, 377
 T cell immunomodulation approaches
  immunoregulatory cytokines 213
  T helper balance modulation 213, 222, 223
 therapeutic targeting 246

Deoxyribonuclease, see Pulmozyme
Diurnal variation, bronchodilator responsiveness 32, 33
Dopamine D_2 receptor
 agonism rationale in airway nerve modulation 68
 dual β_2-adrenoreceptor agonist, see Viozan
Dry-powder inhaler, overview of pulmonary delivery 21, 22

Elastase, see Macrophage elastase, Neutrophil elastase
Emphysema
 alveolar structure and function assessment 33, 34
 gene therapy 375
 immunopathology 26, 27
 retinoid therapy 353, 354
Endothelin-1
 discovery 141
 distribution in lung 141
 levels in lung disease
  allergic rhinitis 143
  asthma 143
  chronic obstructive pulmonary disease 143
 mimicry of lung disease features
  allergic rhinitis 143
  asthma 142, 143
  chronic obstructive pulmonary disease 143
  pulmonary hypertension 143
 processing 141
 receptors
  antagonism benefits 143, 144
  lung 141
Eosinophil
 cytokines in asthma 244, 245
 G protein-coupled receptors
  agonist effects on eosinophils
   Guinea pig 317–320
   humans 317
  subunits 316
  types 317
 interleukin-5, eosinophilia role 265, 266
 recruitment 316
EPI-2010, respirable antisense oligonucleotide 363, 367
Erythromycin, mucus hypersecretion management 161, 162
Estrogen receptor antagonist, see 2-Methoxyestradiol
Exercise performance, assessment 33
Exhaled breath analysis
 breath condensate 46
 carbon monoxide 45
 hydrocarbons 46
 hydrogen peroxide 46
 8-isoprostane 46
 leukotrienes 46
 lipids 47
 nitric oxide 44, 45
 oxynitrogen intermediates 46
 prostaglandins 46
 proteins 46, 47

FK506
 administration routes 238, 239
 animal studies 238
 clinical trials 239, 240
 mechanism of immunosuppression 237, 238
 rationale for asthma treatment 237
Fluocortin butylester
 inactivation by ubiquitous esterases 95
 lung esterases 96, 97
Forced expiratory vital capacity
 alveolar structure and function assessment 33, 34
 interpretation 32
 measurement 30–32, 34
 reference values 32
Formoterol
 clinical use
  asthma 61, 62
  chronic obstructive pulmonary disease 62
 corticosteroid interactions 61
 non-smooth muscle effects 61
 receptor pharmacology 60, 61
 smooth muscle response 61
FR173657
 clinical studies 139
 preclinical studies 138, 139
Functional residual capacity, hyperinflation assessment 33

GATA-3
 asthma
  expression levels 224, 225
  targeting in therapy 225
 negative regulation of Th1 development 223, 224
 T cell development role 223

GATA-3 (continued)
    Th2 specificity and control 223, 224
    transcription factor activity in T cells 223
Gene therapy, *see also* Antisense oligonucleotides, Ribozyme therapy
    asthma
        airway remodeling interference 377, 378
        cytokine overexpression 376, 377
        glucocorticoid receptor overexpression 377
        overview 375, 376
    chronic obstructive pulmonary disease 375
    cystic fibrosis transmembrane conductor, pulmonary delivery of gene therapy vector 22, 374, 375
    emphysema 375
    heritable components of lung disease 358, 359
    vectors 374, 375
Genetic polymorphism
    effect on treatment response 15
    interleukin-4 and receptor in asthma 257
    interleukin-13 in asthma 263
    phase II clinical trials in elucidation 18
    respiratory drug targets
        β_2-adrenoreceptor 16
        glucocorticoid receptor 17
        histamine H_1 receptor 17
        5-lipoxygenase 17
        muscarinic M_2 receptor 16, 17
Glucocorticoid receptor
    genetic polymorphism 17
    transactivation 90, 98, 99
    transrepression 90, 99–101
Good clinical practice, clinical studies 48
Granulocyte-macrophage colony-stimulating factor
    antagonist development 253, 254
    functions 251, 252
    pulmonary alveolar proteinosis role 252, 253
    receptor and signal transduction 251
    transgenic mouse models of disease 253

Histamine H_1 receptor
    antagonists
        anti-allergenic activity 129, 130, 134
        clinical indications 130
        combined H_1/H_3 blockade 134–136
        inverse antagonism 128
        pharmacokinetics 129
        preclinical pharmacology 128
        safety 131
        skin, nose, and bronchi receptor antagonism 129
    genetic polymorphism 17
    structure 128
Histamine H_3 receptor
    antagonists
        allergic rhinitis treatment 133, 134
        combined H_1/H_3 blockade 134–136
        autonomic response modulation 133
        nasal blood flow and resistance modulation 134, 135
Histone acetylation/deacetylation, *see* Chromatin modification
Hydrocarbons, exhaled breath analysis 46
Hydrogen peroxide, exhaled breath analysis 46
Hyperinflation, assessment 33

Icatibant
    clinical studies 139
    preclinical studies 138, 139
IMM125, development status 238, 240
Immunoglobulin E
    allergic response role 201, 204
    anti-immunoglobulin E therapy
        animal studies of E25 202, 203
        clinical trials 203, 204
        development of antibodies 201
        overview 184
        pulmonary delivery 22
        safety 202
    CD23 interactions 206–208
Immunotherapy, *see* Allergen immunotherapy, Mycobacterial immunization, Peptide immunotherapy, Recombinant allergens, Specific immunotherapy
Inducible costimulator, T cell activation 218, 219
Inducible nitric oxide synthase, *see* Nitric oxide synthase
INS365
    clinical studies 167, 168
    pulmonary delivery 166, 167
    toxicology 166
Intercellular adhesion molecule-1
    antagonism
        animal studies 311, 312
        clinical approaches 312, 313
        rationale 310, 311
    function 298–300
    inflammation role 310, 311
Interferon-γ
    functions 274–276
    respiratory disease treatment
        administration routes 277
        animal models 276
        clinical studies 276, 277
        prospects 277, 278
        rationale 276
Interleukin-4
    allergic inflammation role 256

    antagonism for asthma treatment
        approaches 257
        preclinical studies 257
        soluble receptor
            clinical studies of Nuvance 258, 259
            structure 257, 258
    antisense targeting 367, 368
    levels in allergy 257
    mutations in human signaling pathway 348
    polymorphisms in asthma 257
    receptor, pulmonary delivery 22
    STAT6 activation 346, 347
    T cell apoptosis inhibition 256, 257
Interleukin-5
    antagonism
        antibodies 267
        clinical studies of monoclonal antibody treatment 267, 268
        mutant interleukin-5 267
        production inhibitors 266, 267
        receptor antagonists 267
        soluble receptor 267
    antisense targeting 367, 368
    eosinophilia role 265, 266
    levels in asthma 266
Interleukin-8, *see* Chemokines
Interleukin-10
    functions 269, 270
    knockout mouse studies 270, 271
    respiratory disease treatment
        asthma 271
        chronic obstructive pulmonary disease 272
        clinical studies 271
        cystic fibrosis 271, 272
    tissue distribution 269
    receptor and signal transduction 269
Interleukin-12
    functions 274–276
    respiratory disease treatment
        administration routes 277
        animal models 276
        clinical studies 276, 277
        prospects 277, 278
        rationale 276
Interleukin-13
    animal model studies of allergy and inflammation 262, 263
    functions 260–262
    polymorphism in asthma 263
    receptors and signal transduction 260
    soluble receptor antagonism 262, 263
    STAT6 activation 346, 347
Interleukin-18
    functions 274–276
    respiratory disease treatment
        administration routes 277
        animal models 276

clinical studies 276, 277
    prospects 277, 278
    rationale 276
ISIS-2302, intercellular adhesion molecule-1 antagonism 312, 313
8-Isoprostane, exhaled breath analysis 46
Itrocinonide
    inactivation by ubiquitous esterases 95
    lung esterases 96, 97

Kinin receptor
    airway pathophysiology modulation 137, 138
    antagonists
        clinical studies 139
        preclinical studies 138, 139
    kinin processing 137
    types 137

Leukotrienes
    biosynthesis 108, 109, 115
    cysteinyl leukotriene antagonists
        asthma efficacy studies 113, 114
        clinical evaluation 112
        history of development 111, 112
    eosinophil receptor and agonist effects 317–320
    exhaled breath analysis 46
    inhibitors
        5-lipoxygenase inhibition, see 5-Lipoxygenase
        overview 109, 110
    leukotriene B_4 antagonists
        functions and effects of leukotriene B_4 121
        rationale for therapy
            asthma 122
            chronic obstructive pulmonary disease 122
            cystic fibrosis 122
            inflammatory diseases 122
        types and studies 122–124
    types and discovery 108, 111
Levalbuterol, see Albuterol
5-Lipoxygenase
    genetic polymorphism 17
    inhibitors
        asthma efficacy studies
            bronchoprovocation studies 116, 117
            chronic treatment 117, 118
            pharmacology 115, 116
            side effects 115
        leukotriene biosynthesis 108, 109, 115
Loteprednol etabonate
    inactivation by ubiquitous esterases 95
    lung esterases 96, 97
LY 293111 Na, leukotriene B_4 antagonism and effects 123

Macrophage elastase
    emphysema role 177, 178, 180
    inhibitors
        design 178, 179
        smoke-induced emphysema inhibition 179, 180
    knockout mouse 180
Matrix metalloproteinases, see also Macrophage elastase
    classification 178
    structural features 177, 178
Maximum expiratory flow volume, measurement 30–32, 34
Metered dose inhaler, overview of pulmonary delivery 21
2-Methoxyestradiol
    cell culture effects 103
    mechanism of action 105
    metabolic product of estrogen 103
    potential anti-asthma properties 104
    smooth muscle proliferation inhibition 104, 105
Mitogen-activated protein kinase, see p38 mitogen-activated protein kinase
MLD987, development status 238, 240
Montelukast
    asthma efficacy studies 113, 114
    development 112
Mucus hypersecretion
    asthma 160
    chronic obstructive pulmonary disease 160
    drug treatment
        anticholinergics 163
        antisense oligonucleotides 163
        cytokine antagonists 162
        erythromycin 161, 162
        mucoactive drugs 161, 162
        myristoylated alanine-rich C kinase substrate 162
        neural inhibitors 163
        overview 160, 161
        proteinase inhibitors 162
        tachykinin receptor antagonists 163
    regulation 161, 162
Muscarinic M_2 receptor, genetic polymorphism 16, 17
Mycobacterial immunization
    asthma atopy relationship with exposure 226, 227
    BCG vaccination as asthma cure 4, 227
    prospects 228
    T helper cell balance effects 226
Myristoylated alanine-rich C kinase substrate, mucus hypersecretion management 162

Nebulizer, overview of pulmonary delivery 21
Neurokinins, see Tachykinins

Neutrophil elastase
    emphysema role 173, 174
    hypersecretory disease role 173
    inhibitor therapy
        delivery 174
        goals 174
        indications 176
        safety 176
        types of inhibitors 174–176
Nitric oxide
    beneficial actions in lung 156
    deleterious actions in lung 157
    exhaled breath analysis 44, 45
Nitric oxide synthase
    inducible enzyme
        inhibition in animal models of asthma 157, 158
        lung damage 157
    types 156
Nuclear factor-κB
    levels in lung 337
    lung disease-related gene control 337, 338
    signaling pathway
        overview 339–341
        targeting
            rationale 337
            strategies 341
    structure 340

ONO-4047, leukotriene B_4 antagonism and effects 123
OX40, T cell activation 219
Oxidative stress
    antioxidant levels in BAL fluid 151, 152
    chronic obstructive pulmonary disease
        inflammatory gene induction 152, 153
        systemic oxidative stress 152
        therapeutic options
            anti-inflammatory agents 153
            enhancement of lung antioxidants 153, 154
    proteinase/antiproteinase imbalance induction 151
    smoking 151

$P2Y_2$ receptor agonists
    clinical studies 167, 168
    mechanism of action 165
    pulmonary delivery 166, 167
    sputum expectoration enhancement 167
    toxicology 165, 166
p38 mitogen-activated protein kinase
    asthma activity 344
    chronic obstructive pulmonary disease activity 344, 345
    functions 342–344

p38 mitogen-activated protein kinase (continued)
  inhibition
    rationale 342–344
    SB 203580 344
    SB 239063 344, 345
  isoforms 342
PD-1, T cell activation 219
Peak expiratory flow
  diurnal variation 32, 33
  interpretation 32
  measurement 30–32, 34
Peptide immunotherapy
  animal studies 193
  mechanism of action 193
  peptides and fragments 183, 184
  safety 193, 194
  T cell activation studies 192–194
Phosphodiesterase-4 inhibitors
  animal model studies 323
  cellular effects 322, 323
  class-associated side effects 323
  drugs in development 323, 324
  rationale 322, 323
  SB 207499 trials
    asthma 324
    chronic obstructive pulmonary disease 324
  toxicology 323
Polymorphism, see Genetic polymorphism
Potassium channel openers
  airway hyperreactivity
    animal studies 79
    clinical studies 80
    rationale for use 78, 79
  mechanism of action 77
  types 77, 78
Pranlukast
  asthma efficacy studies 113, 114
  development 112
Prostaglandins, exhaled breath analysis 46
Proteinase-3, emphysema role 173, 174
Pulmonary delivery system
  clinical applications 22
  dry-powder inhaler 21, 22
  formulation issues 21
  inhaled particles, factors affecting deposition 21
  metered dose inhaler 21
  nebulizer 21
  rationale and attributes 20
  soft-mist inhaler 21
  Spiros device 22
Pulmozyme, pulmonary delivery 22
Purinergic receptors, see $P2Y_2$ receptor agonists

Rapamycin
  administration routes 238, 239
  animal studies 238
  clinical trials 239, 240
  mechanism of immunosuppression 237, 238
  rationale for asthma treatment 237
Recombinant allergens
  component-resolved diagnosis 195
  epitope determination 196
  hypoallergenic derivatives
    evaluation 198, 199
    genetic engineering and synthesis 197, 198
  immunotherapy trials 199
  production 196
  selection of allergen sources 195, 196
  structure analysis 196, 197
Retinoids
  binding proteins 351
  lung development role 351
  receptor classes 350
  therapeutic application
    acute respiratory distress syndrome 353
    approved uses 354
    bronchopulmonary dysplasia 352
    chronic obstructive pulmonary disease in animal models 351, 352
    emphysema 353, 354
    toxicology 352
  types 350
Ribozyme therapy
  efficacy
    animal models 372
    clinical studies 373
  modifications for stability 371
  natural ribozymes 370
  pharmacokinetics 371, 372
  rationale 371
  specificity 370, 371
  toxicology 372, 373
RS-113456, smoke-induced emphysema inhibition 179, 180
RS-132908, smoke-induced emphysema inhibition 179, 180
RU 24858, mechanism of action 100

Salmeterol
  clinical use
    asthma 61, 62
    chronic obstructive pulmonary disease 62
  corticosteroid interactions 61
  non-smooth muscle effects 61
  receptor pharmacology 60, 61
  smooth muscle response 61
SB 203580, p38 mitogen-activated protein kinase inhibition 344
SB 207499, clinical trials 324
SB 209247, leukotriene B_4 antagonism and effects 123

SB 239063, p38 mitogen-activated protein kinase inhibition 344, 345
SB 265610
  effects on lipopolysaccharide-induced airway neutrophilia 294, 295
  pharmacology 294
SC 53228, leukotriene B_4 antagonism and effects 124
Selectin
  antagonism
    administration routes 308
    clinical trials 308
    consequences 307
    Cylexin 307, 308
    rationale 307
    recombinant soluble P-selectin glycoprotein ligand-1 307, 308
    TBC1269 308
  function 298–300
  inflammation role 306
  types 306
Smoking immunopathology
  chronic bronchiolitis 25, 26
  chronic bronchitis 24, 25
  emphysema 26, 27
Smooth muscle
  airway remodeling 52
  bronchodilator effects on non-airway smooth muscle 57, 58
  contraction mechanisms in airway 55
  genetic variation 58
  long-acting β_2-agonist response 61
  2-methoxyestradiol, proliferation inhibition 104, 105
Sodium chromoglycate, asthma treatment 8
Soft-mist inhaler, overview of pulmonary delivery 21
Specific immunotherapy, see also Allergen immunotherapy, Peptide immunotherapy, Recombinant allergens
  allergens and allergoids 183, 189
  overview 182, 183
  peptides and fragments 183, 184
  second-generation immunotherapy 183
  targets in allergic disease 184
Spiros device, overview of pulmonary delivery 22
STAT6
  activation by interleukin-4 and interleukin-13 346–348
  antisense targeting 368
  asthma therapy targeting 348
  domains 346
  Th2 differentiation role 347
Substance P, see Tachykinins

T cell activation
  costimulatory molecules
    CD28 and B7-1 217, 218
    CTLA-4 and B7-2 217, 218

inducible costimulator and B7-1 218, 219
interleukin-1 receptor superfamily members 219, 220
OX40 and ligand 219
PD-1 and B7H-1 219
peptide immunotherapy 192–194
T cell immunomodulation
allergen immunotherapy 214
approaches
co-stimulation 213
cytokines
immunoregulatory cytokines 213
T helper balance modulation 213, 222, 223
immunosuppression 214, 237–240
T helper surface marker targeting 214
Th2 co-stimulation blockade 214
Th2-specific transcription factors 213
CD4 cells in asthma etiology 222
CD8 cells
animal models of pulmonary disease 235
anti-CD8 antibody therapy 235
asthma role 234
chronic obstructive pulmonary disease role 235, 284
desensitization 235
drug modulation 235
functions 233, 234
chronic obstructive pulmonary disease 215
CpG oligodeoxynucleotides 229–232
GATA-3 role 223–225
mycobacterial immunization 226–228
rationale 212, 213
regulatory T cells 214, 215
STAT6, Th2 differentiation role 347
T helper cell, see Chemokines, T cell immunomodulation
Tachykinins
distribution in lung 146
historical perspective of research 145
levels in lung disorders
asthma 148
chronic obstructive pulmonary disease 148, 149
pathophysiology in lung disease 149
processing 145, 146
receptors
antagonists
mucus hypersecretion management 163
therapeutic benefit 149
types 146, 147

lung 146, 147
modulation of lung disease features
NK-1R 147, 148
NK-2R 148
NK-3R 148
types and affinities 146
types 145
TBC1269, selectin antagonism 308
Theophylline
asthma treatment 7, 8
phosphodiesterase inhibition 321
side effects 2
Tiotropium
chronic obstructive pulmonary disease trials 75, 76
delivery device 74
formulation 74
mechanism of action 72
pharmacokinetics 74, 75
preclinical pharmacology and toxicology 73, 74
Transcription factors, see also specific factors
asthma pathogenesis factors
drug response modification 330
inflammation modulation 330
T helper differentiation modulation 330
types 329
chromatin modification 329
chronic obstructive pulmonary disease factors 331
glucocorticoid inhibition 328
inflammation role 328, 329
Tryptase
airway effects 170
APC 366 inhibition
clinical studies 171, 172
preclinical studies 170
Tumor necrosis factor
inhibitor therapy
administration routes 249
adverse events 249
lung disease studies 249, 250
monoclonal antibodies 249
rheumatoid arthritis trials 249
soluble receptors 249
roles in lung disease
asthma 247, 248
chronic obstructive pulmonary disease 247, 248

Urodilatin
administration route 82
animal studies 81, 82
clinical studies 81
formulation 82
mechanisms of action 81
therapeutic benefits
asthma 83, 84
heart failure 82, 83
renal failure 83
UTP
clinical studies 167, 168
pulmonary delivery 166, 167
sputum expectoration enhancement 167
toxicology 165, 166

Vascular cell adhesion molecule-1 (VCAM-1)
antagonism
animal studies 311, 312
clinical approaches 312, 313
rationale 310, 311
function 298–300
inflammation role 310, 311
Viozan
β_2-adrenoceptor-mediated properties 70
clinical studies 70
development 69
dopamine D_2 receptor-mediated properties 70
mechanism of action 71
receptor pharmacology 69
therapeutic index 70
VLA-4
antagonism
monoclonal antibodies 303
multiple sclerosis trials 304
peptide analogs 303
small-molecule inhibitors 303–305
asthma role 302, 303
biochemical properties 303
function 302

Zafirlukast
asthma efficacy studies 113, 114
development 112
Zileuton
asthma efficacy studies
bronchoprovocation studies 116, 117
chronic treatment 117, 118
pharmacology 115, 116
side effects 115

Abbreviations

ACh	Acetylcholine	ERK	Extracellular signal regulated
AHR	Airway hyperreactivity	ET-1	Endothelin-1
ADP	Adenosine diphosphate		
AMP	Adenosine monophosphate	FcεRI	High-affinity receptor for IgE
ANP	Atrial natriuretic polypeptide	FcεRII	Low-affinity receptor for IgE
AP-1	Activating protein-1	FcγRI	High-affinity receptor for IgG
APC	Antigen-presenting cell	FcγRII	Low-affinity receptor for IgG
APL	Antiphospholipid	FDA	Federal Drug Administration
$α_1$-AT	$α_1$-Antitrypsin	FEV_1	Forced expiratory volume in 1 s
ATP	Adenosine triphosphate	FGF	Fibroblast growth factor
		FGFR	Fibroblast growth factor receptor
BABIM	Bis(5-amidino-2-benzimidazolyl)methane	FRC	Functional residual capacity
BAL	Bronchoalveolar lavage	FVC	Forced vital capacity
BCG	Bacillus Calmette-Guérin		
bFGF	Basic fibroblast growth factor	GATA-3	Gene activator of TCR-α
BHR	Bronchial hyperreactivity	GCP	Good clinical practice
BLT, BLTR	Leukotriene B_4 receptor	GCP-2	Granulocyte chemotactic protein-2
BTPS	Body temperature pressure-saturated	G-CSF	Granulocyte colony-stimulating factor
		GM-CSF	Granulocyte-macrophage colony-stimulating factor
cAMP	Cyclic adenosine monophosphate		
CBP	CREB-binding protein	GM-CSFR	Granulocyte-macrophage colony-stimulating factor receptor
C/EBPβ	CCAAT box/enhancer binding protein-β		
cGMP	Cyclic guanosine monophosphate	GR	Glucocorticoid receptor
CGRP	Calcitonin-gene-related peptide	GSH	Reduced glutathione
CHO	Chinese hamster ovary cells		
COPD	Chronic obstructive pulmonary disease	H_1	Histamine type 1 receptor
COX-2	Cyclooxygenase-2	HAT	Histone acetyl transferase
CREB	cAMP-responsive element binding protein	HDAC	Histone deacetylase
CT	Computerized tomography		
CTGF	Connective tissue growth factor	ICAM	Intracellular adhesion molecule
CTL	Cytotoxic T lymphocyte	ICS	Inhaled corticosteroid
		IFN-γ	Interferon-γ
DBD	DNA binding domain	Ig	Immunoglobulin
D_L	Lung diffusion capacity	IGF-1	Insulin-like growth factor-1
DNA	Deoxyribonucleic acid	I-κBα	Inhibitor of the transcription factor NF-κB
DPT	*Dermatophagoides pteronyssinus*	IL	Interleukin
		iNOS	Inducible nitric oxide synthase
EGF	Epidermal growth factor	IP_3	Inositol-1,4,5-trisphosphate
EGFR	Epidermal growth factor receptor		
ELISA	Enzyme-linked immunosorbent assay	JAK	Janus kinase
EMEA	European Agency for the Evaluation of Medicinal Products	JNK	Jun N-terminal kinase

K_{ATP}	Potassium ATP-sensitive channels
KCO	Potassium channel openers
LABA	Long-acting β_2-adrenoceptor agonist
LBD	Ligand-binding domain
5-LO	5-Lipoxygenase
LPS	Lipopolysaccharide
LT	Leukotriene
MAdCAM-1	Mucosal adressin cell adhesion molecule-1
MAPK	Mitogen-activated protein kinase
MCP	Monocyte chemoattractant protein
M-CSFR	Macrophage-colony-stimulating factor receptor
MDC	Macrophage-derived chemokine
MEF	Maximal expiratory flow
MEFV	Maximal expiratory flow-volume
MGSA/Gro	Melanoma growth stimulatory activity/growth-regulated protein
MHC	Major histocompatibility complex
MIP	Macrophage inflammatory protein
MLCK	Myosin light-chain kinase
MMP	Matrix metalloproteinase
MRI	Magnetic resonance imaging
NANC	Non-adrenergic, non-cholinergic
NAP	Neutrophil-activating peptide
NE	Neutrophil elastase
NF-AT	Nuclear factor of activated T cells
NF-κB	Nuclear factor-κB
NGF	Nerve growth factor
NK	Neurokinin
NMR	Nuclear magnetic resonance
NO	Nitric oxide
NOS	Nitric oxide synthase
NSAID	Non-steroid anti-inflammatory drug
PAF	Platelet-activating factor
$PaCO_2$	Arterial dioxide tension
PaO_2	Arterial oxygen tension
PBMC	Peripheral blood mononuclear cell
PC_{20}	Provocative concentration to cause a 20% fall in FEV_1
PD_{20}	Provocative dose to cause a 20% fall in FEV_1
PDE	Phosphodiesterase
PDGF	Platelet-derived growth factor
PDGFR	Platelet-derived growth factor receptor
PEF	Peak expiratory flow
PEFR	Peak expiratory flow rate
PG	Prostaglandin
PK	Protein kinase
PL	Phospholipase
PMN	Polymorphonuclear neutrophils
PPAR-α	Peroxisome-proliferator-activated receptor-α
PCR	Polymerase chain reaction
PECAM	Platelet endothelial cell adhesion molecule
RANTES	Regulated on activated normal T cell expressed
SaO_2	Arterial oxygen saturation
SCF	Stem cell factor
SIRS	Systemic inflammatory response syndrome
SH2	src homology 2
SNP	Single nucleotide polymorphism
SP	Substance P
SRF	Serum response factor
STAT	Signal transducer and activator of transcription
TARC	Thymus and activation regulated chemokine
TBARS	Thiobarbituric acid-reactive substances
TCR	T cell receptor
TGF-β	Transforming growth factor-β
Th1, Th2	T helper type 1 and type 2 cells
TLC	Total lung capacity
TL_{CO}	Diffusion capacity (transfer factor) for carbon monoxide
TNF-α	Tumour necrosis factor-α
TNFR	Tumour necrosis factor receptor
VCAM	Vascular cell adhesion molecule
VEGF	Vascular endothelial growth factor
VEGFR	Vascular endothelial growth factor receptor
V_D	Volume of distribution
VIP	Vasoactive intestinal peptide
VLA-4	Very late (activation) antigen-4